The description of experimental allergic neuritis by Waksman, whose historical account introduces this book, revealed the likely connection between immunological events and peripheral neuropathy. Subsequent work, involving many other contributors to this, the first volume to be dedicated to the subject, has confirmed the immunopathological basis of a range of peripheral nerve diseases, so that immunological methods of diagnosis and treatment are now increasingly available to clinicians.

There are five sections, dealing with biology and epidemiology, patient evaluation, immune-mediated neuropathies, neuropathies caused by infection, and therapy and management, including rehabilitation.

Neurologists and clinicians in other specialities will welcome this comprehensive review of the field, which provides an authoritative overview of the pathogenesis, diagnosis and treatment of infectious and immune-mediated neuropathies. It is directly relevant to the everyday management of patients, and will also meet the needs of the basic immunological researcher seeking a general overview.

NORMAN LATOV is Professor of Neurology in the Department of Neurology, College of Physicians and Surgeons of Columbia University, New York

JOHN H.J. WOKKE is Professor of Neuromuscular Diseases in the Department of Neurology, University of Utrecht

JOHN J. KELLY, JR is Professor and Chairman, Department of Neurology, The George Washington University, Washington, DC

IMMUNOLOGICAL AND INFECTIOUS DISEASES OF THE PERIPHERAL NERVES

Immunology and Infectious Diseases of the Peripheral Nerves

Edited by
N. Latov
John H. J. Wokke
John J. Kelly, Jr

CAMBRIDGE
UNIVERSITY PRESS

PUBLISHED BY THE PRESS SYNDICATE OF THE UNIVERSITY OF CAMBRIDGE
The Pitt Building, Trumpington Street, Cambridge CB2 1RP, United Kingdom

CAMBRIDGE UNIVERSITY PRESS
The Edinburgh Building, Cambridge CB2 2RU, United Kingdom
40 West 20th Street, New York, NY 10011-4211, USA
10 Stamford Road, Oakleigh, Melbourne 3166, Australia

First published 1998

Printed in the United Kingdom at the University Press, Cambridge

Typeset in Adobe Minion 9½/13pt [SE]

A catalogue record for this book is available from the British Library

Library of Congress Cataloguing in Publication data

Immunological and infectious diseases of the peripheral nerves /
edited by N. Latov, John H.J. Wokke, John J. Kelly.
p. cm.
Includes bibliographical references.
ISBN 0 521 46265 7 (hardback)
1. Nerves, Peripheral – Diseases – Immunological aspects.
2. Nerves, Peripheral – Infections. I. Latov, Norman. II. Wokke,
John H.J. (Johannes Hendricks Josephus), 1952– . III. Kelly,
John J. (John Joseph), 1943– .
[DNLM: 1. Peripheral Nervous System Diseases – etiology.
2. Peripheral Nervous System Diseases – therapy. 3. Immunologic
Diseases – complications. 4. Communicable Diseases – complications.
WL 500 I33 1997]
RC409.I46 1997
616.8′7079 – dc21 97-9494 CIP
DNLM/DLC
for Library of Congress

ISBN 0 521 46265 7 hardback

Contents

List of contributors *ix*
Preface *xii*
The way things were: the discovery of experimental 'allergic' neuritis *xiv*
B.H. Waksman

PART I **Biology and epidemiology**

1 Immune interactions in the peripheral nervous system *1*
C.L. Koski

2 Epidemiology of autoimmune polyneuropathies *29*
J.J. Kelly Jr

3 Immune-mediated experimental neuropathies *36*
J.D. Pollard

PART II **Patient evaluation**

4 Clinical evaluation and differential diagnosis *55*
J.H.J. Wokke and N.C. Notermans

5 Electrophysiological studies *73*
H. Franssen

6 Immunopathological studies in immune-mediated neuropathies *81*
M. Corbo and A.P. Hays

PART III **Immune-mediated neuropathies**

7 Guillain-Barré syndrome and variants *99*
F.G.A. van der Meché

8 Chronic inflammatory demyelinating polyneuropathy *111*
M. Vermeulen

9 Acute and chronic sensory neuronopathy *126*
G. Sobue

10 Acute and chronic autonomic neuropathies *138*
G.A. Suarez and P.A. Low

11 Vasculitic neuropathies *158*
G. Said

12 Neuropathies associated with anti-MAG antibodies and IgM monoclonal gammopathies *168*
E. Nobile-Orazio

13 Motor neuropathies associated with anti-GM1 ganglioside antibodies *190*
T. Kuntzer and A.J. Steck

14 Neuropathies associated with anti-sulfatide and other glycoconjugate antibodies *201*
L.H. van den Berg

15 Paraneoplastic peripheral neuropathy *208*
P.S. Smitt and J.B. Posner

16 Polyneuropathies associated with myeloma, POEMS, and non-malignant IgG and IgA monoclonal gammopathies *225*
J.J. Kelly Jr

17 Neuromyotonia and the Lambert–Eaton myasthenic syndrome *238*
J. Newsom-Davis

18 Toxin- and drug-induced immune neuropathies *251*
N.L. Rosenberg

PART IV **Neuropathies caused by infection**

19 The post-polio syndrome *269*
M.C. Dalakas

20 Peripheral neuropathy in HIV-1 infection *285*
T.H. Brannagan III, T. McAlarney and N. Latov

21 Lyme neuropathy *308*
P.K. Coyle and M.A. Kaufman

22 Neuropathy in leprosy *319*
F.G.I. Jennekens and W.H. van Brakel

23 Neuropathies associated with herpes virus infections *340*
I. Steiner and D. Wolf

PART V **Therapy and management**

24 Immunosuppression and immunomodulation *357*
A. Brand

25 Management of paralytic neuropathy in the intensive care unit *377*
C.F. Bolton

26 Diagnosis and symptomatic therapy of nerve pain *389*
Ch.J. Vecht and P.L.I. Dellemijn

27 Medical rehabilitation *415*
G.W. van Dijk, N.C. Notermans and J. Gerritsen

Index *426*

Contributors

C.F. Bolton, MD FRCP
Department of Clinical Neurological Sciences
Victoria Hospital
375 South Street
London, Ontario N4G 5
Canada

A. Brand, PhD
Bloedbank Leidsenhage
Academisch Ziekenhuis (E3-Q)
PO Box 2184
2301 CD Leiden
The Netherlands

T.H. Brannagan III, MD
Department of Neurology
College of Physicians and Surgeons of Columbia University
Columbia Presbyterian Medical Center
710 W 168th Street
New York, NY 10032
USA

M. Corbo, MD
IRCCS H.S. Raffaele
Clinica Neurologica
Via Orlgettina 60
20132 Milan
Italy

P.K. Coyle, MD
Department of Neurology
SUNY at Stony Brook
Stony Brook, NY 11794
USA

M.C. Dalakas, MD
National Institutes of Health
NINCDS Bldg 10, Rm 4N248
9000 Rockville Pike
Bethesda, MD 20892
USA

P.L.I. Dellemijn, MD
St Joseph Hospital
De Run 4600
5500 HB Veldhoven
The Netherlands

H. Franssen, MD, PhD
Department of Clinical Neurophysiology
University of Utrecht
PO Box 85500
3508 GA Utrecht
The Netherlands

J. Gerritsen, MD
Department of Rehabilitation Medicine
University of Utrecht
PO Box 85500
3508 GA Utrecht
The Netherlands

A.P. Hays, MD
Department of Pathology
Division of Neuropathology
College of Physicians and Surgeons of Columbia University
New York, NY 10032
USA

F.G.I. Jennekens, MD
Department of Neurology
University of Utrecht
PO Box 85500
3508 GA Utrecht
The Netherlands

M.A. Kaufman, MD
Department of Neurology
SUNY at Stony Brook
Stony Brook, NY 11794
USA

J.J. Kelly, Jr, MD
Department of Neurology
George Washington University
2150 Pennsylvania Ave NW, Suite 7-404
Washington, DC 20037
USA

C.L. Koski, MD
Department of Neurology
University of Maryland School of Medicine
22 South Greene Street
Baltimore, MD 20892
USA

T. Kuntzer, MD
Department of Neurology
University of Lausanne
Centre Universitaire Vaudois Hospitalier
CH-1011 Lausanne
Switzerland

N. Latov, MD PhD
Department of Neurology
College of Physicians and Surgeons of Columbia University
Columbia Presbyterian Medical Center
710 W 168th Street
New York, NY 10032
USA

P.A. Low, MD
Department of Neurology
Mayo Clinic
200 First Street SW
Rochester, MN 55905
USA

T. McAlarney, MD
Department of Neurology
College of Physicians and Surgeons of Columbia University
Columbia Presbyterian Medical Center
710 W 168th Street
New York, NY 10032
USA

J. Newsom-Davis, FRS
Neurosciences Group
Institute of Molecular Medicine
John Radcliffe Hospital
Oxford OX3 9DU
UK

E. Nobile-Orazio, MD
Institute of Clinical Neurology
University of Milan
Ospedale Maggiore – Policlinico
Via F. Sforza 35
Milan 20122
Italy

N.C. Notermans, MD
Department of Neurology
University of Utrecht
PO Box 85500
3508 GA Utrecht
The Netherlands

J.D. Pollard
Department of Medicine
The University of Sydney
Camperdown
Sydney, NSW 2006
Australia

J.B. Posner, MD
Department of Neurology
Memorial Sloan-Kettering Cancer Center
1275 York Ave
New York, NY 10021
USA

N.L. Rosenberg, MD
Division of Clinical Pharmacology and Medical Toxicology
University of Colorado School of Medicine and Center for Occupational Neurology and Neurotoxicology
Colorado Neurological Institute
450 West Jefferson Ave
Englewood, CO 80110-3536
USA

G. Said, MD
Department of Neurology
Hôpital de Bicêtre
78 rue due General Leclerc
Le Kremlin-Bicêtre Cedex 94270
France

P.S. Smitt, MD
Department of Neurology
Memorial Sloan-Kettering Cancer Center
1275 York Ave
New York, NY 10021
USA

G. Sobue, MD
Division of Neurology
Fourth Department of Medicine
Aichi Medical University
Nagakute, Aichi 480-11
Japan

A.J. Steck
Nagoya University School of Medicine
Nagoya
Japan

I. Steiner, MD
Department of Neurology
Hebrew University and Hadassah Medical School
PO Box 12000
Jerusalem 91120
Israel

G.A. Suarez, MD
Department of Neurology
Mayo Clinic
200 First Street SW
Rochester, MN 55905
USA

W.H. van Brakel, MD MSc PhD
International Nepal Fellowship Leprosy Project
Western Region
Post Box No. 5
Pokhara 33701
Nepal

L.H. van den Berg, MD
Department of Neurology
University of Utrecht
PO Box 85500
3508 GA Utrecht
The Netherlands

F.G.A. Van der Meché, MD
Department of Neurology
Academic Hospital Rotterdam Dijkzigt
Dr Molewaterplein 40
3015 GD Rotterdam
The Netherlands

G.K. Van Dijk, MD
Department of Neurology
University of Utrecht
PO Box 85500
3508 GA Utrecht
The Netherlands

Ch.J. Vecht, MD
Dr Daniel den Hoed Kliniek
Groene Hilledijk 301
3075 EA Rotterdam
The Netherlands

M. Vermeulen, MD
Department of Neurology
Academisch Medisch Centrum
Meiberdreef 9
3015 AS Amsterdam
The Netherlands

B.H. Waksman
Foundation for Microbiology
300 E 54th Street
New York, NY 10022
USA

J.H.J. Wokke, MD
Department of Neurology
University of Utrecht
PO Box 85500
3508 GA Utrecht
The Netherlands

D. Wolf, MD
Department of Clinical Microbiology and Infectious Diseases
Hebrew University and Hadassah Medical School
PO Box 12000
Jerusalem 91120
Israel

Preface

The study of peripheral nerve diseases has gone through several distinct stages over the decades. This book concerns the latest stage: the era of neuroimmunology and molecular biology.

The first chapter in this development was centered in the late 1800s and the first half of this century until the end of World War II and was mainly directed towards categorizing neuromuscular diseases. Based on clinical signs, fledgling physiology and pathology, patients were segregated into large groups such as myopathies and neuropathies. Neurology in those days was still mostly descriptive. There was poor understanding of disease mechanisms and little or no treatment available.

After World War II, technical advances and the ready accessibility of peripheral nerves for study allowed the development of more advanced physiological techniques led by Buchthal, Lambert and their colleagues. At the same time, morphological and histopatholical techniques were pioneered by Dyck, Thomas, Asbury and others. This led to an explosion of information on the peripheral nervous system. Investigators were now able to further subcategorize the neuropathies into axonal and demyelinating types, and begin to speculate on etiology. This led to a rapid growth in the field as clinicians were able to readily detect neuropathy using electrophysiological techniques and to study the morphology and pathology of nerve disease using sural nerve biopsy. Classical descriptions of inherited neuropathies, acute and chronic inflammatory neuropathies and others soon followed. Still, little was known about the basic mechanisms of these disorders and treatment was based on theoretical and empirical constructs.

The most recent advance, which has taken us beyond morphology and neurophysiology, was conditioned by advances in the fields in neuroimmunology and molecular biology. The description of experimental allergic neuritis by Waksman and colleagues was the first example of the likely connection between immunological events and peripheral neuropathy. Further work by many of the collaborators in this book and others have shown a direct connection between immunological events and nerve damage in humans. We now know that several, and likely many more, neurological and peripheral nerve diseases are directly due to immunological attacks on nervous tissue antigens and can be modified by immunosuppressive treatment.

We are now in the midst of this current stage and it is unclear how far it will take us. Many unexplained neurological and peripheral nerve syndromes are undoubtedly related to, or at least modified by, immunological mechanisms and hence modifiable by immunological treatment. This book provides both the interested researcher and the clinician a perspective on the current state of this fascinating field of neurology.

N. Latov
John H.J. Wokke
John J. Kelly

The way things were: the discovery of experimental 'allergic' neuritis

Byron H. Waksman, MD

I wish to present a somewhat impressionistic picture of the circumstances surrounding my discovery (in collaboration with Raymond Adams) of the model disease known as experimental 'allergic' neuritis (EAN). This discovery was an almost inevitable outcome of the research associated with my first job.

I had been hired, in the fall of 1949, by a neuropathologist at the Massachusetts General Hospital, L. Raymond Morrison, to study experimental allergic encephalomyelitis (EAE) in rabbits, a model he had described in 1947. I was an inexperienced immunologist, fresh from postdoctoral training with Michael Heidelberger at Columbia-Presbyterian Medical School and with no prior knowledge of neuroimmunological questions. Scientists interested in EAE at that time could be numbered on the fingers of one hand; the best known were Ferraro and his colleagues and Alvord on the neurological/neuropathological side, and Kabat and Freund who were basic immunologists. The field thus was relatively unencumbered.

It is difficult for immunologists or neuroscientists working today to imagine the immediate post-World War II scene in the two fields. Before 1950, antibody was known for its role in antimicrobial immunity and as the principal mediator in immunopathological lesions of anaphylactic or Arthus type. Also it was known that antibody is made by plasma cells. Cell-mediated immunity was recognized only in the specific instances of 'infectious' allergy (including tuberculin sensitivity) and contact allergy. It was associated with a characteristic delayed-type skin reaction and could be transferred adoptively by living lymphoid cells from sensitized donors to naive recipients. The relationship between lymphocytes, macrophages, and plasma cells was unclear – many investigators considered lymphocytes as macrophage precursors! The central role of these cells and of the thymus in immune responses was to remain a mystery for another decade. Indeed some leading immunologists (Kabat, Karush) thought that delayed type hypersensitivity (DTH) might be mediated by an unusual high-affinity antibody.

Neuropathologists in 1950 viewed demyelinative diseases as toxic/degenerative/possibly infectious processes affecting myelin, with macrophages (Gitter cells) arising locally by activation of resident microglia as a response to injury and serving simply as scavengers to clean up the products of myelin/tissue breakdown. The medical research community had not accepted autoimmunity as a significant pathogenetic mechanism or pattern, in spite of published reports describing experimental autoimmune diseases affecting the central nervous system (EAE) and eye (phakogenic uveitis, autoallergic uveitis) and Dameshek's studies of the autoimmune hemolytic anemias.

Add to all this the absence of most of the experimental tools that we take for granted today: no plastics, no purified proteins, no chromatographic methods, and few or no reagents to exchange. Immunologists could use serological and immunochemical technology (and electrophoresis and ultracentrifugation) and gel diffusion was just appearing. There were no acceptable ways to handle cells (except for passive transfer). One had to work with whole animals. Inbred animals were not in general use, and there was in any case no tradition that recognized the relevance of animal models for human diseases. For pathological investigations, analytic chemical and histochemical methods were available and immunofluorescence techniques were just being introduced, but ultrastructural investigation lay in the future.

Perhaps most important of all, there was no one to talk to. Except for the immunochemists (a small and rather inbred group), scientists who addressed immunological problems related to disease called themselves microbiologists, pathologists, hematologists, neurologists, ophthalmologists, dermatologists, or tumor biologists, published in their own specialty journals, and for the most part failed to communicate with those in other specialties. In all of Boston in 1950, there were barely a half dozen people who called themselves immunologists. I was lucky that Louis Dienes was the hospital bacteriologist at MGH. He had studied delayed reactivity to purified proteins in the 1920s and had been a mentor and colleague of Jules Freund (even to helping develop the adjuvant that carries Freund's name). He undoubtedly contributed to the evolution of my own thinking about the problem of experimental 'autoallergic' diseases.

Thus it was that my first paper (with Morrison) in 1951 showed that EAE in rabbits was associated with typical skin and corneal reactions of delayed type to myelin antigens and the disease and this hypersensitivity were closely related in degree and time (Waksman & Morrison 1951). Since several investigators had failed to transfer EAE with serum from diseased animals, it became my working hypothesis that EAE itself was a new kind of delayed or tuberculin-type reaction, occurring in the nervous system.

This first paper was followed by a demonstration that the effective component of the Freund adjuvant was wax D (or Pmko), a substance that had recently been shown (S. Raffel, N. Choucroun) to intensify the induction of tuberculin-type sensitivity (Waksman & Adams 1953). Unfortunately Morrison died shortly after my arrival in the laboratory; however, Raymond Adams had taken an interest in EAE-related studies and collaborated on histological aspects of the work at this time and over the next several years.

The next step was the demonstration (in collaboration with Marjorie Lees and Jordi Folch-Pi) that proteolipids of myelin, discovered by this group in 1951, were effective encephalitogens (Waksman et al. 1954). This work, first reported at the American Association of Immunologists' meeting in 1953, confirmed and extended findings of C. Tal and P.K. Olitsky in mice (1952) and N.P. Goldstein and his collaborators in guinea pigs (1953) and preceded the discovery of myelin basic protein as an encephalitogen (by M.W. Kies, E. Roboz, and E.C. Alvord Jr) by several years. Proteolipids elicited striking DTH reactions, closely correlated with the EAE process (Waksman 1956).

Thus the stage was set for an exploration of different parts of the nervous system as possible inducers of unique autoimmune diseases. It must be added parenthetically that, in parallel with this exploration of the nervous system, our laboratory engaged in a systematic study of delayed/tuberculin-type hypersensitivity as such, work which contributed to the new view of such reactions that emerged in the 1960s, as studies began to be reported on the role of the thymus, on lymphocytes, and on cytokines.

At the time that we initiated our study of EAN, there had been no report of immunologically mediated autoimmune disease limited to the peripheral nervous system. Lumsden (1949), in fact, had reported that immunization of guinea pigs with homologous peripheral nerve and adjuvant resulted in typical EAE. On the other hand, EAE was frequently accompanied by lesions of the spinal nerve roots and, in sheep and monkeys given homologous brain, by lesions in spinal ganglia and peripheral nerve (Innes 1951; Ferraro & Roizin 1954).

Our study was reported in preliminary form at the AAI meeting in 1955 and in definitive papers in 1955 and 56 (Waksman & Adams 1954, 1956). We found that rabbits immunized with homologous or heterologous sciatic nerve and adjuvant developed a symmetric ataxic paresis of the extremities with retention of bowel and bladder sphincter control, accompanied by elevated protein but a normal cell count (albumino-cytologic dissociation) in the cerebrospinal fluid (CSF). The lesions showed primary (segmental) demyelination together with an almost exclusively mononuclear inflammatory process in the dorsal roots, spinal ganglia, and peripheral nerves, and showed a focal, largely perivenous localization. In severe disease, there was also some neuronal death in the ganglia and some Wallerian degeneration among nerve fibers in the peripheral nerve. The histological character of the lesions set them off sharply from other experimental lesions affecting peripheral nervous system (PNS) myelin (produced by such agents as triorthocresyl phosphate, diisopropyl fluorophosphate, Mipafox) which were essentially noninflammatory.

EAN was clearly distinct from EAE, in which the central nervous system (CNS) (brain, optic nerves, spinal cord, meninges) were affected, with flaccid paralysis, loss of sphincter control and greatly increased cell counts in the CSF. A spontaneous infectious or other process could be ruled out on a number of grounds. While both antibodies and DTH to neural antigens were present, neither showed a clear correlation with the disease process, unlike the situation in EAE. At the same time the histological changes were essentially identical with those of EAE, suggesting that a similar pathogenic process might be at work in the two diseases. The difference in distribution of the lesions could be attributed almost certainly to the differing distribution of the myelin antigens involved.

The possible usefulness of this experimental disease as a model for human disease was clear from the start: 'EAN provides the first experimental model of a reproducible noninfectious inflammatory disease of the peripheral nervous system.' The human disorder which it most closely resembled was variously known as Landry's paralysis, acute febrile polyneuritis, acute 'infectious' polyneuritis, and the Guillain-Barré syndrome (GBS). 'The resemblances are sufficiently impressive to justify a further exploration of the possibility that acute "infectious" polyneuritis may have an immunological base.' In fact the possibility that the GBS (nowadays AIDP) has an immunological base was already recognized, e.g. by Krücke (1955) following Pette's earlier suggestion (1928) that multiple sclerosis and other demyelinative diseases might be immunological/hyperergic.

Our second EAN paper explored the rather striking difference in lesion distribution in EAE and EAN of different species, the basic histological lesion being always the same. CNS immunization in rabbits resulted in disease affecting the CNS exclusively in about one-quarter of instances and disease of both CNS and PNS in about 3/4; PNS immunization gave lesions exclusively in the PNS (except for occasional mild meningitis related to involvement of nerve roots. In guinea pigs, after CNS immunization, half the animals had CNS disease only and half lesions of both systems; after PNS immunization, a small proportion showed disease limited to the PNS and the rest lesions of both CNS and PNS. In mice the lesion distribution patterns resembled those seen in rabbits. These differences were explained by the involvement of multiple overlapping (and possibly cross-reacting) myelin antigens. The occurrence of peripheral lesions in human demyelinating diseases of the CNS (PVE, PIE, multiple sclerosis) finds a model in rabbit and guinea pig EAE.

A second aspect of lesion distribution was brought out by the comparison of EAN in the different animal species. In rabbits and mice, dorsal root and ganglion lesions were numerous and intense, even diffuse, while nerve lesions were focal and rare; in guinea pigs the lesions in roots and ganglia were mild, while peripheral nerves were diffusely involved. Here, clearly, another factor intervened which proved later to depend on the character of the local vascular network and blood–tissue barriers in the various regions of the PNS.

Our studies of EAN were part of a systematic search for regional differences in nervous tissue antigenicity and the ability to induce distinctive autoimmune syndromes. Immunization with optic nerve resulted in typical EAE; however, in rabbits, EAE frequently included a severe optic neuritis accompanied by secondary uveitis (Bullington & Waksman 1958). Models of phakogenic uveitis and sympathetic ophthalmia (autoimmune uveitis) had been described by Burky in 1934 and Collins in 1949, respectively. The association of uveitis with inflammatory disease of the CNS, however, provided a new model for such entities as the Vogt–Koyanagi syndrome and Harada's disease, as well as sympathetic ophthalmia. We were also successful in showing that EAN in guinea pigs could follow a chronic course, with both relapses and progression (Waksman 1961a), thus providing a possible model for chronic demyelinative inflammatory neuropathy (CIDP) in humans. B.G.W. Arnason, who came to our laboratory in 1959, showed a few years later that another distinctive neuroimmunological syndrome could be induced in the sympathetic nervous system by autoimmunization (Appenzeller et al. 1965).

The general rules uncovered in our EAE/EAN work were shown subsequently to apply equally to autoimmune inflammatory ('autoallergic') diseases affecting nonneural tissues, notably the eye, thyroid, adrenal, and testis (Waksman 1959b). In all cases, lesions were found to occur only in tissue containing the same antigen used for immunization, to be made up from the start exclusively of mononuclear cells (lymphocytes, monocytes/macrophages, plasma cells), and to show destruction of parenchyma in the inflammatory zone, what we chose to call an 'invasive destructive lesion.' These proved to be defining elements in many reactions of cell-mediated (delayed-type, tuberculin-type) hypersensitivity, the tuberculin and contact allergic reactions, allograft rejection (skin), the experimental 'autoallergies,' and delayed reactions to pure proteins (Waksman 1960a); thus we were led to the hypothesis that all such reactions are initiated by a reaction of specifically 'sensitized' lymphocytes in the circulation with antigen in the tissue. (This is the prevailing view of these reactions today.) It also became clear, before the 1950s were over, that EAE and EAN could serve equally as models for acute monophasic disorders, such as postvaccinal and postinfectious encephalomyelitis and GBS, and for chronic relapsing-remitting or progressive diseases such as MS and CIDP.

At the time I went to medical school (the early 1940s) diphtheritic polyneuritis was generally regarded as immunological, because it followed diphtheritic infection by a long symptom-free interval and showed many clinical features like those of the GBS; this view was still widespread in 1950. Histological studies, however, published at the time we were working on EAN, described the PNS lesions as showing primary demyelination without inflammation (Scheid & Peters 1952; Fisher & Adams 1956). We found ourselves in an ideal position to compare this disease in a model system with EAN (Waksman et al. 1957). Rabbits or guinea pigs injected with underneutralized toxin-antitoxin mixtures developed a progressive ataxic paresis with albumino-cytologic dissociation in the CSF indistinguishable from EAN. Histologically, however, the PNS of the affected animals showed pure segmental demyelination without axis cylinder damage or any sign of inflammation. Immunological studies of our diphtheria model proved to be noncontributory, and we concluded that the lesions were produced by direct action of the toxin on Schwann cells and were nonimmunological. This was confirmed by studies that showed toxic/metabolic effects beginning at 24 hours (Majno et al. 1960), while Schwann cell/myelin changes appeared only after 6–7 days, as seen in phase and electron microscopic studies (Webster et al. 1961).

Perhaps the most interesting outcome of the diphtheria study was the demonstration that the lesions were distributed in the PNS in patterns that precisely mimicked those seen in EAN: the rabbit lesions were largely limited to the spinal roots and ganglia (much like the lesions in human diphtheritic disease) while in the guinea pig, lesions predominated in the peripheral nerves. In a final study (Waksman 1961b) related to both EAN and diphtheritic polyneuritis, it turned out that large anionic dyes like Trypan blue stained roots and ganglia intensely but failed to stain nerve in rabbits and monkeys, while in guinea pigs the nerves were diffusely stained. The same patterns were observed with diphtheria toxin and other proteins (ovalbumin, human serum albumin), traced by radiolabelling and/or immunofluorescence, and could be related to the nature of the endoneurial vascular plexus. Leakage of toxin (or dye) and perivascular diapedesis of inflammatory cells occurred only where there were numerous small veins and not where the vascular plexus consisted entirely of capillaries, as in rabbit and monkey nerve. Here there appeared to exist a blood–nerve barrier, comparable in some degree to the blood–brain barrier in the CNS and capable of limiting the access of blood-borne agents including cells. We were able to generalize this finding and show the permissive role of veins in a series of autoimmune inflammatory diseases affecting other tissues (lens, uvea, thyroid, adrenal, testis) (Waksman 1960b).

In conclusion, our EAN studies and the related work on EAE, in addition to providing a convenient model for deeper investigations of AIDP and CIDP, contributed to several striking 'paradigm shifts' taking place in the 1950s and 1960s: the recognition of autoimmunity as a common mechanism underlying neuroimmunological and other disorders; the identification of inflammatory autoimmune diseases as a major category within the larger group of cell-mediated immune reactions; and recognition of the central role of hematogenous lymphocytes and macrophages in producing invasive-destructive lesions of target tissues such as the CNS and PNS.

References

Appenzeller, O., Arnason, B.G., and Adams, R.D. (1965). Experimental autonomic neuropathy: An immunologically induced disorder of reflex vasomotor function. *J. Neurol. Neurosurg. Psychiatry* **25**: 510–515.

Bullington, S.J. and Waksman, B.H. (1958). Uveitis in rabbits with experimental allergic encephalomyelitis. Results produced by injection of nervous tissue and adjuvants. *Arch. Ophthalnicol* **59**: 435–445.

Ferraro, A. and Roizin, L. (1954). Neuropathologic variations in experimental allergic encephalomyelitis. Hemorrhagic encephalomyelitis, perivenous encephalomyelitis, diffuse encephalomyelitis, patchy gliosis. *J. Neuropath. Exp Neurol.* **13**: 60–89.

Innes, J.R.M. (1951). Experimental 'allergic' encephalomyelitis: attempts to produce the disease in sheep and goats. *J. Comp. Path. Ther.* **61**: 241–250.

Krücke, W. (1955). Erkrankungen der peripheren Nerven. In *Handbuch der speziellen pathologischen Anatomie und Histologie*, vol. 13/5, pp. 1–248. Springer, Berlin.

Lumsden, C.E. (1949). Experimental 'allergic' encephalomyelitis. *Brain* **72**: 198–226.

Majno, G., Waksman, B.H., and Karnovsky, L.M. (1960). Experimental study of diphtheritic polyneuritis in the rabbit and guinea pig. II. The effect of diphtheria toxin on lipide biosynthesis by guinea pig nerve. *J. Neuropath exp. Neurol.* **19**: 7–24.

Pette, H. (1928). Klinische und anatomische Studien und die Pathogenese der multiplen Sklerose. *Deut. Zschr. Nervenheilk.* **105**: 76–132.

Waksman, B.H. (1956). Further study of skin reactions in rabbits with experimental allergic encephalomyelitis. *J. Infect. Dis.* **99**: 258–269.

Waksman, B.H. (1959a). Experimental allergic encephalomyelitis as prototype of the class of autoallergic diseases. In: *Mechanisms of Hypersensitivity*, In: International Symposium of the Henry Ford Hospital, Detroit, H. Shaffer et al. Little Brown, pp. 679–691.

Waksman, B.H. (1959b). Experimental allergic encephalomyelitis and the 'autoallergic' diseases. *Int. Arch. Allergy Appl. Immunol.* 14 (Suppl.): 1–87.

Waksman, B.H. (1960a). A comparative histopathological study of delayed hypersensitive reactions. In: *Ciba Foundation Symposium on Cellular Aspects of Immunity*. Churchill, London, pp. 280–322.

Waksman, B.H. (1960b). The distribution of experimental auto-allergic lesions. Its relation to the distribution of small veins. *Am. J. Pathol.* **37**: 673–683.

Waksman, B.H. (1961a). Experimentelle immunologische Erkrankungen des peripheren Nervensystems. In: *Immunopathologie in Klinik und Forschung* ed. P. Miescher and K.O. Vorlaender, pp. 540–564. Immunologische Untersuchungen bei der Polyneuritis und bei Entmarkungskrankheiten, 2d., Geo. Thieme, Verlag.

Waksman, B.H. (1961b). Experimental study of diphtheritic polyneuritis in the rabbit and guinea pig. III. The blood–nerve barrier in the rabbit. *J. Neuropath. Exp. Neurol.* **20**: 35–77.

Waksman, B.H. and Adams, R.D. (1953). Tubercle bacillus lipopolysaccharide as adjuvant in the production of experimental allergic encephalomyelitis in rabbits. *J. Infect. Dis.* **93**: 21–27.

Waksman, B.H. and Adams, R.D. (1955). Allergic neuritis: an experimental disease of rabbits induced by the injection of peripheral nervous tissue and adjuvants. *J. Exp. Med.* **102**: 213–236, (Preliminary report in *Fed. Proc.* **13**: Abstr. 1692, 1954).

Waksman, B.H. and Adams, R.D. (1956). A comparative study of experimental allergic neuritis in the rabbit, guinea pig, and mouse. *J. Neuropath. Exp. Neurol.* **15**: 293–333.

Waksman, B.H., Adams, R.D., and Mansmann, H.C. Jr (1957). Experimental study of diphtheritic polyneuritis in the rabbit and guinea pig. I. Immunologic and histopathologic observations. *J. Exp. Med.* **105**: 591–614.

Waksman, B.H. and Morrison, L.R. (1951). Tuberculin type sensitivity to spinal cord antigen in rabbits with isoallergic encephalomyelitis. *J. Immunol.* **66**: 421–444.

Waksman, B.H., Porter, H., Lees, M.D., Adams, R.D., and Folch, J. (1954). A study of the chemical nature of components of bovine white matter effective in producing allergic encephalomyelitis in the rabbit. *J. Exp. Med.* **100**: 451–471.

Webster, H. deF., Spiro, D., Waksman, B.H., and Adams, R.D. (1961). Phase and electron microscopic studies of experimental demyelination. II. Schwann cell changes in guinea pig sciatic nerves during experimental diphtheritic neuritis. *J. Neuropath. Exp. Neurol.* **20**: 5–34.

PART I Biology and epidemiology

1 Immune interactions in the peripheral nervous system

C.L. Koski

Interaction of the immune system with peripheral nerves either underlies or contributes to the development of an ever increasing variety of inflammatory, infectious or paraneoplastic neuropathies. In many, participation of immune effectors provides a rational for acute interventional therapy. The effectors of both cellular and humoral immune system are implicated and include T cells, NK cells, macrophages, antibodies and complement proteins. In addition, there is a growing recognition of the role of cytokines and neurotransmitters which provide bidirectional signaling and communication between cells of the immune system and primary cells of the endoneurium. The mechanisms by which peripheral nerve tissues interact with these cells and soluble factors govern the pathogenesis of these largely inflammatory neuropathies. Alteration of the blood–nerve barrier which sequesters the endoneurial compartment is an initial step that facilitates the penetration of cells and inflammatory mediators. Then, lymphocytes and antibodies may target the tissues of the endoneurial compartment through specific recognition of protein or carbohydrate epitopes. It should be noted that once inflammatory effectors are brought to the endoneurium, tissue damage, especially myelin damage, can occur even in the absence of a specific immune response directed against myelin. Myelin, which lacks several complement-inhibitory membrane proteins, is particularly susceptible to complement-mediated damage.

The endoneurial compartment consists of axons of varying diameters which are supported by Schwann cells and collagen matrices. Also present are fibroblasts, a population of resident macrophages, occasional mast cells, vascular endothelium and sensory dorsal root ganglia. The motor neurons, although functionally a part of the motor unit, lie within the spinal cord and are supported and maintained by the glia of the central nervous system (CNS). Specific or bystander injury of endoneurial constituents by factors generated through the cellular or humoral immune responses disrupts complex physiological interactions required for the function of peripheral nerve.

The Schwann cell is a principal glial cell of the peripheral nervous system (PNS), capable of secreting numerous tropic factors which include nerve growth factor (NGF) (Rush 1984; Matsuoka et al. 1991; Yamamoto et al. 1993), ciliary nerve trophic factor (CNTF) (Friedman et al. 1992; Rende et al. 1992) and glia derived neurotrophic factor (GDNF) (Henderson et al. 1994) that contribute to axonal out growth, sprouting and neuronal survival. Schwann cells synthesize and produce peripheral nerve myelin, extracellular matrix, and express neural cell adhesion molecules (N-CAM and L1). In addition to secreting cytokines and inflammatory mediators, Schwann cells may also act as antigen presenting cells. Schwann cells differentiate from progenitors derived from neural ectoderm. On embryonic day 16 (E16) in rats, cells in response to growth factors including fibroblast growth factor, begin to express the glial marker, S-100, an intracellular Ca^{2+} binding protein (Jessen & Mirsky 1991; Jessen et al. 1994). Shortly thereafter, on E16 and E17, Schwann cells express the 04 sulfatide antigen, and those destined to form myelin express galactocerebroside. Nonmyelinating, immature Schwann cells express low affinity receptors for NGF (NGFr p75) (Taniuchi et al. 1986) and N-CAM, and a subpopulation of Schwann cells in contact with axons of smaller diameter express a species of glial fibrillary acid protein (GFAP) (Mokuno et al. 1989). Although unmyelinated, smaller axons up to 2.4 μm in diameter in human nerve maintain intimate contact with Schwann cells lying within invaginated cell membranes. Schwann cells in contact with larger axons myelinate a segment of axon with compacted spiral layers of myelin membranes formed by the apposition of the cytoplasmic faces of Schwann cell plasmalemma. Myelinating Schwann cells are negative for NGFr and N-CAM but continue to express S-100, a Fc gamma receptor and CR1, a complement receptor for activated fragments of complement protein C3 and C4, C3b and C4b (Vedeler & Matre, 1990; Vedeler et al. 1989a,b). Axonal contact of the myelin internode, formed by a single Schwann cell, stimulates neurofilament phosphorylation and segregates the axonal sodium channels at the nodes of Ranvier, which contributes to the electrophysiological characteristics of the axon including saltatory conduction. Demyelination or loss of the myelinated internode exposes internodal potassium channels, decreases the conduction efficiency of the ion impulse by blocking the spread of passive depolarization to produce failure of impulse propagation (Waxman & Ritchie 1993). Degeneration of the distal axon by inflammation or trauma allows reversion of Schwann cells to a nonmyelinating phenotype and divestment and/or vesiculation of myelin. After axonal degeneration, surviving columns of Schwann cells are thought to express adhesion molecules, such as L1 and NGFr p75, a permissive receptor for NGF and CNTF, that provide pathways for the regrowth of motor and sensory fibers (Martini 1994). L1 is a heavily glycosylated 200–230 kDa membrane protein, a member of the immunoglobulin supergene family whose expression is restricted to the nervous system. The interaction of L1, expressed on neuronal and Schwann cell surfaces, is enhanced when N-CAM is coexpressed (Kadmon et al. 1990).

Myelin, a specialized membrane produced by fully differentiated Schwann cells, expresses diverse membrane molecules that are important as structural components of the myelin and in maintaining homeostasis of myelin–axon interactions. These molecules can also be antigenic, thus inducing specific immune responses to target peripheral nerve. Within the endoneurium, the 100 kDa myelin associated glycoprotein (MAG), the 30 kDa major glycoprotein of compact myelin (Po), PMP-22 and two basic proteins P2 and P1, are myelin proteins that are, for all practical purposes, not detectable on the surface of the Schwann cell body. MAG is a heavily glycosylated integral membrane protein with a significant homology to N-CAM (Arquint et al. 1987). Its expression in endoneurium is limited to myelin at the internodal loops, the inner and outer mesaxon, the Schmidt–Lantermann incisures and at points of axonal contact. About 95% of MAG in peripheral nerve myelin (PMN) contains a 67 kDa peptide which is produced by alternative splicing (Frail & Braun 1984; Inuzuka et al. 1991). MAG mediates homotypic interaction between Schwann cells and heterotypic interaction of Schwann cells with axons (Martini 1994). The heterotypic ligands for MAG are reported to include heparin sulfate, collagen and chondroitin sulfate (Sadoul et al. 1990). Po, a 30 kDa transmembrane glycoprotein expressed only in compact myelin (Lemke et al. 1988), also forms both homotypic and heterotypic dimers. Although the nature of axonal ligand(s) has not been characterized, its interaction may be responsible for recognition between axon and myelinating Schwann cells at the onset of myelination (Schneider-Schaulies et al. 1990). Genetic deficiency of Po results in a loss of compact myelin. PMP 22 is encoded by a growth arrest specific gene, GAS-3.

Genetic deficiency in rodents is associated with development of a tomaculous neuropathy. Point mutations and reduplications in the Po and PMP-22 genes result in hereditary dysmyelinating neuropathies such as Charcot Marie Tooth syndrome, Dejerine Sottas disease and an inherited tendency to pressure palsies (Suter & Patel 1994). The HNK or L2 carbohydrate epitope expressed on MAG, Po, L1 and other myelin proteins, is implicated in the binding of the paraprotein to peripheral nerve in some patients with monoclonal gammopathy and neuropathy (Latov et al. 1988; van den Berg et al. 1990). A 170 kDa Schwann associated glycoprotein (SAG) is upregulated on both the myelin forming Schwann cell body and myelin membrane itself. P1 and P2 are two basic proteins of 22 kDa and 18 kDa, respectively. They are located at the dense interperiod line of myelin lamellae. P1, which is similar in sequence to the myelin basic protein of central myelin, is proposed to participate in forming compact myelin through dimer formation; however, animals immunized with purified P1 protein develop inflammatory CNS disease. In contrast, immunization with the peripheral myelin produces an inflammatory neuropathy which suggests that P1 is presented in an immunologically different fashion in the PNS compared with myelin basic protein (MBP) in the CNS. P2 predominantly found in association with peripheral nerve structures can also be detected in small amounts in spinal cord. Immunization with P2 induces a T cell mediated subacute inflammatory neuropathy (Brostoff et al. 1972; Kadlubowski & Hughes 1979; Hughes & Powell 1984).

Although proteins such as Po and P2 are the most studied T cell antigens due to their specificity of endoneural expression, there is also a wide variety of acidic and neutral glycolipids within this compartment that are implicated as targets for immunological autoreactivity, especially autoantibody production. In many cases these lipids are not exclusive for endoneurial tissue but instead are shared by cells of intravascular compartment, CNS and other organs. For example, LM1 is a principal ganglioside of human PMN, and also a component of human erythrocyte membrane (Fong et al. 1976; Svennerholm & Friedman 1990). The acidic glycolipid GM1, implicated as an antigen in multifocal motor neuropathy and possibly some axonal or pure motor forms of Guillain-Barré syndrome (GBS), is expressed preferentially on motor axolemma but is also a component of CNS myelin and axolemma (Corbo et

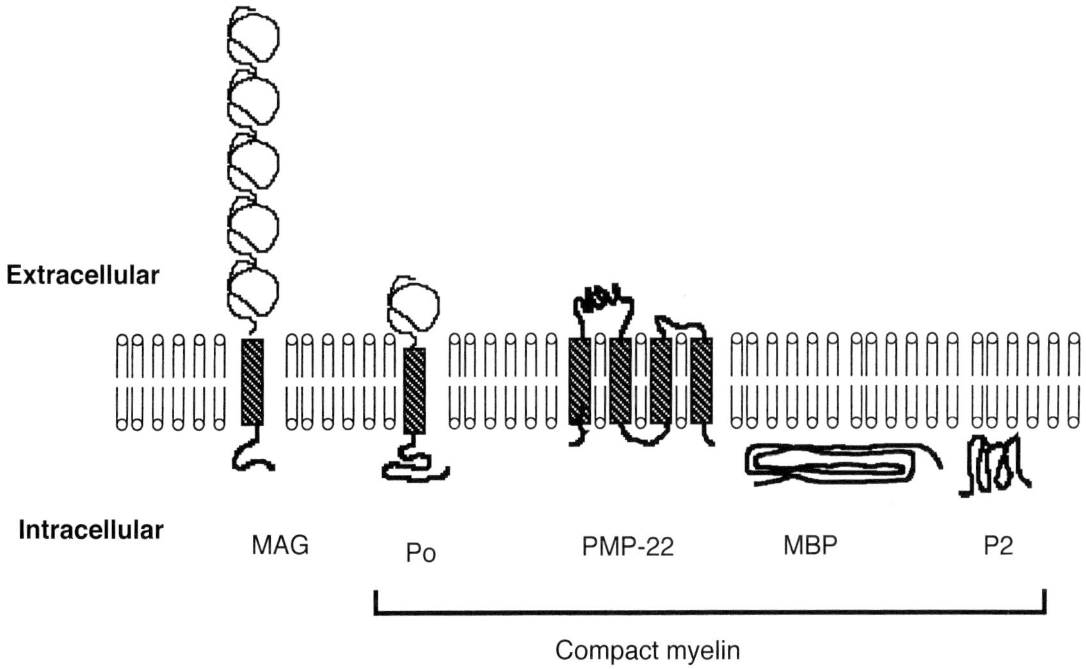

Figure 1.1 *Molecular organization of myelin proteins in peripheral myelin. MAG: myelin associated protein.*

al. 1992, 1993). Anti-GM1 antibody injected endoneurially binds to the node of Ranvier in rabbits and the presynaptic rat neuromuscular junction where it is associated with conduction block and altered neurotransmitter release (Thomas et al. 1991; Santoro et al. 1992). Another acidic glycolipid, GQ1b, appears to be preferentially located at the nodes of oculomotor peripheral nerves and possibly cerebellar tissue (Chiba et al. 1992, 1993). Antibodies to this glycolipid are associated with the Miller Fisher variant of GBS and Bickerstaff's brainstem encephalitis (Yuki et al. 1993a,b). The targeting of specific antigens representative of individual areas of PNS may underlie the development of specific clinical syndromes. Even though these antigens may be expressed elsewhere, penetration of the endoneurium by antibody to bind to specific epitopes on glycolipid antigens may facilitate interaction with effector arms of both the cellular and humoral immune system.

Blood–nerve barrier

The endoneurial compartment is sequestered by a blood–nerve barrier which consists of perineurial connective tissue and the endothelial cells of the endoneurial blood vessels. Although these endothelial cells do not have tight junctions as are expressed by the vascular endothelium of the brain, they are second only to the CNS in their ability to sequester peripheral nerve from plasma constituents. The integrity of this barrier can be altered as a result of immune stimulation, inflammatory vasculitis, immune complex disease, primary infection of the nerve, as well as crush or pressure injuries. Proximally, at the level of the spinal roots, and distally, at the level of the motor end plates, the barrier is less effective. These areas are frequently involved early during the inflammatory demyelination associated with GBS, possibly diabetic neuropathy, and may be the primary sites of injury in the axonal forms of acute motor neuropathy as proposed in the Chinese paralytic syndrome or acute motor axonal neuropathy.

Trafficking of lymphocytes or neutrophils into the endoneurial compartment is influenced by changes induced in the endothelial vessels by a series of chemokines and cytokines. Leukocyte extravasation occurs primarily in the postcapillary venules. Initially cells will roll over the endothelial surface and develop weak tethering through lymphocyte surface molecules including the constitutively expressed L-selectin, and the rapidly induced early adhesion molecule, E-selectin (Shimizu et al. 1992). This weak adhesion, characterized by lymphocyte margination and rolling, is a passive event. Following an appropriate cytokine signal, increased expression of the intercellular adhesion molecule (ICAM) and upregulation of the vascular cell adhesion molecule, VCAM, and platelet endothelial cell adhesion molecule, PECAM, enhances leukocyte flattening and adhesion to the endothelial cells (Lo et al. 1989; Lawrence & Springer 1991). Change in leukocyte shapes permits interendothelial migration and extravasation (Lo et al. 1989; Lawrence & Springer 1991). T cells migrate into sequestered organs such as brain and peripheral nerve in a random manner, stay briefly and migrate back into the circulation (Lassmann et al. 1993). Once in the peripheral nerve, interaction of the T cell receptor with specific peptide presented in the context of MHC class II molecules on cells such as resident macrophages (less likely Schwann cells) is proposed to lead to prolonged sequestration of T cells in endoneural compartment, proliferation of T cells in situ, and local production of cytokines and chemokines. Cytokines such as IL-1, IFN-γ and TNFα and chemokines such as RANTES and IP-10 upregulate adhesion molecules including ICAM as well as class I and II major histocompatibility (MHC) molecules on vascular endothelium. Enhanced expression of these adhesion molecules, in turn, further enhances adhesion of T cells and monocytes/macrophages through ligands which include the lymphocyte function associated antigen-1 (LFA-1) and complement receptor 3 (CR3) (Hartung et al. 1990b). Increased levels of soluble E-selectin (Hartung et al. 1994), ICAM (Jander et al. 1993) and PCAM can be detected in the serum of patients with GBS and chronic inflammatory polyneuritis, which suggests an alteration of endothelial barriers in these diseases. Blocking antibodies to ICAM (Archelos et al. 1993) or to its ligands LAF-1 and CR3 (Archelos et al. 1994) can reduce inflammation of the nerve, as shown in animals with delayed hypersensitivity to peripheral nerve or experimental allergic neuritis (EAN). Enhanced barrier permeability would permit penetration of the endoneurial compartment by intravascular components of inflammatory and immune effectors, which include smaller molecular size factors like cytokines and lipid-derived inflammatory mediators as well as large molecular proteins like antibodies and complement components.

Changes in the endothelial barrier are evident in many other forms of immune interaction with the nerve. Increased expression of ICAM and class I and class II MHC molecules can be detected in the peripheral nerve biopsy of patients with systemic and focal forms of vasculitis (Panegyres et al. 1992) as well as primary infections in peripheral nerve associated with *Mycobacterium leprae* (Cowley et al. 1990) and *Borrelia burgdorferi.* MHC molecules are upregulated on the surface of endothelial cells by proinflammatory cytokines like IFNγ, TNFα and IL1β. Vascular endothelium appears to be the principal immunological target in some of these conditions mediated by sensitized T cells (Kissel et al. 1989), soluble immune complexes (Cochrane & Koffler 1973; Franklin 1980) or by specific antibodies (Kaneko et al. 1994). Additional factors affecting vascular permeability such as complement-derived anaphylatoxin C3a and C5a, and those released from mast cells and basophils such as histamine, platelet activating factor and leukotrienes also contribute to the increased permeability of small blood vessels.

Naturally occurring antiendothelial cell antibodies in human, that affect xenograft rejection, could also theoretically increase blood–nerve barrier permeability in Arthus reaction, serum sickness, vasculitis associated with anticardiolipin antibodies or even in monoclonal gammopathies. Heparan sulfate which acts as a tether for superoxide dismutase on the endothelial cell surface, is released by antiendothelial antibodies and C5a and leads to thrombus formation and oxidative injury (Platt et al. 1991). Antibody-mediated activation of complement forming sublytic numbers of terminal complement complexes C5b-7, C5b-8, C5b-9 in endothelial cells can cause transient intercellular gaps by affecting endothelial cytoskeletal proteins (Saadi & Platt 1995). It is therefore obvious that diverse mechanisms which include a variety of cells like T cells, neutrophils and mast cells and the factors released from them, such as cytokines, chemokines, vasoactive amines, as well as activated complement proteins (C3a, C5a, C5b-8 and C5b-9), can contribute to altering the endothelial permeability barriers, thus allowing greater access of cellular and humoral factors into the endoneurium.

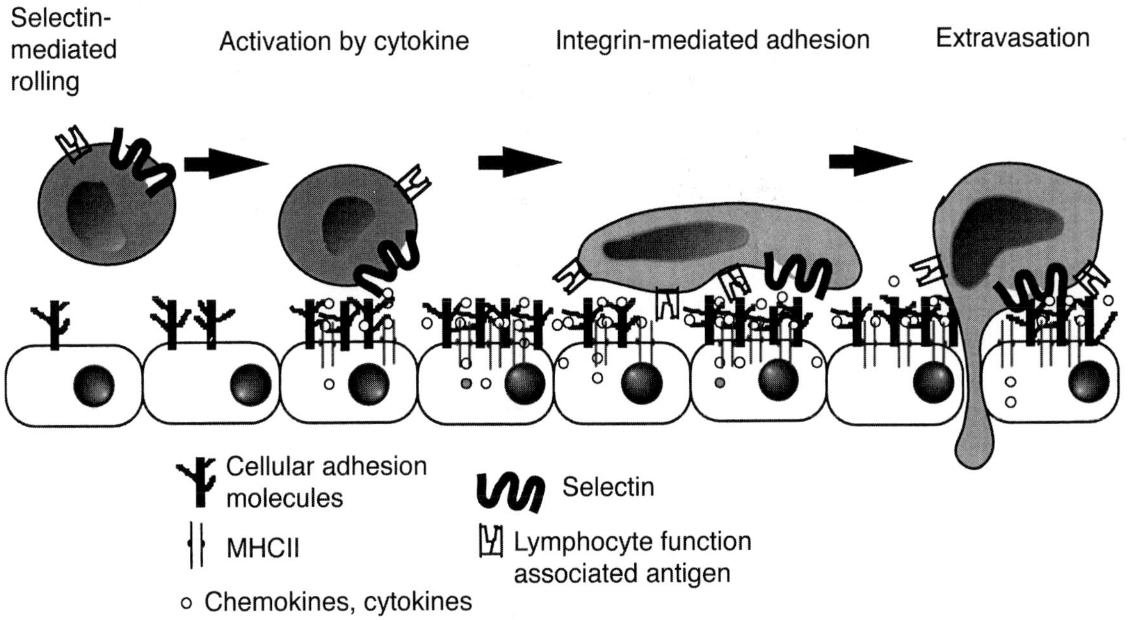

Figure 1.2 *Extravasation of lymphocytes through endothelial barriers.*

Participation of the cellular immune system

Sensitization of T lymphocytes to the peripheral nerve implies a recognition of peptides whose antigenic epitopes are expressed within the endoneurium. In addition to recognizing antigenic epitopes by the antigen receptor, induction of specific T cell response is also regulated through a complex adhesion apparatus which includes costimulatory signals from the antigen presenting cells. Foreign antigens are taken up by antigen presenting cells in which antigens are processed in lysosomal compartment and peptides of antigenic epitopes are then loaded onto appropriate haplotypes of MHC class II molecules in acidic endosomes to be transported to the cell surface where the peptides interact with $CD4^+$ T cell receptors in a MHC restricted manner (Unanue 1993). For induction of an immune response as opposed to peripheral tolerance to a given antigen, a costimulatory signal is required between B7-1 and B7-2 ligands of antigen presenting cells and CD28 receptors on T cells (June et al. 1990). Specific interactions between such receptors and ligands induce antigen presenting cells to produce IL-1. In synergy with IL-6, it increases IL-2 production and causes $CD4^+$ T cell to increase high affinity IL-2r expression to achieve proliferation in response to IL-2. Activated T cells then secrete sets of multiple cytokines that can affect B cell activation and antibody production, generation of cytotoxic T cells and the capacity of monocytes and macrophages to kill intracellular organisms and mobilize inflammatory responses. Based on studies of murine T cell clones, two major subsets of $CD4^+$ T cells have been defined according to the types of cytokines they produce (Mosmann et al. 1986). One is Th1. These cells produce predominantly IL-2 and IFNγ, and are most frequently associated with the development of cell-mediated hypersensitivity reaction and the production of complement-fixing and opsonizing antibodies. Th2 cells produce predominantly IL-4, IL-6, IL-10 and IL-13 among which IL-4 is known to enhance the development of Th2 cells that facilitate the memory B cell development while inhibiting the Th1 generation. IL-12 and IFNγ stimulate the generation of Th1 instead of Th2.

Perhaps one of the best examples of cell-mediated immunity to peripheral nerve antigens is EAN, an animal model for human subacute inflammatory neuropathy. EAN can be induced in a wide variety of animal species by sensitization with peripheral nerve, peripheral nerve myelin, purified P2 basic protein (Brostoff 1972; Kadlubowski & Hughes 1979), the Po glycoprotein (Milner et al. 1987), peptides of P2, Po and with galactocerebroside (Saida et al. 1979). Depending on the route and immunization protocol, animals develop a monophasic illness of ataxia and paralysis within 1 and 4 weeks. Inbred strains vary in their susceptibility to T cell mediated peripheral nerve inflammation. Lewis rats are more susceptible to EAN than the Brown Norway or Sprague Dawley rats (Hoffman et al. 1980; Steinman et al. 1981). The peripheral nerves of EAN animals are infiltrated by mononuclear cells, consisting primarily of Ia positive macrophages but also include T cells (Olsson et al. 1984). The earliest phenotype of T cells infiltrating the peripheral nerves of EAN animals are $CD4^+$ (Brosnan et al. 1985). Later infiltrates, after the peak of clinical disease and during the recovery, are primarily effector/cytotoxic $CD8^+$ T cell which recognize autoantigen in the context of class I MHC (Ota et al. 1987; Strigard et al. 1987). The CD8 subset also includes suppressor cells that protect against autoimmune responses. A role for the CD8 receptor on T cells in clinical EAE was demonstrated using genetically engineered mice (Koh et al. 1992). Mice negative for the CD8 gene had more frequent relapses of CNS inflammation than mice that expressed CD8. The ability to passively transfer disease to naive rats by lymphoid cells of animals with EAN (Hughes et al. 1981), or $CD4^+$ T cell lines specific for either P2 (Linington et al. 1984; Rostami et al. 1985), a basic protein of peripheral nerve myelin, or Po, the major glycoprotein of PNM, supported the T cell dependence of EAN (Linington et al. 1995). Even in the genetically resistant Brown Norway rat, T cell clones reactive to P2 can be detected, isolated and used to passively confer EAN to naive Brown Norway recipients (Linington et al. 1986). Resistance to EAN in certain inbred strains of rodents may be associated with a number of different factors including the inability to produce IFNγ, resulting in the tendency to default to a Th2 cellular response instead of Th1, or the production of adrenal corticotropic hormone (ACTH), through stimulation of the pituitary axis by cytokines. Treatment of EAN in Lewis rats with T cell modulators such as cyclosporin (Hartung et al. 1987b) which blocks both IL-2 production and IL-2 receptor expression, blocking antibodies to the IL-2 receptor expressed on activated T cells (Hartung et al. 1987a), or blocking antibodies to IFNγ (Strigard et al. 1989; Hartung et al. 1990b), inhibits or modulates the disease as does treatment with corticosteroids (Hartung et al. 1988a). The corticosteroid effect may be largely dependent on its ability to downregulate production of cytokines such as IL-1.

Evidence which supports a role for T cells in GBS is the presence of increased numbers of activated T cells in the circulation of patients as shown by expression of high levels of IL-2 receptor, transferrin receptor, class II antigen, the release of soluble IL-2 receptors into the surrounding medium and by proliferation of T cells during an autologous mixed lymphocyte response in GBS patients (Kamin-Lewis et al. 1994). Using an enzyme-linked immunosorbent assay (ELISA), elevated levels of soluble IL-2 receptors were more uniformly detectable in the circulation of GBS patients and less frequently in patients with CIDP when compared with other disease controls (Hartung et al. 1990a). IL-2 receptors and the autologous mixed lymphocyte response (MLR) were highest when GBS patients first presented with neurological symptoms and decreased gradually over 1–3 months. In one study many of these early circulating activated T cells were $CD8^+$ and postulated to represent a response to previous viral infection (Dahle et al. 1994).

Unlike EAN where the phenotype of earliest infiltrating T cells are $CD4^+$ and later infiltrates at the peak of peripheral nerve inflammation are primarily $CD8^+$, the T cells in the peripheral nerves of GBS patients are both $CD4^+$ and $CD8^+$ in a ratio similar to that present in the circulation (Cornblath et al. 1990). The lack of a specific class of infiltrating T cells in human neural biopsies may reflect an enhanced chemotaxic recruitment of cells into the endoneurium that may mask a more specific earlier infiltrate.

The prevalence of specific autoreactive T cells to myelin protein(s) in the circulation of GBS and chronic idiopathic demyelinating neuropathy (CIDP) patients and the role these cells play in demyelination are not well studied because of a lack of a well-defined target antigen. A recent study suggested that the antigens recognized by GBS patient T cells were heterogeneous as peripheral blood lymphocytes from 12 of 19 GBS patients and six of 13 CIDP patients proliferated to either the Po glycoprotein, the P2 protein or fragments of these proteins (Khalili-Shirazi et al. 1992). Some of the 19 GBS patients responded to a peptide of bovine Po (amino acids: 70–85) normally exposed at the intraperiod or plasmalemma face of myelin membrane and six others responded to a fragment derived from the cytoplasmic portion of the molecule (amino acids: 180–199). No reactivity to either fragment was detected in normal controls. In contrast the frequency of response to P2 among normal controls and the patient group was not significantly different. If P2 reactive T cell clones participate significantly in inflammatory neuropathy, one would have to propose a temporal disorder of the normal mechanisms which suppress their activation in the circulation of normal individuals. Further support for such a hypothesis contributing to induction of GBS may be derived from multiple incidences of subacute and chronic inflammatory neuritis reported in immunosuppressed patients undergoing organ transplantation, patients with recent seroconversion for human immunodeficiency virus (HIV) and lymphoproliferative disorders (Arnason & Soliven, 1993). The transient responses to Po described in the study by Khalili-Shirazi et al. were detectable earlier in the clinical course of GBS patients than those to P2 which persisted for up to 146 days. The responses to the glycoprotein appeared to correlate better with development of clinical symptoms while that to P2 may have represented a response to an antigen exposed by previous myelin damage. Although this report was encouraging, a subsequent study of a more limited group of four GBS patients found no reaction to synthetic bovine Po peptides (Pette et al. 1994). They were, however, able to clone T cells lines from each of eight healthy subjects which reacted with Po-peptides 1–20 (14%), 19–38 (74%), 56–71 (2%), 150–169 (6%), 165–184 (8%), 194–208 (4%). Five of Po-specific T cell lines reactive to 19–38 from bovine Po did not react with 19–38 of human Po. These results reaffirm the importance of the use of autologous antigen and the requirement for further studies to determine the role of Po in human myelin autoreactivity.

Many of the antigens implicated in the humoral autoantibody response in patients with acute inflammatory neuropathies to peripheral nerve are glycolipids and the epitope specificity often resides in the carbohydrate moieties. IgM antibodies generated to these largely T cell independent antigens require only 'bystander' amounts of T cell cytokines. The deposition of complement on the surface of infectious particles in the patient's blood enhances B cell response to suboptimal amounts of antigens by stimulation of the specific antigen receptor along with CR2 or CR1 receptors on B lymphocytes (Carter et al. 1988; Carter & Fearon 1992). For T cells to provide specific help to carbohydrate reactive IgG secreting memory B cells they would most likely bind to a protein peptide of a glycoprotein which coexpressed the carbohydrate epitope to which the B cell reacted. Under such circumstances cross-linking and internalization of the glycopeptide through specific immunoglobulin receptors on the surface of a B cell might enhance peptide antigen presentation to T cells in context of class II or Ia molecules. Specific T cells would then secrete cytokines to enhance B cell proliferation, differentiation, affinity maturation and immunoglobulin secretion. More recently, some evidence suggests that lipid antigens can be recognized by CD1 restricted T cells which express neither CD4 nor CD8 (Beckman et al. 1994). Antigen presenting function also has been proposed for the non-MHC-encoded CD1 molecules, a family of nonpolymorphic, β2 microglobulin-associated glycoproteins expressed on most professional antigen presenting cells. This phenomenon has not been investigated in clinical autoimmune disease but may bear relevance to the human inflammatory neuropathies.

Like EAN the perivascular infiltrates in peripheral nerves of GBS patients although including T cells are primarily composed of activated Ia positive macrophages (Prineas 1981; Raine 1985) which also express Fc and complement receptors including CR1 and CR3. Most evidence supports the macrophage as being the primary effector of peripheral nerve demyelination in both EAN, human inflammatory neuropathies and even Wallerian degeneration. Electron microscopic and immunohistochemical analysis in both conditions demonstrate the adherence of Ia and CR3 positive macrophages to myelinated nerve axons and subsequent stripping of normal appearing myelin from these axons (Ballin & Thomas 1968; Lampert 1969; Prineas 1972). Macrophages, attracted to the endoneurium by either gamma interferon (IFN-γ) produced by activated T cells or complement activation fragments such as C5a, can interact with targets opsonized by IgG and fragments of complement component C3. Interaction through specific receptors for the Fc portion of certain IgG, C3b, iC3b or C3dg promotes phagocytosis and release of cytokines, TNFα, IL-6 and IL-1 as well as injurious molecules such as oxygen radicles (Ravetch & Kirit 1991; Suzuki 1991; Krych et al. 1992) and proteases which cleave Po and MBP molecules that are involved in myelin compaction (Cammer et al. 1981). Various agents that block or regulate the expression of CR3 on the macrophages surface, systemically deplete macrophages from the circulation, or inhibit metabolic production of inflammatory mediators such as prostaglandins or cyclooxygenases, abrogate or modulate clinical disease and demyelination in animals with EAN (Tansey & Brosnan 1982; Draggs et al. 1984; Hartung et al. 1988a,b; Heininger et al. 1988). The cytokine production and release of oxygen radicles and membrane destructive enzymes by macrophages have the potential to damage tissue in their immediate vicinity and are the most likely source of bystander injury to axons frequently seen in association with most cases of inflammatory demyelinating neuropathy.

Cellular infiltrates are also characteristic of vasculitis involving peripheral nerve. In contrast to that seen in the inflammatory neuropathies, up to 71% of these cells are T cells, a principal portion of which are $CD8^+$ (Kissel et al. 1989). The remaining cells were primarily macrophages with surprisingly few polymorphonuclear cells, natural killer cells or B cells. Although these series of biopsies were obtained from patients with both systemic vasculitis and that limited to peripheral nerve, many features of the pathology were the same suggesting that the mechanism of vascular damage and inflammation were similar despite the different etiologies. Surprisingly the lack of PMN and the association of antibody and complement deposition with only more prominent perivascular cellular infiltrates suggested a primary role for a T cell dependent cell-mediated injury and that humoral factors served a secondary enhancing role.

Even in type II diabetes mellitus where neuropathy has been linked to abnormal glucose metabolism, increased endoneurial edema and vascular ischemia, both acute and chronic forms of inflammatory nerve damage are being identified with increased frequency. A limited study of 20 patients with mononeuritis multiplex, distal or proximal polyneuropathy showed increased numbers of $CD8^+$ T cells infiltrating the perineurium, endoneurium, as well as around vessels in a perivascular distribution (A.P. Hays 1995, personal communication).

Schwann cells are rarely the target of direct invasion by pathogens with an exception of *Mycobacterium leprae* and a limited number of herpes viruses in some experimental models. Within the peripheral nerve, Schwann cells are primarily infected by *M. leprae*, sparing fibroblasts and neurons. Adhesion of *M. leprae* to Schwann cells involves a lipoarabinomannan complex in the organism cell wall to an unknown receptor (Choudhury et al. 1989). A selective anergy of T cells to *M. leprae* antigens appears to underlie the inability of patients with the lepromatous form of leprosy to mount a cellular immune response to the organism (Mehra & Modlin 1990; Kaplan & Cohn 1991), as there is no evidence of delayed hypersensitivity on skin tests of patients with *M. leprae* or T cell proliferation to *M. leprae* antigens in vitro. Foamy macrophages containing numerous bacilli infiltrate the peripheral nerve of these patients (Dastur et al. 1982; Mshana et al. 1983; Shetty et al. 1988; Job 1989). Cytokine production by macrophages and T cells in these patients are reduced (Ottenhoff & DeVries 1990). Supplementation with IL-2 and IFNγ corrects the inability of patient lymphocytes to mediate killing of the microorganism (Kaplan & Cohn 1991). The decreased IL-2 may inhibit expansion of cytotoxic, IFNγ-producing T cells. As the cellular immune system is compromised, the actual peripheral nerve destruction does not occur until late in the disease. In contrast, the nerves of patients with tuberculoid leprosy contain a paucity of *M. leprae* organisms and are involved by giant cell granuloma which damage both myelin and axons (Dastur et al. 1982; Jacobs et al. 1987; Shetty et al. 1988). The MHC class I expression on Schwann cells is enhanced by IFNγ and Schwann cell cytolysis has been demonstrated in the presence of $CD8^+$ T cells sensitized to *M. leprae* (Samuel et al. 1987; Steinhoff & Kauffmann 1988: Kingston et al. 1989). Recognition of heat shock epitopes shared by *M. leprae* and host Schwann cells or a hypersensitivity to *M. leprae* antigens may cause an attack by T cells on Schwann cells (Kaufmann et al. 1990).

It has been postulated that Schwann cells and resident macrophages can function as antigen presenting cells within the endoneurium to stimulate T cell reactivity during inflammation of peripheral nerve. Schwann cells do have some of the properties necessary for accessory cells because in vitro they express MHC class II molecules after 3 days of treatment with IFNγ (Samuel et al. 1987; Kingston et al. 1989) and are also capable of secreting IL-1 in response to soluble antigens of *M. leprae* and lipopolysaccharide (Bergsteinsdsottir et al. 1991). Presentation of MBP by Schwann cells to a T cell line specific for MBP in vitro resulted in Schwann cell death (Wekerle et al. 1986; Argall et al. 1992). It is likely that Schwann cells are unable to induce a primary immune response involving naive T cells, possibly from an inability to express costimulatory molecules like B7, required by the T cell for activation and proliferation. If antigen presentation occurs within the peripheral nerve, it most likely occurs in the context of resident macrophages fully competent as an antigen presenting cell. Schwann cells through antigen release may participate in the development of antigen-specific immune responses, both during the initial phase of the immune response and also during the chronic phase of the reaction by continuously providing the antigen. Chimera experiments in which experimental allergic encephalitis (EAE) animals were reconstituted with bone marrow cells from animals of a different histocompatibility background, confirmed that the antigen presenting cells that initiated the disease processes were derived from the bone marrow, not peripheral nerve (Lassman et al. 1993).

Participation of the humoral immune system

Evidence suggests that antibodies binding to specific antigen epitopes can target the endoneurium and mediate damage through activation of either complement or antibody-dependent cytolytic cells. The antibody isotype affects the ease with which it penetrates the endoneurial compartment and the effector mechanism recruited in damaging the membrane. IgM is a pentameric molecule of 970–1150 kDa which does not normally penetrate the endoneurium unless the barrier is disrupted by trauma, vasoactive agents such as 5-hydroxy tryptamine or cytokines including IFNγ or TNFα (Spies et al. 1993; G.K. Harvey & J.D. Pollard, personal communication). These IgM antibodies generally have low affinity for antigen as they are formed prior to affinity maturation. A polyvalent nature of antigens expressed on pathogenic organisms and the multiple antigen-binding sites on a single IgM molecule can contribute to achieve higher avidity, therefore resulting in an effective binding to the target surface. Once bound to antigen, IgM is most efficient in activating complement as a single IgM can fix C1q to induce conformational changes, which facilitate activation and cleavage of C1r and C1s dimers to initiate complement cascade activation (Wright et al. 1990). Antigen-bound IgM can also indirectly mediate phagocytosis by activating complement. Fixation of C4b, C3b or iC3b on target membranes facilitates macrophage interaction through surface complement receptors CR1 and CR3. IgG (150 kDa), since it is smaller than IgM, has limited access to enter the endoneurium through an intact blood–nerve barrier (Heininger et al. 1984; Seiz et al. 1985). Among human IgG, IgG3 activates complement more efficiently than IgG1 while IgG2 and IgG4 activate little if any (Bruggermann et al. 1987). IgG2 and IgG4 lack appropriate amino acids near the hinge region of IgG that permit binding of C1q (Duncan & Winter 1988; Sandlie & Michaelson 1991). For IgG1 and IgG3 to cause the required conformational changes in C1q, the Fc regions of minimally three IgG molecules must be in close apposition. Therefore, when antigen epitope density is low, even in the presence of IgG antibody bound to antigen, complement may not be activated. IgG can mediate phagocytosis by macrophages and granulocytes and antibody-dependent cellular cytotoxicity through lymphocytes and natural killer cells. The functions are mediated through Fcγ-specific receptors on the effector cells. Individual specific receptors exist for all four IgG subclasses. Signals transmitted through Fcγ receptors effect not only tissue destruction but modulate the immune response by facilitating antigen presentation, stimulation of effector cells and the release of cytokines and chemokines. IgG1 and IgG3 isotypes are the IgG isotypes interacting with Fcγ receptors of monocytes (Bruggermann et al. 1987; Michaelson et al. 1992). Circulating IgE (190 kDa) is bound to the specific high affinity receptors (FcεR1) expressed on mast cells and basophils. Capping IgE antibodies on mast cells and basophils by antigens crosslinks Fcε receptors, resulting in degranulation with release of vasoactive amines and the generation of arachidonic acid-derived inflammatory mediators. This response participates in the clearance of certain pathogenic organisms as well as allergy and anaphylaxis in atopic patients. IgA (160 and 400 kDa) exists in a monomeric or dimeric form, comprising 10–15% of serum immunoglobulin. The dimer is the dominant immunoglobulin secreted through the mucosa and acts as a first line of defense against invading pathogens. The serum and secretory IgA are produced by B lymphocytes of separate pools. IgA can also cause tissue damage by several mechanisms. It opsonizes macrophage targets by interaction with FcαR, and induces degranulation of eosinophils. Although IgA does not activate complement through the classical pathway, it does activate the alternate pathway by a yet unknown mechanism, possibly through aggregation.

Experimental and clinical evidence suggest that antibody plays a role in paraneoplastic, inflammatory and vasculitic neuropathies by contributing to both subacute and chronic demyelination, and also to the development of axonal destruction, focal conduction block and neuromuscular blockade. Many of these antibodies are IgM and recognize carbohydrate epitopes on several glycolipids and glycoproteins. Specific antigens, GM1 and GQ1b, have been proposed to act as specific targets for motor axons and ocular motor nerves, respectively. Recent in vitro studies demonstrated the ability of antibodies to these gangliosides to inhibit neuromuscular transmission as well as block peripheral conduction (Santoro et al. 1992; Roberts et al. 1994; Takigawa et al. 1995). Other antigens enriched in PMN include LM1, GD1a and GD1b, a series of neutral glycolipids with a ceramide backbone bearing either three, four or five glycosyl polysaccharide moieties which define the immunospecific epitope. Indirect evidences suggest that antibodies to these carbohydrate antigens of PMN may interact with antigenic epitopes of infectious agents due to their shared structures. Specifically GM1 and GQ1b epitopes are described on the core sugars that are included in the lipopolysaccharide (LPS) coat of *Campylobacter jejuni* isotypes, a flagellated organism which is associated with outbreaks of human diarrhea (Yuki et al. 1993b, 1994; Jacobs et al. 1995). A pentosyl ceramide associated with human PNM shares a common epitope with Forssman antigen, a neutral glycolipid associated with Epstein–Barr virus and a variety of bacteria and parasites (Koski et al. 1989). These antibody responses do not appear to represent a chronic autoimmune response as those associated with myasthenia gravis or possibly chronic inflammatory demyelinating polyneuritis. They more likely represent a self-limited host response to an infectious viral or bacterial agent that expresses or shares epitopes in common with a surface/accessible antigen of peripheral nerve.

Chronic and more sustained clinical progression seen in patients with chronic inflammatory polyneuritis is associated with the prevalence of certain human lymphocyte antigen (HLA) types, AW30, AW31, B8, DW3, and glyoxalase 1 (Adams et al. 1979; Stewart et al. 1978). An association of such HLA types indicates a genetic predisposition to develop a chronic autoimmune response to PMN. Antigens implicated in these chronic forms of polyneuropathy and paraprotein-associated neuropathy include GM1, GD1b, chondroitin sulfate, sulfatide, LM1, the HNK or L2 epitope expressed on a variety of glycoproteins and glycolipids, as well as intracellular proteins such as tubulin. High levels of anti-GM1 antibodies are believed to be characteristic for a lower motor neuron syndrome associated with focal conduction block designated as multifocal motor neuropathy.

It would be inaccurate to imply that all antibody responses to peripheral nerve in patients with demyelinating neuropathy or paraprotein-associated neuropathy are IgM in nature. IgG responses to peripheral nerve antigens are less frequent, but are reported in patients with GBS from the UK, Japan, and Netherlands (Yuki et al. 1990; Walsh et al. 1991; Gregson et al. 1993) who developed subacute weakness in association with preceding *Campylobacter jejuni* infection. The IgG responses are limited to IgG1 and IgG3 subclasses (Guijo et al. 1992; Willison & Veitch 1994). This finding contrasts with previous work which suggested that the IgG response to LPS was generally restricted to an IgG2 subclass (Hammarström & Smith 1986). The IgG response in these GBS patients has been proposed to correlate with particularly severe forms of subacute neuropathy in which axonal damage is prominent and recovery is particularly poor. IgG1 and IgG3 would presumably have better access to endoneurium than IgM and these antibodies can fix complement and interact with Fc receptors of macrophages and NK cells. Large series of patients with a similar clinical picture are reported in China, Mexico, Paraguay, as well as in other areas. The incidence is seasonal, affecting predominantly young children (McKhann et al. 1993). In Chinese paralytic syndrome, serologic evidence suggests an association with prior *C. jejuni* infection (Blaser et al. 1991) and one report suggested an increased frequency of antibody to GM1.

Electromyographic and pathological findings support direct damage to axons at the ventral spinal nerve root and the presynaptic neuromuscular junction. Similar large series of studies of GBS patients in the USA and Germany were unable to link the GM1 antibody response to preceding *C. jejuni* infection or to axonal neuropathy (Enders et al. 1993; Vriesendorp et al. 1993). The difference may have reflected a lower frequency of *C. jejuni* positive serology associated neuropathy (10 of 58 and 15 of 38 patients, respectively) (Enders et al. 1993; Vriesendorp et al. 1993), differences in HLA association within the geographical population or assay techniques.

Earlier studies with GBS patients showed no genetic linkage of class I and class II alleles to disease susceptibility. Recent studies of patients with antecedent *C. jejuni* infection, however, linked disease development to class I HLA-B35 in six of six Japanese patients (Yuki et al. 1991) and to class II HLA-DQB3 in 25 of 30 English patients (R.A.C. Hughes, personal communication). Since the class I association could not be verified by others and the statistical frequency in the English study was reached only after pooling alleles within the DQB3 group, further work is required to determine whether T cell restrictions occur in GBS associated with *C. jejuni* or whether the haplotype is preferentially found in a group of patients susceptible to *Campylobacter* infection, but not necessarily inflammatory neuropathy.

IgG monoclonal gammopathy can be identified in patients with rare osteosclerotic myeloma associated with a demyelinating peripheral neuropathy and a POEMS syndrome (Laven Stein et al. 1979; Resnick et al.

1981; Kelly et al. 1983). Endocrine dysfunction in some of these patients may reflect the presence of specific antibodies to neuroendocrine tissues of the pituitary axis (Reulecke et al. 1988).

Not all subacute episodes of demyelination are associated or triggered by preceding infection. Increased frequency or outbreaks of GBS are, at times, noted following administration of influenza, polio and hepatitis vaccines (Arnason & Soliven 1993). Immunosuppressed patients with HIV, lymphoma or organ transplant can also develop GBS or CIDP. The incidence of GBS in certain transplant centers may reach as high as 6% of all organ transplants (B. Triggs, personal communication). Although these patients are adequately immunosuppressed, presumably altered suppressor mechanisms may lead to T cell independent activation of polyclonal B cells and produce IgM antibodies that bind carbohydrate epitopes on a variety of infectious agents (Casali & Notkins 1989; Kipps 1989). When some of these antibodies, which can also be generated as a primary immune response to invading microorganisms, penetrate the endoneurium, they can cause membrane damage or cell death by activating effector arms of the immune system or by signaling a cell to initiate apoptosis. Antibody-induced apoptosis has not been directly demonstrated in endoneurial cells. Extensive in vitro and in vivo studies suggest that antibody in patients with inflammatory or paraneoplastic neuropathies can mediate demyelination or axonal damage by activating complement or mediating cytotoxicity by NK cells or monocytes/macrophages (Feasby et al. 1982; Saida et al. 1982; Sumner et al. 1983; Harrison et al. 1984; Sawant-Mane et al. 1991; Thomas et al. 1991; Santoro et al. 1992). Without induction of any one of these mechanisms, the presence of antibody in patients with neuropathy may only represent an epiphenomenon that serves as a disease marker.

It is less clear that other autoreactive antibodies have any functional significance. Many autoantibodies reported include those recognizing intracellular regulatory enzymes, cytoskeletal proteins, heat shock proteins and cytoplasmic as well as nuclear elements. For example, anti-Hu antibodies are present in some but not all patients with small cell carcinoma of lung associated with a paraneoplastic sensory neuropathy involving the dorsal root ganglia (Croft et al. 1965; Horwich et al. 1977; Chalk et al. 1992). These antibodies are however not specific for dorsal root ganglia but stain the nucleus and cytoplasm of all neurons (Graus et al. 1985; Dick et al. 1988; Altermatt et al. 1991). It is interesting that target antigens appear to be a family of 35–40 kDa RNA binding proteins which regulate posttranscriptional processing of RNA. As antibody binding to a protein can, under certain circumstances serve as a catalyst for enzyme activation, one can speculate that antibodies taken up through a synaptic mechanism could affect protein synthesis at the posttranscriptional level and influence neuronal function or survival. This hypothesis is less likely because of the apparent selectivity of the process for dorsal root ganglion cells and the occurrence of the disorder in patients with Sjögren's syndrome who do not express anti-Hu antibodies (Griffin et al. 1990). Antineutrophil cytoplasmic antibodies are associated with certain types of vasculitis (van der Woude et al. 1985). The antibodies bind both cytoplasmic and perinuclear antigen, and are associated with Wegener's granulomatosis and polyarteritis or other inflammatory disorders, respectively. Patients with primary infection of peripheral nerves with *M. leprae* develop antibodies to heat shock protein antigens shared by the organism and peripheral nerve (Launois et al. 1992). Whether these antibodies to intracellular antigens are involved in disease pathogenesis is currently unknown. They do however serve as a marker of a disease process and as such can be helpful for diagnosis.

Vascular deposition of immune complexes in patients with autoimmune vasculitis, serum sickness and Arthus reaction is associated with the formation of soluble immune complexes in circulation or in situ (Park & Richardson 1953; Lewis & Philpott 1956; Sams et al. 1975; Ronco et al. 1983; Lawley et al. 1984). Immune complex vasculitis, that can damage the blood–nerve barrier, occasionally causes GBS. Circulating immune complexes not eliminated by normal clearance mechanisms through C3b and C1q receptors on erythrocytes and reticuloendothelial phagocytes, can precipitate subendothelially and cause complement activation and chemotactic factor release. Migration of polymorphonuclear leukocytes and macrophages into the vessel followed by release of proteolytic enzymes and free oxygen radicals directly contribute to tissue damage, further inflammation and thrombosis. Antiphospholipid IgG is

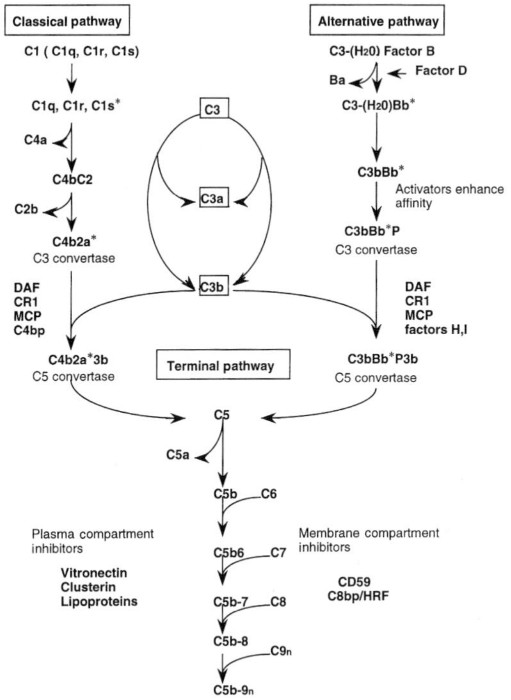

Figure 1.3 *Activation cascade of complement.*

linked to a prothrombotic state in systemic lupus erythematosus with a focal involvement of small endoneurial blood vessels. Antibody binding to endothelium may require a cofactor, β_2-glycoprotein-1 or apolipoprotein H, naturally occurring anticoagulants whose binding may alter its function and contribute to the prothrombotic state.

Complement

Complement consists of more than 19 proteins which include ones that regulate complement cascade activation. The complement system can be activated by the classical or alternative pathway. The classical pathway is activated most frequently through immune complex formation and the activation requires Ca^{2+}. Human IgM, IgG1 and IgG3 (Müller-Eberhard & Calcott 1966; Augener et al. 1971; Schumaker et al. 1976) are capable of activating the pathway although with different affinities for C1q. A single molecule of C1q binds the CH3 domain of IgM Fc. Affinity for the Fc-CH2 domain of IgG antibody is increased by the number of immunoglobulins with which C1q can react (Müller-Eberhard and Calcott 1966; Wright et al. 1980; Doekes et al. 1982) and is affected by epitope density and antigen/antibody ratios. Binding of a C1q to the Fc domain of complement-fixing immunoglobulins in immune complexes, changes the intramolecular distances between the globular headgroups of the C1q molecule and causes activation of C1r dimers, which in turn cleave C1s dimers which express potent esterase activity. The C1s esterase in turn cleaves C4 and C2. Activation of the complement system produces a cascade of enzyme–substrate interaction which generates a series of activation products that can induce inflammation and cell death. Cleavage of C3 by the C3 convertase C4b,2a, produces C3a and C3b. C3a enhances vascular permeability and activates mast cells and basophils. C3b contributes to the formation of C5 convertase C4b,2a,3b, enhances antigen presentation to T cells and opsonizes the activating particles for receptor mediated interaction with macrophages, NK cells and platelets.

The complement cascade can also be activated via the alternative pathway in the absence of specific antibody. This pathway serves as an initial line of defense against foreign organisms prior to the generation of specific antibody. In the alternative pathway, C3b is generated by a C3 convertase Bb, formed by the change of factor B by serum enzyme, factor D. In blood a small amount of C3 (0.005%) continuously undergoes spontaneous cleavage. The thiol radical thus formed reacts with H_2O. The C3-H_2O transiently binds factor B in the presence of Mg^{2+} and allows factor D, a highly specific serine protease, to cleave a single arginyl-lysyl bond in factor B to generate the Bb enzyme. Factor B is only susceptible to factor D cleavage when complexed with C3. The efficiency of this process is dependent on the stability of the C3-H_2O, B complex which is stabilized by protein (P) to generate a longer-lasting enzyme which cleaves C3 to C3b. The C3b produced covalently binds to membranes or particles in the vicinity. Factor B associates with membrane bound C3b and is cleaved by D. The C3 convertase C3b,Bb in association with P is more stable and hence more potent than C3-H_2O, Bb,P and leads to the formation of the alternative pathway C5 convertase by cleavage and binding of a further C3 to yield C3b,Bb,P,3b. IgG can enhance this process by most likely providing a site for covalent linkage of C3b that protects it from decay. Alternative pathway activation is strictly regulated by factors H and I. Factor H dissociates Bb from C3b permitting the cleavage of C3b by I to yield iC3b which cannot participate in convertase function. Alternative pathway activators generally have repeating carbohydrate structures on their surface, such as LPS. In peripheral myelin, Po protein is capable of activating the alternative pathway facilitating C3b,Bb production (Koski et al. 1985). As will be discussed later, PNM does not express CD35, CD46 or CD55 of all which are regulatory molecules of C3/C5 convertases that can also serve as a cofactor for factor I, like factor H. Such deficiencies of regulatory proteins would enhance the ability of PNM to activate the alternative pathway.

Cleavage of C5 generates a chemotactic and anaphylatoxic fragment of C5a and C5b fragment which initiates the activation cascade of terminal complement proteins to form channel forming complexes C5b-8 and C5b-9 in the membrane. These complexes, capable of ionic conductance and cytolysis, do not cause cell death when the number of complexes formed is limited. Sublytic numbers of C5b-9 channels can induce diverse cellular responses which include generation of superoxide radicals, arachidonic acid, leukotrienes and prostaglandins (Hallet et al. 1981; Imagawa et al. 1983; Hansch et al. 1984; Shirazi et al. 1989).

Complement activation on target membranes is down regulated by a diverse group of membrane proteins. CRI (CD35), a receptor for C3b and C4b ligands, acts as a cofactor for factor I to enzymatically degrade C4b and C3b (Ahearn & Fearon 1989). Decay accelerating factor, DAF (CD55), and membrane cofactor protein, MCP (CD46), inhibit the C3 and C5 convertase formation (Nicholson-Weller et al. 1982; Medof et al. 1984; Cole et al. 1985). CD59 and homologous restriction factor (HRF)/C8-binding protein (C8-bp) are capable of inhibiting incorporation of C8 and C9, and polymerization of C9 during the assembly of terminal complement complexes (TCC) (Schonermark et al. 1986; Sugita et al. 1988). CD55, CD59 and C8-bp, GPI-anchored membrane proteins of human cells, are widely expressed on cells of hemopoietic lineage where they serve as important inhibitors of autologous complement activation. The expression deficiency of these membrane proteins, especially CD55 and CD59, is the cause of episodic hemolysis in patients with paroxysmal nocturnal hemoglobinuria due to enhanced lytic susceptibility of their erythrocytes to complement (Rosse 1989). In addition to regulating cell lysis by homologous complement, these molecules participate in other activities of the cell which include cell activation, transmembrane signaling and adhesion (Kroczek et al. 1986; Anderson et al. 1993; Morgan et al. 1993). CD46, also called MCP, is the receptor for measles virus, *Trypanosoma cruzii* and the M protein of group A streptococcus (Naniche et al. 1993; Atkinson et al. 1994).

Data from our own laboratory showed Schwann cells derived from adult human sural nerve express a number of these complement regulatory proteins, which include DAF (CD55), MCP (CD46), CR1 (CD35) and CD59. Interestingly, myelin membrane, formed by the apposition of the cytoplasmic faces of the glial cell plasma membranes, expressed only CD59, a regulator of the terminal complement cascade, and failed to express significant quantities of CR1 (CD35), DAF (CD55) and MCP (CD46). The lack of expression of C3/C5 convertase inhibitors on compact myelin may serve to enhance the efficiency of complement-mediated opsonization of myelin during demyelination initiated either by antibody-dependent or independent processes. PNM activates the alternative pathway of complement in the absence of specific antibodies and the Po is, in part, responsible for the activation (Koski et al. 1985). Lack of CD46 and CD55 would contribute to the sustained formation of the alternative pathway C3 and C5 convertases on the surface of myelin. The differential expression of complement regulatory proteins, DAF, MCP, CR1 and CD59, on myelinating cells and myelin would protect glial cells from the complement attack during inflammation while facilitating efficient opsonization, formation of C5b-9 and membrane vesiculation mediated by C5b-9. These results would be enhanced phagocytosis and clearance of damaged myelin by macrophages. Macrophages as previously mentioned are critical effector cells of demyelination in inflammatory neuropathies associated with GBS, its animal model EAN and also in myelin clearance in Wallerian degeneration (Bruck & Friede 1991; Arnason & Soliven 1993).

Complement-fixing antibodies to peripheral nerve and PMN (anti-PNM) can be detected in the serum of up to 95% of GBS patients (Latov et al. 1981; Koski et al. 1985, 1990). Lower titers of similar antibodies can be detected in 20–27% of normal controls. Elevated serum titers of anti-PNM antibody also correlated with current episodes of inflammatory polyneuritis but could only be detected in 20% of patients with progressive or chronic polyneuritis. Detection of such antibodies during the disease course of GBS patients correlated with the development of neurological symptoms and clearance, both during the natural course of disease (Koski et al. 1986) and following plasma exchange (Vriesendorp et al. 1991), correlated with improvement in muscular strength and pulmonary vital capacity. Immunoabsorption and precipitation studies suggested that the immunoglobulin isotype detected by the C1 fixation and transfer assay was primary IgM (Koski et al. 1985).

Several lines of evidence indicate ongoing complement activation in GBS patients. Levels of C4 are depleted in cerebrospinal fluid (Sano 1985) while activation products of both the early and late complement cascade including C3a, C5a (Hartung et al. 1987e) and SC5b-9 are increased (Sanders et al. 1986). C5b-9 has also been found on myelinated fibers of multiple spinal, peripheral and cranial nerves of a GBS patient (Koski et al. 1987). Preliminary studies suggest that like EAN, C5b-9 can be detected on Schwann cells and the surface of myelin internodes of GBS patients prior to the appearance of mononuclear cell infiltrates (C. Macko, personal communication). The kinetics of SC5b-9 appearance in serum which peaked 3–5 days after peak anti-PNM antibody detection and cleared by 30 days suggested that anti-PNM antibody mediated complement activation in these patients. Passive transfer studies in vitro and in vivo vary in the ability of serum from GBS and CIDP patients to produce demyelination. Such findings reflect the dependency of these experimental models on multiple factors including antibody titers and the activity of serum complement used in the studies. Anti-PNM Ab titers in individual GBS serum correlated with the ability of that serum to mediate complement dependent-demyelination of dissociated dorsal root ganglion cultures (Sawant-Mane et al. 1991). In this in vitro system, demyelination was dependent on the C5b-9 generation as the use of a human serum depleted of C7 prevented demyelination. Reconstitution of the serum with purified C7 allowed formation of C5b-9 and demyelination.

Complement is also implicated as an effector in a variety of inflammatory neuropathies, peripheral nerve vasculitis and paraprotein-associated neuropathies. C3 and C5b-9 deposition on the vascular endothelium was noted in peripheral nerve biopsies of both the systemic vasculitides and those vasculitides focal to the peripheral nerve (Kissel et al. 1989). As deposition of immunoglobulin and complement was limited to vessels with more prevalent cellular infiltrates, it was suggested that complement activation by immune complexes may have a secondary role by enhancing the severity of vasculitis. Complement deposition including C3d, C1q and C5b-9 is also described in the peripheral nerves of demyelinating neuropathies associated with acquired monoclonal gammopathy in which the paraprotein binds the HNK epitope of 100 kDa MAG, Po and L1 and acidic sulfated glycolipids (Hays et al. 1987, 1988).

Influx of Ca^{2+} through C5b-8 or C5b-9 channels in the multilamellar myelin membrane activates endogenous neutral proteases such as calpain to which molecules such as Po and MBP are sensitive (Cammer et al. 1986; Shin & Koski 1992). As both MBP and Po are involved in compaction of myelin lamellae, their cleavage at the cytoplasmic face would lead to intralamellar splitting and subsequent vesiculation of the internode. C5b-9 insertion into target membranes also stimulates phospholipase A_2 activity leading to generation of lysolecithin which itself can cause demyelination (Imagawa et al. 1983).

Although most complement components are produced by the liver and monocytes/macrophages, several endoneurial cells are also capable of production of complement components. It is likely that most of the complement proteins may be produced by endoneurial cells which include the resident and invading macrophages, fibroblasts and Schwann cells. Whether local production of these proteins participates in the pathophysiology of endoneurial damage in a biologically meaningful way is not yet known. It is however provocative that deposition of C5b-9 on Schwann cells and myelin has been detected in EAN animals and some GBS patients prior to cellular infiltration and also in the presence of presumably intact blood–nerve barrier.

Activation of complement within the nervous system is proposed to contribute to the pathophysiology of Alzheimer's disease and possibly amyloid neuropathy. C1, C3, and C5b-9 are detected in association with and around amyloid deposits (Eikenbloom et al. 1989; McGeer et al. 1989).

C3 is an important pivotal protein in the complement cascade. C3 contributes to formation of C5 convertases of both the classical and alternative pathway of complement, and its cleavage products are ligands for CR1, CR3 or CR2. Production of C3 by Schwann cells in vitro is enhanced by IFNγ and TNFα, cytokines that usually downregulate C3 production by macrophages and fibroblasts (Dashiell et al. 1993). Schwann cells therefore may be an important source of C3 during endoneurial inflammation. Schwann cells also express a complement receptor CRI, which binds C3b and C4b (Vedeler et al. 1989a). The role of such ligand interaction on Schwann cells located in a sequestered nervous tissue has not been defined; however, such an interaction may contribute to cell–cell adhesion, cytokine production or regulation of C3 convertases formed on neighboring cells. C3b ligands can activate macrophages by crosslinking CR1, by downregulating complement receptors on cell surface and enhancing IL-1 secretion.

EAN as discussed earlier is a model of inflammatory demyelination of peripheral nerve in which disease can be passively transferred with T cells. Although antibodies can frequently be detected in these animals, particularly in the passive transfer models, they are not thought to participate in disease development; however, this concept can be challenged. Complement proteins and their activation products including C5b-9, have been detected in myelinated fibers and Schwann cells of peripheral nerve prior to cellular infiltration (Stoll et al. 1991) and introduction of cobra venom factor into the animal can affect the clinical course of EAN (Feasby et al. 1987; Vriesendorp et al. 1995). Cobra venom factor, a form of cobra C3b which forms stable C3 convertase, effectively depletes serum C3, thereby blocking the generation of C5b-8/C5b 9. Cobra venom factor treatment of Lewis rats delayed the onset of clinical signs of EAN induced by bovine PNS. Most significant changes were noted in animals immunized with lower amounts of myelin and with less severe clinical disease. The most striking change was reflected in reduced or absent CR3 macrophages (Vriesendorp et al. 1995). These data suggest that even in a disease model thought to be T cell dependent, complement may still participate in the effector phase of myelin damage. Complement may be involved in T cell induced EAN by either regulating $CR3^+$ on macrophages or by myelin opsonization to enhance the CR3/CR1-mediated phagocytosis by macrophages.

Detectable levels of complement-fixing anti-PNM antibody exist in patients not associated with endoneurial damage (Koski et al. 1985; Koski 1990). Enhanced blood–nerve barrier affected by cytokines produced by activated T cells would allow the penetration of high molecular weight proteins such as IgM and C1 during pathological conditions such as those seen in GBS, chronic inflammatory polyneuritis, serum sickness vasculitis or leprosy. An elevated albumin level in the spinal fluid of patients with inflammatory demyelinating neuropathies reflects the breakdown of the blood–nerve barrier, permitting penetration of the endoneurium by serum components, otherwise sequestered. Recent experiments demonstrated that T cells, antibody and complement can synergistically contribute to PNS demyelination in naive rats. Antigalactocerebroside antibodies or serum of EAN animals significantly augmented demyelination of peripheral nerve by limited numbers of passively transferred P2 specific T cells (Harvey & Pollard 1992; Hahn et al. 1993). Intraneural injection of cytokines, IFNγ, TNFα and/or IL-1 during passive transfer of EAN serum also resulted in peripheral nerve demyelination that did not occur in the absence of either cytokines or immune sera (Spies et al. 1993). Finally, activated T cells specific for irrelevant antigens like ovalbumin, could also facilitate demyelination in naive rats receiving EAN serum when 1 μg of ovalbumin was injected intraneurally into the sciatic nerve (Pollard et al. 1995).

It is likely that cytokines such as IFN-γ, TNFα and IL-1 produced by activated lymphocytes and macrophages are involved in inflammatory demyelination through their pleiotropic activities. For example, these cytokines enhance expression of adhesion molecules on endothelial cells of blood–nerve barrier that can, in turn, enhance adhesion and migration of immunocompetent T cells.

Cytokines

Cytokines are biologically potent peptides produced by activated cells in a transient manner. They are capable of modulating cell–cell communication, cell activation differentiation and growth. They can induce cell death and affect tissue remodeling. They are produced by cells of the immune system, cells of hematopoietic origin and cells derived from epithelial as well as mesenchymal origin. The converse may also be true that most cells may respond to cytokines through respective specific receptors. The array of biological interactions between cytokines and cells of the nervous system is likely to be complex because (1) many cytokines have overlapping biological activities, (2) production of a cytokine and the cellular response to it is regulated in cell-specific manner that is determined by both the cell type, and its state of differentiation, and (3) the presence of other cytokines, hormones and chemicals can either inhibit or enhance cytokine production as well as the cellular response to a cytokine.

IL-1α, IL-1β, IL-6 and TNFα are proinflammatory cytokines sharing a wide range of biomodulatory activities, both immunological and nonimmunological in nature (Strober & James 1989). They stimulate hematopoiesis, synthesis of acute phase proteins by hepatocytes and effect tissue remodeling. They can stimulate the hypothalamic–pituitary–adrenal axis, act as pyrogens and induce sleep. Their functions also include their mutual regulation. For example, IL-1α stimulates macrophages to produce TNFα, IL-6 and other inflammatory mediators such as C3. IL-1β or IL-6 can induce TNFα in astrocytes and these activities are enhanced by IFNγ.

Peripheral nerve injury by trauma, inflammation or ischemia is associated with endoneurial infiltration of lymphocytes and macrophages capable of producing a variety of cytokines including IL-1α, IL-1β, IL-6, IFNγ, TNFα, and TGFβ. Cells within the endoneurium can enhance the cytokine production of infiltrating lymphoid cells through release of substance P and calcitonin gene related peptide from sensory afferent fibers (Lotz et al. 1988; Ansel et al. 1993; Sakagami et al. 1993). Stimulation of sympathetic nerve upregulates β-adrenergic receptors on lymphocytes resulting in IL-6 production (Nakamura et al. 1993). Neutralizing antibodies to TNFα and IFNγ significantly reduced the degree of inflammation and severity in clinical symptoms in EAE and EAN (Selmaj & Raine 1988; Hartung 1990b).

IL-1β stimulates Schwann cells in both an autocrine and paracrine manner to secrete C3 and can serve as a cofactor for Schwann cell mitosis (S. Dashiell & C.L. Koski, unpublished observation 1995). Schwann cells have the type 2 IL-1β receptors and express mRNA encoding IL-1r antagonist under specific circumstances (R.P. Lisak, personal communication). IL-1β in association with TNFα and IFNγ has profound effects on vascular endothelium; they enhance ICAM and MHC expression, increase neutrophil adherence and cause degranulation which promote vasodilatation and increased permeability (Okusawa et al. 1988).

As described above, TNFα also affects both immune and nonimmune cells (Vassalli 1992) and the biological activities of TNFα overlap extensively with those of IL-1 and IL-6. As TNFα and IL-1 can induce the synthesis of each other, it is often difficult to determine the unique role of one specific cytokine in vivo, unless the activity is abrogated by monospecific antibodies. TNFα is, however, one of the most potent proinflammatory cytokines which affect the vascular endothelium. Intravenous infusion produces septic shock in rodents and rabbits. TNFα production appears to be particularly relevant to subacute inflammatory neuropathy as elevated levels of plasma TNFα can be detected in 20–50% of GBS patients and is associated with greater disease severity with respiratory dependence (Sharief et al. 1993). The high affinity TNFα receptor has homology with receptors for NGF and the Fas ligand. Stimulation of Fas is involved in lymphocyte apoptosis and possible peripheral immune tolerance (Wantanabe et al. 1992). TNFα can induce apoptosis in oligodendrocytes and in vitro demyelination (Robbins et al. 1987; Selmaj et al. 1991); however, it does not directly cause Schwann cell death or PNM demyelination in vitro (Mithen et al. 1990). Intraneural injection of TNFα in animals produced variable results. Axonal damage was noted in mice whereas limited demyelination with altered nerve conduction was reported in rats. Intraorbital inoculation of TNFα in rabbits interfered with impulse propagation along axons (Brosnan et al. 1989). TNFα alone did not alter the mRNA or protein expression of MAG and Po in an immortalized Schwann cell line; however, MAG and Po mRNA was decreased in a dose-dependent fashion with increasing amounts of IFNγ in the presence of TNFα (Schneider-Schaulies et al. 1991; Dashiell et al. 1993). Other Schwann cell marker molecules such as L1 and NCAM were not affected under the same condition that increased MHC class II expression. Treatment of cocultured Schwann cells and neurons with TNFα and IFN gamma reduced neurite outgrowth that was directly related to the reduced MAG expression. Unlike its effect on monocytes and fibroblasts, TNFα in association with IFNγ, upregulates both the expression of C3 mRNA and the protein synthesis and enhances IL-1 secretion by Schwann cells (Dashiell et al. 1993). The production of IL-1 and TNFα by infiltrating inflammatory cells stimulate the secretion and release of endoneurial growth factors such as NGF and PDGF which contribute to neurite outgrowth and Schwann cell mitogenesis (Lindholm et al. 1987; Hattori et al. 1993). The ability of TNFα and IFNγ to downregulate transcription of myelin genes such as MAG and Po and stimulate the production of classical growth factors including CNTF, PDGF and TGFβ are biologically significant, because they can contribute to the growth and repair of damaged nerves.

TGFβ produced by T_H2 T cells and nonlymphoid cells like Schwann cells (Mews & Meyer 1993) can participate in inflammation as regulatory molecule (Sporn & Roberts 1992). TGFβ is chemotactic for T cells, neutrophils and macrophages. It stimulates fibroblasts and Schwann cells to proliferate. During ongoing inflammation, TGFβ can inhibit T cells and IFNγ-activated macrophages to downregulate inflammation. It also stimulates Schwann mitogenesis, decreases or inhibits the expression of myelin proteins and the low affinity NGF receptor, P75 (Mews & Meyer 1993). Systemic administration of TGFβ decreases the severity of EAE in mice (Gregorian et al. 1994a).

IL-10 and IL-12 mRNA can also be expressed by Schwann cells (J.L. Rutkowski, personal communication 1995). IL-10 and IL-12 modulate cytokine production. IL-10 has antiinflammatory effects on macrophages and T cells and inhibits the production of TNFα, IL-1, IL-6, IL-8, and IL-2 (Dewaal Malefyt et al. 1991). As TNFα is itself a potent inducer of IL-10 (Wanidworanun & Strober 1993), IL-10 may function as a regulatory factor for TNFα through an inhibitory feedback loop to decrease TNFα production by infiltrating monocytes. IFNγ production by T cells and NK cells induced by IL-12 is also inhibited by IL-10 (Chan et al. 1991; Manetti et al. 1993).

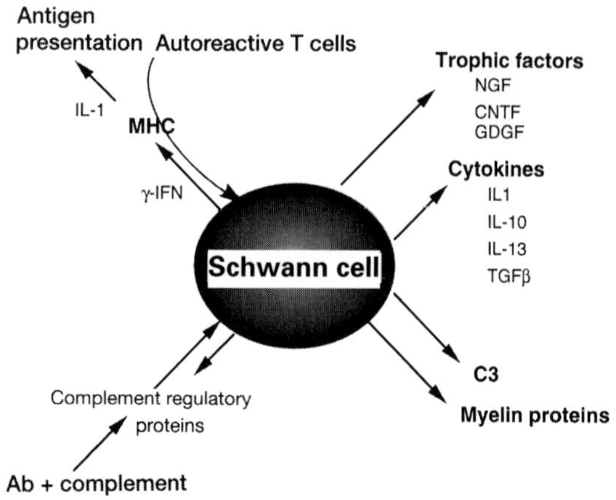

Figure 1.4 *Schwann cells although targets of immune attack can modulate inflammation through antigen presentation as well as production of cytokines and acute phase reactants.*

Recognition of the participants derived from diverse immune and inflammatory responses in the development of peripheral nerve diseases has significantly advanced our ability to treat an increasing number of neuropathies. Pharmacological agents including immunoglobulin, cytotoxic drugs, corticosteroids and intervention therapies such as plasma exchange, although temporally limited, can modulate or arrest disorders thereby reducing morbidity and mortality of patients previously treated with more conservative supportive therapies. The effectiveness of these agents that affect the host immune and inflammatory responses will be greatly improved when we understand the mechanisms of their activities in each disease pathogenesis.

References

Adams, D., Festenstein, H., Gibson, J.D., and Jaraquemada, J. (1979). HLA antigens in chronic relapsing idiopathic inflammatory polyneuropathy. *J. Neurol. Neurosurg. Psychiatry* **42**: 184–186.

Ahearn, J.M. and Fearon, D.T. (1989). Structure and function of the complement receptor, CR1 (CD35) and CR2 (CD21). *Adv. Immunol.* **46**: 183–219.

Altermatt, H.J., Rodriquez, M., Scheithauer, B.W., and Lennon, V.A. (1991). Paraneoplastic anti-Purkinje and type I antineuronal nuclear autoantibodies bind selectively to central, peripheral, and autonomic nervous system cells. *Lab. Invest.* **65**: 412–420.

Anderson, D.J., Abbott, A.F., and Jack, R.M. (1993). The role of complement component C3b and its receptors in sperm–oocyte interaction. *Proc. Natl. Acad. Sci. USA* **90**: 10051–10055.

Ansel, J.C., Brown, J.R., Payan, D.G., and Brown, M.A. (1993). Substance P selectively activates TNF-alpha gene expression in murine mast cells. *J. Immunol.* **150**: 4478–4485.

Archelos, J.J., Maurer, M., Jung, S., Toyka, K.V., and Hartung, H.P. (1993). Suppression of experimental allergic neuritis by an antibody to the intracellular adhesion molecule ICAM-1. *Brain* **116**: 1043–1058.

Archelos, J.J., Maurer, M., Jung, S., Miyasaka, M., Tamatani, T., Toyka, K.V., and Hartung, H.P. (1994). Inhibition of experimental autoimmune neuritis by an antibody to the lymphocyte function-associated antigen-1. *Lab. Invest.* **70**: 667–675.

Argall, K.G., Armati, P.J., Pollard, J.D., Watson, E., and Bonner, J. (1992). Interactions between Cd4$^+$ T cells and rat Schwann cells in vitro. 1. Antigen presentation by Lewis rat Schwann cells to P2-specific CD4$^+$ T cells lines. *J. Neuroimmunol.* **40**: 1–18.

Arnason, B.G.W. and Soliven, B. (1993). *Acute inflammatory demyelinating polyradicules neuropathy* (W.B. Sanders Company, Philadelphia).

Arquint, M., Roder, J., Chia, L.S., Down, J., Wilkinson, D., Bayley, H., Braun, P., and Dunn, R. (1987). Molecular cloning and primary structure of myelin-associated glycoprotein. *Proc. Natl. Acad. Sci. USA* **84**: 600–604.

Atkinson, J.P., Krych, M., Nickells, M., Birmingham, D., Subramanian, V.B., Clemenza, L., Alvarez, J., and Liszewski, K. (1994). Complement receptors and regulatory proteins: immune adherence revisited and abuse by micro-organisms. *Clin. Exp. Immunol.* **97** (Suppl. 2): 1–3.

Augener, W., Grey, H.M., Cooper, N.R., and Muller-Eberhard, H.J. (1971). The reaction of monomeric and aggregated immunoglobulin with C1. *Immunochemistry* **8**: 1011–1020.

Ballin, R.H.M. and Thomas, P.K. (1968). Electron microscope observations on demyelination and remyelination in experimental allergic neuritis. Part I. Demyelination. *J. Neurol. Sci.* **8**: 1–18.

Beckman, E.M., Porcelli, S.A., Morita, C.T., Behar, S.M., Furlong, S.T., and Brenner, M.B. (1994). Recognition of a lipid antigen by CD1-restricted $\alpha\beta^+$ T cells. *Nature* **372**: 691–694.

Bergsteinsdsottir, K., Kingston, A., Mirsky, R., and Jessen, K.R. (1991). Rat Schwann cells produce interleukin-1. *J. Immunol.* **34**: 15–33.

Blaser, M.J., Olivares, A., Taylor, D.N., Cornblath, D.R., and McKhann, G.M. (1991). *Campylobacter* serology in patients with chinese paralytic syndrome. *Lancet* **338**: 308 (letter).

Brosnan, C.F., Litwak, M.S., Schroeder, C.E., Selmaj, K., Raine, C.S., and Arezzo, J.C. (1989). Preliminary studies of cytokine-induced functional effects of the visual pathways in the rabbit. *J. Neuroimmunol.* **25**: 227–239.

Brosnan, J.V., Fellowes, R., Craggs, R.I., King, R.H., Bowley, T.J., and Thomas, P.K. (1985). Changes in lymphocyte subsets during the course of experimental allergic neuritis. *Brain* **108**: 315–334.

Brostov, S.W., Burnett, P., Lamper, P.W., and Eylar, E.H. (1972). Isolation and characterization of a protein from sciatic nerve myelin responsible for experimental allergic neuritis. *Nature New Biol.* **235**: 210–212.

Bruck, W. and Friede, R.L. (1991). The role of complement in myelin phagocytosis during PNS Wallerian degeneration. *J. Neurologic. Sci.* **103**: 182–187.

Bruggermann, M., Williams, G.T., Bindon, C.I., Clark, M.R., Walker, M.R., JeVeris, R., Waldmann, H., and Neuberger, M.S. (1987). Comparison of the effector functions of human immunoglobulins using a matched set of chimeric antibodies. *J. Exp. Med.* **166**: 1351–1361.

Cammer, W., Brosnan, C.F., and Boom, B.K. (1981). Degradation of the Po, P1 and Pr proteins in peripheral nervous system myelin by plasmin: implications regarding the role of macrophages in demyelinating diseases. *J. Neurochem.* **36**: 1506–1514.

Cammer, W., Brosnan, C., Basile, C., Bloom, B.R., and Norton, W.T. (1986). Complement potentiates the degradation of myelin proteins by plasmin: implications for a mechanism of inflammatory demyelination. *Brain Res.* **364**: 91–101.

Carter, R.H., Spycher, M.O., Ng, Y.C., Hovman, H., and Fearon, D.T. (1988). Synergistic interaction between complement receptor type 2 and membrane IgM on B lymphocytes. *J. Immunol.* **141**: 457–463.

Carter, R.H. and Fearon, D.T. (1992). CD19: lowering the antigen threshold for antigen receptor stimulation of B lymphocytes. *Science* **256**: 105–107.

Casali, P. and Notkins, A.L. (1989). Probing the human B-cell repertoire with EBV: polyreactive antibodies and CD5$^+$ B lymphocytes. *Ann. Rev. Immunol.* **7**: 513–535.

Chalk, C.H., Windebank, A.J., Kimmel, D.W., and McManis, P.G. (1992). The distinctive clinical features of parenoplastic sensory neuronopathy. *Can. J. Neurol. Sci.* **19**: 346–351.

Chan, S.H., Perussia, B., Gupta, J.W., Kobayashi, M., Pospisil, M., Young, H.A., Wolf, S.F., Young, D., Clark, S.C., and Trinchieri, G. (1991). Induction of interferon-γ production by natural killer cell stimulatory factor: characterization of the responder cells and synergy with other inducers. *J. Exp. Med.* **173**: 869–879.

Chiba, A., Kusunoki, S., Shimizu, T., and Kanazawa, I. (1992). Serum IgG antibody to ganglioside GQ1b is a possible marker of Miller Fisher syndrome. *Ann. Neurol.* **31**: 677–679.

Chiba, A., Kusunoki, S., Obata, H., Machinami, R., and Kanazawa, I. (1993). Serum anti-GQ1b IgG antibody is associated with ophthalmoplegia in Miller Fisher syndrome and Guillain-Barré syndrome: clinical and immunohistochemical studies. *Neurology* **43**: 1911–1918.

Choudhury, A., Mistry, N.F., and Antia, N.H. (1989). Blocking of mycobacterium leprose adherence to dissociated Schwann cells by antimycobacterial antibodies. *Scand. J. Immunol.* **30**: 505–509.

Cochrane, C.G. and Koffler, D. (1973). Immune complex disease in experimental animals and man. *Adv. Neurol.* **16**: 185–264.

Cole, J.L., Housley, Jr., Dykman, T.R., MacDermott, R.P., and Atkinson, J.P. (1985). Identification of an additional class of C3 binding membrane proteins of human peripheral blood leukocytes and cell lines. *Proc Natl. Acad. Sci. USA* **82**: 859–863.

Corbo, M., Quattrini, A., Lugaresi, A., Santoro, M., Latov, N., and Hays, A.P. (1992). Patterns of reactivity of human anti-GM1 antibodies with spinal cord and motor neurons. *Ann. Neurol.* **32**: 487–493.

Corbo, M., Quattrini, A., Latov, N., and Hays, A.P. (1993). Localization of GM1 and Gal(beta 1–3)GalNAc antigenic determinants in peripheral nerve. *Neurology* **43**: 809–814.

Cornblath, D.R., Griffin, D.E., Welch, D., GriYn, J.W., and McArthur, J.C. (1990). Quantitative analysis of endoneurial T cells in human sural nerve biopsies. *J. Neuroimmunol.* **26**: 113–118.

Cowley, S.A., Gschmeissner, S.E., Negesse, Y., Curtis, J., and Turk, J.L. (1990). Major histocompatibility complex class II antigen expression in nerves in leprosy; an immunoelectronmicroscopial study. *Int. J. Leprosy & Other Mycbact. Dis.* **58**: 560–565.

Craggs, R.I., King, R.H., and Thomas, P.K. (1984). The effect of suppression of macrophage activity on the development of experimental allergic neuritis. *Acta Neuropathol. (Berl.)* **62**: 316–323.

Croft, P.B., Henson, R.A., Urich, H., and Wilkinson, P.C. (1965). Sensory neuropathy with bronchial carcinoma: a study of four cases showing serological abnormalities. *Brain* **88**: 501–514.

Dahle, C., Vrethem, M., and Ernerudh, J. (1994). T lymphocyte subset abnormalities in peripheral blood from patients with the Guillain-Barré syndrome. *J. Neuroimmunol.* **53**: 219–225.

Dashiell, S., Vanguri, P., and Koski, C.L. (1997). Cytokines and dibutyrol cyclic AMP induce C3 production in rat Schwann cells. GLIA, in press.

Dastur, D.K., Porwal, G.L., Shah, J.S., and Revankar, C.R. (1982). Immunological implications of necrotic, cellular, and vascular changes in leprous neuritis: light and electron microscopy. *Lepr. Rev.* **53**: 45–65.

Dewaal Malefyt, R., Abrams, J., Bennett, B., Figdor, C.G., and de Vries, J.E. (1991). IL-10 inhibits cytokine synthesis by human monocytes: an autoregulatory role for IL-10 produced by monocytes. *J. Exp. Med.* **174**: 1209–1220.

Dick, D.J., Harris, J.G., Falkous, G., Foster, J.B., and Xuerb, J.H. (1988). Neuronal anti-nuclear antibody in paraneoplastic sensory neuronopathy. *J. Neurol. Sci.* **85**: 1–8.

Doekes, G., Vanes, L.A., and Daha, M.R. (1982). Influence of aggregate size on the binding and activation of the first component of human complement by soluble IgG aggregates. *Immunology* **45**: 705–713.

Duncan, A.R. and Winter, G. (1988). The binding site for C1q on IgG. *Nature* **332**: 738–740.

Eikelenboom, P., Hack, C.E., Rozemuller, J.M., and Stam, F.C. (1989). Complement activation in amyloid plaques in Alzheimer's dementia. *Virchows Arch. (Cell Pathol.)* **56**: 259–262.

Enders, U., Karch, A., Toyka, K.V., Michels, M., Zielasek, J., Pette, M., Heesemann, J., and Hartung, H.P. (1993). The spectrum of immune responses to *Campylobacters jejuni* and glycoconjugates in Guillain-Barré syndrome and in other neuro immunological disorders. *Ann. Neurol.* **34**: 136–144.

Feasby, T.E., Gilbert, J.J., Hahn, A.F., and Neilson, M. (1987). Complement depletion suppresses Lewis rat experimental allergic neuritis. *Brain Res.* **419**: 97–103.

Feasby, T.E., Hahn, A.F., and Gilbert, J.J. (1982). Passive transfer studies in Guillain-Barré polyneuropathy. *Neurology (NY)* **32**: 1159–1167.

Friedman, B., Scherer, S.S., Rudge, J.S., Helgren, M., Morriscy, D., Mclain, J., Wang, D.Y., Wiegand, S.J., Furth, M.E., and Lindsay, R.M. (1992). Regulation of ciliary neurotrophic factor expression in myelin-related Schawnn cells in vivo. *Neuron* **9**: 295–305.

Fong, J.W., Ledeen, R.W., Kundu, S.K., and BrostoV, S.W. (1976). Gangliosides of peripheral nerve myelin. *J. Neurochem.* **26**: 175–162.

Frail, D.E., Webster, H.D., and Braun, P.E. (1985). Developmental expression of the myelin-associated glycoprotein in the peripheral nervous system is different from that in the central nervous system. *J. Neurochem.* **45**: 1308–1310.

Frail, D.E. and Braun, P.E. (1984). Two developmentally regulated messenger RNAs differing in their coding region may exist for the myelin-associated glycoprotein. *J. Biol. Chem.* **259**: 14 857–14 862.

Franklin, E.C. (1980). The role of cryoglobulins and immune complexes in vasculitis. *J. Alergy Clin. Immunol.* **66**: 269–273.

Gordon, N. (1994). Chinese paralytic syndrome or acute motor axonal neuropathy. *Arch. Dis. Childhood* **70**: 64–65.

Graus, F., Cordon-Cardo, C., and Posner, J.B. (1985). Neuronal antinuclear antibody in sensory neuronopathy from lung cancer. *Neurology* **35**: 538–543.

Gregorian, S.K., Lee, W.P., Beck, L.S., Rostami, A., and Amento, E.P. (1994a). Regulation of experimental autoimmune neuritis by transforming growth factor beta 1. *Cell. Immunol.* **156**: 102–112.

Gregson, N.A., Koblar, S., and Hughes, R.A.C. (1993). Antibodies to gangliosides in Guillain-Barré syndrome: specificity and relationship to clinical features. *Q. J. Med.* **86**: 111–117.

Griffin, J.W., Cornblath, D.R., Alexander, E., Campbell, J., Low, P.A., Bird, S., and Feldman, E.L. (1990). Ataxic sensory neuropathy and dorsal root ganglionitis associated with Sjögren's syndrome. *Ann. Neurol.* **27**: 304–315.

Guijo, C.G., Garcia-Merino, A., Rubio, G., Guerrero, A., Martinez, A.C., and Apra, J. (1992). IgG anti-ganglioside antibodies and their subclass distribution in two patients with acute and chronic motor neuropathy. *J. Neuroimmunol.* **37**: 141–148.

Hahn, A.F., Feasby, T.E., Wilkie, L., and Lovgren, D. (1993). Antigalactocerebroside antibodies increases demyelination in adoptive transfer experimental allergic neuritis. *Muscle Nerve* **16**: 1174–1180.

Hallet, M.B., Luizio, J.P., and Campbell, A.K. (1981). Stimulation of Ca^{2+} dependent chemiluminescence in rat polymorphonuclear leukocytes by polystyrene beads and the nonlytic action by complement. *Immunology* **44**: 569–576.

Hammarström, L., and Smith, C.I.E. (1986). IgG subclasses in bacterial infections. *Monogr. Allergy* **19**: 122–123.

Hansch, G.M., Seitz, M., Martinotti, G., Betz, M., Rauterberg, E.W., and Gemsa, D. (1984). Macrophages release arachidonic acid, and prostaglandin E_2 and thromboxane in response to late complement components. *J. Immunol.* **133**: 2145–2150.

Harrison, B.M., Hansen, L.A., Pollard, J.D., and McLeod, J.G. (1984). Demyelination induced by serum from patients with Guillain-Barré syndrome. *Ann. Neurol.* **115**: 163–170.

Hartung, H.P., Schafer, B., Diamantstein, T., Fierz, W., Heininger, K., and Toyka, K.V. (1987a). Suppression of P2-T cell line-mediated experimental autoimmune neuritis by interleukin-2 receptor targeted monoclonal antibody ART 18. *Brain Res.* **489**: 120–128.

Hartung, H.P., Schafer, B., Fierz, W., Heininger, K., and Toyka, K.V. (1987b). Cyclosporin A prevents P2 T-cell line-mediated experimental autoimmune neuritis (AT-EAN) in rat. *Neurosci. Lett.* **83**: 195–200.

Hartung, H.P., Schwenke, C., Bitter-Suermann, D., and Toyka, K.V. (1987c). Guillain-Barré syndrome: activated complement components C3a, C5a in CSF. *Neurology* **37**: 1006–1009.

Hartung, H.P., Schafer, B., Heininger, K., Stoll, G., and Toyka, K.V. (1988a). The rat of macrophages and eicosanoids in the pathogenesis of experimental allergic neuritis. Serial clinical, electrophysiological, biochemical and morphological observations. *Brain* **111**: 1039–1059.

Hartung, H.P., Schafer, B., Heininger, K., and Toyka, K.V. (1988b). Suppression of experimental autoimmune neuritis by the oxygen radical scavengers superoxide dismutase and catalase. *Ann. Neurol.* **23**: 453–460.

Hartung, H.P., Hughes, R.A.C., Taylor, W.A., Heininger, K., and Toyka, K.V. (1990a). T cell activation in Guillain-Barré syndrome and in MS: elevated serum levels of soluble IL-2 receptors. *Neurology* **40**: 215–218.

Hartung, H.P., Schafer, B., van der meide, P.H., Fierz, W., Heininger, K., and Toyka, K.V. (1990b). The role of interferon-gamma in the pathogenesis of experimental autoimmune disease of the peripheral nervous system. *Ann. Neurol.* **27**: 247–257.

Hartung, H.P., Reiners, K., Michels, M., Hughes, R.A.L., Heidenreich, F., Zielasek, J., Enders, U., and Toyka, K.V. (1994). Serum levels of soluble E-selectin (ELAM-1) in immune-omediated neuropathies. *Neurology* **44**: 1153–1158.

Harvey, G.K. and Polland, J.D. (1992). Peripheral nervous system demyelination from systemic transfer of experimental allergic neuritis serum. *J. Immunol.* **41**: 159–166.

Hattori, A., Tanaka, E., Murase, K., Ishida, N., Chatani, Y., Tsujimoto, M., Hayashi, K., and Kohno, M. (1993). Tumor necrosis factor stimulates the synthesis and secretion of biologically active nerve growth factor in non-neuronal cells. *J. Biol. Chem.* **268**: 2577–2582.

Hays, A.P., Latov, N., Takatsu, M., and Sherman, W.H. (1987). Experimental demyelination of nerve induced by serum of patients with neuropathy and an anti-MAG IgM M-protein. *Neurology* **37**: 242–256.

Hays, A.P., Lee, S.S., and Latov, N. (1988). Immune reactive C3d on the surface of myelin sheaths in neuropathy. *J. Neuroimmunol.* **18**: 231–244.

Heininger, K., Liebert, U.G., Toyka, K.V., Haneveld, F., Schwendemann, G., Kolb-Bachofen, V., and Ross, H.G. (1984). Chronic inflammatory polyneuropathy. Reduction of nerve conduction velocities in monkeys by systemic passive transfer of immunoglobulin G. *J. Neurol. Sci.* **66**: 1–14.

Heininger, K., Schafer, B., Hartung, H.P., Fierz, W., Linington, C., and Toyka, K.V. (1988). The role of macrophages in experimental autoimmune neuritis induced by a P2-specific T-cell line. *Ann. Neurol.* **23**: 326–331.

Henderson, C.E., Phillips, H.S., Pollock, R.A., Davies, A.M., Lemeulle, C., Armanini, M., Simpson, L.C., MoVet, B., Vandlen, R.A., Koliatsos, V.E., and Rosenthal, A. (1994). GDNF: a potent survival factor for motoneurons present in peripheral nerve and muscle. *Science* **266**: 1062–1064.

Hoffman, P.M., Powers, J.M., Weise, M.J., and Brostoff V, S.W. (1980). EAN: 1. Rat strain differences in the response to bovine myelin antigens. *Brain Res.* **195**: 355–362.

Horwich, M.S., Cho, L., Porro, R.S., and Posner, J.B. (1977). Subacute sensory neuropathy: a remote effect of carcinoma. *Ann. Neurol.* **2**: 7–19.

Hughes, R.A.C., Kadlubowski, M., Gray, I.A., and Leibowitz, S. (1981). Immune responses in experimental allergic neuritis. *J. Neurol. Neurosurg. Psychiatry* **44**: 565–569.

Hughes, R.A.C. and Powell, H.C. (1984). Experimental allergic neuritis: demyelination induced by P2 alone and non-specific enhancement by cerebroside. *J. Neuropathol. Exp. Neurol.* **43**: 154–161.

Imagawa, D.K., Osifchin, N.E., Paznekas, W.A., Shin, M.L., and Mayer, M.M. (1983). Consequences of cell membrane attack by complement: release of arachidonate and formation of inflammatory derivatives. *Proc. Natl. Acad. Sci. USA* **80**: 6647–6651.

Inuzuka, T., Fujita, N., Sato, S., Baba, H., Ishiguro, H., and Miyatake, T. (1991). Expression of the large myelin-associated glycoprotein isoform during the development in the mouse peripheral nervous system. *Brain Res.* **562**: 173–175.

Jacobs, B.C., Endtz, H., van der Meche, F.G., Hazenberg, M.P., Achtereekte, H.A., and van Doorn, P.A. (1995). Serum anti-GQ1b IgG antibodies recognize surface epitopes on *Campylobacter jejuni* from patients with Miller Fisher syndrome. *Ann. Neurol.* **37**: 260–264.

Jacobs, J.M., Shetty, V.P., and Antia, N.H. (1987). Myelin changes in leprous neuropathy. *Acta Neuropathol. (Berl.)* **74**: 75–80.

Jander, S., Heidenreich, F., and Stoll, G. (1993). Serum and CSF levels of soluble intercellular adhesion molecule-1 (1CAM-1) in inflammatory neurologic diseases. *Neurology* **43**: 1809–1813.

Jessen, K.R., Brennan, A., Morgan, L., Mirsky, R., Kent, A., Hashimoto, Y., and Gavrilovic, J. (1994). The Schwann cell precursor and its fate: a study of cell death and differentiation during gliogenesis in rat embryonic nerves. *Neuron* **12**: 509–527.

Jessen, K.R. and Mirsky, R. (1991). Schwann cell precursors and their development. *GLIA* **4**: 185–194.

Job, C.K. (1989). Nerve damage and leprosy. *Int. J. Lepr.* **57**: 532–539.

June, C.H., Ledbetter, J.A., Linsley, P.S., and Thompson, C.B. (1990). Role of the CD28 receptor in T cell activation. *Immunol. Today* **11**: 211–216.

Kadlubowski, M. and Hughes, R.A.C. (1979). Identification of the neuritogen for experimental allergic neuritis. *Nature* **277**: 140–141.

Kadmon, G., Kowitz, A., Altevogt, P., and Schachner, M. (1990). The neural cell adhesion molecule N-CAM enhances L1-dependent cell-cell interactions. *J. Cell Biol.* **110**: 193–208.

Kamin-Lewis, R.M., Karasanyi, N., Koski, C.L., and Lewis, G.K. (1994). Adherence-mediated T cell activation in multiple sclerosis and other neurologic disorders. *J. Neuroimmunol.* **53**: 163–171.

Kaneko, K., Savage, C.O., Pottinger, B.E., Shah, V., Pearson, J.D., and Dillon, M.J. (1994). Antiendothelial cell antibodies can be cytotoxic to endothelial cells without cytokine pre-stimulation and correlate with ELISA antibody measurement in Kawasaki disease. *Clin. Exp. Immunol.* **98**: 264–269.

Kaplan, G. and Cohn, Z.A. (1991). Leprosy and cell-mediated immunity. *Curr. Opin. Immunol.* **3**: 91–96.

Kaufmann, S.H.E., Schoel, B., Wand-Wurttenberger, A., Steinhoff, U., Munk, M.E., and Koga, T. (1990). T cells, stress proteins, and pathogenesis of mycobacterial infections. *Curr. Top. Microbiol. Immunol.* **155**: 125–141.

Kelly, J.J., Kyle, R.A., Miles, J.M., and Dyck, P.J. (1983). Osteosclerotic myeloma and peripheral neuropathy. *Neurology* **33**: 202–210.

Khalili-Shirazi, A., Hughes, R.A., Brostoff, S.W., Linington, C., and Gregson, N. (1992). T cell responses to myelin proteins in Guillain-Barré syndrome. *J. Neurologic Sci.* **111**: 200–203.

Kingston, A.E., Bergsteinsdottir, K., Jessen, K.R., van der meide, P.H., Colston, M.J., and Mirsky, R. (1989). Schwann cells co-cultured with stimulated T cells and antigen express major histocompatibility complex (MHC) class II determinants without interferon-Γ pretreatment: synergistic effects of interferon-Γ and tumor necrosis factor on MHC class II induction. *Eur. J. Immunol.* **19**: 177–183.

Kipps, T.J. (1989). The CD5 B cell. *Adv. Immunol.* **47**: 117–185.

Kissel, J.T., Riethman, J.L., Omerza, J., Rammohan, K.W., and Mendell, J.R. (1989). Peripheral vasculitis: immune characterization of the vascular lesions. *Ann. Neurol.* **25**: 291–297.

Koh, D.R., Fung Leung, W.P., Ho, A., Gray, D., Acha-Orbea, H., and Mark, T.W. (1992). Less mortality but more relapses in experimental allergic encephalomyelitis in CD8-/-mice. *Science* **256**: 1210–1213.

Koski, C.L., Humphrey, R., and Shin, M.L. (1985). Anti-peripheral myelin antibody in patients with demyelinating neuropathy. Quantitative and kinetic determination or serum antibody by complement fixation. *Proc. Natl. Acad. Sci. USA* **82**: 905–909.

Koski, C.L., Gratz, E., Sutherland, J., and Mayer, R.F. (1986). Clinical correlation with anti-peripheral nerve myelin antibodies in Guillain-Barré syndrome. *Ann. Neurol.* **19**: 573–577.

Koski, C.L., Sanders, M.E., Swoveland, P.T., Fawley, J.T., Shin, M.L., Farnk, M.M., and Joiner, K.A. (1987). Activation of terminal components of complement in patients with Guillain-Barré syndrome and other demyelinating neuropathies. *J. Clin. Invest.* **80**: 1492–1497.

Koski, C.L., Chou, D.K.H., and Jungalwala, F.B. (1989). Anti-peripheral nerve myelin antibodies in Guillain-Barré syndrome bind a neutral glycolipid of peripheral myelin and cross-react with Forssman antigen. *J. Clin. Invest.* **84**: 280–287.

Koski, C.L. (1990). Characterization of complement-fixing antibodies to peripheral nerve myelin in Guillain-Barré syndrome. *Ann. Neurol.* **27** (Suppl.), S44–S47.

Koski, C.L., Vanguri, P., and Shin, M.L. (1985). Activation of the alternative pathway of complement by human peripheral nerve myelin. *J. Immunol.* **134**: 182–187.

Kroczek, R.A., Gunter, K.C., Germain, R.N., and Shevach, E.M. (1986). Thy-1 functions as a signal transduction molecule in T lymphocytes and transfected B lymphocytes. *Nature* **322**: 181–184.

Krych, M., Atkinson, J.P., and Holers, V.M. (1992). Complement receptors. *Curr. Opin. Immunol.* **4**: 8–13.

Lampert, P.W. (1969). Mechanisms of demyelination in experimental allergic neuritis. Electronmicroscopic studies. *Lab. Invest.* **20**: 127–138.

Lassmann, H., Schmied, M., Vass, K., and Hickey, W.F. (1993). Bone marrow derived elements and resident microglia in brain inflammation. *GLIA* **7**: 19–24.

Lassmann, H., Zimprich, F., Rossler, R., and Vass, K. (1991). Inflammation in the nervous system: basic mechanisms and immunological concepts (Review). *Rev. Neurol.* **147**: 763–781.

Latov, N., Gross, R.B., Kastelman, J. et al. (1981). Complement-fixing anti-peripheral nerve myelin antibodies in patients with inflammatory polyneuritis and with polyneuropathy and paraproteinemia. *Neurology* **31**: 1503–1534.

Latov, N., Hays, A.P., and Sherman, W.H. (1988). Peripheral neuropathy and anti-MAG antibodies. *Crit. Rev. Neurobiol.* **3**: 301–332.

Launois, P., N'Diaye, M., Sarthou, J.L., Millan, J., and Bach, M.A. (1992). Anti-peripheral nerve antibodies in leprosy patients recognize an epitope shared by the *M. Leprae* 65 kDa heat shock protein. *J. Autoimmun.* **5**: 745–757.

Laven Stein, B., Dalakas, M., and Engel, W.K. (1979). Poly neuropathy in 'non secretory' osteosclerotic multiple myeloma with immunoglobulin deposition in peripheral nerve tissue. *Neurology* **29**: 611 (abstract).

Lawley, T.J., Bielory, L., Gascon, P., Yancey, K.B., Young, N., and Frank, M.M. (1984). A prospective clinical and immunologic analysis of patients with serum sickness. *N. Engl. J. Med.* **311**: 1407–1413.

Lawrence, M.B. and Springer, T.A. (1991). Leukocytes roll on a selectin at physiologic flow rates: distinction from and prerequisite for adhesion through integrins. *Cell* **65**: 859–873.

Lemke, G. (1988). Unwrapping the genes of myelin. *Neuron* **1**: 535–543.

Linington, C., Mann, A., Izumo, S., Uyemura, K., Suzuki, M., Meyermann, R., and Wekerle, H. (1986). Induction of experimental allergic neuritis in the BN rat: P2 protein-specific T-cells overcome resistance to actively induced disease. *J. Immunol.* **137**: 3826–3831.

Lewis, I.C. and Philpott, M.G. (1956). Neurological complications in the Schonlein-Henoch syndrome. *Arch. Dis. Child.* **31**: 369–371.

Lindholm, D., Heumann, R., Meyer, M., and Thoenen, H. (1987). Interleukin-1 regulates synthesis of nerve growth factor in non-neuronal cells in rat sciatic nerve. *Nature* **330**: 658–659.

Linington, C., Izumo, S., Suzuki, M., Uyemura, K., Meyermann, R., and Wekerle, H. (1984). A permanent rat T cell line that mediates experimental allergic neuritis in the Lewis rat in vivo. *J. Immunol.* **133**: 1946–1950.

Linington, C., Lassmann, H., and Kosin, S. (1995). Experimental allergic neuritis in the Lewis rat: induction by Po protein specific T cell lines. *Eur. J. Immunol.* (in press).

Lo, S.K., Detmers, P.A., Levin, S.M., and Wright, S.D. (1989). Transient adhesion of neutrophils to endothelium. *J. Exp. Med.* **169**: 1779–1793.

Lotz, M., Vaughan, J.H., and Carson, D.A. (1988). Effect of neuropeptides on production of inflammatory cytokines by human monocytes. *Science* **241**: 1218–1221.

Manetti, R., Parronchi, P., Giudizi, M.G., Piccinni, M.P., Maggi, E., Trinchieri, G., and Romagnani, S. (1993). Natural killer cell stimulatory factor (interleukin-12) induces T helper type 1 (Th1)-specific immune responses and inhibits the development of IL-4-producing Th cells. *J. Exp. Med.* **177**: 1199–1204.

Martini, R. (1994). Expression and functional roles of neural cell surface molecules and extracellular matrix components during development and regeneration of peripheral nerves. *J. Neurocytol.* **23**: 1–28.

Matsuoka, I., Meyer, M., and Thoenen, H. (1991). Cell-type-specific regulation of nerve growth factor (NGF) synthesis in non-neuronal cells: comparison of Schwann cells with other cell types. *J. Neurosci.* **11**: 3165–3177.

McGeer, P.L., Akiyama, H., Itagaki, S., and McGeer, E.G. (1989). Immune system response in Alzheimer's disease. *Can. J. Neurol. Sci.* **16**: 516–527.

McKhann, G.M., Cornblath, D.R., Griffn, J.W., Ho, T.W., Li, C.Y., Jiang, Z., Wu, H.S., Zhaori, G., Liu, Y., and Jou, L.P. (1993). Acute motor axonal neuropathy: a frequent cause of acute flaccid paralysis in china. *Ann. Neurol.* **33**: 333–342.

Medof, M.E., Kinoshita, T., and Nussenzzwig. V. (1984). Inhibition of complement activation on the surface of cells after incorporation of decay-accelerating factor (DAF) into their membranes. *J. Exp. Med.* **160**: 1558–1578.

Mehra, V. and Modlin, R.L. (1990). T-lymphocytes in leprosy lesions. *Curr. Top. Microbiol. Immunol.* **155**: 97–109.

Mews, M. and Meyer, M. (1993). Modulation of Schwann cell phenotype by TGF-β1: Inhibition of Po mRNA expression and downregulation of the low affinity NGF receptor. *GLIA* **8**: 208–217.

Michaelson, T.E., Aase, A., Norderhaug, L., and Sandlie, I. (1992). Antibody dependent cell-mediated cytotoxicity induced by chimeric mouse-human IgG subclasses and IgG3 antibodies with altered hinge region. *Mol. Immunol.* **29**: 319–326.

Milner, P., Lovelidge, C.A., Taylor, W.A., and Hughes, R.A.C. (1987). Po myelin protein produces experimental allergic neuritis in Lewis rats. *J. Neurol. Sci.* **79**: 275–285.

Mithen, F.A., Colburn, S., and Berchem, R. (1990). Human alpha tumor necrosis factor does not damage cultures containing rat Schwann cells and sensory neurons. *Neurosci. Res.* **9**: 59–63.

Mokuno, K., Kamholz, J., Behrman, T., Black, C., Feinstein, D., Lee, V., and Pleasure, D. (1989). Neuronal modulation of Schwann cell glial fibrillary acidic protein (GFAP). *J. Neurosci. Res.* **23**: 396–405.

Morgan, B.P., van den Berg, C.W., Davies, V., Hallet, M.B., and Horejsi, V. (1993). Cross-linking of CD59 and of other phosphatidylinositol-anchored molecules on neutrophils triggers cell activation via tyrosine kinase. *Eur. J. Immunol.* **23**: 2841–2850.

Mosmann, T.R., Cherwinski, H., Bond, M.W., Giedlin, M.A., and Koffman, R.L. (1986). Two types of murine helper T cell clone. I. Definition according to profiles of lymphokine activities and secreted proteins. *J. Immunol.* **136**: 2348–2357.

Mshana, R.N., Humber, D.P., Harboe, M., and Belehu, A. (1983). Demonstration of mycobacterial antigens in nerve biopsies from leprosy patients using peroxidase-antiperoxidase immunoenzyme technique. *Clin. Immunol. Immunopathol.* **29**: 359–368.

Müller-Eberhard, H.J. and Calcott, M.A. (1966). Interaction between C1q and G-globulin. *Immunochemistry* **3**: 500–512.

Nakamura, A., Kohsaka, T., and Johns, E.J. (1993). Differential regulation of interleukin-6 production in the kidney by the renal sympathetic nerves in normal and spontaneously hypertensive rats. *J. Hypertens.* **11**: 491–497.

Naniche, D., V-Kreshnan, G., Cernoi, F., Wild, T.F., Rossi, B., Radurdim-Combe, C., and Gerlier, D. (1993). Human membrane cofactor protein (CD46) acts as a cellular receptor for measles virus. *J. Virol.* **67**: 6025–6032.

Nicholson-Weller, A., Burge, J., Fearon, D.T., Weller, P.F., and Austen, K.F. (1982). Isolation of a human erythrocyte membrane glycoprotein with decay accelerating activity for C3-convertases of the complement system. *J. Immunol.* **129**: 184–189.

Okusawa, S., Gelfand, J.A., Ikejima, T., Connolly, R.J., and Dinarello, C.A. (1988). Interleukin-1 induces a shock-like state in rabbits. Synergism with tumor necrosis factor and the effect of cyclooxygenase inhibition. *J. Clin. Invest.* **81**: 1162–1172.

Olsson, T., Holmdahl, R., Klareskog, L., Forsum, U., and Kristensson, K. (1984). Dynamics of Ia-expressing cells and T lymphocytes of different subsets during experimental allergic neuritis in Lewis rats. *J. Neurol Sci.* **66**: 141–149.

Ota, K., Irie, H., and Takahashi, K. (1987). T cell subsets and Ia-positive cells in the sciatic nerve during the course of experimental allergic neuritis. *J. Neuroimmunol.* **13**: 283–292.

Ottenhoff, T.H.M. and de Vries, R.R.P. (1990). Antigen reactivity and autoreactivity: two sides of the cellular immune response induced by mycobacteria. *Curr. Top. Microbiol. Immunol.* **155**: 111–121.

Panegyres, P.K., Faul, R.J., Russ, G.R., Appleton, S.L., Wangel, A.G., and Blumbergs, P.C. (1992). Endothelial cell activation in vasculities of peripheral nerve and skeletal muscle. *J. Neurol. Neurosurg. Psychiatry* **55**: 4–7.

Park, A.M. and Richardson, J.C. (1953). Cerebral complications of serum sickness. *Neurology* **3**: 227–283.

Pette, M., Linington, C., Gengaroli, Gross-Wilde, H., Toyka, K.V., and Hartung, H.P. (1994). T lymphocyte recognition sites on peripheral nerve myelin Po protein. *J. Neuroimmunol.* **54**: 29–34.

Platt, J.L., Dalmasso, A.P., Lindman, B.J., Ihrcke, N.S., and Bach, F.H. (1991). The role of C5a and antibody in the release of heparan sulfate from endothelial cells. *Eur. J. Immunol.* **21**: 2887–90.

Pollard, J.D., Waterland, K.W., Harvey, G.K., Jung, S., Bonner, J., Spies, J.M., Toyka, K.V., and Hartung, H.P. (1995) Activated T cells of non neural specificity open the blood–nerve barrier to circulating antibody. *Ann. Neurol.* **37**: 467–475.

Prineas, J.W. (1972). Acute idopathic polyneuritis: an electron microscope study. *Lab. Invest.* **26**: 133–147.

Prineas, J.W. (1981). Pathology of the Guillain-Barré syndrome. *Ann. Neurol.* **9** (Suppl.), 6–19.

Raine, C.S. (1985). Experimental allergic encephalomyelitis and experimental allergic neuritis, Vinken, P.J., et al., eds. Elsevier, Amsterdam.

Ravetch, J.V. and Kiret, J.P. (1991). Fc receptors. *Ann Rev. Immunol.* **9**: 457–492.

Rende, M., Nuir, D., Ruoslahti, E., Hagg, T., Varon, S., and Manthorpe, M. (1992). Immuno-localization of ciliary neuronotrophic factor in adult rat sciatic nerve. *GLIA* **5**: 25–32.

Resnick, D., Greenway, G.D., Bardwick, P.A., Zvaiffer, N.J., Gill, G.N., and Newman, D.R. (1981). Plasma cell dyscrasia with polyneuropathy, organomegaly, endocrinopathy, M-protein, and skin changes: the POEMS syndrome. Distinctive radiographic abnormalities. *Radiology* **140**: 17–22.

Reulecke, M., Dumas, M., and Meier, C. (1988). Specific antibody activity against neuroendocrine tissue in a case of POEMS syndrome with IgG gammopathy. *Neurology* **614**: 614–616.

Robbins, D.S., Shirazi, Y., Drysdale, B.E., Lieberman, A., Shin, H.S., and Shin, M.L. (1987). Production of cytotoxic factor for oligodendrocytes by stimulated astrocytes. *J. Immunol.* **139**: 2593–2597.

Roberts, M., Willison, H., Vincent, A., and Newsom-Davis, J. (1994). Serum factors in Miller Fisher variant of Guillain-Barré syndrome and neurotransmitter release. *Lancet* **343**: 454–455.

Ronco, P., Verroust, P., Mignon, F., Kourilsky, O., Vanhille, P., Meyrier, A., Mery, J.P., and Morel-Maroger, L. (1983). Immunopathological studies of polyarteritis nodosa and Wegener's granulomatosis: a report of 43 patients and 51 renal biopsies. *Q. J. Med.* **52**: 212–223.

Rosse, W.F. (1989). Paroxysmal nocturnal hemoglobinuria: the biochemical defects and the clinical syndrome. *Blood Rev.* **3**: 192–200.

Rostami, A.J., Burns, J.B., Brown, M.J., Rosen, J., Zweiman, B., Lisak, R.P., and Pleasure, D.E. (1985). Transfer of experimental allergic neuritis with P2-reactive T-cell lines. *Cell. Immunol.* **91**: 354–361.

Rush, R.A. (1984). Immunohistochemical localization of endogenous nerve growth factor. *Nature* **312**: 364–367.

Saadi, S. and Platt, J.L. (1995). Transient perturbation of endothelial integrity induced by natural antibodies and complement. *J. Exp. Med.* **181**: 21–31.

Sadoul, R., Fahrig, T., Bartsch, U., and Schachner, M. (1990). Binding properties of lyposomes containing the myelin-associated glycoprotein MAG to neural cell cultures. *J. Neurosci, Res.* **25**: 1–13.

Said, G. and Hontebeyrie-Joskowicz, M. (1992). Nerve lesions induced by macrophage activation. *Res. Immunol.* **143**: 589–599.

Saida, T., Saida, K., Dorfman, S.H. et al. (1979). Experimental allergic neuritis induced by sensitization with galactocerebroside. *Science* **204**: 1103–1106.

Saida, T., Saida, K., Lisak, R.P., Brown, M.J., Silberberg, D.H., and Asbury, A.K. (1982). In vivo demyelinating activity of sera from patients with Guillain-Barré syndrome. *Ann. Neurol.* **11**: 69–75.

Sakagami, Y., Girasole, G., Yu, X.P., Boswell, H.S., and Manolagas, S.C. (1993). Stimulation of interleukin-6 production by either calcitonin gene-related peptide or parathyroid hormone in two phenotypically distinct bone marrow-derived murine stromal cell lines. *J. Bone Mineral Res.* **8**: 811–816.

Sams, W.M., Jr., Claman, N.H., Kohler, P.F., McIntosh, R.M., Small, P., and Mass, M.F. (1975). Human necrotizing vasculitis: immunoglobulins and complement in vessel walls of cutaneous lesions and normal skin. *J. Invest. Dermatol.* **64**: 441–445.

Samuel, N.M., Mirsky, R., Grange, J.M., and Jessen, K.R. (1987). Expression of major histocompatibility complex class I and class II antigens in human Schwann cell cultures and effects of infection with *Mycobacterium leprae. Clin. Exp. Immunol.* **68**: 500–509.

Sanders, M.E., Koski, C.L., Robbins, D., Shin, M.L., Frank, M.M., and Joiner, K.A. (1986). Activated terminal complements in cerebro-spinal fluid in Guillain-Barré syndrome and multiple sclerosis. *J. Immunol.* **136**: 4456–4459.

Sandlie, I. and Michaelson, T.E. (1991). Engineering monoclonal antibodies to determine the structural requirements for complement activation and complement mediated lysis. *Mol. Immunol.* **28**: 3161–3168.

Sano, Y. (1985). Studies on the complement system in cerebrospinal fluid. *Acta Med. Univ. Kagoshima* **27**: 1–16.

Santoro, M., Uncini, A., Corbo, M., Staugaitis, S.M., Thomas, F.P., Hays, A.P., and Latov, N. (1992). Experimental conduction block induced by serum from a patient with anti-GM1 antibodies. *Ann. Neurol.* **31**: 385–390.

Sawant-Mane, S., Clark, M.B., and Koski, C.L. (1991). In vitro demyelination by serum antibody from patients with Guillain-Barré syndrome requires terminal complement complexes. *Ann. Neurol.* **29**: 397–404.

Schneider-Schaulies, J., von Brunn, A., and Schachner, M. (1990). Recombinant peripheral myelin protein Po confers adhesion and neurite out-growth-promoting properties. *J. Neurosci. Res.* **27**: 286–297.

Schonermark, S., Rauterberg, E.W., Shin, M.L., Lore, S., Roelcke, D., and Hansch, G.M. (1986). Homologous species restriction in lysis of human erythrocytes: a membrane derived protein with C8-binding capacity functions as an inhibitor. *J. Immunol.* **136**: 1772–1776.

Schumaker, V.N., Calcott, M.A., Speigelberg, H.L., and Muller-Eberhard, H.J. (1976). Ultracentrifuge studies of the binding of IgG of different subclasses to the C1q subunit of the first component of complement. *Biochemistry* **15**: 5175–5181.

Seiz, R.J., Heininger, K., Schwendemann, G., Toyka, K.V., and Wechsler, W. (1985). The mouse blood–brain barrier and blood–nerve barrier for IgG: a tracer study by use of the avidin-biotin system. *Acta Neuropathol. (Berlin)* **68**: 15–21.

Selmaj, K., Raine, C.S., and Cross, A.H. (1991). Anti-tumor necrosis factor therapy abrogates autoimmune demyelination. *Ann. Neurol.* **30**: 694–700.

Selmaj, K.W. and Raine, C.S. (1988). Tumor necrosis factor mediates myelin and oligodendrocyte damage in vitro. *Ann. Neurol.* **23**: 339–346.

Sharief, M.K., McLean, B., and Thompson, E.J. (1993). Elevated serum levels of tumor necrosis factor-α in Guillain-Barré syndrome. *Ann. Neurol.* **33**: 591–596.

Shetty, V.P., Antia, N.H., and Jacobs, J.M. (1988). The pathology of early leprous neuropathy. *J. Neurol. Sci.* **88**: 115–131.

Shimizu, Y., Newman, W., Tanaka, Y., and Shaw, S. (1992). Lymphocyte interactions with endothelial cells. *Immunol. Today* **13**: 106–112.

Shin, M.L. and Koski, C.L. (1992). *The complement system in demyelination.* R. Martenson, CRC Press, Boca Raton, pp. 801–831.

Shirazi, Y., McMorris, F.A., and Shin, M.L. (1989). Arachidonic acid mobilization and phosphoinositide turnover by the terminal complement complex, C5b-9, in rat oligodendrocytes×C6 glioma hybrids. *J. Immunol.* **142**: 4385–4391.

Spies, J.M., Westland, K.W., Bonner, J.G., and Pollard, J.D. (1993). The role of T cells and their products in opening the blood–nerve barrier. *J. Neuroimmunol.* **43**: 212 (abstract).

Sporn, M.B. and Roberts, A.B. (1992). Transforming growth factor β: recent progress and new challenges. *J. Cell Biol.* **119**: 1017–1021.

Steinhoff, U. and Kaufmann, S.H.E. (1988). Specific lysis by $CD8^+$ T cells of Schwann cells expressing Mycobacterium leprae antigens. *Eur. J. Immunol.* **18**: 969–972.

Steinman, L., Smith, M.E., and Forno, L.S. (1981). Genetic control of susceptibility to experimental allergic neuritis and the immune response to P2 protein. *Neurology* **31**: 950–954.

Stewart, G.L., Pollard, J.D., McLeod, J.D., and Wolnizer, C.M. (1978). HLA antigens in the Landry-Guillain-Barré syndrome and chronic relapsing polyneuritis. *Ann. Neurol.* **4**: 285–289.

Stoll, G., Schmidt, B., Sebastian, J. et al. (1991). The presence of the terminal complement complexes (C5b-9) precedes myelin degradation in immune mediated demyelination of rat peripheral nervous system. *Ann. Neurol.* **30**: 147–155.

Strigard, K., Brismar, T., Olsson, T., Kristensson, K., and Klareskog, L. (1987) T lymphocyte subsets, functional deficits and morphology in sciatic nerves during experimental allergic neuritis. *Muscle Nerve* **10**: 329–337.

Strigard, K., Holmdahl, R., van der Meide, P.H., Klareskog, L., and Olsson, T. (1989). In vivo treatment of rats with monoclonal antibodies against gamma interferon effects on experimental allergic neuritis. *Acta Neurol. Scand.* **80**: 201–207.

Strober, W. and James, S.P. (1989). The interleukins. *Pediatr Res.* **24**: 549–557.

Sugita, Y., Nakano, Y., and Tomita, M.I. (1988). Isolation from human erythrocytes which inhibits the formation of complement transmembrane channels. *J. Biochem. (Japan)* **104**: 633–637.

Sumner, A.J., Lisak, R.P., Brown, M.J., and Asbury, A.K. (1983). Demyelinating activity of Guillain-Barré syndrome (GBS) serum. *Neurology* **33**: 81 (abstract).

Suter, U. and Patel, P.I. (1994). Genetic basis of inherited peripheral neuropathies. *Hum. Mut.* **3**: 95–102.

Suzuki, T. (1991). Signal transduction mechanisms through FcΓ receptors on the mouse macrophage surface. *FASEB J.* **5**: 187–193.

Svennerholm, L. and Friedman, P. (1990). Antibody detection in Guillain-Barré syndrome. *Ann. Neurol.* **27**: S36–S40.

Swant-Mane, S., Clark, M.B., and Koski, C.L. (1991). In vitro demyelination by serum antibody from patients with Guillain-Barré syndrome requires terminal complement complexes. *Ann. Neurol.* **29**: 397–404.

Takigawa, T., Yasuda, H., Kikkawa, R., Shigeta, Y., Saida, T., and Ritasato, H. (1995). Antibodies against GM1 ganglioside affect K^+ and Na^+. Currents in isolated rat myelinated nerve fibers. *Ann. Neurol.* **37**: 436–442.

Taniuchi, M., Clark, H.B., and Johnson, Jr (1986). Induction of nerve growth factor receptor in Schwann cells after axotomy. *Proc. Natl. Acad. Sci. USA* **83**: 4094–4098.

Tansey, F.A. and Brosnan, C.F. (1982). Protection against experimental allergic neuritis with silica quartz dust. *J. Neuroimmunol.* **3**: 169–179.

Thomas, F.P., Trojaborg, W., Nagy, C., Santoro, M., Sadiq, S.A., Latov, N., and Hays, A.P. (1991). Experimental autoimmune neuropathy with anti-GM1 antibodies and immunoglobulin deposits at the nodes of Ranvier. *Acta Neuropathol.* **82**: 378–383.

Unanue, E.R. (1993). *Macrophages antigen-presenting cells and the phenomena of antigen handling and presentation.* William E. Paul, Raven Press, New York.

Van den Berg, L.H., Sadiq, S.A., Thomas, F.P., and Latov, N. (1990). Characterization of HNK-1 bearing glycoproteins in human peripheral nerve myelin. *J. Neurosci. Res.* **25**: 295–299.

Van der Woude, F.J., Rasmussen, N., Labatto, S., Wiik, A., Permin, H., van Es, L.A., van der Giessen, M., van der Hem, G.K., and The, T.H. (1985). Autoantibodies against neutrophils and monocytes: tool for diagnosis and marker of disease activity in Wegener's granulomatosis. *Lancet* **1**: 425–429.

Vassalli, P. (1992). The pathophysiology of human tumor necrosis factors. *Ann. Rev. Immunol.* **10**: 411–453.

Vedeler, C.A., Matre, R., and Fischer, E. (1989a). Isolation and characterization of complement receptors CRI from human peripheral nerves. *J. Neuroimmunol.* **23**: 215–221.

Vedeler, C.A., Nilsen, R., and Matre, R. (1989b). Localization of Fcγ receptors and complement receptors CR1 on human peripheral nerve fibers by immune electron microscopy. *J. Neuroimmunol.* **23**: 29–33.

Vedeler, C.A. and Matre, R. (1990). Peripheral nerve CR1 limit complement-mediated hemolysis. *J. Neuroimmunol.* **30**: 95–98.

Vriesendorp, F.J., Mayer, R.F., and Koski, C.L. (1991). Kinetics of anti-peripheral nerve myelin antibody in patients with Guillain-Barré syndrome treated and not treated with plasmapheresis. *Arch. Neurol.* **48**: 858–861.

Vriesendorp, F.J., Mishu, B., Blaser, M.J., and Koski, C.L. (1993). Serum of antibodies to GM1, GD1b, peripheral nerve myelin and *Campylobacter jejuni* in patients with Guillain-Barré syndrome and controls: correlation and prognosis. *Ann. Neurol.* **34**: 130–135.

Vriesendorp, F.J., Flynn, R.E., Pappolla, M.A., and Koski, C.L. (1995). Complement depletion affects demyelination and inflammation in experimental allergic neuritis. *J. Neuroimmunol.* **50**: 157–165.

Walsh, F.S., Cronin, M., Koblar, S., Doherty, P., Winer, J., Leon, A., and Hughes, R.A.C. (1991). Association between glycoconjugate antibodies and *Campylobacter* infection in patients with Guillain-Barré syndrome. *J. Neuroimmunol.* **34**: 43–51.

Wanidworanun, C. and Strober, W. (1993). Predominant role of tumor necrosis factor-α in human monocyte IL-10 produced by synthesis. *J. Immunol.* **151**: 6853–6861.

Wantanabe, F.R., Brannan, C.I., Copeland, N.G., Jenkins, N.A., and Nagata, S. (1992). Lymphoproliferation disorder in mice explained by defects in Fas antigen that mediates apoptosis. *Nature* **356**: 314.

Waxman, S.G. and Ritchie, J.M. (1993). Molecular dissection of the myelinated axon. *Ann. Neurol.* **33**: 121–136.

Wekerle, H., Schwab, M., Linington, C., and Meyermann, R. (1986). Antigen presentation in the peripheral nervous system: Schwann cells present endogenous myelin autoantigens to lymphocytes. *Eur. J. Immunol.* **16**: 1551–1557.

Willison, H.J. and Veitch, J. (1994). Immunoglobulin subclass distribution and binding characteristics of anti-GQ1b antibodies in Miller Fisher syndrome. *J. Neuroimmunol.* **50**: 159–165.

Wright, J.F., Shulman, M.J., Isenman, D.E., and Painter, R.H. (1990). C1 binding by mouse IgM. The effect of abnormal glycosylation at position 402 resulting from a serine to asparagine exchange at residue 406 of the mu-chain. *J. Biol. Chem.* **265**: 10 506–10 513.

Wright, J.K., Tschopp, J., Jaton, J.C., and Engel, J. (1980). Dimeric, trimeric, and tetrameric complexes of immunoglobulin G fix complement. *Biochem. J.* **187**: 775–780.

Yamamoto, M., Sobue, G., Li, M., Arakawa, Y., Mitsuma, T., and Kimata, K. (1993). Nerve growth factor (NGF), brain-derived neurotrophic factor (BDNF) and low-affinity nerve growth factor receptor (LNGFR) mRNA levels in cultures rat Schwann cells; differential time-and-dose-dependent regulation by cAMP. *Neurosci. Lett.* **152**: 37–40.

Yuki, N., Yoshino, H., Sato, S., and Miyatake, T. (1990). Acute axonal polyneuropathy associated with anti-GM1 antibodies following campylobacter enteritis. *Neurology* **40**: 1900–1902.

Yuki, N., Sato, S., Itoh, T., and Miyatake, T. (1991). HLA-B35 and acute axonal polyneuropathy following *Campylobacter* infection. *Neurology* **41**: 1561–1563.

Yuki, N., Sato, S., Tsuji, S., Hozumi, I., and Miyatake, T. (1993a). An immunologic abnormality common to Bickerstaff's brain stem encephalitis and Fisher's syndrome. *J. Neurologic. Sci.* **118**: 83–87.

Yuki, N., Taki, T., Inagaki, F., Kasama, T., Takahashi, M., Saito, K., Handa, S., and Miyatake, T. (1993b). A bacterium lipopolysaccharide that elicits Guillain-Barré syndrome has a GM-1 ganglioside like structure. *J. Exp. Med.* **178**: 1771–1775.

Yuki, N., Taki, T., Takahashi, M., Saito, K., Yoshino, H., Tai, T., Handa, S., and Miyatake, T. (1994). Molecular mimicry between GQ1b ganglioside and lipopolysaccharides of *Campylobacter jejuni* isolated from patients with Fisher's syndrome. *Ann. Neurol.* **36**: 791–793.

2 Epidemiology of autoimmune polyneuropathies

J.J. Kelly, Jr

Introduction

Over the last 15–20 years, there has been an explosion of knowledge about autoimmune polyneuropathies. These disorders can be divided roughly into two groups: those associated with underlying systemic autoimmune diseases such as systemic lupus erythematosus or periarteritis nodosa, infectious diseases such as Lyme borreliosis or human immunodeficiency virus (HIV) and those primary to the peripheral nervous system such as Guillain-Barré syndrome (GBS) and chronic inflammatory demyelinating polyradiculoneuropathy (CIDP). The natural history, histopathology and electrophysiology of these conditions are now well characterized in many cases. With a few exceptions, however, accurate epidemiological data are lacking, especially for those disorders primary to the peripheral nervous system (PNS). This chapter will focus on this latter group as the epidemiology of the former is largely that of the underlying systemic disease.

Epidemiological studies of polyneuropathies, as pointed out by Alter (1990), are difficult for a number of reasons. First, there are many etiologies in an unselected group of polyneuropathies and severity and disability varies markedly depending on etiology and even within etiologies. Thus, there is little to be learned by describing the epidemiology of an unselected group of polyneuropathy patients. Second, even if one well-defined category of polyneuropathy is investigated, there is often no agreement on diagnostic criteria. Thus, incidence and prevalence will vary greatly depending on whether the neuropathy is investigated prospectively or retrospectively. In addition, the use of laboratory criteria such as electromyography (EMG) and quantitative sensory and motor testing greatly increases the detection of polyneuropathies. When patients with carcinoma were screened for polyneuropathy, for instance, the diagnosis rate increased from a few percent in retrospective studies using only clinical criteria to up to 50–60% in prospective studies adding laboratory tools (Kelly 1987).

Despite these misgivings, epidemiological studies of the autoimmune polyneuropathies are valuable for a number of reasons. First of all, most of these disorders, especially GBS and CIDP, have clear onsets and are easily recognized using clinical and laboratory tools. Thus, it is possible to assemble a relatively homogeneous group prospectively or retrospectively using predetermined diagnostic criteria (NINCDS Ad Hoc Committee, 1978).

Second, epidemiological studies of these disorders have given us valuable clues concerning etiology. For example, the association of GBS with swine flu vaccination (Centers for Disease Control, 1976; Kennedy et al. 1978; Hurwitz et al. 1981; Kaplan et al. 1983; Beghi et al. 1985) and, later, with *Campylobacter jejuni* gastroenteritis (Griffin & Ho 1993; Chapter 6), has led to further immunological investigations which promise to help us to understand better the immunopathogenesis of this disorder. Similarly, the association of idiopathic polyneuropathies with monoclonal gammopathies (Kelly et al. 1981) helped pave the way for the description of a number of distinct polyneuropathy syndromes etiologically associated with plasma cell dyscrasias.

The following sections summarize the current knowledge of the epidemiology of the most common of the polyneuropathies due to primary autoimmune diseases of the peripheral nervous system.

Guillain-Barré syndrome

There have been a number of studies in recent years which have described the epidemiologic characteristics of GBS (Table 2.1). These studies have varied greatly in numbers of patients, diagnostic criteria, and other factors, and it is thus surprising that for the most part the incidence rates are in such close agreement. This is likely because GBS is easily diagnosed in most cases and is rarely confused with other disorders.

One of the most complete and reliable studies was undertaken in Rochester, Minnesota, where case acquisiton and data collection were high due to the linked medical records system at the Mayo Clinic for all of Olmsted County, Minnesota (Kennedy et al. 1978; Beghi et al. 1985). Forty-eight patients were identified who met the NINCDS criteria (NINCDS Ad Hoc Committee, 1978). The incidence in these 48 patients was 1.7 per 100 000 person-years. Incidence in males was slightly higher than in females and the incidence in older patients (3.4 per 100 000 person-years in those greater than 60 years old) was higher than in younger patients (0.8 per 100 000 person-years in those less than 18 years old). Epidemiological studies of GBS have also pointed out the association of antecedent or triggering events with the onset of GBS (Alter 1990). Most commonly, these take the form of nonspecific upper respiratory or 'flu-like' illnesses which are relatively mild. Other patients report mild gastrointestinal upsets with nausea and diarrhea. These generally antedate the onset of neurological illness by up to 4 weeks and more commonly in the range of 1–3 weeks; however, some studies have suggested that the risk from preceding illness may stretch for as long as 8 weeks (Hurwitz et al. 1981; Kaplan et al. 1983). Despite this association, which has held true in a number of studies, there seems to be no seasonal predeliction for GBS. Case control studies have also shown a possible association with cytomegalovirus (Dowling et al. 1977) but no association with prior immunization, allergic or metabolic disorders or exposure to toxins (Kennedy et al. 1978). More recently, a suggested association between GBS, particularly severe axonal forms of GBS sometimes associated with antiganglioside antibodies, and *Campylobacter jejuni* gastroenteritis infection has been reported (Griffin and

Table 2.1 *Incidence rates of Guillain-Barré syndrome in well-defined populations*

Area*	Years	Number	Average annual incidence (per 100 000)
Iceland	1954–63	13	0.7
England	1955–61	3	0.6
Guam	1960–66	5	1.9
Olmsted City			
Minnesotta	1935–76	40	1.7
California	1972–76	18	1.2
Israel	1969–72	89	0.8
Norway	1957–77	112	1.2
U.S.	1976–77		
Vaccinated		432	1.3
Unvaccinated		516	3.4

Source: *See original article for references. Modified from Schoenberg BS (1978): Epidemiology of Guillain-Barré syndrome. In *Neurological Epidemiology: Principles and Clinical Applications.* B.S. Schoenberg ed.: New York, Raven Press, p. 249. Reprinted by permission.

Ho 1993). If verified, this raises intriguing possibilities as *C. jejuni* is a bacterium confined to the gastrointestinal tract and thus unlikely to perturb systemic immune function. The mechanism of autoimmunity in this case may be 'molecular mimicry' with cross-reaction between antibodies directed at antigens, possible gangliosides, shared by the bacterium and peripheral nerve.

One of the most intriguing 'experiments of nature' in modern times occurred with the national program in 1976–77 to mass-inoculate against the A/New Jersey strain of flu (swine flu). Following inoculation, there was an upsurge in reported cases of GBS and preliminary reports suggested a greatly increased incidence in those inoculated (Centers for Disease Control 1976). Subsequent studies showed that the rate in vaccinated individuals was approximately 1.4 times greater than the average risk (Centers for Disease Control, 1976; Kennedy et al. 1978; Hurwitz et al. 1981; Kaplan et al. 1983; Beghi et al. 1985). Later inoculation programs with different strains of virus were not associated with increased risk of GBS (Beghi et al. 1985), suggesting that there might have been something unusual about the 1976–77 inoculum.

Thus, on the basis of epidemiologic studies, it is now widely accepted that GBS can be triggerred by a variety of preceding events and illnesses in the preceding 4–8 weeks. This has led to important theories concerning the pathogenesis of this disorder and has helped to direct further studies.

Chronic inflammatory demyelinating polyradiculoneuropathy

Although individual cases and small groups of patients with probable chronic inflammatory demyelinating polyradiculoneuropathy (CIDP) had been described in the literature over the past 100 years, credit for bringing this syndrome to light in the modern era is usually given to Austen (1956, 1958), who described 32 patients with 'hypertrophic' neuropathy who had a relapsing and remitting course and were steroid responsive. The most influential paper, however, was by Dyck and colleagues (1975) who analysed 53 patients, detailed their clinical features, and provided diagnostic criteria. These criteria have recently been refined by Barohn and colleagues (1989) and a panel of experts (Ad Hoc Subcommittee of the ANA AIDS Task Force, 1991), who described a large series of patients. Unfortunately, publicized series are all highly selective and from large tertiary care institutions and therefore give no good estimates of the true incidence or prevalence of this disorder. Most neuromuscular centers find that, of the inflammatory neuropathies, GBS is the most frequent and CIDP relatively infrequent; however, because of its protracted nature, the prevalence of CIDP is likely greater than that of GBS. Studies of the prevalence and incidence of this disorder are needed to assess its impact on society.

Dysproteinemic polyneuropathies

The first report of the cooccurrence of a plasma cell dyscrasia and polyneuropathy appeared in 1937 when Davison and Balser reviewed the neurological complications associated with multiple myeloma and described a peripheral neuropathy in a 39-year-old woman with multiple myeloma. The neuropathy was mainly sensory in type and on postmortem examination evidence of axonal degeneration was found in the posterior roots and in the brachial plexus. Since then, there have been multiple reports of single patients or groups of patients describing myeloma neuropathy (Scheinker 1938; Victor et al. 1958; Walsh 1971; Davis and Drachman 1972; Kelly et al. 1981; McLeod et al. 1984) or osteosclerotic myeloma neuropathy (Waldenström et al. 1978; Driedger and Pruzanski 1979; Bardwick et al., 1980; Kelly et al. 1983). These reports suggested strongly that while polyneuropathy associated with multiple myeloma was quite heterogeneous in type and seemed to run an independent course from the underlying disease, that associated with osteosclerotic myeloma was strikingly homogeneous in character and closely associated with the course of the malignancy.

Early reports of amyloid polyneuropathy began to appear in the 1930s (De Navasquez & Treble 1938), followed by later reports (Chambers et al. 1958; Thomas & King 1974; Benson et al. 1975; Cohen & Benson 1984). The natural history of this disorder was then described in detail, and it was shown that primary systemic or light chain derived amyloid polyneuropathy appeared to be homogeneous in nature (Trotter et al. 1977; Kelly et al. 1979).

The first reports of polyneuropathy linked to a nonmalignant plasma cell dyscrasia and not associated with amyloid appeared later (Logothetis et al. 1968; Forsman et al. 1973; Read & Warlow 1978; Dalakas & Engel, 1981). These reports suggested that these polyneuropathies were heterogeneous in type without a common clinical and pathological thread, except perhaps for those neuropathies associated with IgM gammopathies. Thus, the exact relationship between these 'benign' gammopathies, later renamed monoclonal gammopathy of undetermined significance (MGUS) on the one hand, and neuropathy on the other hand remained unclear, as the natural history and the pathological picture of these neuropathies varied widely and no mechanism for nerve fiber damage was apparent. As a result, until the late 1970s, the importance of these reports was difficult to judge. There was convincing evidence for a histopathological relationship between light chain derived amyloidosis and polyneuropathy, but solid epidemiological data were lacking and the mechanism of nerve fiber damage was unknown in the other disorders.

A series of studies were then published which helped to clarify these relationships. In 1980, Kahn and colleagues reviewed their experience with monoclonal gammopathies and polyneuropathies between 1975 and 1978. During this period, they examined 14 000 sera for monoclonal proteins. Out of this group, 56 were detected in patients without evidence of malignant plasma cell dyscrasias. Sixteen of these patients, who were felt to have benign monoclonal gammopathy, were found to have a polyneuropathy. In addition, the authors found a significant association between polyneuropathies with 'very slow nerve conduction velocities' and IgM kappa gammopathies. In 1982, Osby, Noring and colleagues reported 21 consecutive outpatients with so-called benign monoclonal gammopathy. On careful clinical examination, 15 were found to have some evidence of polyneuropathy. Based on these two studies, polyneuropathies appeared to be overrepresented in patients with benign monoclonal gammopathy.

In 1981, Kelly and colleagues presented evidence which showed that the prevalence of monoclonal gammopathy was statistically increased in patients with idiopathic polyneuropathies compared with controls and that monoclonal gammopathies were four times more common in patients with idiopathic polyneuropathies as opposed to patients with a likely underlying cause. The study was a prospective assessment of serum proteins in patients with polyneuropathies presenting to the Mayo Clinic over a 1-year period between 1978 and 1979. Patients were identified in the EMG laboratory and were examined for evidence of a clinically significant neuropathy. Patients were categorized as having a secondary neuropathy if the evaluation revealed a likely cause and idiopathic if no cause was found after routine screening which did not include serum protein studies. Serum protein electrophoretic patterns were performed in all and immunoelectrophoresis was performed if a localized band was seen. If an M-protein was found, full hematological workup was carried out including urine immunoelectrophoresis or immunofixation, bone marrow aspirate and biopsy, tissues biopsies for amyloid, and metastatic skeletal surveys. Based on these studies, patients were placed in diagnostic categories such as multiple myeloma, osteosclerotic myeloma, Waldenstrom's macroglobulinemia, primary systemic amyloidosis, gamma heavy-chain disease, or MGUS.

In all, a clinically significant polyneuropathy was recognized in 692 patients over the 1-year period (Table 2.2). Of these, 358 had an underlying disease or

Table 2.2 *Etiology of polyneuropathy in 692 patients with polyneuropathy*

Type	Number	Percentage
Idiopathic	334	48
Secondary	358	52
Cause of secondary cases		
Diabetes	217	31
Inherited	47	7
Alcohol	26	4
Vitamin deficiency or toxin	21	3
Collagen-vascular disease	16	2
Uremia	14	2
Malignancy	12	2
Other	5	1

Source: Reprinted with permission from Kelly, J.J. Jr, Kyle, R.A., and Latov, N. (1987) *Polyneuropathies associated with monoclonal gammopathies.* Martinus-Nijhoff, Boston.

Table 2.3 *Final clinical diagnosis of 28 patients with monoclonal gammopathy and peripheral neuropathy*

	Subclassification of protein by heavy and light chains							
	Number	IgGk	IgGl	IgAk	IgMk	IgMl	kappa	lambda
MGUS	16	5	4	3	2	1	0	1
PSA	7	1	2	0	0	0	2	2
MM	3	3	0	0	0	0	0	0
WM	1	0	0	0	0	1	0	0
Gamma-HCD	1	0	0	0	0	0	0	0
Total	28							

Note:
Legend: k: kappa light chain; l: lambda. MGUS: monoclonal gammopathy of undetermined significance; PSA: primary systemic (light chain derived) amyloidosis; MM: multiple myeloma, both lytic and osteosclerotic; WM: Waldenström's macroglobulinemia; gamma-HCD: gamma heavy chain disease.
Source: Reprinted with permission from Kelly, J.J. Jr (1981) Prevalence of monoclonal protein in peripheral neuropathy. *Neurology* **31**:1480–1483.

condition which likely caused the neuropathy (secondary neuropathy), and 334 had no apparent explanation for the neuropathy (idiopathic neuropathy). Approximately 80% of the patients in each group had serum protein electrophoretic studies. In the idiopathic group, 10% had an M-protein compared with 2.5% in the secondary group and 1–2% in age-matched community control, a figure which corresponds to the frequency of monoclonal gammopathy in community studies (Axelsson et al. 1966; Kyle et al. 1972). Patients were then classified by hematologic diagnosis and M-protein type (Table 2.3).

This study supported previous work and suggested, at least in these large referral centers, an increased prevalence, approaching 10%, of plasma cell dyscrasias in patients with idiopathic polyneuropathies. Whether this data can be translated to other hospitals is unclear. Other less rigorously controlled studies with smaller samples showed either no increase in polyneuropathy in patients with monoclonal gammopathy (Read et al. 1978; Straaten et al. 1985) or no increase in gammopathy in patients with idiopathic neuropathy (Nusselt et al. 1971; Fagius 1983); however, other small series suggested a link between IgM monoclonal gammopathies and polyneuropathy, especially of the demyelinating type and with prominent sensory loss and ataxia (Nobile-Orazio et al. 1987; Gosselin et al. 1991; Suarez & Kelly, 1993).

More evidence appeared in the 1980's with the publication by Latov and colleagues of a series of papers (Abrams et al. 1982; Braun et al. 1982; Latov et al. 1980, 1988) showing that in many patients with benign monoclonal gammopathy of IgM type, the immunoglobulin was found by direct immunofluorescent staining to be deposited on the myelin sheaths of nerve fibers. These studies showed that the monoclonal protein was bound to myelin associated glycoprotein (MAG) and other simpler carbohydrate groups on the myelin sheath. This reaction appears to be specific for this neuropathy. Although the role of the monoclonal IgM antibodies in nerve fiber damage in these neuropathies is still unclear, this reactivity is at least a powerful marker and establishes the specificity of this disease and its relationship to the underlying plasma cell dyscrasia and serum monoclonal protein. The prevalence of anti-MAG neuropathy has been estimated by Latov (Latov et al. 1988). It is known that approximately 0.2% of adults have an IgM monoclonal gammopathy and that 8–50% of these have an associated polyneuropathy. As about 50% of these have been shown to be anti-MAG in type, Latov has estimated the prevalance at between 1 and 5 per 10 000 adults.

These studies established the important association between plasma cell dyscrasias and their peripheral blood products, monoclonal gammopathies, with idiopathic polyneuropathies. It is now known that there is a clear etiological link between plasma cell dyscrasias and some of these polyneuropathies, including light chain amyloidosis, osteosclerotic myeloma, anti-MAG polyneuropathy and perhaps others, especially patients with IgM monoclonal gammopathies. For others, such as IgG and IgA-MGUS associated polyneuropathies, the nature of the relationship and whether it is a meaningful one, is still unclear. The epidemiological studies, starting with single and small group case reports, and culminating with controlled statistical studies, helped to focus attention on these disorders and led to subsequent neurochemical and immunological studies which are establishing the immunopathogenesis of these disorders.

Conclusion

As shown in this review, epidemiological studies can suggest not only a statistical link between disorders but can also suggest possible etiological relationships. They can certainly serve as a stimulus for more directed research into the nature of the relationships uncovered. In the case of GBS, the epidemiological studies are beginning to shed new light on the immunopathogenesis of this devastating polyneuropathy. In the case of neuropathies associated with plasma cell dyscrasias, epidemiological studies have established a strong relationship between specific diseases and polyneuropathies and, at least in the case of anti-MAG polyneuropathy, have helped to encourage research which led to the discovery of the immune mechanisms underlying this disorder and, ultimately, to treatment.

References

Abrams, G.R., Latov, N., Hays, A.P. Sherman, W., and Zimmerman, E.A. (1982). Immunocytochemical studies of human peripheral nerve with serum from patients with polyneuropathy and paraproteinemia. *Neurology (NY)* **32**: 821–826.

Ad Hoc Subcommittee of the American Academy of Neurology AIDS Task Force. (1991). Research criteria for the diagnosis of chronic inflammatory demyelinating polyradiculoneuropathy (CIDP). *Neurology* **41**: 617–618.

Alter, M. (1990). The epidemiology of Guillain-Barré syndrome. *Neurology* **27**(Suppl.): S7–S12

Austen, J.H. (1956). Observations on the syndrome of hypertrophic neuritis (the hypertrophic institial radiculoneuropathies). *Medicine (Balt.)* **35**: 187.

Austen, J.H. (1958). Recurrent polyneuropathies and their corticosteroid treatment with five-year observation of a placebo-controlled case treated with corticotorphin, cortisone, and prednisone. *Brain* **81**: 157–192.

Axelsson, U., Bachman, R., and Hallen, J. (1966). Frequency of pathological proteins (M components) in 6995 sera from an adult population. *Acta Med Scand.* **179**: 235–247.

Bardwick, P.A., Zvaifler, N.G., Gill, G.N., Newman, D., Greenway, G.D., and Resnick, D.L. (1980). Plasma cell dyscrasia with polyneuropathy, organomegaly, endocrinopathy, M-protein, and skin changes: the POEMS syndrome. *Medicine (Balt.)* **59**: 311–322.

Barohn, R.J., Kissel, J.T., Warmolts, J.R., and Mendell, J.R. (1989). Chronic inflammatory polyradiculoneuropathy. Clinical characteristics, course, and recommendation for diagnostic criteria. *Arch. Neurol.* **46**: 878–884.

Beghi, E., Kurland, L.T., Mulder, D.W., and Widerholt, W.C. (1985). Guillain-Barré syndrome: clinicoepidemiologic features and effect of influenza vaccine. *Arch. Neurol.* **42**: 1053–1057.

Benson, M.D., Cohen, A.S., Brandt, K.D., and Cathcart, E.S. (1975). Neuropathy, M-components, and amyloid. *Lancet* **1**: 10–12.

Braun, P.E., Frail, D.E., and Latov, N. (1982). Myelin associated glycoprotein is the antigen for monoclonal IgM in polyneuropathy. *J. Neurochem.* **39**: 1261–1265.

Centers for Disease Control: Guillain-Barré syndrome-United States. (1976). M.M.W.R., **25**: 401.

Chambers, R.A., Medd, W.E., and Spencer, H. (1958). Primary amyloidosis: with special reference to involvement of the nervous system. *Q. J. Med* **27**: 207–226.

Cohen, A.S. and Benson, M.D. (1984). Amyloid neuropathy. In: *Peripheral neuropathy*, 2nd edn, P.J. Dyck, P.K. Thomas, E.H. Lambert, R. Bunge (eds). W.B. Saunders, Philadelphia. pp. 1866–1898.

Dalakas, M.C. and Engel, WK. (1981). Polyneuropathy with monoclonal gammopathy: studies of 11 patients. *Ann. Neurol.* **10**: 45–52.

Davis, L.E. and Drachman, D.B. (1972). Myeloma neuropathy: successful treatment of two patients and review of cases. *Arch. Neurol.* **27**: 507–511.

Davison, C. and Balser, B.H. (1937). Myeloma and its neural complications. *Arch. Surg.* **35**: 913–936.

De Navasquez, S. and Treble, H.A. (1938). A case of primary generalized amyloid disease with involvement of the nerves. *Brain* **61**: 116–128.

Dowling, P., Menonna, J., and Cook, S. (1977). Cytomegalovirus complement fixation antibody in Guillain-Barré syndrome. *Neurology* **27**: 1153–1156.

Driedger, H. and Pruzanski, W. (1979). Plasma cell neoplasia with osteosclerotic lesions: a study of five cases and a review of the literature. *Arch. Intern. Med.* **139**: 892–896.

Dyck, P.J., Lais, A.C., Ohta, M., Bastron, J.A., Okazaki, H., and Grooves, R.V. (1975). Chronic inflammatory polyradiculoneuropathy. *Mayo Clin. Proc.* **50**: 621.

Fagius, J. (1983). Chronic cryptogenic polyneuropathy. The search for a cause. *Acta Neurol. Scand.* **67**: 173–180.

Forsman, O., Bjorkman, G., Hollender, A., and Englund, N.E. (1973). IgM-producing lymphocytes in peripheral nerve in a patient with benign IgM monoclonal gammopathy. *Scand. J. Haematol.* **11**: 332–335.

Gosselin, S., Kyle, R.A., and Dyck, P.J. (1991). Neuropathy associated with monoclonal gammopathies of undetermined significance. *Ann. Neurol.* **30**: 54–61.

Griffin, J.W. and Ho, T.W.H. (1993). The Guillain-Barré syndrome at 75: the *Campylobacter* connection. *Ann. Neurol.* **34**: 125–127.

Hurwitz, E.S., Schonberger, L.B., Nelson, D.B., and Holman, R.C. (1981). Guillain-Barré syndrome and the 1978–1979 influenza vaccine. *N. Engl. J. Med.* **304**: 1557–1561.

Kahn, S.N., Riches, P.G., and Kohn, J. (1980). Paraproteinemia in neurological disease: incidence, association, and classification of monoclonal immunoglobulins. *J. Clin. Pathol.* **33**: 617–621.

Kaplan, J.E., Schonberger, L.B., Hurwitz, E.S., and Katona, P. (1983). Guillain-Barré syndrome in the United States, 1978–1981: additional observations from the national surveillance system. *Neurology* **33**: 633–637.

Kelly, J.J. Jr. (1987). Polyneuropathies associated with malignancies and plasma cell dyscrasias. In: *Clinical electromyography*, Brown, W.F. and Bolton, C.F. (eds), Butterworth, Stoneham, pp. 305–319.

Kelly, J.J. Jr, Kyle, R.A., Miles, J.M., O'Brien, P.C., and Dyck, P.J. (1981). The spectrum of peripheral neuropathy in myeloma. *Neurology (NY)* **31**: 24–31.

Kelly, J.J. Jr, Kyle, R.A., Miles, J.M., and Dyck, P.J. (1983). Osteosclerotic myeloma and peripheral neuropathy. *Neurology (NY)* **33**: 202–210.

Kelly, J.J. Jr, Kyle, R.A., O'Brien, P.C., and Dyck, P.J. (1979). The natural history of peripheral neuropathy in primary systemic amyloidosis. *Ann. Neurol.* **6**: 1–7.

Kelly, J.J. Jr, Kyle, R.A., O'Brien, P.C., and Dyck, P.J. (1981). Prevalence of monoclonal protein in peripheral neuropathy. *Neurology (NY)* **31**: 1480–1483.

Kennedy, R.H., Danielson, M.A., Mulder, D.W., and Kurland, L.T. (1978). Guillain-Barré syndrome: a 41-year epidemiologic and clinical study. *Mayo Clin. Proc.* **53**: 93.

Kyle, R.A., Finkelstein, S., Elveback, L.R., and Kurland, L.T. (1972). Incidence of monoclonal proteins in a Minnesota community with a cluster of multiple mydoma. *Blood* **40**: 719–724.

Latov, N.R., Hays, A.P., and Sherman, W.H. (1988). Peripheral neuropathy and anti-MAG antibodies. *CRC Crit. Rev. Neurobiol.* **3**: 301.

Latov, N., Sherman, W.H., Nemni, R., Galassi, G., Shyong, I.S., Penn, A.S., Chess, L., Olarte, M.R., Rowland, L.P., and Osserman, E.F. (1980). Plasma cell dyscrasia and peripheral neuropathy with monoclonal antibody to peripheral nerve myelin. *N. Engl. J. Med.* **303**: 618–621.

Logothetis, J., Kennedy, W.R., Ellington, A., et al. (1968). Cryoglobulinemic neuropathy. *Arch. Neurol.* **19**: 389–397.

McLeod, J.G., Walsh, J.C., and Pollard, J.C. (1984). Neuropathies associated with paraproteinemias and dysproteinemias. In: *Peripheral neuropathy*, 2nd edn, P.J. Dyck, P.K. Thomas, E.H. Lambert, R. Bunge. eds. W.B. Saunders, Philadelphia, pp. 1847–1865.

National Institute for Neurological and Communicative Disorders and Stroke Ad Hoc Committee. (1978). Criteria for diagnosis of Guillian-Barré syndrome. *Ann. Neurol.* **3**: 565–566.

Nobile-Orazio, E., Marmiroli, P., Baldini, L., Spagnol, G., Barbieri, S., Moggio, M., Polli, N., Polli, E., and Scarlato, G. (1987). Peripheral neuropathy in macroglobulinemia: incidence and antigen specificity of M-protein. *Neurology* **37**: 1506–1514.

Nusselt, L., Rieder, H.P., and Kaeser, H.E. (1971). Serum proteinveranderungen bei polyneuritis. *Schweizer Med. Wochenschr.* **101**: 1479–1482.

Osby, L.E., Noring, L., Hast, R., Kjellin, K.G., Knutsson, E., and Siden, A. (1982). Benign monoclonal gammopathy and peripheral neuropathy. *Br. J. Haematol.* **51**: 531–539.

Read, D. and Warlow, C. (1978). Peripheral neuropathy and solitary plasmacytoma. *J. Neurol. Neurosurg. Psychiatry* **47**: 177–184.

Read, D.J., Van Hegan, R.I., and Mathews, W.B.(1978). Peripheral neuropathy and benign IgG paraproteinemia. *J. Neurol. Neurosurg. Psychiatry* **41**: 215–218.

Scheinker, L. (1938). Mylom und Nervensystem. *Deutsch. Zeits. Nervenheilanstalt.* **147**: 247–273.

Straaten, M.J.K., Agerstaff, R.G.A., and De Matt, C.E.M. (1985). Peripheral polyneuropathy and monoclonal gammopathy of undetermined significance. *J. Neurol. Neurosurg. Psychiatry* **48**: 706–708.

Suarez, G.A. and Kelly, J.J. Jr. (1993). Polyneuropathy associated with monoclonal gammopathy of undetermined significance: further evidence that IgM-MGUS neuropathies are different than IgG-MGUS. *Neurology* **43**: 1304–1308.

Thomas, P.K. and King, R.H.M. (1974). Peripheral nerve changes in amyloid neuropathy. *Brain* **97**: 395–406.

Trotter, L., Engel, W.K., and Ignaczak, T.F. (1977). Amyloidosis with plasma cell dyscrasia: an overlooked cause of adult onset sensorimotor neuropathy. *Arch. Neurol.* **34**: 209–214.

Victor, M., Banker, B.C., and Adams, R.D. (1958). The neuropathy of multiple myeloma. *J. Neurol. Neurosurg. Psychiatry* **21**: 73–78.

Waldenström, J.G., Adner, A., Gydell, K., et al. (1971). Osteosclerotic 'plasmacytoma' with polyneuropathy, hypertrichosis, and diabetes. *Acta Med. Scand.* **203**: 297–303.

Walsh, J.C. (1971). The neuropathy of multiple myeloma: an electrophysiological and histological study. *Arch. Neurol.* **25**: 404–414.

3 Immune-mediated experimental neuropathies

J.D. Pollard

Introduction

Experimental models of immune-mediated neuropathies have indubitably contributed in a major way to our understanding of the human diseases which they represent. Although the etiology of the autoimmune demyelinating neuropathies remains unknown, certain mechanisms of disease production have been elucidated from a study of experimental allergic neuritis (EAN) and therapeutic stratagems have been devised. In this particular animal model, disease suppression may be achieved by several therapeutic maneuvres and it is likely that these will be applied to human disease over the subsequent few years. A similiar process is currently occurring in regard to experimental allergic encephalomyelitis (EAE) and the major human demyelinating disease, multiple sclerosis, with exciting results and the introduction of new therapies which for the first time have positively influenced the disease course.

Experimental allergic neuritis

Experimental allergic neuritis (EAN) was described by Waksman and Adams (1955, 1956) who demonstrated that animals of several species injected with peripheral nerve and Freund's adjuvant, develop flaccid paralysis which progressed over several days, following a latent period of about 2 weeks. Animals which survived the paralytic period eventually recovered. The pathological changes were shown to be characterized by invasion of nerves and nerve roots by inflammatory cells and the presence of primary demyelination within these inflammatory cell foci. The close resemblance of these clinical and pathological features to the Guillain-Barré syndrome (GBS) was recognized.

EAN may be induced by whole nerve homogenate, myelin, the myelin proteins P_2 and Po or peptides derived from these. Neuritogenic T cell epitopes for P_2 and Po have been defined; amino acid sequences 61–70 for P_2 and sequences 56–71 in the extracellular domain of Po and a second epitope Po 180–199 located within the cytoplasmic carboxyl terminal domain of the protein. (Uyemura et al. 1982, Olee et al. 1989; Linington et al. 1992). EAN may also be induced by adoptive transfer of T cell lines specific for P_2, Po and the neuritogenic peptides described above (Linington et al. 1984; Rostami et al. 1991; Linington and Brostoff 1993).

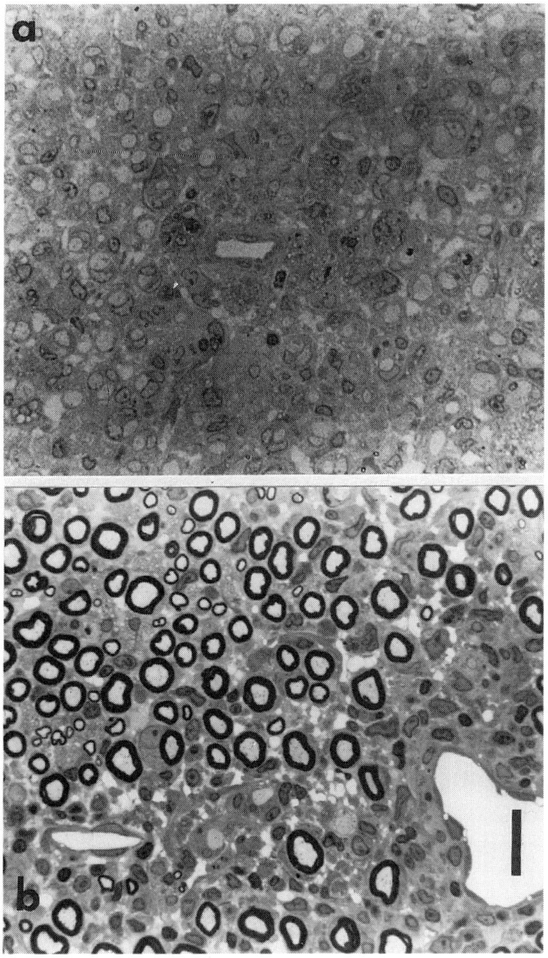

Figure 3.1 *Transverse section of L4 nerve root of Lewis rats with experimental allergic neuritis, stained with toluidene blue. (a) Following active immunization. (b) Following passive transfer of 2×10⁶ P2 reactive T cells. Note widespread demyelination in (a) but only occasional demyelinated fibers in (b). Bar: 20 μm.*

Clinical features

Animals develop weakness and ataxia 12–16 days following active immunization or 4–6 days after passive T cell transfer. In the most commonly studied animal, the Lewis rat, weakness is first manifest in the tail, which droops. Thereafter hind leg weakness occurs, followed by forelimb weakness. Paralysis of the feet is a common early sign and loss of righting reflexes. Complete paralysis including the respiratory muscles may occur, with consequent death of the animal. Weight loss is an almost invariable sign and usually begins before weakness is manifest. In the monkey, cranial nerve involvement particularly of the facial nerve, is an early sign. In all species progression of disease occurs for about 5–7 days and then following a plateau period of a similar time span, recovery occurs. EAN was formerly regarded as an uniphasic disease as animals were usually sacrificed in the acute disease phase. If animals are allowed to recover a percentage will undergo spontaneous relapses and remissions (see Chronic EAN).

Immunopathology

The characteristic pathological features of EAN are multifocal inflammatory lesions in nerve roots and peripheral nerve with demyelination most prominent in perivascular regions, within these inflammatory foci. Ultrastructural studies have shown that demyelination is closely related to the presence of macrophages. Ballin and Thomas (1968) demonstrated a vesicular dissolution of myelin and consequent myelin phagocytosis by macrophages, and Lampert (1969) first reported stripping of myelin lamellae by macrophage processes and macrophage phagocytosis of myelin of normal appearance was reported in the nerve roots of rabbits with EAE by Wisniewski et al. (1969).

The pathological changes in EAN induced by passive transfer of autoreactive T cells is also characterized by similar multifocal inflammatory lesions with demyelination (Linington et al. 1984; Izumo et al. 1985); however, it needs to be emphasized that the amount of demyelination obtained by passive cell transfer is considerably less than that obtained by active immunization (Spies et al. 1995) (Figure 3.1). The attempt to induce more severe disease by the administration of larger cell numbers causes more severe axonal degeneration rather than more demyelination (Heininger et al. 1986). The degree of demyelination induced by passive transfer of T cells can be enhanced by the co-administration of systemic antimyelin antibody (Hahn et al. 1993; Spies et al. 1995).

It is likely that the extensive demyelinating lesions seen in EAN induced by active immunization result from both T cell and B cell activation.

Cell-mediated immunity

T cells

An important role for T cells was established by early studies in which the injection of EAN lymph node cells either intravenously (Astrom and Waksman 1962) or intraneurally caused demyelination (Arnason and Chelmika-Szorca 1972). More recent studies have confirmed these findings (Hughes et al. 1981a; Hodgkinson et al. 1994). Passive transfer studies using $CD4^+$ T cell lines, generated against P_2 protein (Linington et al. 1984; Rostami et al. 1985) and more recently against Po protein (Linington et al. 1992) have established the importance of T cell induction.

The means by which T cells cause demyelination remains unknown. Studies by Spies et al. (1995) in which $CD4^+$, EAN inducing T cells were injected intraneurally showed a powerful effect on opening of the blood–nerve barrier but no demyelination. It appears therefore that these $CD4^+$ cells do not themselves directly cause demyelination but they may provide specific helper cell function for the activation and recruitment of host $CD8^+$ cells and/or macrophages. It may be that they provide help for the activation of B cells to produce antimyelin antibodies. Activated T cells appear to possess the capacity to traverse endothelial barriers (Wekerle et al. 1986) (Figure 3.2). Antigen specific $CD4^+$ T cells having traversed the blood–nerve barrier presumably interact with perivascular antigen presenting cells (APC) displaying the appropriate neuritogenic epitope in association with major histocompatibility (MHC) class II (Figure 3.3). This interaction initiates an inflammatory response orchestrated by cytokines which results in T cell proliferation and recruitment of host effector cells and changes to the blood–nerve barrier. Activated T cells which do not find their antigen presumably leave the endoneurium and re-enter the circulation (Wekerle et al. 1986; Pollard et al. 1994).

Immunocytochemical studies have shown the presence of $CD4^+$ T cells within nerve before the onset of clinical disease (Schmidt et al. 1993). One of the important cytokines involved in these processes is interferon gamma (IFN-γ); T cells showing IFN-γ immunoreactivity have been demonstrated in nerve lesions prior to disease expression (Hartung et al. 1990). IFN-γ can induce MHC molecules on macrophages and Schwann cells and induces macrophages to release toxic oxygen radicals, proteases and other proinflammatory molecules (Tsai et al. 1991; Hartung et al. 1993); it participates in cell recruitment and induces adhesion molecules on endothelial cells and other leucocytes. Administration of IFN-γ to EAN rats enhances disease and antibody to IFN-γ inhibits EAN (Hartung et al. 1990). Other cytokines are indubitably involved but their roles are yet to be defined.

Macrophages

Macrophages are the dominant cellular species within the inflammatory lesions of EAN and ultrastructural studies have shown that they are the major effector cells in myelin dissolution and removal (Ballin and Thomas 1968; Lampert 1969; Wisniewski et al. 1969). The precise mechanism by which macrophages are directed to destroy the myelin sheath is unknown; opsonization by antimyelin antibody and/or complement activation providing a ligand for the CR3 receptor may be involved. Stoll et al. (1991) have shown the deposition of terminal complement complex C5b-9 (TCC) in nerve on myelin sheaths and Schwann cell membranes at day 11, before clinical disease expression. In that study, macrophages congregated preferentially in regions of strong TCC staining.

Many studies designed to inactivate macrophages have underlined the important effector role of these cells (Tansey and Brosnan 1983; Craggs et al. 1984; Hartung et al. 1988a,b). Activated macrophages produce toxic oxygen radicals and treatment of EAN animals with oxygen radical scavengers such as superoxide dismutase and catalase, caused disease suppression (Hartung et al. 1988b). Macrophages also produce proteinases such as trypsin which when injected intraneurally causes demyelination (Watson et al. 1994) and proteinase inhibitors delay disease onset (Schabet et al. 1991). It is of particular interest that the injection of trypsin induced perivenous demyelination in all regards similar to that seen in EAN.

Macrophages are a major source of tumor necrosis factor (TNF) which has been implicated in myelinolysis in vitro; however, intraneurial injection of very large quantities of TNF-alpha (10 000 IU) in the Lewis rat has not produced demyelination (Spies et al. 1995). Macrophages also release complement (Hartung and Hadding 1985).

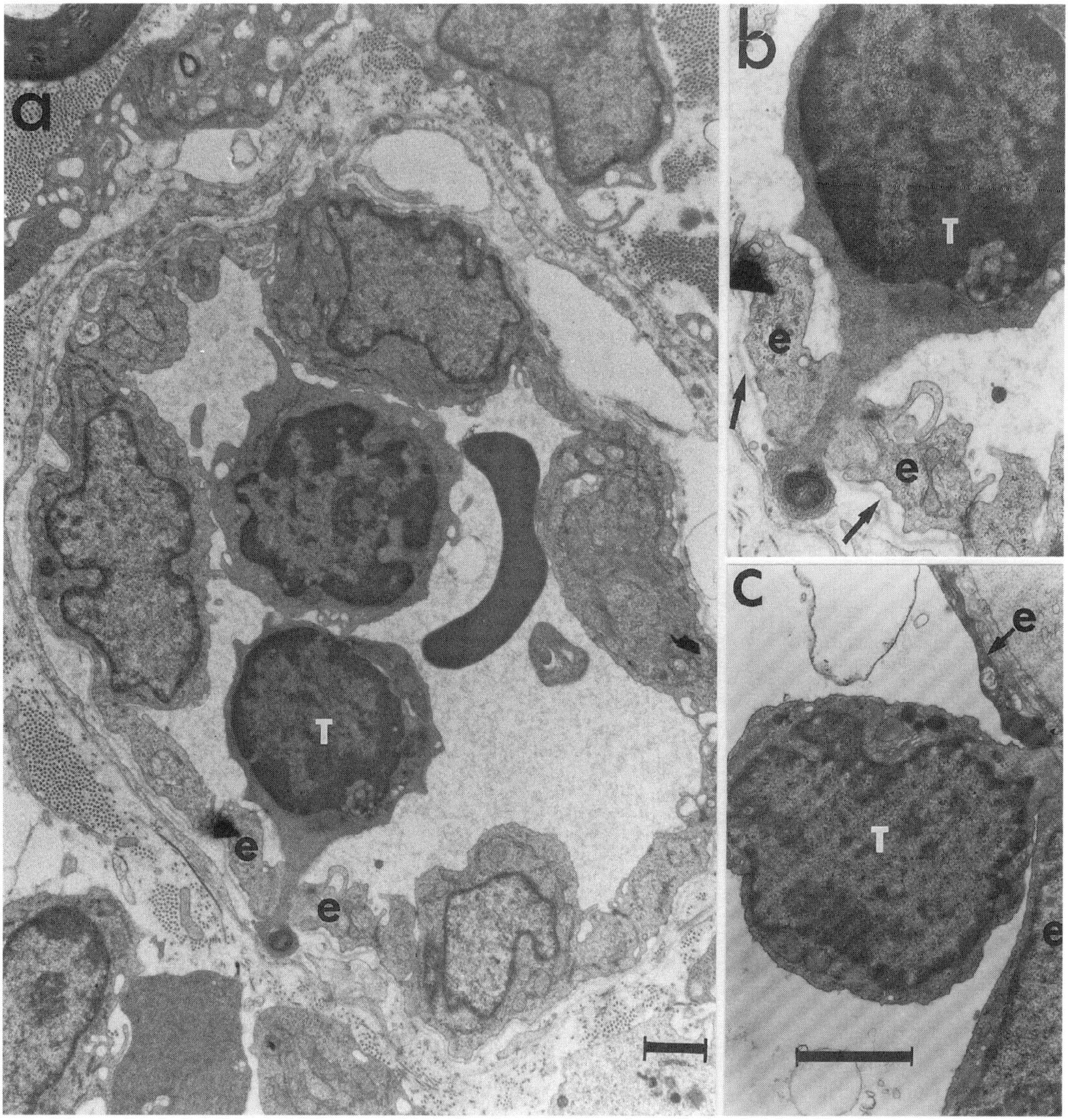

Figure 3.2 *(a) Transendothelial migration of activated T cells. An endoneurial capillary contains two T cells, one of which (T) has extruded a process through endothelial cell (e). Bar: 2 μm. (b) Higher power of T showing T cell process has penetrated endothelial wall (e) and basal lamina. Bar: 1 μm. (c) T cell (T) beginning to pass between/endothelial cells (e), at the interendothelial cell junction. Bar: 1 μm.*

Humoral immunity

In the Lewis rat with EAN, antibodies to P_2 protein have been demonstrated but their titer does not correlate with disease activity (Hughes et al. 1981a; Rostami et al. 1985). In the rabbit, however, there is substantial evidence of an important role for antibody. Saida et al. (1978) showed that the serum of rabbits given EAN by immunization with myelin, produced profound conduction block and demyelination when injected into rat sciatic nerve (Figure 3.4). This demyelinating activity was shown to be largely due to antibody to galactocerebroside (GC) (Saida et al. 1978,

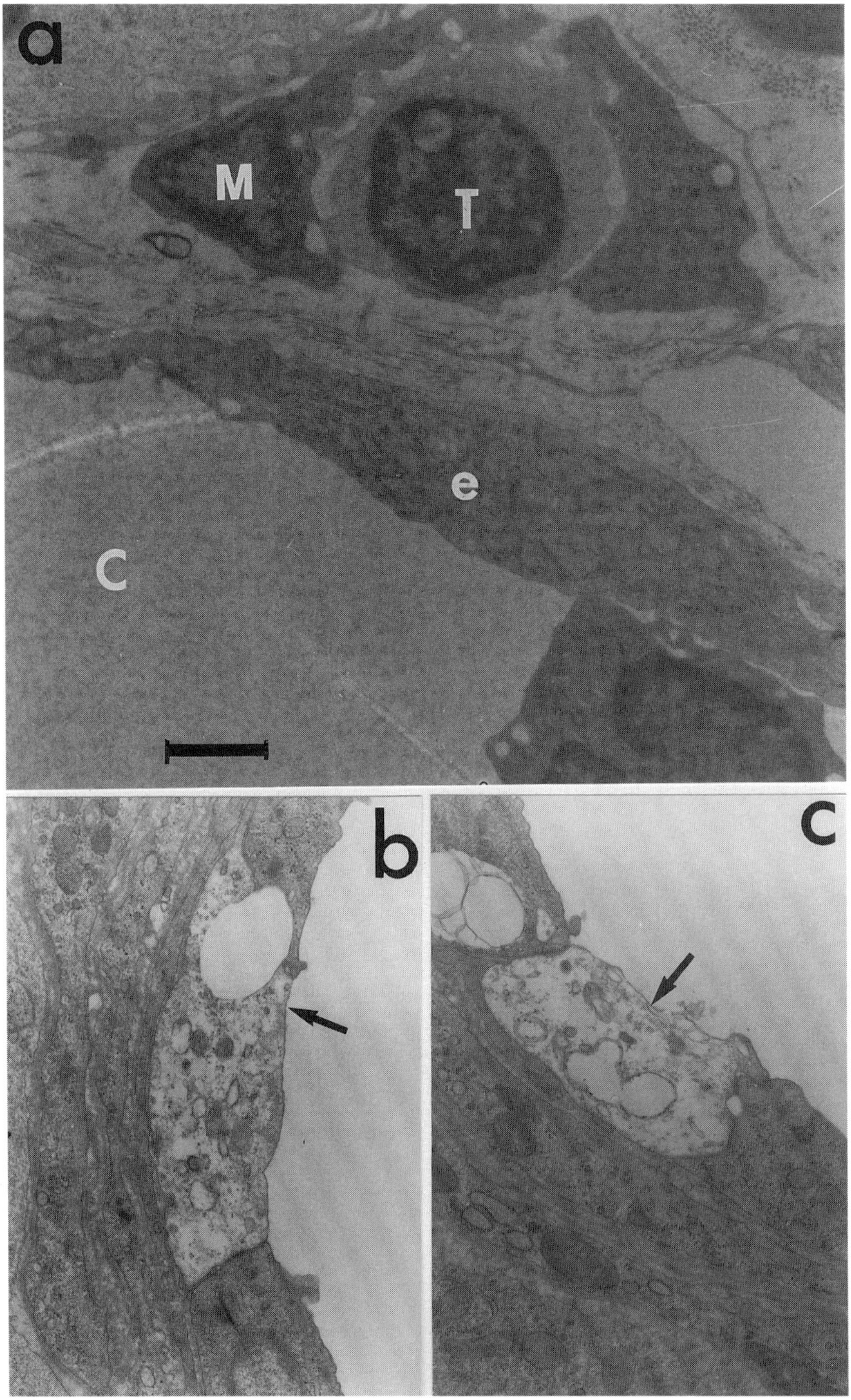

Figure 3.3 *(a) T cell (T) which has migrated from capillary (c) into endoneurium is interreacting with perivascular monocyte (M). The intimate intercellular contact suggests antigen presentation. (b) and (c) Edematoaus vacuolated endothelial cells following T cell migration. Note lack of interendothelial cell tight junctions. Bar: 2 μm.*

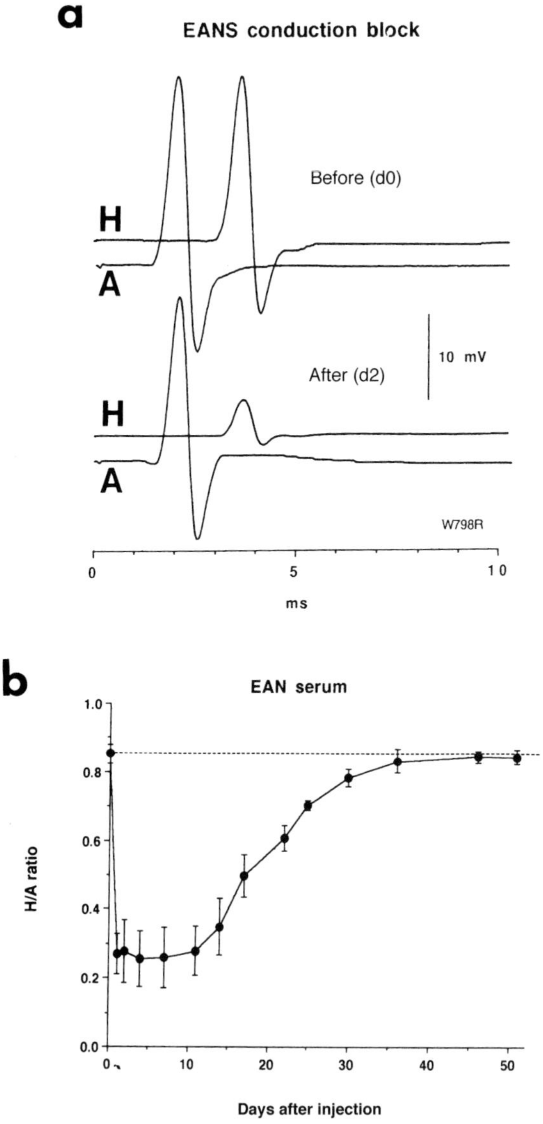

Figure 3.4 *Conduction block following intraneural injection into rat sciatic nerve of rabbit experimental allergic neuritis (EAN) serum. (a) Compound muscle action potentials (CMAP) recorded from small muscles of the feet following stimulation of sciatic nerve at ankle (A) and hip (H). Note marked drop in CMAP amplitude from hip stimulation on day 2 representing conduction block. (b) Time course of conduction block following EAN serum injection.*

1979; Pollard et al. 1994). The clinical course of rabbit EAN may be stabilized by removal of antimyelin antibody by plasma exchange and the presence of abundant antimyelin antibody can be demonstrated within the endoneurium by immunohistochemistry (Harvey et al. 1987, 1988)(Figure 3.5).

Repeated injection of rabbits with GC was shown to produce elevated levels of circulating anti-GC antibodies and to produce a multifocal demyelinating neuropathy with lesions in nerve roots, dorsal root ganglia, proximal nerves and less frequently distal nerves (Saida et al. 1981). These regions of pathology corresponded to areas of deficient blood–nerve barrier and Saida et al. (1981) proposed that the demyelination was mediated primarily by circulating antibodies to GC.

Antibody to Po also produces demyelination (Hughes et al. 1985) and could contribute to the demyelinating effect of rabbit EAN serum. Complement may also play a role in demyelination. Feasby et al. (1987) showed that depletion of complement by cobra venom suppressed EAN. Particularly compelling evidence has been provided from the immunocytochemical studies on ultracryosections by Stoll et al. (1991). C5b-9 terminal complement complex was shown on Schwann cell membranes and myelin sheaths prior to disease onset. Macrophages were shown to accumulate particularly in areas of TCC staining.

The blood–nerve barrier

The nerve endoneurium containing myelinated fibres is protected from myelinotoxic circulating factors by an intact blood–nerve barrier and by the perineurial barrier. The blood–nerve barrier consists of the tight junctions between endothelial cells, a low rate of transendothelial endocytosis and high electrical resistance. Perineurial cells are also joined by tight junctions (Thomas, et al. 1993). The blood–nerve barrier is to some degree deficient at the proximal and distal ends (in the region of the nerve roots, dorsal root ganglia and peripheral nerve terminals) and this deficiency has been demonstrated by intravenous injection of protein binding dyes (Olsson 1968). These areas of relative deficiency are also the regions of maximum pathology in EAN and it is likely that these two findings are causally related (Harvey and Pollard 1992b).

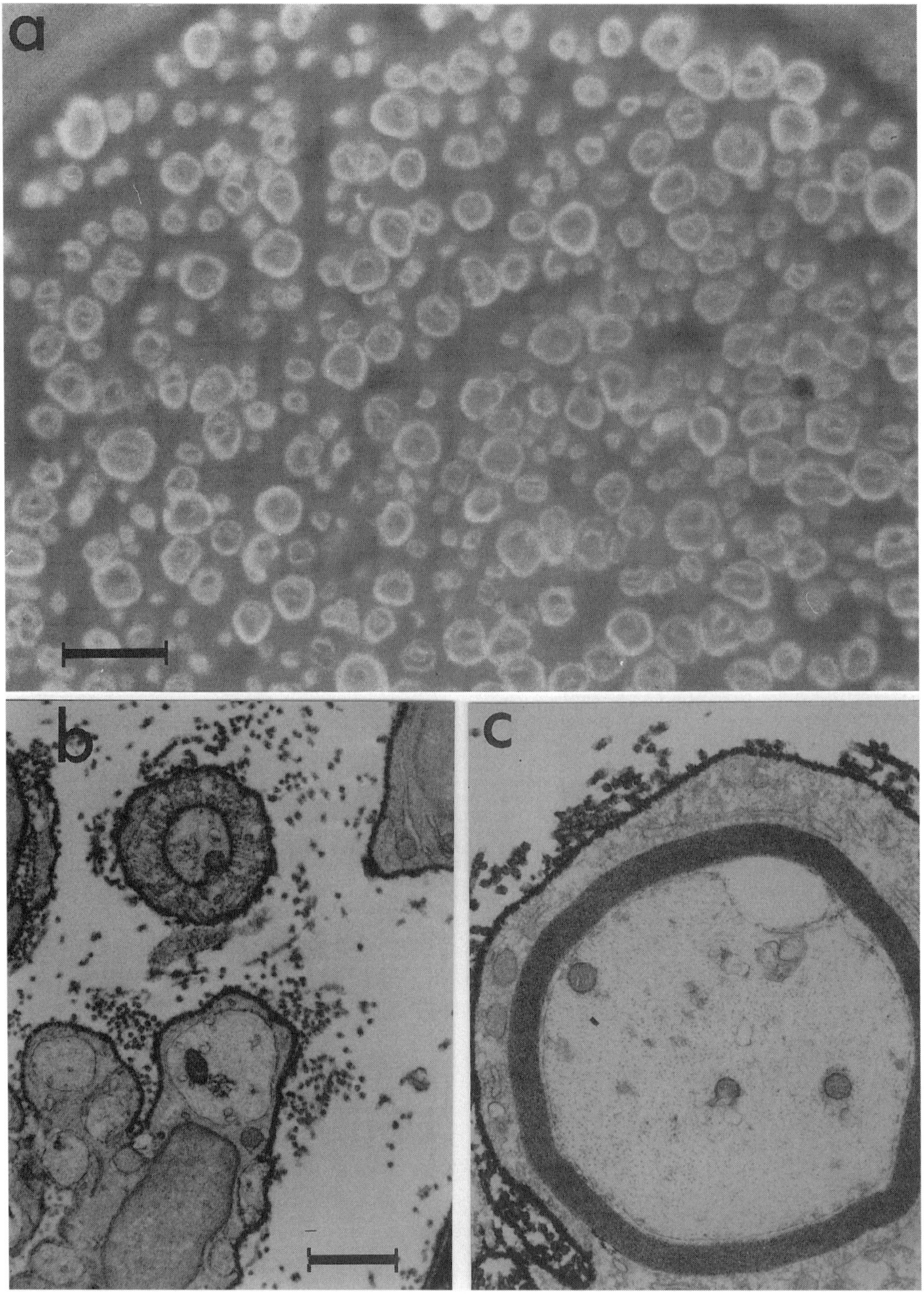

Figure 3.5 *Transverse section of rat sciatic nerve has been incubated with rabbit experimental allergic neuritis (EAN) serum followed by fluorescein labeled goat anti-rabbit IgG. Immunofluorescence, showing antimyelin IgG binding to nerve fibers. Bar: 20 μm. (b) and (c) Immunoelectron microscopy of sciatic nerve from a rabbit with chronic EAN. Immunoperoxidase stain showing IgG bound to external surface of Schwann cells. Bar: 1 μm.*

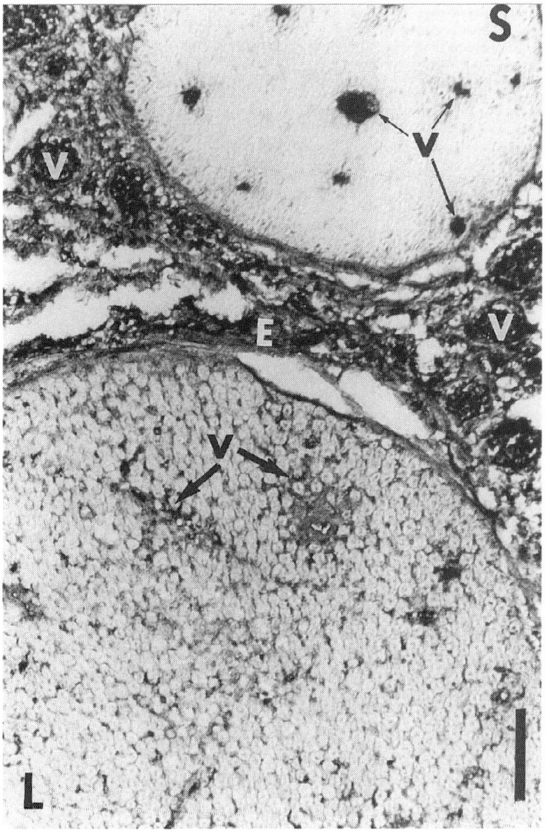

Figure 3.6 *Activated T cells cause breakdown of blood–nerve barrier. Rat sciatic nerve following intravenous horseradish peroxidase, given 2 days after injection of P_2 reactive T cells into the large fascicle. Note peroxidase staining (black) contained within blood vessels of small fascicle (S), but diffusing from vessels (V) throughout endoneurium of large fascicle (L). Absence of tight junctions in epineurial vessels (V) allows peroxidase into epineurial tissue (E). Bar: 100 μm.*

The efficacy of the blood–nerve barrier to circulating antimyelin antibody has been clearly demonstrated by several studies in which passive transfer of rabbit EAN serum or monoclonal or polyclonal IgG directed against Po, P_2 or M.A.G. failed to produce evidence of demyelination (Toyka and Heininger, 1989; Harvey and Pollard 1993; Spies et al. 1995). Harvey and Pollard (1993) showed that when rats treated with systemic rabbit EAN serum (containing high titres of GC antibody) were injected intraneurally with a minute quantity of the vasoactive amino 5-hydroxytryptamine, conduction block and demyelination were evident at the site of injection due to a focal opening of the blood–nerve barrier. An even more profound local increase in blood–nerve barrier permeability was demonstrated by Spies et al. (1995) by the intraneural injection of activated P_2 reactive T cells (Figure 3.6). In these experiments, vasoactive amine alone, or T cells alone, caused no demyelination; only in animals with circulating antibody and local blood–nerve barrier breakdown could conduction block and demyelination be demonstrated. In recent studies, T cells of non-neural specificity (ovalbumen (OVA) reactive) were induced to accumulate in nerve following passive transfer intravenously, by prior injection of OVA antigen into the sciatic nerve (Pollard et al. 1994). In such animals a focal blood–nerve barrier breakdown was shown 3 days after cell transfer, as T cells began to accumulate in nerve, and in animals with circulating GC antibody focal demyelination occurred (Pollard et al. 1994) (Figure 3.7). Morphological correlates of blood–nerve barrier breakdown included loss of tight junctions between endothelial cells and endothelial cell damage following T cell transmigration (Figure 3.3). Clearly the accumulation of activated T cells of any specificity within nerve and their interaction with local antigen presenting cells activates focal opening of the blood–nerve barrier and it is likely that cytokines including TNF alpha and INF gamma are involved in this process (Spies et al. 1995). Powell et al. (1991) have beautifully illustrated morphological changes associated with blood–nerve barrier breakdown in passive transfer EAN by showing loss of tight junctions and separation between endothelial cells in regions of T cell traffic.

Synthesis

Clearly there are many potential T cell epitopes on the peripheral nervous system (PNS) myelin–Schwann cell complex, and following immunization with myelin, T cells reactive to one or more of these epitopes may circulate enter the endoneurium and accumulate in nerve. Interaction of these T cells with their antigen presented in the contest of MHC class II on perivascular APCs issues in a cytokine orchestrated inflammatory response with T cell and macrophage recruitment, local blood–nerve barrier breakdown and consequent nerve fiber damage. It seems likely that

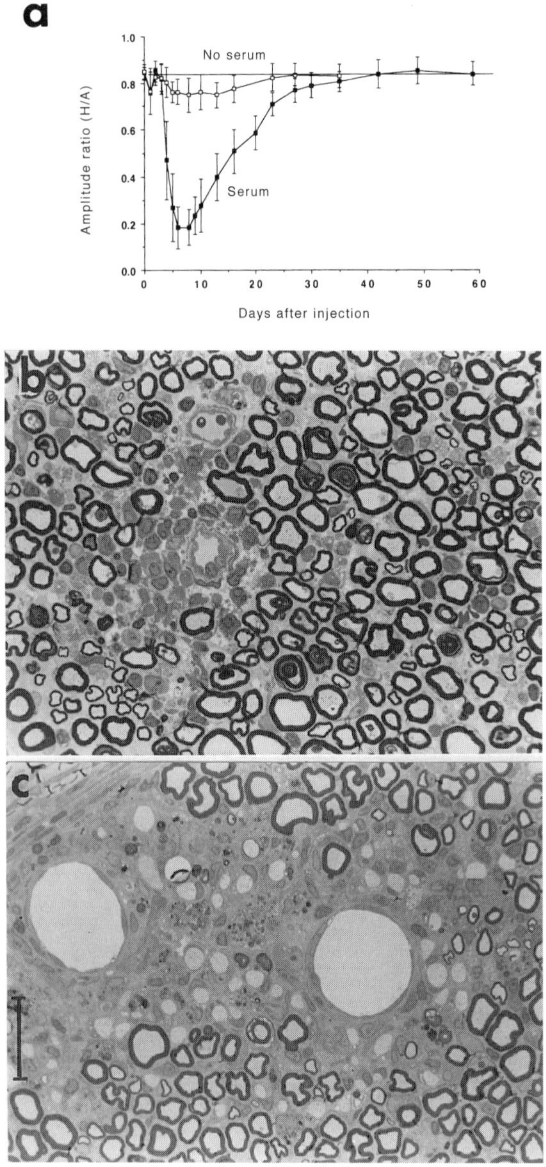

Figure 3.7 *(a) CMAP hip/ankle amplitude ratio (a measure of conduction block) plotted against time following intravenous infusion of ovalbumen reactive T cells and intraneural injection of ovalbumen. (■) Animals given daily intraperitoneal anti-GC serum. (□) Control animals without serum. Note rapid onset conduction block beginning day 3 only in animals given GC serum. (b) Transverse section of tibial nerve from control animal at day 5. Note marked perivascular accumulation of T cells without demyelination. (c) Transverse section of tibial nerve at day 5 from a serum-treated animal. Note perivascular T cells and marked demyelination. Bar: 20 μm.*

following active immunisation, B cell activation will result with consequent antibody production and circulation. The diffuse demyelination seen in actively induced EAN using myelin antigen would appear to be a synergistic response between T and B cell responses, with one important T cell effect, disruption of the blood–nerve barrier. In passive transfer EAN, blood–nerve barrier breakdown occurs with local T cell and macrophage recruitment, and cytokine production, but in the absence of antibody little demyelination is seen. Since demyelination characterises the common form of GBS, actively induced EAN is a better animal model than the passive transfer disease.

The final mechanism by which the myelin sheath is destroyed remains unknown. Macrophages are clearly involved but whether as primary effector cells or non-specific phagocytes following prior Schwann cell damage has not been determined. T cells play an essential role in EAN and in vitro, $CD4^+$ EAN inducing P_2 specific T cells are cytotoxic to Schwann cells (Argall et al. 1992). Evidence of such cytotoxicity in vivo is lacking and direct intraneural injection of these activated T cell lines does not cause demyelination (Spies et al. 1995); nor is there convincing evidence at this time for demyelination resulting from damage induced by the cytokines produced by T cells.

The studies of Stoll et al. (1991) showing complement deposition in nerves prior to demyelination, suggests this may be one mechanism by which macrophages can be directed to the myelin–Schwann cell complex. Similarly, antimyelin antibody (anti GC, anti-Po) could guide macrophages via Fc receptor mechanisms. Antibody to GC is well established in rabbit EAN but in the rat antimyelin antibody has not been demonstrated in situ; however, the studies of Hahn et al. (1993) and Spies et al. (1995) have shown that the infusion of antimyelin antibody into rats with passively transferred T cell disease results in a degree of demyelination in these animals similar to that found in animals with actively induced disease. This does not prove but it strongly suggests that actively induced EAN involves T cell and humoral (antibody) components.

The neurophysiological studies of La Fontaine et al. (1982) and Sumner et al. (1982) in which GC antibody induced conduction block within 1 hour, suggest that these antibodies can induce Schwann cell lysis and consequent myelin damage of rapid onset. Other antibodies or complement components may effect myelin damage through attracting macrophages. There are several mechanisms by which these cells may demyelinate. Apart from phagocytosing opsonized myelin, macrophages may produce proteinases or toxic oxygen radicals, or other proinflammatory components, damaging to myelin.

Electrophysiological changes

Cragg and Thomas (1964) first demonstrated slowing of motor nerve conduction velocity and conduction block in EAN. Harvey and Pollard (1992b) studied patterns of conduction failure in actively induced EAN in the Lewis rat and found in some animals a length dependent conduction block and progressive decline in the compound muscle action potential (CMAP) amplitude as the stimulating electrode was moved proximally. In other animals a small CMAP was found even with distal stimulation or no significant CMAP decrement was obtained. Histological evidence of demyelination was found in most animals of both groups in nerve roots and in distal nerve segments. In the former group of animals nerve lesions were more severe in these areas with more involvement of intervening sciatic nerve. These findings suggested that in mild disease there is lesion formation initially in areas of blood–nerve barrier permeability, i.e. roots and distal motor nerves, but when more severe disease exists lesions also occur in disseminated foci between these areas.

Distal latencies may be prolonged, CMAPs dispersed or reduced, conduction velocity slowed and abnormalities of F waves or spinal evoked potentials occur (Tuck et al. 1981; Heininger et al. 1986; Harvey and Pollard 1992a). Prolongation of the spinal evoked response following lower limb stimulation is the earliest electrophysiological abnormality seen and correlates closely with the onset of weakness and pathological changes in nerve roots (K. Westland, personal communication). Dispersion of the CMAP is usually seen in animals with chronic EAN or in the recovery phase of acute EAN.

Similar patterns of conduction failure are seen following passive transfer disease but the degree of abnormality and time course are dependent on the number of T cells transferred (Heininger et al. 1986). When high cell numbers are given a disease of more rapid onset occurs with severe CMAP reduction indicating severe axonal degeneration. It is of considerable importance that the marked intraneural T cell accumulation following this procedure is not accompanied by demyelination but rather destruction of myelin, Schwann cell and axon.

The intraneural injection into rat sciatic nerve of serum from EAN rabbits produces profound focal conduction block and demyelination (Saida et al. 1978; Sumner et al. 1982). The demyelinating factor is mostly antibody to GC (Saida et al. 1979; Pollard et al. 1994). Antibody to GC, produced by repeated innoculation of rabbits with GC has a similar effect on intraneural injection or when applied intrathecally onto nerve roots (La Fontaine et al. 1982) and rapidly evolving conduction block within 3 hours is seen. Morphological correlates of these early electrophysiological changes to GC serum include mild paranodal demyelination and widening of Schmidt–Lanterman incisures. In this model of acute demyelination, the distal CMAP remained of normal amplitude, but that obtained from stimulating above the injection site progressively declined in amplitude without dispersion (Figure 3.4). Little or no conduction slowing was seen. This important study demonstrated that conduction block, rather than slowing of conduction was the major electrophysiological consequence of acute demyelination.

Spies et al. (1995) produced focal demyelinating lesions within rat sciatic nerve by the intraneurial injection of activated T cells in animals given systemic EAN serum (anti-GC antibodies). T cell injections induced blood–nerve barrier breakdown, and focal demyelination over a 1 cm region was demonstrated by inching studies using platinum wire electrodes moved along the surface of the nerve. The physiological changes in EAN and in the human disorder which it represents presumably result from multifocal lesions of this type.

Therapeutic intervention

As the complex network of pathogenic mechanisms involved in the demyelinating process of EAN has been demonstrated, so have many experiments been reported of diverse ways to interrupt the disease process. It is the hope and design of this research that such studies will lead to better therapy for the human inflammatory demyelinating neuropathies.

Treatment of animals with T cell monoclonal antibodies may inhibit EAN. Strigard et al. (1988) showed disease inhibition with antibodies to CD4 and CD8 T cells, and Jung et al. (1992) used an antibody to the αβ T cell receptor which markedly suppressed disease expression.

Macrophages have been targeted in several ways and their important role in demyelination amply demonstrated. Tansey and Brosnan (1985) and Craggs et al. (1984) gave intraperitoneal silica dust to divert and inhibit monocytes and showed almost complete disease suppression. Hartung et al. (1988a, b) blocked specific macrophage metabolic pathways; they used inhibitors of arachadonic acid metabolism, indomethacin and BW755c and oxygen radical scavengers, superoxide dismutase and catalase and found similar disease suppression.

Mast cells were depleted of their vasoactive amine 5-hydroxytryptamine by Tansey and Brosnan (1984) in an experiment in which rats were injected with reserpine. This treatment delayed disease onset. The mast cell stabilizing drug Nedocramil has also been shown to attenuate EAN (Seeldrayers et al 1989).

Antibody to the important cytokine IFN-gamma almost completely suppressed EAN (Strigard et al. 1989; Hartung et al. 1990) and antibody to TNF-alpha reduced disease severity (Stoll et al. 1993). Cyclosporin A which effectively impairs cytokine production by T cells also suppressed EAN (King et al. 1983). EAN may also be suppressed by an antibody to the intercellular adhesion molecular 1 (ICAM-1), a molecule which mediates T cell traffic from the capillary into nerve (Archelos et al. 1993). Monoclonal antibody to MHC class II molecules, which play a central role in antigen presentation and recognition, has also suppressed EAN (Strigard et al. 1989).

Treatment directed towards humoral mechanisms has also been shown to be effective. Feasby et al. (1987) delayed disease onset and reduced demyelination by depleting complement with cobra venom. Plasma exchange and IgG immunoabsorption reduced disease severity in association with lowering antimyelin immunoglobulin (Antony et al. 1981; Gross et al. 1983; Harvey et al. 1988, 1989).

Finally, corticosteroids which act on many components of the immune response are effective in suppressing both active and passive transfer EAN (Hughes et al. 1981a, b, Heininger et al. 1988).

Chronic experimental allergic neuritis (CEAN)

CEAN is the animal model of CIDP. Pollard et al. (1975) injected outbred guinea pigs with monthly injections of nerve homogenate in Freund's adjuvant. The majority of animals suffered typical monophasic EAN and were resistant to second and later injections but 12% of animals relapsed when reinjected. Animals given a single injection were kept alive following recovery from EAN and 10% of animals were found to develop spontaneously chronic progressive or relapsing disease. Animals which developed chronic disease (progressive or relapsing) were found to develop hypertrophic 'onion-bulb' changes in nerve similar to those found in patients with CIDP (Pollard and Selby 1978). Wisniewski et al. (1974) induced EAN in monkeys and found that some animals pursued a relapsing course following a single immunization and hypertrophic changes were also evident in the nerves of some animals. If Lewis rats are allowed to recover from EAN and are followed by clinical examination, spontaneous recurrences may occur (Craggs et al. 1986; Brosnan et al. 1987; Adam et al. 1989). Brosnan et al. (1987) found relapses were more commonly seen when immature animals were immunized. A majority of rabbits given a single immunizing injection of a large dose of antigen, followed for a prolonged period, will pursue a chronic relapsing or progressive course (Harvey et al. 1987). These animals provide an excellent model for CIDP as their clinical course is similar to that seen in patients; the electrophysiological findings are characterized by marked slowing of motor conduction velocity and dispersion of compound muscle action potentials and within nerve roots extensive hypertrophic changes with onion bulb formation is evident (Figure 3.8). High levels of antimyelin IgG and IgM are present in these animals (Harvey et al. 1987, 1989) of which a major portion is anti GC antibody (Pollard et al. 1994). From these studies of normal animals it is apparent that factors which predispose to chronic disease include:

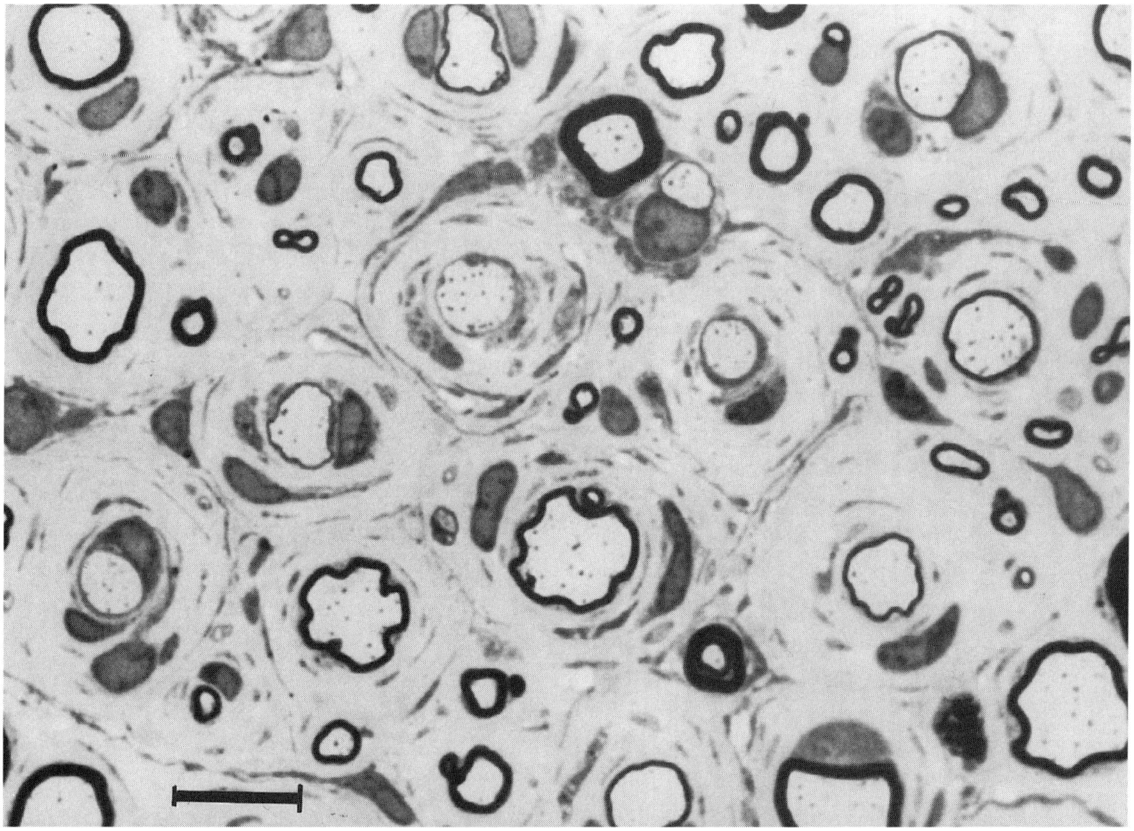

Figure 3.8 *Hypertrophic neuropathy in chronic experimental allergic neuritis (EAN). Transverse section from the L4 nerve root of a rabbit with chronic EAN showing marked onion bulb formation. Bar: 10 μm.*

1. Genetic predisposition.
2. Antigen dose.
3. Immature age of animals.
4. Repeated exposure.

In addition, if Lewis rats are given low dose cyclosporin A following immunization, a chronic relapsing disease results (McCombe et al. 1990). Attempts to produce CEAN by repeated transfer of P_2 reactive T cells has resulted in a neuropathy characterized by severe axonal damage but without onion-bulb formation (Lassmann et al. 1991). Their finding highlights the propensity of passive transfer EAN to cause nerve inflammation rather than extensive demyelination.

Finally, immunization of rabbits with sulfogluceronyl paragloboside (SGPG) has produced a mild CEAN (Yu et al. 1990) and antibodies to SGPG cause demyelination on intraneural injection (Maeda et al. 1991a). Although GC-induced EAN is often referred to as a model of human CIDP neither relapsing and remitting clinical course nor onion bulb formation have been described in GC-EAN rabbits. Nevertheless, CG-EAN is an important animal model as it is the prototype of neuropathy associated with antibody to glycolipid. Antibodies to glycolipids and gangliosides are currently under intense investigation as mediators of the pathological changes in inflammatory demyelinating neuropathy and other lower motor neuron syndromes.

Experimental paraprotein neuropathy

Neuropathies associated with paraproteinemias have received much attention following the seminal description by Latov et al. (1980) of a patient with a benign IgM paraprotein in whom the paraprotein was shown to exhibit antimyelin activity. The same group demonstrated the binding of the protein to myelin associated glycoprotein (MAG) and later work from several laboratories recognized that the antigenic target was a carbohydrate epitope common to MAG, two acidic glycolipids, Po and several neural cell adhesion molecules (Pollard 1993). Despite strong evidence of an association between the IgM paraproteins and the neuropathy, attempts to prove a causal relationship by passive transfer were disappointing, (Steck et al. 1985; Toyka and Heininger 1987). Recent studies have shown that this and other attempts to transfer neuropathy by systemic administration of immunoglobulin in most laboratory animals were doomed to failure because of an intact blood–nerve barrier (Pollard et al. 1994; Spies et al. 1995). The blood–nerve barrier was bypassed in studies by Hays et al. (1987), in which anti MAG IgM M protein was injected intraneurally. This study demonstrated demyelination in the presence of exogenous complement.

Tatum (1993) performed passive transfer studies into new born chicks with monoclonal 1gM from a patient with neuropathy. New born chicks lack an effective blood–nerve barrier, moreover chick MAG expresses abundant HNK-1 epitope as does human MAG but not that from rodents. Peripheral nerve demyelination characteristic of the human syndrome was demonstrated. The experimental lesion consisted of segmental demyelination and remyelination with little evidence of inflammation and widening of myelin lamellae. Antibody was demonstrated particularly within Schmidt–Lanterman incisures and nodes of Ranvier, regions of uncompacted myelin where MAG is know to be concentrated. This study therefore provides strong evidence that the demyelination seen in patients with these IgM paraproteins, is indeed antibody mediated. Although the mechanism of demyelination in this condition may be unique, this finding does support the view that antibodies to neural components present in other peripheral nerve disorders may also be pathogenic (Tatum 1993).

Peripheral neuropathy is also rarely associated with multiple myeloma. A relationship between the M protein and the neuropathy is less certain than it is with the anti MAG antibodies described above. Besinger et al. (1981) injected mice daily with purified IgG or Fab fragments from patients with myeloma or benign monoclonal gammopathy. The mice developed a demyelinating neuropathy with slowing of motor nerve conduction velocities. There is evidence that unlike rat, the mouse blood–nerve barrier is incomplete (Arvidson 1977). Nemni et al. (1987) induced monoclonal immunoglobulin producing tumors in BalbC mice by the intraperitoneal injection of mineral oil or pristane. One-third of the mice developed neuropathy but no immunoglobulin or light chains could be shown within the endoneurium. No subsequent studies have illustrated the mechanism of these neuropathies associated with myeloma and no new target epitopes have been defined.

Experimental Chagas' disease

The neurological manifestations of Chagas' disease are dominated by the occurrence of autonomic neuropathy at the chronic stage of the disease. Peripheral neuropathy is not common (Said 1994). Humans are infected with *Trypanosoma cruzi* most commonly by blood sucking bugs. The disease is common in South America and has been estimated to affect 20 million people (Said 1994). Experimental models of Chagas' disease have illuminated the mechanism of nerve and muscle damage in humans.

In a series of experiments Said et al. (1985) inoculated mice with the trypanomastigote form of *T. cruzi* and demonstrated mild inflammatory infiltrates throughout the sciatic nerve and the presence of the organism within macrophages. At the chronic stage prominent inflammatory infiltrates resembling granulomas were present adjoining endoneurial capillaries; these were composed of T cells, monocyte macrophages and mast cells. Within these lesions amastigotes were difficult to localize but *T. cruzi* antigen was demonstrated by immunohistochemistry. Associated with these lesions, focal areas of demyelination were found and distal axonal degeneration. Delayed type hypersensitivity was favored over antibody mediation of these lesions as intraneural injection of serum from chronically infected mice produced no disease whereas injection of trypanomastigotes caused local inflammation and demyelination similar to that seen in infected animals. Hontebeyrie-Joskowiez et al. (1987) showed that CD4$^+$ T cells from infected mice could passively transfer intraneural granulomas whether given systematically or intraneurally. T cell lines able to transfer disease were specific for either *T. cruzi* antigen or peripheral nerve antigen, although there was some evidence for T cell recognition of determinants shared between nerve and *T. cruzi*. In this regard it is of interest that van Voorkis and Eisen (1989) have shown that antibodies to a 160 KDa flagellum associated protein cross-react with a 48 KDa protein of peripheral nerve. The respective role of autoantibodies and T cells in this model have yet to be resolved (Said 1994).

Acknowledgments

This work was supported by grants from the National Health and Medical Research Council of Australia and from the National Multiple Sclerosis Society of Australia.

References

Adam, A.M., Atkinson, P.F., Hall, S.M., Hughes, R.A.C., and Taylor, W.A. (1989). Chronic experimental allergic neuritis in Lewis rat. *Neuropathol. Appl. Neurobiol.* **15**: 249–264.

Antony, J.H., Pollard, J.D., and McLeod, J.G. (1981). Effects of plasmapheresis on the course of experimental allergic neuritis in rabbits. *J. Neurol. Neurosurg. Psychiatry* **44**: 1124–1128.

Archelos, J.J., Maurer, M., Jung, S., Miyasaka, M., Tamatani, T., Toyka, K.V., and Hartung, H. (1993). Inhibition of experimental autoimmune neuritis by an antibody to the lymphocyte function-associated antigen 1. *Lab. Invest.* **70**: 667–675.

Argall, K.G., Armati, P.J., Pollard, J.D., & Bonner, J.G. (1992). Interactions between CD4$^+$ T cells and rat Schwann cells in vitro. 2. Cytotoxic effects of P2–specific CD4$^+$ T cell lines on Lewis rat Schwann cells. *J. Neuroimmunol.* **40**: 19–30.

Arnason, B.G.W. and Chelmicka-Szorc, E. (1972). Passive transfer of experimental allergic neuritis in Lewis rats by direct injection of sensitized lymphocytes into sciatic nerves. *Acta Neuropath. (Berl.)* **22**: 1–6.

Arvidson, B. (1977). Cellular uptake of exogenous horseradish peroxidase in mouse peripheral nerve. *Acta Neuropathol. (Berl.)* **37**: 35–42.

Astrom, K.E. and Waksman, B.H. (1962). The passive transfer of experimental allergic encephalomyelitis and neuritis with living lymphoid cells. *J. Pathol. Bacteriol.* **83**: 89–106.

Ballin, R.H.M. and Thomas, P.K. (1968). Electron microscope observations on demyelination and remyelination in experimental allergic neuritis. Part.1. Demyelination. *J. Neurol. Sci.* **8**: 1–12.

Besinger, U.A., Toyka, K.V., and Anzil, A.P. (1981). Myeloma neuropathy passive transfer from man to mouse. *Science* **213**: 1027–1030.

Brosnan, J.V., Craggs, R.I., King, R.H.M., and Thomas, P.K. (1987). Reduced susceptibility of T cell deficient rats to induction of experimental allergic neuritis. *J. Neuroimmunol.* **14**: 267–282.

Cragg, B.G. and Thomas, P.K. (1964). Changes in nerve conduction in experimental allergic neuritis. *J. Neurol. Neurosurg. Psychiatry* **27**: 106–115.

Craggs, R.I., Brosnan, J.V., King, R.H., and Thomas, P.K. (1986). Chronic relapsing experimental allergic neuritis in Lewis rats: effects of thymectomy and splenectomy. *Acta Neuropathol. (Berl.)*, **70**: 22–29.

Craggs, R.I., King, R.H.M., and Thomas, P.K. (1984). The effect of suppression of macrophage activity on the development of experimental allergic neuritis. *Acta Neuropathol. (Berl.)*, **62**: 316–323.

Feasby, T.E., Gilbert, J.J., Hahn, A.F., and Neilson, M. (1987). Complement depletion suppresses Lewis rat experimental allergic neuritis. *Brain Res.* **419**: 97–103.

Gross, M.L.P., Craggs, R.I., King, R.H.M., and Thomas, P.K. (1983). The treatment of experimental allergic neuritis by plasma exchange. *J. Neurol. Sci.* **61**: 149–160.

Hahn, A.F., Feasby, T.E., Wilkie, L., and Lovgren, D. (1993). Antigalactocerebroside antibody increases demyelination in adoptive transfer experimental allergic neuritis. *Muscle Nerve* **16**: 1174–1180.

Hartung, H. and Hadding, U. (1985). Synthesis of complement macrophages and modulation of their functions through compliment activation. In *Complement*, ed. H.J. Müller-Eberhard and A. Miescher, pp. 279–322. Berlin: Springer.

Hartung, H., Schafer, B., Heininger, K., Stoll, G., and Toyka, K.V. (1988a). The role of macrophages and eicosanoids in the pathogenesis of experimental allergic neuritis. Serial clinical, electrophysiological, biochemical, and morphological observations. *Brain* **111**: 1039–1059.

Hartung, H., Schafer, B., Heininger, K., and Toyka, K.V. (1988b). Suppression of experimental autoimmune neuritis by the oxygen radical scavengers superoxide dismutase and catalase. *Ann. Neurol.* **23**: 453–460.

Hartung, H., Schafer, B., van der Meide, P.H., Fierze, W., Heininger, K., and Toyka, K.V. (1990). The role of interferon-gamma in the pathogenesis of experimental autoimmune disease of the peripheral nervous system. *Ann. Neurol.* **27**: 247–257.

Hartung, H., Stoll, G., and Toyka, K.V. (1993). Immune reactions in the peripheral nervous system. In *Peripheral Neuropathy*, ed. P.J. Dyck, P.K. Thomas, J.W. Griffin, P.A. Low and J.F. Poduslo, pp. 418–444. Philadelphia: Saunders.

Harvey, G.K. and Pollard, J.D. (1992a). Peripheral nervous system demyelination from systemic transfer of experimental allergic neuritis serum. *J. Neuroimmunol.* **41**: 159–166.

Harvey, G.K. and Pollard, J.D. (1992b). Patterns of conduction impairment in experimental allergic neuritis. An electrophysiological and histological study. *J. Neurol. Neurosurg. Psychiatry* **55**: 909–915.

Harvey, G.K., Pollard, J.D., Schindhelm, K., and Antony, J.H. (1987). Chronic experimental allegic neuritis. An electrophysiological and histological study in the rabbit. *J. Neurol. Sci.* **81**: 215–225.

Harvey, G.K., Schindhelm, K., Antony, J.H., and Pollard, J.D. (1988). Membrane plasma exchange in experimental allergic neuritis: effect on antibody levels and clinical course. *J. Neurol. Sci.* **88**: 207–218.

Harvey, G.K., Schindhelm, K., and Pollard, J.D. (1989). IgG immunoadsorption in experimental allergic neuritis: effect on antibody levels and clinical course. *J. Neurol. Neurosurg. Psychiatry* **52**: 865–870.

Hays, A.P., Latov, N., Takatsu, M., and Sherman, W.H. (1987). Experimental demyelination of nerve induced by serum of patients with neuropathy and an anti-MAG IgM M-protein. *Neurology* **37**: 242–256.

Heininger, K., Schafer, B., Hartung, H., Fierz, W., Linington, C., and Toyka, K.V. (1988). The role of macrophages in experimental allergic neuritis induced by a P_2 specific T cell line. *Ann. Neurol.* **23**: 326–331.

Heininger, K., Stoll, G., Linington, C., Toyka, K.V., and Wekerle, H. (1986). Conduction failure and nerve conduction slowing in experimental allergic neuritis induced by P_2 specific T cell lines. *Ann. Neurol.* **19**: 44–49.

Hodgkinson, S.J., Pollard, J.D., and McLeod, J.G. (1994). Demyelination due to intraneural injection of EAN T-cells. *J. Neurol. Sci.* **123**: 162–172.

Hontebeyrie-Joskowicz, M., Said, G., Milon, G., Marchal, G., and Eisen, H. (1987). $L3T4^+$ T cells able to mediate parasite-specific delayed type hypersensitivity play a role in the pathology of experimental Chagas' disease. *Eur. J. Immunol.* **17**: 1027–1033.

Hughes, R.A.C., Kadlubowski, M., Gray, I.A., and Leibowitz, S. (1981a). Immune responses in experimental allergic neuritis. *J. Neurol. Neurosurg. Psychiatry* **44**: 565–569.

Hughes, R.A.C., Kadlubowski, M., and Hufschmidt, A. (1981b). Treatment of acute inflammatory polyneuropathy. *Ann. Neurol.* **9**(suppl.): 125–133.

Hughes, R.A.C., Powell, H.C., Braheny, S.L., and Brostoff, S.W. (1985). Endoneurial injection of antisera to myelin antigens. *Muscle Nerve* **8**: 516–522.

Izumo, S., Linington, C., Wekerle, H., and Meyermann, R. (1985). Morphologic study on experimental allergic neuritis mediated by T cell line specific for bovine P2 protein in Lewis rats. *Lab. Invest.* **53**: 209–218.

Jung, S., Kramer, S., Schluesener, H.J., Hunig, T., Toyka, K.V., and Hartung, H. (1992). Prevention and therapy of experimental autoimmune neuritis by an antibody against T-cell receptors-alpha/beta. *J. Immunol.* **148**: 3768–3775.

King, R.H.M., Craggs, R.I., and Gross, M.L.P. (1983). Suppression of experimental allergic neuritis by cyclosporin A. *Acta Neuropathol.* **59**: 262–268.

LaFontaine, S., Rasminsky, M., Saida, T., and Sumner, A.J. (1982). Conduction block in rat myelinated fibres following acute exposure to anti-galactocerebroside serum. *J. Physiol.* **323**: 287–306.

Lampert, P.W. (1969). Mechanisms of demyelination in experimental allergic neuritis – electronmicroscopic studies. *Lab. Invest.* **20**: 127–138.

Lassmann, H., Fierz, W., Neuchrist, C., and Meyermann, R. (1991). Chronic relapsing experimental allergic neuritis induced by repeated transfer of P_2-protein reactive T cell lines. *Brain* **114**: 429–442.

Latov, N., Sherman, W.H., and Nemi, R. (1980). Plasma-cell dyscrasia and peripheral neuropathy with a monoclonal antibody to peripheral nerve myelin. *N. Engl. J. Med.* **303**: 618–621.

Linington, C. and Brostoff, S.W. (1993). Peripheral nerve antigens. In *Peripheral Neuropathy* ed. P.J. Dyck, P.K. Thomas, J.W. Griffin, P.A. Low and J.F. Poduslo, pp. 404–417. Philadelphia: W.B.Saunders.

Linington, C., Izumo, S., Suzuki, M., Uyemura, K., Meyermann, R., and Wekerle, H. (1984). A permanent rat T cell line that mediates experimental allergic neuritis in the Lewis rat in vivo. *J. Immunol.* **133**: 1946–1950.

Linington, C., Lassmann, H., Ozawa, K., Kosin, S., and Mongan, L. (1992). Cell adhesion molecules of the immunoglobulin supergene family as tissue-specific autoantigens: Induction of experimental allergic neuritis (EAN) by Po protein-specific T cell lines. *Immunology* **22**: 1813–1817.

Maeda, Y., Bigbee, J.W., Maeda, R., Miyatani, N., Kalb, R.G., and Yu, R.K. (1991a). Induction of demyelination by intraneural injection of antibodies against sulfoglucuronyl paragloboside. *Ex. Neurol.* **113**: 221–225.

Maeda, Y., Brosnan, C.F., Miyatani, N., and Yu, R.K. (1991b). Preliminary studies on sensitization of Lewis rats with sulfated glucuronyl paragloboside. *Brain Res.* **S41**: 257–264.

McCombe, P.A., van der Kreek, S.A., and Pender, M.P. (1990). The effects of prophylactic cyclosporin A on experimental allergic neuritis (EAN) in the Lewis rat. Induction of relapsing EAN using low dose cyclosporin A. *J. Neuroimmunol.* **28**: 131–136.

Nemni, R., Fazio, R., Corbo, M., Sacchi, C., Smirne, S., and Canal, N. (1987). Peripheral neuropathy associated with experimental plasma cell neoplasm in the mouse. *J. the Neurol. Sci.* **77**: 321–329.

Olee, T., Weise, M., Powers, J., and Brostoff, S.W. (1989). A T cell epitope for experimental allergic neuritis is an amphipathic alphabetical structure. *J. Neuroimmunol.* **21**: 235–241.

Olsson, Y. (1968). Topographical differences in the vascular permeability of the peripheral nervous system. *Acta Neuropathol (Berl.)*, **10**: 26–34.

Pollard, J.D. (1993). Neurological complications of the plasma cell dyscrasias. In *Handbook of Clinical Neurology*, ed. P.J. Vinken, G.W. Bruyn and H.L. Klawans, pp. 391–411. Amsterdam: Elsevier Press.

Pollard, J.D. and Selby, G. (1978). Relapsing neuropathy due to tetanus toxoid. *J. the Neurol. Sci.* **37**: 113–125.

Pollard, J.D., King, R.H.M., and Thomas, P.K. (1975). Recurrent experimental allergic neuritis. An electron microscope study. *J. Neurol. Sci.* **24**: 365–383.

Pollard, J.D., Westland, K.W., Harvey, G.K., Jung, S., Spies, J.M., Toyka, K.V., and Hartung, H. (1995). Activated T cells of non-neural specificity open the blood nerve barrier to circulating antibody. *Ann. Neurol.* **37**: 467–476.

Powell, H.C., Olee, T., Brostoff, S.W., and Mizisin, A.P. (1991). Comparative histology of experimental allergic neuritis induced with minimum length neuritogenic peptides by adoptive transfer with sensitized cells or direct sensitization. *J. Neuropathol. Exp.Neurol.* **50**: 658–674.

Rostami, A.M. and Gregorian, S.K. (1991). Peptide 53–78 of myelin P_2 protein is a T cell epitope for the induction of experimental autoimmune neuritis. *Cell Immunol.* **132**: 433–436.

Rostami, A., Burns, J.B., Brown, M.J., Rosen, J., Zweiman, B., Lisak, R.D., and Pleasure, D.E. (1985). Transfer of experimental allergic neuritis with P_2 reactive T-cell lines. *Cell Immunol.* **91**: 354–361.

Said, G. (1994). Inflammatory neuropathies associated with known infections (HIV, leprosy, Chagas' disease, Lyme disease). In *Bailliere's Clinical Neurology* ed. J.G. McLeod, pp. 149–171. London: Bailliere Tindall, WB Saunders.

Said, G., Joskowicz, M., Barreira, A., and et.al. (1985). Neuropathy associated with experimental Chagas' disease. *Ann. Neurol.* **18**: 676–683.

Saida, K., Saida, T., Brown, M.J., and Silberberg, D.H. (1979). Peripheral nerve demyelination induced by intraneural injection of antigalactocerebroside serum. A morphological study. *Am. J. Pathol.* **95**: 99–110.

Saida, T., Saida, K., Silberberg, D.H., and Brown, M.J. (1978). Transfer of demyelination by intraneural injection of experimental allergic neuritis serum. *Nature* **272**: 639–641.

Saida, T., Saida, K., Silberberg, D.H., and Brown, M.J. (1981). Experimental allergic neuritis induced by galactocerebroside. *Ann. Neurol.* **9**(suppl.): 87–101.

Schabet, M., Whitaker, J.N., Schott, K., Stevens, A., Zurn, A., Buhler, R., and Wietholter, H. (1991). The use of protease inhibitors in experimental allergic neuritis. *J. Neuroimmunol.* **31**: 265–272.

Schmidt, B., Stoll, G., van der Meide, P.H., Jung, S., and Hartung, H. (1992). Transient cellular expression of interferon-gamma in experimental autoimmune neuritis. *Brain*: 1633–1646.

Seeldrayers, P.A., Yasui, D., Weiner, H.L., and Johnson, D. (1989). Treatment of experimental allergic neuritis with nedocromil sodium. *J. Neuroimmunol.* **25**: 221–226.

Spies, J.M., Westland, K.W., Bonner, J.G., and Pollard, J.D. (1995). Intraneural activated T cells cause focal breakdown of the blood nerve barrier. *Brain* **118**: 857–868.

Steck, A.J., Murray, N., Justafre, J.C., Meier, C., Toyka, K.V., Heininger, K., and Stoll, G. (1985). Passive transfer studies in demyelinating neuropathy with IgM monoclonal antibodies to myelin associated glycoprotein. *J. Neurol. Neurosurg. Psychiatry* **48**: 927–929.

Stoll, G., Jung, S., Jander, S., van der Meide, P., and Hartung, H. (1993). Tumor necrosis factor-alpha in immune-mediated demyelination and Wallerian degeneration of the rat peripheral nervous system. *J. Neuroimmunol.* **45**: 175–182.

Stoll, G., Schmidt, B., Jander, S., Toyka, K.V., and Hartung, H. (1991). Presence of the terminal complement complex (C5b-9) precedes myelin degradation in immune-mediated demyelination of the rat peripheral nervous system. *Ann. Neurol.* **30**: 147–155.

Strigard, K., Holmdahl, R., van der Meide, P.H., Klareskog, L., and Olson, T. (1989). In vivo treatment of rats with monoclonal antibodies against gamma interferon: effects on experimental allergic neuritis. *Acta Neurol. Scand.* **80**: 201–207.

Strigard, K., Olsson, T., Larsson, P., Holmdahl, R., and Klareskog, L. (1988). Modulation of experimental allergic neuritis in rats by in vivo treatment with monoclonal anti T cell antibodies. *J. Neurol. Sci.* **83**: 283–291.

Sumner, A.J., Saida, K., Saida, T., Silberberg, D.H., and Asbury, A.K. (1982). Acute conduction block associated with experimental antiserum-mediated demyelination of peripheral nerve. *Ann. Neurol.* **11**: 469–477.

Tansey, F.A. and Brosnan, C.F. (1983). Protection against experimental allergic neuritis with silica quartz dust. *J. Neuroimmunol.* **3**: 169–179.

Tatum, A.H. (1993). Experimental paraprotein neuropathy, demyelination by passive transfer of human IgM anti-myelin-associated glycoprotein. *Ann. Neurol.* **33**: 502–506.

Thomas, P.K., Berthold, C.H., and Ochoa, J. (1993). Microscopic anatomy of the peripheral nervous system. In *Peripheral Neuropathy,* ed. P.J. Dyck, P.K. Thomas, J.W. Griffin, P.A. Low and J.F. Poduslo, pp. 28–91. Philadelphia: W.B. Saunders.

Toyka, K.V. and Heininger, K. (1987). Humoral factors in peripheral nerve disease. *Muscle Nerve,* **10**: 222–232.

Tsai, C.P., Pollard, J.D., and Armati, P.J. (1991). Interferon gamma inhibition suppresses experimental allergic neuritis; modulation of major histocompatibility complex expression on Schwann cells in vitro. *J. Neuroimmunol.* **31**: 133–145.

Tuck, R.R., Pollard, J.D., and McLeod, J.G. (1981). Autonomic neuropathy in experimental allergic neuritis: an electrophysiological and histological study. *Brain* **104**: 187–208.

Uyemura, K., Suzuki, M., Kitamura, K., Hovie, K., Ogawa, Y., Matsuyama, H., Nozaki, S., and Muramatsu, I. (1982). Neuritogenic determinant of bovine P_2 protein in peripheral nerve myelin. *J. Neurochem.* **39**: 895–899.

Van Voorhis, W.C. and Eisen, H. (1989). A surface antigen of *Trypanosoma cruzi* that mimics mammalian nervous tissue. *J. Exp. Med.* **169**: 641–652.

Waksman, B.H. and Adams, R.D. (1955). Allergic neuritis: an experimental disease of rabbits induced by injection of peripheral nervous tissue and adjuvants. *J. Exp. Med.* **102**: 213–235.

Waksman, B.H. and Adams, R.D. (1956). A comparative study of experimental allergic neuritis in the rabbit, guinea pig and mouse. *J. Neuropathol. Exp. Neurol.* **15**: 293–332.

Watson, S.L., Westland, K., and Pollard, J.D. (1994). An electrophysiological and histological study of trypsin induced demyelination. *J. Neurol. Sci.* **126**: 116–125.

Wekerle, H., Linington, C., Lassmann, H., and Meyermann, R. (1986). Cellular immune reactivity within the CNS. *Trends Neurosc.* **9**: 271–277.

Wisniewski, H., Prineas, J., and Raine, C.S. (1969). An ultrastructural study of experimental demyelination and remyelination. 1. Acute experimental allergic encephalomyelitis in the peripheral nervous system. *Lab. Invest.* **21**: 105–118.

Wisniewski, H.M., Brostoff, S.W., Carter, H., and Eylar, E.H. (1974). Recurrent experimental allergic polyganglioradiculoneuritis. *Arch. Neurol.* **30**: 347–358.

Yu, R.K., Ariga, T., and Kohriyama, T. (1990). Autoimmune mechanisms in peripheral neuropathies. *Ann. Neurol.* **27**(suppl.), S30.

PART II Patient evaluation

4 Clinical evaluation and differential diagnosis

J.H.J. Wokke and N.C. Notermans

Introduction

The diagnosis of neuropathy is not usually difficult given the motor, sensory, and autonomic symptoms and signs which may lead a patient to seek advice from a physician. The presence of neuropathy in a single nerve, mononeuropathy, can have a variety of causes including compression by a tight transverse carpal ligament, as in the carpal tunnel syndrome. Sometimes mononeuropathy is the initial manifestation of a generalized disease such as vasculitis. In the latter case, patients often present with multiple mononeuritis, which means involvement of at least two different nerves which do not originate in the same nerve root. Plexus neuropathy is diagnosed if there are clinical or electrophysiological abnormalities in at least two different nerves which are branches of a distinct cervicobrachial or lumbosacral plexus. Polyneuropathy is characterized by a more or less symmetrical distribution of sensory and motor abnormalities which are usually more pronounced distally and more so in the legs than in the arms. In vasculitic neuropathy multiple mononeuritis may persist (Dyck et al. 1987; Said et al. 1988; Hawke et al. 1991) or precede asymmetrical polyneuropathy which in turn may evolve to distal symmetrical polyneuropathy (Hawke et al. 1991). Although most polyneuropathies share a mixed sensory-motor pattern of abnormalities, either pattern may predominate or be exclusively present, e.g. the motor deficit in multifocal motor neuropathy (van den Berg et al. 1995), or sensory dysfunction and ataxia in subacute sensory neuronopathy which may accompany small cell lung cancer (Graus et al. 1986).

After a careful workup of a patient with a neuropathy (Notermans et al. 1991; McLeod 1995), in most cases a cause can be identified (Dyck et al. 1995), and only a minority of about 10% of patients remain with idiopathic, usually axonal, neuropathy (Notermans et al. 1993).

The syndrome of neuropathy knows many causes (Dyck et al. 1981; Notermans et al. 1991; McLeod 1995). Finding the cause is fundamental so that the individual patient can be informed about prognosis and possible treatment (McLeod 1995). If common causes such as metabolic dysfunction, vitamin deficiences, and use of toxic substances or drugs have been excluded and a hereditary cause appears unlikely, most neuropathies result from dysfunction of the immune system. In Europe and North America, 5% of adults are estimated to suffer from autoimmune diseases (Steinman 1995). Many of these concern the peripheral nervous system either in combination with systemic disease as in vasculitis, or as the sole manifestation of a systemic abnormality as in monoclonal gammopathy of undetermined significance, or without systemic clues as in inflammatory neuropathy. The immune-mediated peripheral neuropathies show tremendous variation in their clinical manifestations, time course, response to treatment and outcome. We present a concise discussion of the various symptoms and signs of dysfunction of peripheral nerves, and the possible temporary profiles of peripheral neuropathies. Special attention is paid to characteristic features, if present, of immune-mediated peripheral neuropathies, and to the problem of differential diagnosis. Finally, we discuss how to measure the deficit and disability which may result from neuropathy.

Clinical characteristics of neuropathy

Motor symptoms and signs

Symptoms and signs of dysfunction of motor nerves include muscle cramps, spontaneous involuntary movements, weakness and atrophy of skeletal muscles. All of these may be present simultaneously, although atrophy is not usually an early feature. Not infrequently, these features follow in succession.

Muscle cramps

Cramps are painful contractions of a single muscle causing movement; they mostly occur at night causing the subject to wake up, or during the day following volitional contraction (Layzer 1994). They usually last only a few seconds. Nocturnal cramps, especially of the calf muscles and the flexors of the knees and toes, are a physiological phenomenon in young adults. Cramps in other muscles or a recurrence of cramps in middle-aged persons should raise suspicion of dysfunction of motor nerves or neurons. Cramps may also occur in healthy individuals following strenuous exercise, and interestingly in patients with Duchenne and Becker muscular dystrophy. Rarely, exercise-induced myalgia and cramps even at night are the sole manifestations of dystrophinopathy (Gospe et al. 1989). Other features such as a highly elevated activity of serum creatine kinase activity, positive family history and hypertrophy of the calves support a suspicion of muscular dystrophy. Although cramps are most commonly neural in origin (Layzer 1994), they are not a presenting and diagnostic feature of immune-mediated neuropathy. More generalized muscle stiffness at rest occurs in two rare autoimmune diseases: neuromyotonia (Chapter 16) and in axial muscles in the stiff-man syndrome (Layzer 1994); in the latter, spontaneous painful muscle spasms may also be present.

Fasciculations

Fasciculations are spontaneous contractions, or twitches, of muscle fibers belonging to the same motor unit. They are visible through the skin and again may occur in healthy individuals especially in the calf muscles. They are not always noticed by the subject and a careful search should be made for them without hurry when the patient is at rest. They occur following a spontaneous and sporadic action potential and have the dimensions of a motor unit potential which may be normal or abnormal in size and form. Although fasciculations occur frequently as an early sign in motor neuron disease (Swash et al. 1988), the majority arise in terminal motor axons (Roth 1992). A low excitability threshold of the axonal membrane appears to be a condition for the production of fasciculations (Roth 1992).

To understand the distal origin of fasciculations, it should be kept in mind that soon after entering the muscle, the large axons of motor neurons radiate nearby to the individual muscle fibers, which they innervate and which belong to the same motor unit (Wokke et al. 1990). The syndrome of so-called benign fasciculations appears to occur more frequently in patients working in the field of medicine, possibly because of a heightened awareness of a normal phenomenon (Blexrud et al. 1993). Fasciculations and cramps may occur without heralding progressive disease; a viral infection has been hypothesized as a cause of the syndrome (Blexrud et al. 1993). Twenty-one of 312 consecutive patients (6.7%) with amyotrophic lateral sclerosis had fasciculations as the initial and sole manifestation. Other deficits developed within 7 months (range 2–14 months) (Eisen & Stewart 1994). The absence of electrophysiological abnormalities other than fasciculation potentials may distinguish benign fasciculations (Blexrud et al. 1993).

Fasciculations are a prominent feature of neuromyotonia (Sinha et al. 1991); they also occur in post-poliomyelitis progressive spinal muscular atrophy (Cashman et al. 1987), and after the Guillain-Barré syndrome (GBS) (Valisescu et al. 1984), but to date there have been no systematic studies of the occurrence of fasciculations as a residual sign in GBS. The early occurrence of fasciculations and cramps has been observed in a patient with a purely motor demyelinating polyradiculoneuropathy and IgM plasma cell dyscrasia (Rowland et al. 1982), but fasciculations are usually absent from the early and late stages of monoclonal gammopathy of undetermined significance and polyneuropathy (Notermans et al. 1994a).

Fasciculations do occur in multifocal motor neuropathy and may erroneously detract attention from a treatable disease (van den Berg et al. 1995). In all patients with pure lower motor neuron syndromes, the presence of motor nerve conduction abnormalities should be scrutinized, as slowing of motor nerve conduction and conduction block may lead to the diagnosis of multifocal motor neuropathy. It is not known whether the muscular cramp-fasciculation syndrome represents an autoimmune disease (Tahmoush et al. 1991). If so, it may be an abortive and not very incapacitating form of neuromyotonia. As in benign fasciculations, fibrillations and positive sharp waves are absent on electrophysiological testing in this syndrome (Tahmoush et al. 1991).

Myokymia

Myokymia is a continuous, and to some extent rhythmic, quivering or rippling of muscle. The wavelike movement of myokymia contrasts with the brief, single twitches of fasciculations (Albers et al. 1981). Myokymia may originate from repetitive discharges of hyperactive motor units at the site of a peripheral nerve lesion. In case of fatigue, myokymia of the orbicularis oculi muscle can often be observed in healthy individuals. Myokymia is also a prominent feature of neuromyotonia. It rarely occurs in paretic facial muscles in the early stages of GBS (Daube et al. 1979). Rare cases of limb myokymia have been reported in acute inflammatory neuropathy and in vasculitic sensorimotor polyneuropathy (Albers et al. 1981).

In patients with rheumatoid arthritis who receive gold therapy, myokymia and fasciculations sometimes occur, which disappear following cessation of treatment; an autoimmune pathogenesis for these spontaneous movements has been suggested (Mitsumoto et al. 1982).

Hypotonia

Decrease or loss of normal muscle tone may be caused by involvement of lower motor neurons, peripheral motor nerves or muscle, but also occurs following disturbance of proprioceptive pathways, and cerebellar dysfunction. Usually hypo- or areflexia are also present; however, recently the concept of hypotonia as loss of resistance felt during passive movement of an extremity, which is explained by decrease or disappearance of muscle stretch reflexes, has been brought into question. On clinical examination, passive movements only appear to be of value in detecting spasticity or rigidity (van der Meché & van Gijn 1986).

Myotonia

Myotonia is the phenomenon of delayed relaxation after voluntary muscle contraction and is almost exclusively seen in hereditary disorders of the protein kinases or ion channels of the muscle membrane. Myotonia is a myopathic phenomenon, but as patients complain of stiffness, the condition may be confused with neuromyotonia (Chapter 16) which results from repetitive discharges of presynaptic origin (Harper & Rüdel 1994). This problem is, however, purely academic, as there are so many other characteristic abnormalities in patients with either myotonic dystrophy or congenital myotonia (Harper & Rüdel 1994).

Hypertrophy and atrophy

Pseudohypertrophy, especially of the calves, is a common feature of dystrophinopathy (Gospe et al. 1989). Neurogenic muscle hypertrophy of the calves has been observed seldom in anterior horn cell degeneration, in hereditary motor and sensory neuropathy, in S1 radiculopathy, and rarely in the aftermath of GBS (Vasilescu et al. 1984). Hypertropy is never a presymptomatic finding in immune-mediated neuropathy, but enlargement of the muscles of the tongue, back and limbs due to depositions of amyloid may be the initial manifestation in patients with monoclonal gammopathy without neuropathy (Jennekens & Wokke 1987).

Atrophy of muscle may result from myopathy and neuropathy whatever the cause, but also from disuse, cachexia and aging (Jennekens 1992). Neurogenic muscle changes occur gradually throughout the muscular system with aging, but atrophy is not usually present before the eighth decade (Jennekens 1992). These changes can be explained by an age-related loss of motor neuron cells in the spinal cord (Tomlinson & Irving 1977).

Inactivity can lead to considerable muscle atrophy, which is histologically characterized by atrophy of type 2 muscle fibers. These abnormalities are observed in severely ill patients and in selected muscles after enforced immobilization, e.g. following a fracture. The rate of atrophy is slow, although the mean muscle fiber size may decrease by approximately 80% in a period of 8 weeks (Jennekens 1992). A fulminant decrease of muscle tissue caused by massive protein breakdown may occur in critically ill patients (Wokke et al. 1988; Bolton et al. 1993). In this recently recognized condition, axonal neuropathy and myopathy result from an unknown mechanism in patients with mechanical ventilation and multiorgan failure (Zochodne et al. 1987). Muscle weakness prevents ventilatory weaning. This condition can be differentiated from GBS by the rare occurrence of cranial nerve dysfunction, near normal nerve conduction and no conduction block, and consistently reduced amplitudes of compound muscle action potentials and sensory nerve amplitudes (Ropper et al. 1991). Extensive denervation is also an electromyographic feature of critical illness neuropathy (Zochodne et al. 1987).

If atrophy results from denervation, it may occur gradually over a period of months or years as in motor neuron disease (Swash & Ingram 1988), and chronic neuropathy (Notermans et al. 1993, 1994a; van den Berg et al. 1995), or rapidly in weeks as in vasculitic neuropathy (Dyck et al. 1987; Hawke et al. 1991). In the course of chronic and vasculitic neuropathies, atrophy of distal muscles prevails; asymmetry is a feature of motor neuron disease (Swash & Ingram 1988) and of vasculitis (Duck et al. 1987; Said et al. 1988; Hawke et al. 1991). In neuropathy, atrophy is the result of a disturbance of the continuous processes of denervation and reinnervation (Jennekens 1994). The latter can compensate through the mechanism of collateral sprouting of intact axons for partial denervation, but this process cannot proceed unlimited. In motor neuron disease, reinnervation depends on the remaining functional motor neurons (Swash & Ingram 1988), whereas in neuropathy, the limiting factor is the extent of axonal degeneration, primarily as caused by nerve ischemia in vasculitis or secondarily as in inflammatory demyelinating neuropathies. In autoimmune myasthenia gravis, atrophy of muscle is not a prominent feature, probably because only functional, antibody-related, and temporary denervation of a number of muscle fibers within motor units occurs (Jennekens 1994). While deposition and activation of complement produces structural damage of motor end plates, continuously new end plates are being formed nearby (Wokke et al. 1990).

Weakness

The final common pathway of most neuropathies is weakness which motivates the patient to seek urgent advice about treatment and prognosis. Although in neuropathy the origin of weakness is dysfunction of lower motor neurons, severe disturbance of proprioceptive functions may also impede movements, as does pain. In neuropathy, weakness usually affects the distal muscles of the limbs first (Notermans et al. 1991; McLeod 1995), progressing to proximal regions when therapy is impossible or unsuccessful. This is especially so in axonal dying-back neuropathies, as it is the longer axons which the neurons first fail to maintain (Cavanagh 1984). In many immune-mediated neuropathies, such as in vasculitis, inflammatory demyelinating neuropathies and in gammopathy, weakness also often manifests in the distal muscles of the legs (Dyck et al. 1987; Said et al. 1988; Barohn et al. 1989; Hawke et al. 1991; Ropper 1992; Notermans et al. 1994a). In vasculitis and inflammatory demyelinating neuropathies, weakness of the proximal muscles frequently follows, or may even be the first manifestation (Dyck et al. 1987; Said et al. 1988; Barohn et al. 1989; Hawke et al. 1991; Ropper 1992). In patients with the fully developed GBS weakness of facial muscles is seen in 60% and of the oropharynx in 50% of patients (Ropper 1992); in the Miller Fisher variant of GBS, ophthalmoplegia is a predominant abnormality (Fisher 1956). In the chronic variant of inflammatory demyelinating neuropathy (CIDP), facial muscle weakness has been observed in 12–15% of patients (Barohn et al. 1989), and bulbar weakness in 6% (McCombe et al. 1987); weakness of other muscles innervated by cranial nerves is even rarer (McCombe et al. 1987; Barohn et al. 1989). In vasculitis or primary amyloidosis, weakness of muscles innervated by cranial nerves is infrequent (Dyck et al. 1987; Hawke et al. 1991; Traynor et al. 1991). Cranial nerve dysfunction may occur at any point during the course of human immunodeficiency virus (HIV-1) infection and hoarseness resulting from laryngeal nerve mononeuropathy has been observed (Lange 1994).

Sensory symptoms and signs

Most peripheral nerves contain fascicles with large, small and unmyelinated nerve fibers. The latter outnumber the small myelinated nerve fibers which in their part are more numerous than the larger ones. Using the light microscope, a bimodal distribution of myelinated nerve fibers can be observed with peaks at diameters of 3–5 μm and 10 μm (Jacobs & Love 1985; Thomas et al. 1993). This histological difference bears clinical significance as the large myelinated sensory fibers conduct exteroceptive stimuli such as crude and light touch and tactile discrimination, and in addition proprioceptive stimuli, whereas small myelinated and unmyelinated fibers are part of the exteroceptive sensory system and conduct pain and temperature sense (Light & Perl 1993). The autonomic nervous system also conducts through unmyelinated nerve fibers. In many neuropathies both populations of nerve fibers are affected as are motor nerve fibers, but both populations may also be affected separately.

A second reason for a distinction is the organization of the sensory system in the spinal cord. Large myelinated fibers switch over to their secondary sensory neurons in the nucleus gracilis or cuneatus in the medulla oblongata; crossing-over also takes place at this level (House & Pansky 1967). Dysfunction of the dorsal funiculi which may occur in spinal multiple sclerosis (Matthews 1985), cervical myelopathy (Voskuhl & Hinton 1990), or vitamin B_{12} deficiency may therefore mimic to some degree large sensory fiber neuropathy. In contrast, soon after entering the spinal cord, small myelinated and unmyelinated fibers cross and switch over to their secondary neurons; their afferent axons are located in the lateral spinothalamic tracts soon after entry into the spinal cord (House & Pansky 1967). Sensory symptoms can be subdivided into negative and positive. Negative means sensory loss due to impairment of conduction or of axonal degeneration, whereas positive means sensation in the absence of normal stimulation of receptors (Thomas & Ochoa 1993). Both categories are usually present in sensory neuropathy, although to varying degrees depending on cause and course. In the following we shall discuss these phenomena, paying particular attention to dysfunction of small or large myelinated nerve fibers.

Pain, paresthesias, and dysesthesias

In peripheral neuropathy pain originates from stimulation of nociceptors, or from involvement in the disease process of small myelinated and unmyelinated nerve fibers. Burning, aching and lancinating pains are a feature of neuropathy in most patients with systemic or nonsystemic vasculitis (Dyck et al. 1987; Said et al. 1988; Hawke et al. 1991), and in vasculitic neuropathy in cryoglobulinemia (Thomas et al. 1992), or paraneoplastic vasculitic neuropathy (Oh et al. 1991). Pain is also a presenting and prominent feature of neuropathies associated with primary systemic amyloidosis (Kelly et al. 1979). About half of the patients with monoclonal gammopathy of undetermined significance and neuropathy (MGUSP) but no cryoglobulinemia or primary amyloidosis suffer pain; this proportion did not alter in the course of a 5-year follow-up period (Notermans et al. 1994a). Pain may occur in about a quarter of the patients with GBS (Ropper 1992), in whom radicular pain with positive provocation tests can represent an initial feature; in 20% of patients presenting with CIDP, the chief complaint is pain which may range from a sensation of burning feet to aching pain in the muscles (McCombe et al. 1987). In both conditions motor abnormalities usually prevail in the course of the disease, although a sensory variant of CIDP has been reported (Oh et al. 1992). Pain is not usually an incapacitating symptom in ataxic (sub)acute sensory neuropathy, but many patients may experience pain during the course of the disease (Horwich et al. 1977; Windebank et al. 1990; Chalk et al. 1992). This condition occurs with or without malignancy, usually small-cell lung carcinoma or sometimes breast adenocarcinoma, and lymphocytic inflammatory infiltrates in dorsal root ganglia suggest an autoimmune pathogenesis at that level (Horwich et al. 1977; Windebank et al. 1990). Pain can occur in the course of progressive neuropathy and even during the recovery phase; the mechanism of the latter is at present not fully understood (Thomas & Ochoa 1993). Causalgia is a burning pain which occurs spontaneously, associated with hyperpathia after partial nerve injury. In addition the skin of the affected region may be atrophic, cool, reddish in color and may perspire excessively (Thomas & Ochoa 1993). Causalgia is a localized phenomenon and does not occur early on in peripheral neuropathy.

Paresthesias and dysesthesias result from dysfunction of the exteroceptive sensory system and cannot always be easily distinguished from pain as patients do not tend to discern these complaints. A distinction is nevertheless necessary as pain may have so many causes other than neuropathy. By recording a careful medical history with the emphasis on the nature of the unpleasant sensations, localization and time course, a distinction is possible in most cases. Paresthesias are abnormal sensations that the patient experiences in the absense of specific stimulation and include feelings of cold, warmth, numbness, tingling, crawling, heaviness, compression, and itching (Haerler 1992; Thomas & Ochoa 1993). Dysesthesias are distorted, usually painful or electric, interpretations of sensations after tactile or painful stimulation (Thomas & Ochoa 1993). Hyperalgesia and allodynia specifically point to dysfunction of small myelinated and unmyelinated nerve fibers and are detected by neurological examination. Paresthesias and dysesthesias are among the most common heralds of neuropathy. They occur in vasculitic neuropathy, are a presenting feature in 70% of patients with the Guillain-Barré syndrome (Ropper et al. 1991), in 64% of patients with CIDP (McCombe et al. 1987), and in about 80% of patients with MGUSP (Notermans et al. 1994a). Almost all patients with subacute sensory neuronopathy nominate paresthesias and pain as their primary symptoms (Windebank et al. 1990; Chalk et al. 1992). In the latter condition, the upper limbs may be affected first, whereas in vasculitic mononeuritis multiplex the region of disturbed sensation depends on the nerves involved; however as the disease process cannot be stopped, the typical distribution of polyneuropathy usually evolves with severe complaints of the lower limbs. Intermittent paresthesias, usually distal in distribution, but sometimes proximal and quite patchy in upper or lower limbs, have been observed in 54% of patients with Lyme neuroborreliosis (Halperin et al. 1990). Only minimal, if any, distal sensory loss was demonstrated and neurophysiological evidence of a more or less generalized neuropathy was only found in 39% of these patients and was compatible with axonal degeneration.

Hypalgia and hypesthesia

Decrease of pain and tactile senses is evident from clinical examination, which is also necessary to locate the deficit in order to make a distinction between dysfunction of single or multiple peripheral nerves or of dorsal root ganglia, or nerve roots (Haerer 1992). In most polyneuropathies the distal parts of the limbs are more affected compared with proximal areas. This is especially so in MGUSP (Notermans et al. 1994a). In GBS sensory loss is initially present in 40% of the patients increasing to 70% in the fully developed illness (Ropper 1992), and a varying degree of sensory impairment has been reported in 72–86% of CIDP patients (McCombe et al. 1987; Barohn et al. 1989). All patients with subacute sensory neuronopathy have sensory loss and in a large proportion of these one or both sides of the face are affected (Windebank 1990). In vasculitic neuropathy sensory loss depends on the nerves affected (Dyck et al. 1987; Said et al. 1988; Hawke et al. 1991). The neurological manifestations of stage II of Lyme disease, lymphocytic meningoradiculitis, are radicular pain and sensory loss or dysesthesias in areas of affected nerves or nerve roots (Vallat et al. 1987; Halperin 1990). Sural nerve biopsies reveal perivascular infiltrates of mononuclear cells, but no vasculitis (Vallat et al. 1987). In some patients there is electrophysiological evidence of a demyelinating neuropathy (Halperin et al. 1990; Oey et al. 1991).

Loss of proprioception

The senses of motion and position are necessary to maintain the position of the organism in its environment. The receptors are situated in joints, muscles spindles and tendons, the Golgi tendon organs being very important. Impulses are conducted through large myelinated nerve fibers. Dysfunction leads to sensory ataxia and clumsiness of movements, decrease of vibration and joint position and movement senses, and domination of pressure sensation (Haerer 1992). On examination attention should be given to the presence of pseudoathetoid movements. Sensory ataxia can easily be discriminated from cerebellar ataxia, as most cerebellar syndromes also show other features of cerebellar dysfunction such as dysarthria and saccadic pursuit eye movements or nystagmus, which are absent in immune-mediated neuropathy. In nonvasculitic neuropathy, predominant sensory ataxia may occur rarely (Dyck et al. 1987), whereas in systemic vasculitic neuropathy, loss of proprioceptive functions depends upon the degree of axonal degeneration (Hawke et al. 1991). Ataxia is an early phenomenon in 10% of the patients with GBS (Ropper 1992), and is the hallmark of the Miller Fisher variant of GBS (Fisher 1956). A minority of 5–10% of the CIDP patients show a clinically pure sensory neuropathy which may persist and dominate in later stages (McCombe 1987; Oh et al. 1992). Subclinical electrophysiological abnormalities compatible with demyelination of motor nerves are a prerequisite for the diagnosis of CIDP. Profound loss of propriocepsis occurs in all patients with subacute sensory neuronopathy and may lead to wheelchair dependency (Dalakas 1986; Ohnishi & Ogawa 1986; Horwich et al. 1977; Windebank et al. 1990; Chalk et al. 1992). In about half of the patients, the onset of symptoms may occur in the upper limbs (Windebank et al. 1990). At the start of our study of patients with MGUSP about two-thirds had abnormal vibration sense at the malleolus, and 93% had abnormal Romberg tests. After a follow-up period of 5 years, all test results were abnormal (Notermans et al. 1994a).

Postural and action tremors have been reported in neuropathy, but these have not been systematically analysed (Bain 1993). A small minority of the patients with CIDP have tremor (Dalakas et al. 1984; McCombe et al. 1987), as patients with gammopathy may have (Rowland et al. 1982; Ohnishi & Ogawa 1986). No doubt due to their rare occurrence, it is not known whether these tremors result from disturbed propriocepsis.

Dysfunction of autonomic nerves

Dysfunction of autonomic nerves is not mentioned in vasculitic neuropathy (Dyck et al. 1987; Said et al. 1988; Hawke et al. 1991), or CIDP (McCombe et al. 1987). It does occur in a minority of patients with GBS usually as a sphincter dysfunction (Ropper 1992). In some patients with subacute sensory neuronopathy, a systematic search may reveal orthostatic hypotension or anhydrosis as signs of autonomic dysfunction (Chalk et al. 1992). If autonomic dysfunction is associated with monoclonal gammopathy, amyloid depositions in peripheral nerves should be scrutinized (Kelly et al. 1979).

Reflexes

Hyporeflexia or areflexia may result from disturbed conduction along afferent or efferent nerve fibers and is, therefore, a common feature of neuropathy. In healthy subjects mentally induced asymmetry has been observed which may be clinically relevant (Stam et al. 1989). Several scales are used to measure muscle tendon reflexes. Recently, a simple five-point scale was again advocated to standardize the difficult assessment of reflexes (Hallett 1993). In vasculitic neuropathy, reflexes are low or absent in affected regions (Dyck et al. 1987; Said et al. 1988; Hawke et al. 1991). In paraneoplastic subacute sensory neuronopathy, global hyporeflexia or areflexia is the general rule, but in the localized form which may occur without malignancy, as in Sjögren's syndrome, reflexes can be low or absent in affected regions only (Dalakas 1986; Malinow et al. 1986; Ohnishi & Ogawa 1986; Horwich et al. 1977; Windebank et al. 1990; Chalk et al. 1992). GBS areflexia is initially present in 75% of patients and in the fully developed disease in over 90% (Ropper 1992); the same figure is observed in CIDP (Barohn et al. 1989). Tendon reflexes disappear in about 60% of patients with MGUSP in the course of the disease (Notermans et al. 1994a).

Pyramidal features and hyperreflexia are uncommon in immune-mediated neuropathy but have incidentally been reported in vasculitis. Also, patients with rheumatoid arthritis may have superior cervical spine abnormalities which may cause myelopathy. In patients with paramalignant subacute sensory neuronopathy pyramidal features and hyperreflexia may result from metastasis in the brain or spine causing myelopathy. Stage 3 of Lyme disease is characterized by CNS manifestations and symptoms of peripheral neuropathy have by then vanished (Wokke et al. 1987). In patients with AIDS, a painful predominantly sensory axonal neuropathy and loss of ankle reflexes may occur (Lange 1994); pyramidal signs in these patients should raise a suspicion of CNS involvement.

Other diagnostic features

The temporal profile of a neuropathy may in itself provide important diagnostic information. As immune-mediated neuropathy may be a manifestation of systemic disease and symptoms and signs of neuropathy may either precede, coincide or follow, a careful anamnesis and general physical examination paying special attention to evidence of systemic disease, are obligatory in many patients with neuropathy.

We shall first discuss which aspects of the time course of neuropathy are important and next briefly mention which symptoms and signs of other organ systems could help in the diagnosis of immune-mediated neuropathy, especially when occurring as an early manifestation of systemic disease.

The temporal profile of neuropathy

In vasculitic neuropathy, symptoms and deficits may follow the temporal and spatial patterns suggestive of ischemic nerve injury as progression may reach a peak in hours or days (Dyck et al. 1987). In one study symptoms of vasculitic neuropathy commenced at a mean time of 19 weeks prior to the diagnosis being made, whereas other symptoms commenced at a mean of 24 weeks prior to diagnosis (Hawke et al. 1991). If death is related to active vasculitis, patients usually die within 6 months of the onset of illness, and even patients who survive the first year fare worse than the general population (Hawke et al. 1991). Some patients do recover, even if not completely, after a number of years (Dyck et al. 1987; Hawke et al. 1991). GBS symptoms reach their worst within 4 weeks (Asbury et al. 1978). In CIDP the progressive phase may last for weeks or months. A relapsing course has been observed in two-thirds of patients with CIDP (McCombe et al. 1987). Recently subacute idiopathic demyelinating polyradiculoneuropathy was defined by a progressive phase of 4–8 weeks (Hughes et al. 1992); the neuropathy is characterized by a relatively mild course and insidious onset. Differences with GBS are the absence of autonomic failure and the preservation of independent ventilation (Hughes et al. 1992). The rate of evolution of sensory neuronopathy is in the order of weeks to a few months (Horwich et al. 1977; Windebank et al. 1990; Chalk et al. 1992). A fulminant nonparaneoplastic ataxic neuropathy of unknown origin developing within 1–2 weeks has been documented (Sternman et al, 1980; Fernandez et al. 1994). In the majority of patients, paraneoplastic sensory neuropathy precedes the discovery of cancer by a mean interval of about 1 year (Horwich et al. 1977). The longest reported interval between onset of the neuropathy and diagnosis of cancer is 5 years (Horwich et al. 1977). In MGUSP, progression, if prospectively studied, is slow but definite (Donofrio et al. 1989; Notermans et al. 1994a). The clinical course is remitting in some patients (Donofrio et al. 1989). If IgG paraproteinemia is present, this remission may be explained by an alternative diagnosis of CIDP (Bleasel et al. 1993). If the clinical situation of patients with MGUSP deteriorates rapidly, this may either be explained by malignant lymphoid disease (Donofrio et al. 1989; Notermans et al. 1994a), or primary amyloidosis. The first peripheral nerve manifestations of HIV-1 infection may be symptomatic axonal predominantly sensory polyneuropathy, acute, subacute or chronic inflammatory demyelinating neuropathy, or vasculitic neuropathy with or without cryoglobulinemia (Lange 1994).

Clinical evidence of systemic disease

In systemic necrotizing vasculitis and connective tissue diseases, general medical features such as fever, weight loss and malaise, or symptoms and signs of specific tissues or organ tracts such as asthma in allergic angiitis and granulomatosis (Churg-Strauss syndrome) or arthritis in rheumatoid arthritis, occur before neuropathy becomes evident (Shannon & Goetz 1995). Also many patients first experience musculoskeletal or gastrointestinal complaints or skin rashes. In systemic vasculitis cutaneous vasculitis may lead to livedo, necrosis and nodules (Said et al 1988; Hawke et al. 1991). CNS manifestations, which may be focal and result from vasculitis, or global such as aseptic meningitis or cognitive impairment, occur in a substantial number of patients with systemic necrotizing vasculitis or connective tissue disease (Shannon & Goetz 1995). In polyarteritis nodosa, peripheral neuropathy may be the initial manifestation of systemic vasculitis (Hawke et al. 1991). Sjögren's syndrome is defined by the clinical triad of xerophthalmia, xerostomia, and nondeforming arthritis. It is second in prevalence only to rheumatoid arthritis, and peripheral nerve involvement has been reported to occur in 10–32% of patients (Shannon & Goetz 1995). Polyneuropathy may be the first manifestation of Sjögren's syndrome as we found diagnostic labial salivary gland biopsies in some patients with so-called chronic idiopathic axonal polyneuropathy without xerophthalmia or xerostomia (van Dijk et al. 1994). If sensory neuropathy occurs in Sjögren's syndrome this can mimic carcinomatous sensory neuropathy (Asbury & Brown 1990).

Purpura, cyanosis and sometimes ulceration of the skin of the distal limbs are characteristic features of cryoglobulinemia. Cryoglobulins are serum proteins that precipitate when cooled and redissolve when heated. They can either be the isolated monoclonal (type I), as found in paraproteinemia, or mixed including a monoclonal component (type II), or finally polyclonal (type III). Cryoglobulins may occur idiopathically (essential cryoglobulinemia) or secondary to other diseases such as lymphoproliferative disorders, connective tissue disorders, chronic infections or HIV infection (Cavaletti et al. 1990; Gemignani et al. 1992; Stricker et al. 1992). The incidence of neuropathy in cryoglobulinemia may vary from 7 to 60% (Cavaletti et al. 1990). The neuropathy may be caused by frank vasculitis or alternatively by thickening and obliteration of endoneurial vessels (Gemignani et al. 1992; Prior et al. 1992), and may be an early and rarely a solitary manifestation of cryoglobulinemia (Thomas et al. 1992).

Erythema chronicum migrans is a pathognomonic manifestation of stage I of Lyme disease and is not always spontaneously mentioned (Halperin et al. 1990). Patients who did not enter the symptomatic early stage of Lyme disease may manifest with cardiac conduction abnormalities, lymphocytic meningoradiculitis, CNS abnormalities or arthritis. Although peripheral nervous system abnormalities are a regular finding in late Lyme neuroborreliosis, all reported patients also experienced systemic or rheumatological symptoms (Halperin et al. 1990). Given the high prevalence of false positive serological tests in endemic areas, the diagnosis of Lyme neuropathy should only be considered if other diagnostic features of infection with *B. burgdorferi* are present, or if the cerebrospinal fluid shows pleocytosis.

Sarcoidosis is a systemic disease of unknown etiology with immunological alterations (Silberberg 1995). Most patients with early sarcoidosis are diagnosed in an asymptomatic stage after a routine chest radiograph or have respiratory symptoms, often dyspnea, disturbed vision from uveitis or iridocyclitis, or skin changes. The incidence of neurological involvement in sarcoidosis is between 4 and 8% of patients, and peripheral nerves may be involved in a quarter to a half of these patients. Thickening of peripheral nerves or nerve roots but also perineurial infiltrates have been observed and may lead to either symmetrical involvement or multiple mononeuropathy. The symptoms may occur early in the disease and be slight or transient (Silberberg 1990). Peripheral neuropathy appears to be extremely rare, whereas cranial neuropathies, especially of the seventh nerve, were the most frequent manifestation of neurosarcoidosis (Stern et al. 1985).

Skeletal deformities

Chronic neuropathy may lead to contractures and deformity of the joints by disuse and if occurring before cessation of the growth period, by disturbance of the physiological balance between agonists and antagonists. In the young, the presence of deformities of the feet such as pes cavus and clawing of the toes or pes equinovarus should raise a suspicion of a chronic, probably hereditary polyneuropathy (Harding & Thomas 1980). Scoliosis may also result from early onset neuropathy. In adults these abnormalities of the feet may also occur, as may deformities of the fingers. Weakness of the shoulder abductors may lead to the frozen shoulder syndrome.

Differential diagnosis

After the clinical diagnosis of neuropathy has been made, the temporal profile of the neuropathy should be established: acute (maximum of deficit within 4 weeks), subacute ($5<\text{maximum}<12$ weeks), chronic progressive (>12 weeks), chronic relapsing and remitting. Next, the underlying pathology and cause must be identified in order to advise the patient on treatment strategies and prognosis. Given the numerous possible causes of neuropathy, a systematic approach to the diagnosis is necessary (Notermans et al. 1991; McLeod 1995). The need of a careful family history and examination of possibly affected family members must be emphasized. Skeletal deformities in family members may suggest a hereditary cause of the neuropathy (Harding & Thomas 1980). Clinical and previous laboratory evidence of systemic disease should also be taken into account.

Next, the first step is neurophysiological testing in order to discriminate between the primary processes of axonal degeneration, demyelination and motor or sensory neuronopathy (Chapter 4; Asbury & Gilliatt 1984; Notermans et al. 1991; Thomas & Ochoa 1993; McLeod 1995). Nerve conduction studies including analysis of late responses and concentric needle investigations are also necessary to detect subclinical abnormalities in the case of asymmetric clinical syndromes. A distinction between axonal degeneration and demyelination may not always be possible (Thomas & Ochoa 1993). The majority of the neuropathies appear to result from axonal degeneration (Thomas & Ochoa 1993). Neurophysiological testing is not always needed if a likely cause, as for instance diabetes mellitus, renal insufficiency and alcoholism, emerges from the anamnesis (McLeod 1995). Clinical features, temporal profile and neurophysiological characteristics are next combined and the polyneuropathy is classified into a certain category (Figure 4.1) (Thomas & Ochoa 1993; McLeod 1995). The second step is other laboratory testing to establish a cause of the neuropathy. The extent of laboratory analysis depends upon the qualification of the neuropathy with regards to temporal profile and the results of neurophysiological analysis. For instance, in young adults with chronic progressive or nonprogressive demyelinating neuropathy the most likely diagnosis is hereditary motor and sensory neuropathy type IA (Charcot–Marie–Tooth disease IA) and the diagnostic test is a search for a duplication on chromosome 17p (Hoogendijk et al. 1994).

Measurement of deficit and handicap

Quantitative measurement of muscle strength may be required to analyse the topographical distribution of clinical and subclinical weakness and to monitor progression of disease (Goonetillike et al. 1994). The development of therapeutic strategies for many immune-mediated polyneuropathies necessitates accurate measurement and quantification of the deficit and handicap in order to be able to estimate the efficacy of a given treatment. For this purpose, the clinical neurological examination may be not sensitive enough to detect small but significant changes. We shall briefly discuss how to quantify motor and sensory dysfunction. The measurement of autonomic dysfunction is discussed in Chapter 9. Finally, the usefulness of disability scales in patients with polyneuropathy will be discussed.

Quantification of motor function

The strength of individual muscles or muscle groups can easily be measured by estimating, in a standardized way, the counterforce required to overcome the patient's best effort; in clinical practice and in many trials, results are scored by manual muscle testing using the ordinal 6-grade Medical Research Council (MRC) scale (MRC 1975). With this method, the degree and distribution of weakness can rapidly be assessed in a wide range of muscles. Calculating an MRC-sumscore by summation of the scores of selected muscles and muscle groups facilitates quantification of motor performance (Kleyweg et al. 1988; Notermans et al. 1994a). Mild localized weakness may be missed by manual muscle testing and especially the single grade 4 of the MRC scoring system represents a wide range of strength (Andres et al. 1989; Hoogendijk et al. 1994); more objective methods may therefore be required.

Dynamometry provides an alternative for manual muscle testing; results are read from an interval scale (Wiles & Karni 1983; van der Ploeg et al. 1984; Edwards et al. 1987; Mendell & Florence 1990; Wiles et al. 1993; Goonetillike et al. 1994). Fixed dynamometers produce highly reproducible results (Andres et al. 1989; Wiles et al. 1993), but can be inconvenient in disabled patients (Goonetillike et al. 1994). Hand-held devices are extremely usable and are gaining popularity. The examiner just needs to overcome the maximally contracted muscle or muscle group; the force needed to overcome is thus effectively isometric (van der Ploeg et al. 1984, 1991; Goonetillike et al. 1994). Readings are taken at the moment that the subject's force has been overcome. This technique is called the 'careful break test' (van der Ploeg

Figure 4.1 *Diagnostic algorithm for evaluation of polyneuropathy in adults*.*
Immunological diseases of the peripheral nerves are printed in italics.

4.1a. Acute and subacute polyneuropathy

	Predominantly motor	Predominantly sensory	Mixed
EMG			
Demyelinating	Inflammatory *Guillain-Barré syndrome* (axonal degeneration may prevail); van der Meché et al. 1991 *Subacute inflammatory demyelinating polyneuropathy*	Inflammatory *Miller Fisher syndrome* (with ataxia and opthalmoplegia)	Inflammatory *Guillain-Barré syndrome* *Subacute inflammatory demyelinating polyneuropathy*
Axonal	Toxic Nitrofurantoin Lead (also systemic abnormalities) Gold Inorganic mercury (also CNS abnormalities)	Toxic Organic mercury (also CNS abnormalities)	Toxic Arsenic, thallium (also systemic abnormalities)
	Metabolic Diabetic amyotrophy (asymmetrical in lower limbs, painful) Porphyria (neuropathy rarely the first manifestation)	Metabolic Acute painful diabetic neuropathy (rare)	
		Autoimmune (antibody-mediated?) *Subacute sensory neuropathy* (progression in weeks to months)	Probably immune-mediated *Critical illness polyneuropathy*
			Vasculitic neuropathy

**Polyneuropathy in children frequently has a genetic cause; many severe syndromes with autosomal recessive inheritance have been described. †Although the electromyography (EMG) can generally differentiate between primary demyelinating and axonal neuropathies, problems may arise in individual patients in whom no clear distinction is possible. Evolution of the neuropathy in time may be another confusing factor. Several measurements at different moments may be required.*

Figure 4.1 *(cont.)*

4.1b Diagnostic algorithm for evaluation of polyneuropathy in adults.* Chronic polyneuropathy

	Predominantly motor	**Predominantly sensory**	**Mixed**
EMG†			
Demyelinating	Hereditary *HMSN I*		Hereditary *HMSN I*
	Inflammatory *Chronic inflammatory demyelinating polyneuropathy (CIDP)* *Multifocal motor neuropathy*	Inflammatory *CIDP* (rare, abnormal motor nerve conduction)	Inflammatory *CIDP*
		Paraproteinemic‡	Paraproteinemic‡
Axonal	Hereditary HMSN II	Hereditary Hereditary sensory and autonomic neuropathy I (painful, acral mutilation) Refsum disease (retinitis pigmentosa)	Hereditary HMSN II Tangier disease (orange tonsils, low serum cholesterol) Refsum disease (retinitis pigmentosa)
	Metabolic Hypoglycemic (insulinoma)	Metabolic Diabetes (sensory>autonomic> motor) Renal insufficiency (extensive secondary demyelination) Hypothyroidism Primary biliary cirrhosis Acromegaly	
		Deficiency Vitamins B1 (painful), B12, B6 (ataxic), E (ataxic, cerebellar)	
	Toxic Chloroquine (proximal>distal) Dapsone Vincristine	Toxic Almitrine Alcohol? Disulfiram Chloramphenicol Isoniazid Metronidazole Misonidazole Platinum Taxol Vitamin B6 (ataxic)	Toxic Amiodarone (may be predominantly motor and demyelinating Hexacarbons (glue-sniffing; demyelination may evolve Colchicine (provided renal impairment) Lithium carbonate Phenytoin (mild) Suramin

‡Electrophysiological studies of monoclonal gammopathy of undetermined significance (MGUS) neuropathies, especially in the case of IgM-MGUS, show more demyelinating features (Suarez and Kelly 1993); however, pure axonal MGUS-neuropathies may occur.

Figure 4.1b (*cont.*)

Predominantly motor	Predominantly sensory	Mixed
	Infectious *Lyme disease* *Leprosy* *HIV-I*	
	Paraproteinemic‡ Amyloid Familial *Primary*	Paraproteinemic‡ Vasculitic (may occur paraneoplastic) *Cryoglobulinemic*
Autoimmune *Lower motor neuron syndrome with anti-GMI antibodies*	Autoimmune *Sjögren's syndrome*	Autoimmune? *Sarcoidosis* (facial nerve palsy)
	Idiopathic Chronic idiopathic atactic Chronic idiopathic axonal polyneuropathy	Idiopathic Chronic idiopathic axonal polyneuropathy

et al. 1991). The value of fixed and hand-held dynamometry has been particularly analysed in muscular dystrophy and motor neuron disease (Goonetillike et al. 1994). The variability of readings obtained by hand-held dynamometers compares well with that obtained by fixed devices. In a recent study of patients with motor neuron disease the test-retest values of readings with hand-held dynamometry in one patient varied by about 13%. The accuracy of measurement was only influenced to a minor degree by changing examiners. Most investigators agree that a single assessor in the same patient can minimize the variability of readings obtained by hand-held dynamometry applied in the same patient (Andres et al. 1986; Goonetillike et al. 1994). The mean absolute percentage of test-retest variation using a fixed myometer for measuring isometric strength was 6.6% for normal subjects and 8.9% in patients with amyotrophic lateral sclerosis (Andres et al. 1986). Dynamometry readings may be less reproducible in weaker muscles (MRC<4–) (Goonetillike et al. 1994).

Quantification of sensory functions

Using cotton wool, a sharp pin and a tuning fork the surface of the body is examined for regions of abnormal or absent sensation and this method provides satisfactory information about gross sensory loss (Haerer 1992). Summation of results of clinical testing of sensory modalities may be helpful in monitoring the course of the neuropathy in a simple way (Notermans et al. 1994a,b); however, quantification based upon the classical neurological examination may fail to detect small changes. In a consensus report from the Peripheral Nerve Association (1993) a number of instruments have been recommended for quantifying sensory modalities. The computer-assisted sensory examination (CASE) is based on the detection of touch pressure, vibratory and temperature sensation thresholds (Dyck et al. 1993). Knowing the responses in a large series of healthy persons, it is possible to express results in a patient as a percentile specific for age, sex and site. Although the test results are very reliable, the requirement of a specialized testing site and expertise may make the method less easily accessible in a clinical setting. Another quantitative method of testing for thermal cutaneous sensation is based on the measurement of temperature perception thresholds for warmth and cold using a thermode at the ventral side of the wrist (Jamal et al. 1985).

Table 4.1 *A functional grading scale in the Guillain-Barré syndrome*

0	Healthy
1	Minor signs or symptoms of neuropathy but capable of manual work
2	Able to walk without support or a stick but incapable of manual work
3	Able to walk with a stick, appliance, or support
4	Confined to bed or chairbound
5	Requiring assisted ventilation
6	Dead

Note:
Frequently a walking distance is specified in grades 2 and 3, i.e. 5 m (Guillain-Barré Group, 1985), or 10 m (Van der Meché, 1992)
Source: Hughes et al. 1978.

Table 4.2 *The modified Rankin scale*

0	Asymptomatic
1	Nondisabling symptoms that do not interfere with lifestyle
2	Minor disability; symptoms that lead to some restriction of lifestyle, but do not interfere with the patients' capacity to look after themselves
3	Moderate disability; symptoms that significantly interfere with lifestyle or prevent totally independent existence
4	Moderate severe disability; symptoms that clearly prevent independent existence, although patient does not need constant attention
5	Severely disabled; totally dependent requiring constant attention

Source: Van Swieten 1988.

Table 4.3 *A scale for ataxia*

0	Normal-stand on one foot with eyes closed
1	Stand/walk normally with eyes closed
2	Stand/walk with minor swaying with eyes closed, but normally with eyes open
3	Stand/walk with some swaying with eyes open
4	Stand/walk on a large base with eyes open
5	Standing/walking impossible without support

Source: Nobile–Orazio 1988.

Impairment of vibration sense is measured using a vibrameter, a hand-held instrument with which vibration thresholds can be determined at various parts of the body using an electromagnetic vibrator (Goldberg & Lindblom 1979; Elderson et al. 1989; Dyck et al. 1993).

Sensory ataxia can be quantified in a simple way with the tapping test (Notermans et al. 1994c); the device used consists of two push buttons placed at a fixed distance 35 cm apart, connected to an automatic counter. The patient is asked to push the buttons alternately with the dominant limb, as fast as possible, within a given period of time.

Disability scales

To assess the severity and progression of polyneuropathies and to monitor the efficacy of treatment, it is important to measure disability accurately. For this purpose several scales have been developed; the disadvantages of these scales in relation to polyneuropathy may be their lack of specificity and sensitivity (Windebank 1987). Generally, spoken disability scales should be simple, and practical in the clinical setting; they also have to be validated in interobserver studies. In the Guillain-Barré syndrome a six-point functional grading scale devised by Hughes et al. is widely used (Table 4.1) (Hughes et al. 1978). The modified Rankin scale represents another simple and practical method for measuring disability (Table 4.2) (van Swieten et al. 1988) and although this six-point scale was originally validated in patients with stroke, its value has been demonstrated in studies of patients with MGUSP, CIDP and chronic idiopathic axonal polyneuropathy (van Doorn et al. 1990; Notermans et al. 1994a,b). The disability resulting from ataxia can be measured using the scale of Nobile-Orazio et al. (Table 4.3) (Nobile-Orazio et al. 1988). The diabetic neuropathy neurological disability score designed by Dyck et al. represents the sum of separate clinical scores of muscle strength, reflexes and sensation (Dyck et al. 1980), and does not provide direct information on the handicap.

References

Albers, J.W., Allen II, A.A., Bastron, J.A., and Daube, J.R. (1981). Limb myokymia. *Muscle Nerve* **4**: 494–504.

Andres, P.L., Hedlund, W., Finison, L., Conlon, T., Felmus, M., and Munsat, T.L. (1986). Quantitative motor assessment in amyotrophic lateral sclerosis. *Neurology* **36**: 937–941.

Andres, P.L., Skerry, L.M., and Munsat, T.L. (1989). Measurement of strength in neuromuscular diseases. In *Quantification of Neurological Deficit* ed. T.L. Munsat. London: Butterworths. pp. 87–99.

Asbury, A.K., Arnason, B.G.W., Karp, H.R., and McFarlin, D.F. (1918). Criteria for diagnosis of Guillain-Barré syndrome. *Ann Neurol.* **3**: 565–566.

Asbury, A.K. and Brown, M.J. (1990). Sensory neuronopathy and pure sensory neuropathy. *Cur. Opin. Neurol. Neurosurg.* **3**: 708–711.

Asbury, A.K. and Gilliatt, R.W. (1984). The clinical approach to neuropathy. In *Peripheral Nerve Disorders*, ed. A.K. Asbury London: Butterworths. pp. 1–20.

Bain, P. (1993). A combined clinical and neurophysiological approach to the study of patients with tremor. *J. Neurol. Neurosurg. Psychiatry* **69**: 839–844.

Barohn, R.J., Kissel, J.T., Warmolts, J.R., and Mendell, J.R. (1989). Chronic inflammatory demyelinating polyradiculoneuropathy. Clinical characteristics, course, and recommendations for diagnostic criteria. *Arch. Neurol.* **46**: 878–884.

Bleasel, A.F., Hawke, S.H.B., Pollard, J.D., and McLeod, J.G. (1993). IgG monoclonal paraproteinaemia and peripheral neuropathy. *J. Neurol. Neurosurg. Psychiatry* **56**: 52–57.

Blexrud, M., Windebank, A.J., and Daube, J.R. (1993). Long-term follow-up of 121 patients with benign fasciculations. *Ann. Neurol.* **34**: 622–625.

Bolton, C.F., Young, G.B., and Zochodne, D.W. (1993). The neurological complications of sepsis. *Ann. Neurol.* **33**: 94–100.

Cashman, N.R., Maselli, B., Wollman, R., Roos, R., Simon, R., and Antel, J.P. (1987). Late denervation in patients with antecedent paralytic poliomyelitis. *N. Engl. J. Med.* **317**: 7–12.

Cavaletti, G., Petruccioli, M.G., and Crespi, V. (1990). A clinico-pathological and follow-up study of 10 cases of essential type II cryoglobulinaemic neuropathy. *J. Neurol. Neurosurg. Psychiatry* **53**: 886–889.

Cavanagh, J.B. (1984). The problems of neurons with long axons. *Lancet* **i**: 1284–1287.

Chalk, C.H., Windebank, A.J., Kimmel, D.W., and McManis, P.G. (1992). The distinctive clinical features of paraneoplastic sensory neuronopathy. *Can. J. Neurol. Sci.* **19**: 346–351.

Dalakas, M.C. (1986). Chronic idiopathic ataxic neuropathy. *Ann. Neurol.* **19**: 545–554.

Dalakas, M.C., Teräväinen, G., Engel, W.K. (1984). Tremor as a feature of chronic relapsing and dysgammaglobulinemic polyneuropathies. *Arch. Neurol.* **41**: 711–714.

Daube, J.R., Kelly, J.J. Jr., and Martin, R.A. (1979). Facial myokymia with polyradiculoneuropathy. *Neurology(Minneap.)* **29**: 662–669.

Donofrio, P.D. and Kelly, J.J. (1989). AAEE case report no. 17: peripheral neuropathy in monoclonal gammopathy of undetermined significance. *Muscle Nerve* **12**: 1–8.

Dyck, P.J., Karnes, J., O'Brien, P.C., and Zimmerman, I.R. (1993). Detection thresholds of cutaneous sensation in humans. In *Peripheral Neuropathy*, ed. P.J. Dyck, P.K. Thomas, E.H. Lambert and R. Bunge, pp. 706–8. Philadelphia: W.B. Saunders.

Dyck, P.J., Sherman, W.R., Hallcher, L.M., Service, F.J., O'Brien, P.C., Grina, L.A., Palumbo, P.J., and Swanson, C.J. (1980). Human diabetic endoneurial sorbitol, fructose and myo-inositol related to sural nerve morphometry. *Ann. Neurol.* **8**: 590–596.

Dyck, P.J.J., Benstead, T.J., Conn, D.L., Stevens, J.C., Windebank, A.J., and Low, P.A. (1987). Nonsystemic vasculitic neuropathy. *Brain* **110**: 843–854.

Dyck, P.J.J., Oviatt, K.F., and Lambert, E.H. (1981). Intensive evaluation of referred unclassified neuropathies yields improved diagnosis. *Ann. Neurol.* **10**: 222–226.

Edwards, R.H.T., Chapman, S.J., Newman, D.J., and Jones, D.A. (1987). Practical analysis of variability of muscle function measurements in Duchenne muscular **atrophy. *Muscle Nerve* 10: 6–14.**

Eisen, A. and Stewart, H. (1994). Not-so-benign fasciculation. *Ann. Neurol.* **35**: 375.

Elderson, A., Gerritsen van der Hoop, R., Haanstra, W., Neijt, J.P., Gispen, W.H., and Jennekens, F.G.I. (1989). Vibration perception and thermoperception as quantitative measurements in the monitoring of cisplatin-induced neurotoxicity. *J. Neurol. Sci.* **93**: 167–114.

Fernández, J.M., Dávalos, A., Ferrer, I., Cervera, C., Codina, A., and Ochoa, J.L. (1994). Acute sensory neuronopathy: report of a child with remarkable clinical recovery. *Neurology* **44**: 762–764.

Fisher, M. (1956). An unusual variant of acute idiopathic polyneuritis (syndrome of ophthalmoplegia, ataxia and areflexia). *N. Engl. J. Med.* **255**: 57–65.

Gemignani, F., Pavesi, G., Fiocchi, A., Manganelli, P., Ferraccioli, G., and Marbini, A. (1992). Peripheral neuropathy in essential mixed cryoglobulinaemia. *J. Neurol. Neurosurg. Psychiatry* **55**: 116–120.

Goldberg, J.M. and Lindblom, W. (1979). Standardised method of determining vibratory perception thresholds for diagnosis and screening in neurological investigation. *J. Neurol. Neurosurg. Psychiatry* **42**: 793–803.

Goonetillike, A., Modarres-Sadeghi, H., and Guiloff, R.J. (1994). Accuracy, reproducibility, and variability of hand-held dynamometry in motor neuron disease. *J. Neurol. Neurosurg. Psychiatry* **57**: 326–332.

Gospe, S.M., Lazaro, R.P., Lava, N.S., Grootscholten, P.M., Scott, M.O., and Fischbeck, K.H. (1989). Familial X-linked myalgia and cramps: a nonprogressive myopathy associated with a deletion in the dystrophin gene. *Neurology* **39**: 1227–1280.

Graus, F., Elkon, K.B., Cordon-Cardo, C., and Posner, J.B. (1986). Sensory neuronopathy and small cell lung cancer: antineuronal antibodies that also reacts with the tumor. *Am. J. Med.* **80**: 45–52.

Guillain-Barré Syndrome Study Group. (1985). Plasmapheresis and acute Guillain-Barré syndrome. *Neurology* **35**: 1096–1104.

Haerer, A.F. (1992). The sensory system. In *DeJong's Neurological Examination*, 5th edn. Philadelphia: JB Lippincott, pp. 47–76.

Hallett, M. (1993). NINDS Myotatic Reflex Scale. *Neurology* **43**: 2723.

Halperin, J., Luft, B.J., Volkman, D.J., and Dattwyler, R.J. (1990). Lyme neuroborreliosis. Peripheral nervous system manifestations. *Brain* **113**: 1207–1221.

Harding, A. and Thomas, P.K. (1980); The clinical features of hereditary motor and sensory neuropathy types I and II. *Brain* **103**: 259–280.

Harper, P.S. and Rüdel, R. (1994). Myotonic dystrophy. In *Myology*, 2nd edn, ed. A.G. Engel and C. Franzini-Armstrong, pp. 1192–1219. New York: McGraw-Hill.

Hawke, S.H.B., Davies, L., Pamphlett, R., Guo, Y.-P., Pollard, J.D., and McLeod, J.G. (1991). Vasculitic neuropathy. A clinical and pathological study. *Brain* **114**: 2175–2190.

Hoogendijk, J.E., De Visser, M., Bolhuis, P., Hart, A.A.M., and Ongeboer de Visser, B.W. (1994). HMSN type I: clinical and neurographical features of the 17p duplication subtype. *Muscle Nerve* **17**: 1010–1015.

Horwich, M.S., Cho, L., Porro, R.S., and Posner, J.B. (1977). Subacute sensory neuropathy: a remote effect of carcinoma. *Ann. Neurol.* **2**: 7–19.

House, E.L. and Pansky, B. (1967). General somatic afferent system. In *A Functional Approach to Neuronanatomy*, 2nd edn. New York: McGraw-Hill, pp. 152–175.

Hughes, R., Sanders, E., Hall, S., Atkinson, P., Colchester, A., and Payan, P. (1992). Subacute idiopathic demyelinating polyradiculoneuropathy. *Arch Neurol.* **49**: 612–616.

Hughes, R.A.C., Newsom-Davis, J.M., Perkin, G.D., and Pierce, J.M. (1978). Controlled trial of prednisolone in acute polyneuropathy. *Lancet* **II**: 750–735.

Jacobs, J.M. and Love, S. (1985). Qualitative and quantitative morphology of human sural nerve at different ages. *Brain* **108**: 897–924.

Jamal, G.A., Hansen, S., Weir, A.I., and Ballantyne, J.P. (1985). An improved automated method for measurement of the thermal thresholds. 1. Normal subjects. *J. Neurol. Neurosurg. Psychiatry* **48**: 354–360.

Jennekens, F.G.I. and Wokke, J.H.J. (1987). Proximal weakness of the extremities as main feature of amyloid myopathy. *J. Neurol. Neurosurg. Psychiatry* **50**: 1353–1358.

Jennekens, F.G.I. (1992). Disuse, cachexia and aging. In *Skeletal Muscle Pathology*, 2nd edn, F.L. Mastaglia, J.N. Walton, pp. 753–767. Edinburgh: Churchill Livingstone.

Jennekens, F.G.I. (1994). Neurogenic disorders. In *Skeletal Muscle Pathology*, 2nd edn, ed. F.L. Mastaglia and J.N. Walton, pp. 563–597. Edinburgh: Churchill-Livingstone.

Kelly, J.J. Jr, Kyle, R.A., O'Brien, P.C., and Dyck, P.J. (1979). The natural history of peripheral neuropathy in primary systemic amyloidosis. *Ann. Neurol.* **6**: 1–7.

Kleyweg, R.P., van der Meché, F.G.A., and Meulstee, J. (1988). Treatment of Guillain-Barré syndrome with high-dose gammaglobulin. *Neurology* **38**: 1639–1641.

Lange, D.J. (1994). AAEM minimonograph no. 41: neuromuscular diseases associated with HIV-1 infection. *Muscle Nerve* **17**: 16–30.

Layzer, R.B. (1994). Muscle pain, cramps, and fatigue. In *Myology*, ed. A.G. Engel and C. Franzini-Armstrong, pp. 1754–1768. New York: McGraw-Hill.

Light, A.R. and Perl, E.R. (1993). Peripheral sensory systems. In *Peripheral Neuropathy*, 3rd edn, ed. P.J. Dyck, P.K. Thomas, E.H. Lambert and R. Bunge, pp. 149–165. Philadelphia: W.B. Saunders.

Malinow, K., Yannakis, G.D., Glusman, S.M., Edlow, D.W., Griffin, J., Pestronk, A., Powel, D.L., Ramsey-Goldman, R., Eidelman, B.H., Medsger, T.A., and Alexander, E.L. (1986). Subacute sensory neuropathy secondary to dorsal root ganglionitis in primary Sjögren's syndrome. *Ann. Neurol.* **20**: 535–537.

Matthews, W.B. (1985). Differential diagnosis. In *McAlpine's Multiple Sclerosis*, ed. W.B. Matthews, pp. 146–166. Edinburgh: Churchill Livingstone.

McCombe, P.A., Pollard, J.D., and McLeod, J.G. (1987). Chronic inflammatory demyelinating pllyradiculoneuropathy. A clinical and electrophysiological study of 92 cases. *Brain* **110**: 1617–1630.

McLeod, J.G. (1995). Investigation of peripheral neuropathy. *J. Neurol. Neurosurg. Psychiatry* **58**: 274–283.

Medical Research Council (1975). *Aids to the Investigation of The Peripheral Nervous System.* London: Her Majesty's Stationary Office, 45: 1–2.

Mendell, J.R. and Florence, J. (1990). Manual muscle testing. Muscle Nerve **13**: S16–S20.

Mitsumoto, H., Wilbourn, A.J., and Subramony, S.H. (1982). Generalized myokymia and gold therapy. *Arch. Neurol.* **39**: 449–450.

Nobile-Orazio, E., Baldini, L., and Barbieri, S. (1988). Treatment of patients with neuropathy and anti-MAG IgM M-proteins. *Ann. Neurol.* **24**: 93–97.

Notermans, N.C., Wokke, J.H.J., and Jennekens, F.G.I. (1991). Clinical work-up of the patient with a polyneuropathy. In Handbook of Clinical Neurology, vol. 16, ed. De Jong JMBV, pp. 253–270. Amsterdam: Elsevier.

Notermans, N.C., Wokke, J.H.J., Franssen, H., van der Graaf, Y., Vermeulen, M., van den Berg, L.H., Bär, P.R., and Jennekens, F.G.I. (1993). Chronic idiopathic polyneuropathy presenting in middle or old age: a clinical and electrophysiological study of 75 patients. *J. Neurol. Neurosurg. Psychiatry* **56**: 1066–1071.

Notermans, N.C., Wokke, J.H.J., Lokhorst, H., Franssen, H., van der Graaf, Y., and Jennekens, F.G.I. (1994a). Polyneuropathy associated with monoclonal gammopathy of undetermined significance. A prospective study of the prognostic value of clinical and laboratory abnormalities. *Brain* **117**: 1385–1393.

Notermans, N.C., Wokke, J.H.J., van der Graaf, Y., Franssen, H., van Dijk, G.W., and Jennekens, F.G.I. (1994b). Chronic idiopathic axonal polyneuropathy: a five year follow-up. *J. Neurol. Neurosurg. Psychiatry* **57**: 1525–1527.

Notermans, N.C., van Dijk, G.W., van der Graaf, Y., van Gijn, J. and Wokke, J.H.J. (1994c). Measuring ataxia. Quantification based on the standard neurological examination. *J. Neurol. Neurosurg. Psychiatry* **57**: 22–26.

Oey, P.L., Franssen, H., Bernsen, R.A.J.A.M., and Wokke, J.H.J. (1991). Multifocal conduction block in a patient with *Borrelia burgdorferi* infection. *Muscle Nerve* **14**: 375–377.

Oh, S.J., Slaughter, R., and Harrell, L. (1991). Paraneoplastic vasculitic neuropathy: a treatable neuropathy. *Muscle Nerve* **14**: 152–156.

Oh, S.J., Joy, J.L., and Kuruoglu, R. (1992). 'Chronic sensory demyelinating neuropathy': chronic inflammatory demyelinating polyneuropathy presenting as a pure sensory neuropathy. *J. Neurol. Neurosurg. Psychiatry* **55**: 667–680.

Ohnishi, A. and Ogawa, M. (1986). Preferential loss of large lumbar primary sensory neurons in carcinomatous sensory neuropathy. *Ann. Neurol.* **20**: 102–104.

Prior, R., Schober, R., Scharffetter, K., and Wechsler, W. (1992). Occlusive microangiopathy by immunoglobulin (IgM-kappa) precipitation: pathogenetic relevance in paraneoplastic cryoglobulinemic neuropathy. *Acta Neuropathol.* **83**: 423–426.

Peripheral Neuropathy Association (1993). Quantitative sensory testing: a consensus report. *Neurology* **43**: 1050–1052.

Ropper, A.H., Wijdicks, E.F.M., and Truax, B.T. *Guillain-Barré Syndrome.* Philadelphia: F.A. Davis, pp. 223–224.

Ropper, A.H. (1992). The Guillain-Barré syndrome. *N. Engl. J. Med.* **326**: 1130–1136.

Roth, G. (1992). The origin of fasciculations. *Ann. Neurol.* **12**: 542–547.

Rowland, L.P., Defendini, R., Sherman, W., Hirano, A., Olarte, M.R., Latov, N., Lovelace, R.E., Inoue, K., and Osserman, E.F. (1982). Macroglobulinemia with peripheral neuropathy simulating motor neuron disease. *Ann. Neurol.* **11**: 532–536.

Said, G., Lacroix-Ciaudo, C., Fujimura, H., Blas, C., and Faux, N. (1988). The peripheral neuropathy of necrotizing arteritis: a clinicopathological study. *Ann. Neurol.* **23**: 461–465.

Shannon, K.M. and Goetz, C.G. (1995). Connective tissue diseases and the nervous system. In *Neurology and General Medicine*, 2nd edn, ed. M. Aminoff, pp. 447–471. New York: Churchill Livingstone.

Silberberg, H. (1995). Sarcoidosis of the nervous system. In *Neurology and General Medicine* 2nd edn, ed. M. Aminoff, pp. 847–858. New York: Churchill Livingstone.

Sinha, S., Newsom-Davis, J., Mills, K., Byrne, N., Lang, B., and Vincent, A. (1991). Autoimmune aetiology for acquired neuromyotonia (Isaacs' syndrome). *Lancet* **338**: 75–77.

Stam, J., Speelman, H.D., and van Crevel, H. (1989). Tendon reflex asymmetry by voluntary mental effort in healthy subjects. *Arch Neurol.* **46**: 70–73.

Steinman, L. (1995). Escape from 'horror autotoxicus': pathogenesis and treatment of autoimmune disease. *Cell* **80**: 7–10.

Sterman, A.B., Schaumburg, H.H., and Asbury, A.K. (1980). The acute sensory neuronopathy syndrome: a distinct clinical entity. *Ann. Neurol.* **7**: 354–358.

Stern, B.J., Krumholz, A., Johns, C., Scott, P., and Nissim, J. (1985). Sarcoidosis and its neurological manifestations. *Arch. Neurol.* **42**: 909–917.

Stricker, R.B., Sanders, K.A., Owen, W.F., Kiprov, D.D., and Miller, R.G. (1992). Mononeuritis multiplex associated with cryoglobulinemia in HIV infection. *Neurology* **42**: 2103–2105.

Suarez, G.A. and Kelly, J.J. (1993). Polyneuropathy associated with monoclonal gammopathy: further evidence that IgM-MGUS neuropathies are different than IgG-MGUS. *Neurology* **43**: 1304–1308.

Swash, M. and Ingram, D. (1988). Preclinical and subclinical events in motor neuron disease. *J. Neurol. Neurosurg. Psychiatry* **51**: 165–168.

Tahmoush, A.J., Alonso, R.J., Tahmoush, G.P., and Heiman-Patterson, T.D. (1991). Cramp-fasciculation syndrome: a treatable hyperexcitable peripheral nerve disorder. *Neurology* **41**: 1021–1024.

Thomas, F.P., Lovelace, R.E., Ding, X.-S., Sadig, S.A., Petty, G.W., Sherman, W.H., Latov, N., and Hays, A.P. (1992). Vasculitic neuropathy in a patient with cryoglobulinemia and anti-IgM monoclonal gammopathy. *Muscle Nerve* **15**: 891–898.

Thomas, P,K., Berthold, C.-H., and Ochoa, J. (1993). Microscopic anatomy of the peripheral nervous system. Nerve trunks and spinal roots. In *Peripheral Neuropathy*, 3rd edn, ed. P.J. Dyck, P.K. Thomas, E.H. Lambert and R. Bunge, pp. 28–73. Philadelphia: W.B. Saunders.

Thomas, P.K. and Ochoa, J. (1993). Clinical features and differential diagnosis. In *Peripheral Neuropathy*, 3rd edn, P.J. Dyck, P.K. Thomas, E.H. Lambert and R. Bunge, pp. 756–764. Philadelphia: WB Saunders.

Tomlinson, B.E. and Irving, D. (1977). The number of limb motor neurons in human lumbosacral cord throughout life. *J. Neurol. Sci.* **34**: 213–219.

Traynor, A.E., Gertz, M.A., and Kyle, R.A. (1991). Cranial neuropathy associated with primary amyloidosis. *Ann. Neurol.* **29**: 451–454.

Vallat, J.M., Lubeau, M., Leboutet, M.J., Dumas, M., and Desproges-Gotterom. (1987). Tick-bite meningoradiculitis: clinical, electrophysiologic, and histologic findings in 10 cases. *Neurology* **37**: 749–753.

Van den Berg, L.H., Kerkhoff, H., Oey, P.L., Franssen, H., Mollee, I., Vermeulen, M., Jennekens, F.G.I., and Wokke, J.H.J. (1995). Treatment of multifocal motor neuropathy with high-dose intravenous immunoglobulins: a double-blind, placebo-controlled study. *J. Neurol. Neurosurg. Psychiatry* **59**: 248–252.

Van Dijk, G.W., Notermans, N.C., Kruize, A.A., and Wokke, J.H.J. (1994). Diagnostic value of labial salivary gland biopsy in chronic idiopathic axonal polyneuropathy. *J. Neurol.* **241** S: 160.

Van Doorn, P.A., Brand, A., Strengers, P.F.W., Meulstee, J., and Vermeulen, M. (1990). High-dose intravenous immunoglobulin treatment in chronic inflammatory demyelinating polyneuropathy: a double-blind, placebo-controlled, cross over study. *Neurology* **40**: 209–212.

Van der Meché, F.G.A. and van Gijn, J. (1986). Hypotonia: an erroneous clinical concept? *Brain* **109**: 1169–1178.

Van der Meché, F.G.A., Meulstee, J., and Kleyweg, R.P. (1991). Axonal damage in the Guillain-Barré syndrome. *Muscle Nerve* **14**: 997–1002.

Van der Meché, F.G.A., Schmitz, P.I.M., and the Dutch Guillain-Barré Study Group. (1992). A randomized trial comparing intravenous immune globulin and plasma exchange in Guillain-Barré syndrome. *N. Engl. J. Med.* **326**: 1123–1129.

Van der Ploeg, R.J.O., Oosterhuis, H.J.G.H., and Reuvekamp, J. (1984). Measuring muscle strength. *J. Neurol.* **231**: 200–203.

Van der Ploeg, R.J.O., Fidler, V., and Oosterhuis, H.J.G.H. (1991). Hand-held myometry: reference values. *J. Neurol. Neurosurg. Psychiatry* **54**: 244–247.

Van Swieten, J.C., Koudstaal, P.J., Visser, M.C., Schouten, H.J.A., and van Gijn, J. (1988). Interobserver agreement for assessment of handicap in stroke patients. *Stroke* **19**: 604–607.

Vasilescu, C., Alexianu, M., and Dan, A. (1984). Muscle hypertrophy and a syndrome of continuous motor unit hyperactivity in prednisone-responsive Guillain-Barré polyneuropathy. *J. Neurol.* **231**: 276–279.

Voskuhl, R.R. and Hinton, R.C. (1990). Sensory impairment in the hands secondary to spondylitic compression of the cervical spinal cord. *Arch. Neurol.* **47**: 309–311.

Wiles, C.M. and Karni, Y. (1983). The measurement of muscle strength in patients with peripheral neuromuscular disorders. *J. Neurol. Neurosurg. Psychiatry* **46**: 1006–1013.

Wiles, C.M., Mills, K.R., and Edwards, R.H.T. (1993). Quantization of muscle contraction and strength. In *Peripheral Neuropathy*, 3rd edn, ed. P.J. Dyck, P.K. Thomas, E.H. Lambert and R. Bunge, pp. 698–705. Philadelphia: W.B. Saunders.

Windebank, A.J. Blexrud, M.D., Dyck, P.J., Daube, J.R., and Karnes, I.L. (1990). The syndrome of acute sensory neuropathy: clinical features and electrophysiologic and pathologic changes. *Neurology* **40**: 584–591.

Windebank, A.J. (1987). Assessment of symptoms, deficits and neural activity. In *Diabetic Neuropathy*, ed. P.J. Dyck, P.K. Thomas, E.H. Lambert and R. Bunge, pp. 100–106. Philadelphia: W.B. Saunders.

Wokke, J.H.J., Jennekens, F.G.I., van den Oord, C.J.M., Veldman, H., Smit, L.M.E., and Leppink, G.J. (1990). Morphological changes in the human end plate with age. *J. Neurol. Sci.* **95**: 291–310.

Wokke, J.H.J., Jennekens, F.G.I., van den Oord, C.J.M., Veldman, H., and van Gijn, J. (1988). Histological investigations of muscle atrophy and end plates in two critically ill patients with generalized weakness. *J. Neurol. Sci.* **00**: 95–106.

Wokke, J.H.J., van Gijn, J., Elderson, A., and Stanek, G. (1987). Chronic forms of *Borrelia burgdorferi* infection. *Neurology* **37**: 1031–1034.

Zochodne, D.W., Bolton, C.F., Wells, G.A., Gilbert, J.J., Hahn, A.F., Brown, J.D., and Sibbald, W.A. (1987). Critical illness polyneuropathy: a complication of sepsis and multi-organ failure. *Brain* **110**: 819–842.

5 Electrophysiological studies

H. Franssen

Introduction

In the management of patients with (suspected) immune-mediated neuropathy the results of electrophysiological studies are used for confirmation of the diagnosis of polyneuropathy, classification of the polyneuropathy into different categories (motor/sensory, axonal/demyelinating, uniform/multifocal), estimation of the prognosis for recovery, and follow-up. In the case of inflammatory neuropathies, classification is the most important of these items as this will guide the diagnosis and subsequent treatment. The emphasis in this chapter will therefore lie on the distinction between demyelination and axonal damage on the basis of pathophysiological principles and the use of electrodiagnostic protocols and criteria.

Conduction in normal and demyelinated single nerve fibers

Normal fibers

A normal myelinated nerve fiber consists of an axon around which myelin segments are wrapped with a length of approximately 1 mm. The axon diameter, internodal distance, and conduction velocity are mutually related: the larger the diameter, the greater the internodal distance and conduction velocity (Waxman 1980).

There are several types of ion channels, each type having a specific distribution along the axonal membrane. Voltage gated sodium channels are concentrated mainly at the node of Ranvier and in much less quantities at the internodal membrane. Voltage gated slow and fast potassium channels are located at the internodal membrane but are virtually absent at the node of Ranvier (Brismar 1980; Chiu & Ritchie 1981; Neumcke & Stampfli 1982; Elmer et al. 1990). In mammalian nerve fibers the voltage gated sodium channels are essential for the generation of action potentials. This includes the repolarization phase which, contrary to the giant axon of the squid, occurs independent of potassium channels (Waxman & Foster 1980; Kocsis & Waxman 1981). The potassium channels play a role in the stabilization of the axonal membrane and in the generation of action potentials occurring at a high frequency (Ritchie & Chiu 1981; Kocsis et al. 1987; Bostock et al. 1995).

Nerve conduction also depends on the passive

electrical properties of the various parts of a nerve fiber. These properties include the resistance and capacitance (i.e. the ability to store electric charges). The axon cylinder has a low resistance and a high capacitance both of which facilitate the flow of current in the axon. On the other hand, the high resistance and low capacitance of the myelin sheath impair the flow of current through the internode (Koles & Rasminksy 1972).

When depolarization at the node of Ranvier reaches the threshold for action potential generation the voltage gated sodium channels will open resulting in an inward current of sodium ions flowing from extracellular space (for a review see Kandel et al. 1991). Some current will be lost due to minimal leakage through the axon membrane and the myelin sheath and to the slight electrical resistance of the axoplasm. Furthermore, the amount of current is limited by the opening time of sodium channels. Despite the slight loss, the current reaching the next node is more than sufficient (i.e. five to seven times greater than required) to generate a new action potential (Tasaki 1959). The main factor which determines the internodal conduction time is the time needed for the generation of the action potential. The internodal conduction time is about 17–20 μs (Rasminsky & Sears 1972).

When the temperature of the nerve is raised, the sodium channels open faster, but their total opening time shortens. The more rapid sodium activation is accompanied by a shorter action potential rise time and a decreased internodal conduction time (and, consequently, an increased conduction velocity). The more rapid sodium inactivation results in a reduction of current. Above 44°C this reduction is so severe that an inadequate amount of current is available to generate an action potential at the next node of Ranvier. This form of conduction block is known as heat block (Davis et al. 1975).

Demyelinated fibers

The effects of demyelination in single nerve fibers have been studied in animal models and in computer simulations (e.g. McDonald 1963; Koles & Rasminsky 1972; Rasminsky 1973; Schauf & Davis 1974). Complete absence of a myelin segment will result in conduction block. Continuous conduction, as in unmyelinated nerve fibers, will not occur due to the scarcity of sodium channels in the internodal region. Moreover, the membrane potential tends to be hyperpolarized due to the action of the exposed potassium channels.

When only the thickness of the myelin sheath is reduced, conduction will also become impaired, mainly because in damaged myelin capacitance is greater and resistance is smaller than in normal myelin (Schauf & Davis 1974). This results in leakage of current through the damaged myelin. If the reduction in current is not severe enough to cause conduction block it will result in an increased time before the threshold for the generation of an action potential is reached, an increased action potential rise time and an increased internodal conduction time. Under these circumstances an additional reduction in current caused by an increase of the nerve temperature may induce conduction block. Even a slight increment in temperature within the physiological range, e.g. from 36 to 37°C, may produce this effect (Rasminsky 1973).

Electroneurography and electromyography

Nerve conduction studies in patients with a demyelinating neuropathy may reveal the above described effects of demyelination in an indirect manner because compound action potentials (i.e. summated nerve or muscle action potentials) instead of single nerve fiber action potentials are recorded.

Conduction block and temporal dispersion

When there is a focal conduction block in a part of the motor fibers in a nerve the amplitude of the compound muscle action potential (CMAP) after stimulation proximal to the lesion will be reduced whereas the amplitude of the CMAP will be normal after stimulation distal to the lesion. A major problem in the detection of partial conduction block is that such reduction in CMAP amplitude can be caused by several other mechanisms, including temporal dispersion, submaximal stimulation at the proximal site of a nerve segment, Wallerian degeneration, and collateral sprouting. These mechanisms will be discussed.

A nerve consists of fibers of different diameters, so the conduction times of action potentials in these fibers differ. This difference is known as temporal dispersion. In a normal nerve temporal dispersion causes some desynchronization and, consequently, some phase cancellation (i.e. cancellation of the negative phase of one action potential by the positive phase of another) of the motor unit potentials contributing to the CMAP. As the duration of motor unit potentials is considerably greater than the amount of temporal dispersion, the degree of phase cancellation is rather small (Olney et al. 1987). Temporal dispersion and the effects of desynchronization and phase cancellation increase with the distance over which conduction is measured. Thus the CMAP on proximal stimulation of a nerve segment has a slightly reduced amplitude and a slightly increased duration compared with the CMAP on distal stimulation of a nerve segment. In demyelinating neuropathies not all nerve fibers may be affected equally by demyelination. This results in increased temporal dispersion. The reduction in CMAP amplitude and the increase in CMAP duration on proximal versus distal stimulation will then be much greater than in a normal nerve. By means of animal experiments and computer simulations, Rhee et al. (1990) studied the effects of temporal dispersion, conduction distance and different sized motor unit potentials. The results indicated that, with increasing conduction distance, temporal dispersion alone can produce an amplitude reduction of up to 80–90% whereas the reduction in area was maximally 50%. These authors concluded that a CMAP area reduction of more than 50% indicates conduction block in at least some nerve fibers. The effects of temporal dispersion are minimized when conduction is measured across a very short nerve segment of 2–3 cm (inching). An abrupt reduction in CMAP amplitude over such a short segment is considered to be a reliable indicator for conduction block (Cornblath et al. 1991). Unfortunately there are no criteria for the degree of amplitude reduction that is required for this method.

When supramaximal stimulation at the proximal site of a nerve segment is not possible, the amplitude of the CMAP after proximal stimulation is smaller than that after distal stimulation, giving a false impression of conduction block. This can be caused by an increased threshold for electrical stimulation due to demyelination at the proximal stimulation site (Cornblath et al. 1991), and by a relatively deep location of a normal nerve such as the median and ulnar nerve at Erb's point and the tibial nerve at the popliteal fossa.

Demyelination can be accompanied by Wallerian degeneration or subsequent reinnervation. A few days following axonal damage, the axons are unexcitable at a proximal site but still excitable at a more distal site (Gilliatt & Hjorth 1972). Following reinnervation by collateral sprouting, phase cancellation may occur between giant motor unit potentials contributing to the CMAP (Cornblath et al. 1991). Both mechanisms can result in a reduction of CMAP amplitude on proximal versus distal stimulation and can therefore mimick conduction block.

There is no generally accepted electrodiagnostic criterion for conduction block. The suggested criteria include amplitude reduction of 20% (Feasby et al. 1985), amplitude reduction of 30% (Albers et al. 1985), area reduction of 50% (Rhee et al. 1990), and amplitude as well as area reduction of 50% (Lange et al. 1992; van den Berg et al. 1995a,b). The most liberal criterion of 20% is likely to result in false positive findings as this value can also be found in normal subjects (Oh et al. 1994). On the other hand, the most strict criteria may underestimate the presence of conduction block as has been suggested by Barbieri et al. (1996).

Conduction block cannot be assessed reliably by means of sensory nerve conduction studies because, even in a normal nerve, there is a considerable reduction in compound sensory nerve action potential (SNAP) amplitude on proximal versus distal stimulation. This is explained by the fact that the duration of individual nerve action potentials contributing to the SNAP is of the same magnitude as the amount of temporal dispersion (Olney et al. 1987).

The finding of abnormal temporal dispersion can be used as evidence of focal demyelination. An increase in the duration of the CMAP on proximal versus distal stimulation of more than 30% has been considered to be indicative of abnormal temporal dispersion due to demyelination (Lange et al. 1992). This criterion has not been validated by comparing results in patients with demyelinating neuropathy, patients with axonal neuropathy and controls. Moreover, the amount of temporal dispersion which can be found in normal nerves depends on the nerve which is investigated (Oh et al. 1994).

Conduction velocity

An important question is whether it is possible to differentiate axonal damage and demyelination by measuring maximal nerve conduction velocity.

In cats with diphteric neuritis the maximal conduction velocity in mixed and sensory nerves was on average 26% slower than in controls (McDonald 1963). These values could not be explained by loss of fast conducting fibers. During clinical recovery values of 25–35% were found. There was considerable overlap with values in normal animals.

In patients with the hypertrophic type of Charcot–Marie–Tooth neuropathy the maximal sensory and motor conduction velocity in, respectively, the sural and peroneal nerve was slower than 60% of the normal mean whereas in patients with the neuronal type it was always faster than 60% of the normal mean (Buchtal & Behse 1977). In the patients with the hypertrophic type, slowing of motor conduction was 5–12% greater than slowing of sensory conduction. Although distal motor latency was greater in the hypertrophic than in the neuronal type, the values overlapped in both types.

On the basis of these findings criteria were developed for values of conduction velocity and derived variables that are suggestive of demyelination. The criteria of Kelly (1983) include a reduction of maximal motor conduction velocity to less than 60% of the normal mean. The criteria of Cornblath (1990) include a reduction of maximal motor conduction velocity to less than 80% of the lower limit of normal, absent F waves, minimal F wave latency greater than 120% of the upper limit of normal, and distal motor latency greater than 125% of the upper limit of normal. These values were 70, 150, and 150%, respectively, if the CMAP amplitude is less than 80% of the lower limit of normal, probably to account for the effect of axonal degeneration on conduction velocity. When the CMAP amplitude is very small, however, a value in the demyelinating range is unlikely to constitute sufficient evidence of a demyelinating neuropathy because in that case only a few motor units can be investigated. Considering the overlap between distal motor latencies in demyelinating and axonal neuropathies (Buchtal & Behse 1977), it is doubtful whether this variable is useful for the distinction between axonal damage and demyelination. It is nevertheless used in the current criteria for chronic inflammatory demyelinating polyneuropathy (CIDP) and multifocal motor neuropathy (MMN). It must be emphasized that in inflammatory neuropathies, and especially in the acute phase of the Guillain-Barré syndrome, the conduction velocity can be moderately reduced (McDonald 1963; Asbury & Cornblath 1990; Meulstee et al. 1995). Thus a conduction velocity value that does not fulfill the criteria for demyelination cannot be used as an argument against demyelination.

Temperature

For several reasons it is important that nerve temperature is about 37°C. First, the above described criteria for conduction slowing in demyelination are based on investigations performed at about 37°C (McDonald 1963; Buchtal & Behse 1977). Second, the induction of conduction block by temperature increment, as observed in demyelinated single nerve fibers, has recently been confirmed by electroneurography in human patients (Chaudhry et al. 1993; Franssen et al. 1995) (Figure 5.1). This implies that conduction block can be missed when the investigated limb is too cold. Third, in demyelinating neuropathy the increase in maximal conduction velocity per degree centigrade is different from that in normal nerves so that correction factors cannot be used (Davis et al. 1975; Notermans et al. 1994). Fourth, the occurrence of fibrillation potentials diminishes with muscle temperature (Feinstein et al. 1945; Notermans et al. 1994). When the skin temperature at the wrist or the ankle is below 32°C it is likely that the near nerve temperature is reduced. In that case, the limb has to be warmed in water of 37°C for a sufficiently long time to obtain a nerve temperature of about 37°C (Franssen & Wieneke 1994). The necessary warming time depends on the skin temperature. When this lies between 27 and 32°C at least 20 minutes of warming are necessary. Warming by an infrared heater device is insufficient (Geerlings & Mechelse 1985).

Electrodiagnostic protocols

Electrodiagnostic protocols have been formulated for the differential diagnosis or for the evaluation of neuropathies (Donofrio & Albers 1990; Albers 1993). The following protocol is based on those used in the

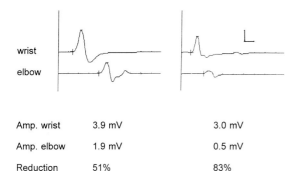

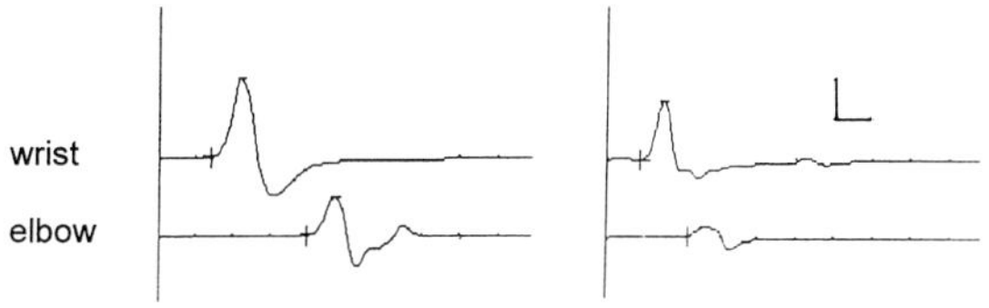

Amp. wrist	3.9 mV	3.0 mV
Amp. elbow	1.9 mV	0.5 mV
Reduction	51%	83%

Figure 5.1 *CMAPs following stimulation of the median nerve in a patient with multifocal motor neuropathy at 25°C (left) and at 40°C (right). The reduction in amplitude on proximal versus distal stimulation is larger at 40°C than at 25°C, indicating that the amount of nerve fibers with conduction block increases with temperature. Time and amplitude scales are 5 ms and 2 mV, respectively. AMP: baseline to negative peak amplitude of the CMAP.*

diagnosis of CIDP and MMN (van den Berg et al. 1995a; Franssen et al. 1997).

Electroneurography and electromyography

After it has been ensured that the limbs are sufficiently warmed, motor conduction to distal muscles is investigated in one of each of the following nerves: median nerve (stimulation at the wrist, elbow, axilla, and Erb's point), ulnar nerve (stimulation at the wrist, 5 cm distal to the elbow, 5 cm proximal to the elbow, axilla, and Erb's point), peroneal nerve (stimulation at the ankle, 5 cm distal to the fibular head and 5 cm proximal to the fibular head), and tibial nerve (stimulation at the ankle and at the popliteal fossa). Sensory conduction following distal stimulation is investigated in one median and one sural nerve. Concentric needle electromyography includes at least a distal and a proximal muscle of one arm and one leg. If this reveals abnormalities the investigation is extended to exclude nerve or root compression. When multifocal motor neuropathy is suspected but no evidence of conduction block can be obtained, the investigation is extended to homologous nerves at the other side and to segments of nerves innervating proximal arm muscles, i.e. musculocutaneous nerve (stimulation at the axilla and Erb's point, recording from the biceps brachii muscle), and median nerve (stimulation at the elbow, axilla, and Erb's point, recording from the flexor carpi radialis muscle). If necessary, high voltage stimulation of cervical roots can be applied to detect proximal conduction block (Lange et al. 1992). In case of suspected conduction block in an arm nerve segment, an attempt is made to localize the block by inching. For nerve segments in the forearm, nerve anastomosis has to be excluded when an amplitude reduction is found. When no responses can be obtained in hand or foot muscles following distal stimulation, conduction is investigated in the median nerve to the flexor carpi radialis muscle and in the peroneal nerve to the tibialis anterior muscle. If no sensory responses can be obtained sensory conduction studies are extended to the ulnar and radial nerves and to nerves at the other side.

The following motor conduction variables are measured: distal CMAP amplitude, reduction in CMAP amplitude and area for each segment, increase in CMAP duration for each segment, conduction velocity in each segment, minimal F wave latency, distal motor latency. The amplitude, area, and duration are measured from the negative part of the CMAP. Sensory conduction variables include SNAP amplitude and conduction velocity.

Criteria for demyelination

The criteria for demyelination include definitive conduction block (area reduction of at least 50%, regardless of conduction distance or amplitude reduction of at least 30% detected by inching), possible conduction block (amplitude reduction of at least 30% for arm nerves or of at least 40% for leg nerves), increased temporal dispersion (duration increase of at least 30%), motor nerve conduction velocity less than 75% of the lower limit of normal, distal motor latency more than 130% of the upper limit of normal, absent F waves, shortest F wave latency more than 130% of the upper limit of normal. For the diagnosis of conduction block the amplitude of the negative part of the CMAP has to be at least 1 mV. For the conduction velocity, distal motor latency and F wave criteria to be valid the amplitude of the negative part of the CMAP, following distal stimulation, has to be at least 0.5 mV.

Criteria for axonal degeneration

Criteria suggestive of axonal damage (Kelly 1983; Notermans et al. 1996) include those that require the absence of demyelination (no evidence of conduction block or abnormal temporal dispersion, conduction velocity and minimal F wave latency and distal motor latency not in the demyelinating range) and those that require positive evidence of axonal neuropathy (spontaneous muscle fiber activity and polyphasic or giant motor unit potentials on concentric needle electromyography, reduced amplitude of CMAP or SNAP after distal stimulation). It must be stressed that the latter can also be caused by very distally located conduction block, although in most instances this is difficult to prove.

Criteria for CIDP and MMN

For the diagnosis of CIDP and MMN different sets of electrophysiological criteria, often in combination with clinical and laboratory criteria have been formulated.

The criteria for CIDP of Barohn et al. (1989) require a motor conduction velocity in the demyelinating range in at least two nerves. The criteria of Albers & Kelly (1989) have been modified by the American Academy of Neurology (1991) and by the Dutch Working group on diagnostic criteria for CIDP and MMN (Franssen et al. 1997). The latter set requires three out of the following items: (1) definitive or possible motor conduction block in at least one nerve segment, (2) motor conduction velocity in the demyelinating range in at least two nerves, (3) distal motor latency in the demyelinating range in at least two nerves, and (4) absent F waves or minimal F wave latency in the demyelinating range in at least one nerve. The criteria for demyelination are those described in Criteria for demyelination. The F wave criterion can only be included if the distal motor latency and conduction velocity in that nerve do not reach values compatible with demyelination. Abnormalities at common compression sites do not count, unless sensory conduction across that site is normal. On the basis of the combined clinical, laboratory, and electrophysiological findings the diagnosis of CIDP is definite (requiring at least three electrophysiological items), probable (requiring at least one electrophysiological item), or possible.

Bromberg (1991) tested the sets of Barohn et al. (1989), Albers & Kelly (1989) and the American Academy of Neurology (1991) by applying them to retrospectively studied patients with CIDP, motor neuron disease, or diabetic polyneuropathy. There was no significant difference in diagnostic sensitivity for CIDP among the three sets, the maximal sensitivity being approximately 66%. Nerve conduction studies were however limited to the lower arm and not every patient underwent the same protocol. It is therefore possible that a greater sensitivity can be achieved with more extended and standard protocols.

The electrophysiological criteria for MMN (Franssen et al. 1997) require at least the presence of motor conduction block, normal or near normal sensory conduction (Corse et al. 1996), and evidence of denervation and reinnervation on concentric needle electromyography. In addition motor conduction velocity, minimal F wave latency, and distal motor latency can be compatible with demyelination. On the basis of combined clinical, laboratory, and electrophysiological findings the diagnosis of MMN is definite (requiring definite conduction block), probable (requiring possible conduction block), or possible (requiring evidence of demyelination without conduction block).

References

Ad hoc Subcommittee of the American Academy of Neurology (1991). Research criteria for diagnosis of chronic inflammatory demyelinating polyneuropathy (CIDP). *Neurology* **41**: 617–618.

Albers, J.W. (1993) Clinical neurophysiology of generalized polyneuropathy. *J. Clin. Neurophysiol.* **10**: 149–166.

Albers, J.W., Donofrio, P.D., and McGonagle, T.K. (1985). Sequential electrodiagnostic abnormalities in acute inflammatory demyelinating polyradiculoneuropathy. *Muscle Nerve* **8**: 528–539.

Albers, J.W. and Kelly, J.J. (1989). Acquired inflammatory demyelinating polyneuropathies: clinical and electrodiagnostic features. *Muscle Nerve* **12**: 435–451.

Asbury, A.K. and Cornblath, D.R. (1990). Assessment of current diagnostic criteria for Guillain-Barré syndrome. *Ann. Neurol.* **27** (suppl.): S21–S24.

Barbieri, S., Cappellari, A., Nobile-Orazio, E., Meucci, N., and Scarlato, G. (1996). Is partial motor conduction block in multifocal motor neuropathy a dynamic entity. *J. Neurol.* **243** (suppl. 2): S5.

Barohn, R.J., Kissel, J.T., Warmolts, J.R., and Mendell, J.R. (1989). Chronic inflammatory demyelinating polyradiculoneuropathy. *Arch. Neurol.* **46**: 878–884.

Bostock, H., Sharief, M.K., Reid, G., and Murray, N.M.F. (1995). Axonal ion channel dysfunction in amyotrophic lateral sclerosis. *Brain* **118**: 217–225.

Brismar, T. (1980). Potential clamp analysis of membrane currents in rat myelinated nerve fibers. *J. Physiol.* **298**: 171–184.

Bromberg, M.B. (1991). Comparison of electrodiagnostic criteria for primary demyelination in chronic polyneuropathy. *Muscle Nerve* **14**: 968–976.

Buchthal, F. and Behse, F. (1977). Peroneal muscular atrophy (PMA) and related disorders. I. Clinical manifestations as related to biopsy findings, nerve conduction and electromyography. *Brain* **100**: 41–66.

Chaudhry, W., Crawford, T.O., and DeRossett, S.E. (1993). Thermal sensitivity in demyelinating neuropathy. *Muscle Nerve* **16**: 301–306.

Chiu, S.Y. and Ritchie, J.M. (1981). Evidence for the presence of potassium channels in the internodal region of acutely demyelinated mammalian single nerve fibers. *J. Physiol.* **313**: 415–437.

Cornblath, D.R. (1990). Electrophysiology in Guillain-Barré syndrome. *Ann. Neurol.* **27** (suppl.): S17–S20.

Cornblath, D.R., Sumner, A.J., Daube, J., Gilliat, R.W., Brown, W.F., Parry, G.J., Albers, J.W., Miller, R.G., and Petajan, J. (1991). Conduction block in clinical practice. *Muscle Nerve* **14**: 869–871.

Corse, A.M., Chaudhry, V., Crawford, T.O., Cornblath, D.R., Kuncl, R.W., and Griffin, J.W. (1996). Sensory nerve pathology in multifocal motor neuropathy. *Ann. Neurol.* **39**: 319–325.

Davis, F.A., Schauf, C.L., Reed, B.J., and Kesler, R.L. (1975). Experimental studies of the effects of extrinsic factors on conduction in normal and demyelinated nerve. I. Temperature. *J. Neurol. Neurosurg. Psychiatry* **39**: 442–448.

Donofrio, P.D. and Albers, J.W. (1990). AAEM minimonograph no. 34: polyneuropathy: classification by nerve conduction studies and electromyography. *Muscle Nerve* **13**: 889–903.

Elmer, L.W., Black, J.A., Waxman, S.G., et al. (1990). The voltage-dependent sodium channel in mammalian PNS and CNS: antibody characterization and immunocytochemical localization. *Brain Res.* **532**: 222–231.

Feasby, T.E., Brown, W.F., Gilbert, J.J., and Hahn, A.F. (1985). The pathological basis of conduction block in human neuropathies. *J. Neurol. Neurosurg. Psychiatry* **48**: 239–244.

Feinstein, B., Pattle, R.E., and Weddell, G. (1945). Metabolic factors affecting fibrillation in denervated muscle. *J. Neurol. Neurosurg. Psychiatry* **8**: 1–11.

Franssen, H., Vermeulen, M., and Jennekens, F.G.I. (1997). Chronic inflammatory neuropathies. In *Diagnostic Criteria for Neuromuscular Disorders*, 2nd edn, ed. A.E.H. Emery. London: Royal Society of Medicine Press.

Franssen, H. and Wieneke, G.H. (1994). Nerve conduction and temperature: necessary warming time. *Muscle Nerve* **17**: 336–344.

Franssen, H., Wieneke, G.H., Notermans, N.C., and Van den Berg, L.H. (1995). Temperature dependent conduction block in peripheral neuropathy. *Neuro-Orthopedics* **17/18**: 75–82.

Geerlings, A.H.C. and Mechelse, K. (1985). Temperature and nerve conduction velocity, some practical problems. *Electromyogr. Clin. Neurophysiol.* **25**: 253–260.

Gilliatt, R.W. and Hjorth, R.J. (1972). Nerve conduction during Wallerian degeneration in the baboon. *J. Neurol. Neurosurg. Psychiatry* **35**: 335–341.

Kandel, E.R., Schwartz, J.H., and Jessell, T.M. (1991). *Principles of Neural Science*, 3rd edn, pp. 66–118; 250–252. New York: Elsevier Science Publishing Co.

Kelly, J.J. (1983). The electrodiagnostic findings in peripheral neuropathy associated with monoclonal gammopathy. *Muscle Nerve* **6**: 504–509.

Kocsis, J.D., Eng, D.L., Gordon, T.R., et al. (1987). Functional differences between 4-aminopyridine and tetraethylammonium-sensitive potassium channels in myelinated axons. *Neurosci. Lett.* **75**: 193–198.

Kocsis, J.D. and Waxman, S.G. (1981). Action potential electrogenesis in mammalian central axons. In *Demyelinating Diseases: Basis and Clinical Electrophysiology*, ed. S.G. Waxman and J.M. Ritchie, pp. 299–312. New York: Raven Press.

Koles, Z.J. and Rasminsky, M. (1972). A computer simulation of conduction in demyelinated nerve. *J. Physiol.* **227**: 351–364.

Lange, D.J., Trojaborg, W., Latov, N., Hays, A.P., Younger, D.S., Uncini, A., Blake, D.M., Hirano, M., Burns, S.M., Lovelace, R.E., and Rowland, L.P. (1992). Multifocal motor neuropathy with conduction block: Is it a distinct clinical entity? *Neurology* **42**: 497–505.

McDonald, W.I. (1963). The effects of experimental demyelination on conduction in peripheral nerve: a histological and electrophysiological study. II. Electrophysiological observations. *Brain* **86**: 501–524.

Meulstee, J., Van der Meché, F.G.A., and the Dutch Guillain–Barré Study Group (1995). Electrodiagnostic criteria for polyneuropathy and demyelination: application in 135 patients with Guillain–Barré syndrome. *J. Neurol. Neurosurg. Psychiatry* **59**: 482–486.

Neumcke. B. and Stampfli R. (1982). Sodium currents and sodium-current fluctuations in rat myelinated nerve fibers. *J. Physiol.* **329**: 163–184.

Notermans, N.C., Franssen, H., Wieneke, G.H., and Wokke, J.H.J. (1994). Temperature dependence of nerve conduction and EMG in neuropathy associated with gammopathy. *Muscle Nerve* **17**: 516–522.

Notermans, N.C., Wokke, J.H.J., Van den Berg, L.H., Van der Graaf, Y., Franssen, H., Teunissen, L.L., and Lokhorst, H.M. (1996). Chronic idiopathic axonal polyneuropathy. Comparison of patients with and without monoclonal gammopathy. *Brain* **119**: 421–427.

Oh, S.J., Kim, D.E., and Kuruoglu, H.R. (1994). What is the best diagnostic index of conduction block and temporal dispersion? *Muscle Nerve* **17**: 489–493.

Olney, R.K., Budingen, H.J., and Miller, R.G. (1987). The effect of temporal dispersion on compound action potential area in human peripheral nerve. *Muscle Nerve* **10**: 728–733.

Rasminsky, M. (1973). The effects of temperature on conduction in demyelinated single nerve fibers. *Arch. Neurol.* **28**: 287–292.

Rasminsky, M. and Sears, T.A. (1972). Internodal conduction in undissected demyelinated nerve fibers. *J. Physiol.* **227**: 323–350.

Rhee, E.K., England, J.D., and Sumner, A.J. (1990). A computer simulation of conduction block: effects produced by actual block versus interphase cancellation. *Ann. Neurol.* **28**: 146–156.

Ritchie, J.M. and Chiu, S.Y. (1981). Distribution of sodium and potassium channels in mammalian myelinated nerve. In *Demyelinating Diseases: Basic and Clinical Electrophysiology*, ed. S.G. Waxman and J.M. Ritchie, pp. 329–342. New York: Raven Press.

Schauf, C.L. and Davis, F.A. (1974). Impulse conduction in multiple sclerosis: a theoretical basis for modification by temperature and pharmacological agents. *J. Neurol. Neurosurg. Psychiatry* **37**: 152–161.

Tasaki, I. (1959). Conduction of the nerve impulse. In *Handbook of Physiology*, Section 1, *Neurophysiology*, vol. 1, ed. J. Field, H. Magoun and V.E. Hall, pp. 75–122. Washington DC: American Physiological Society.

Van den Berg, L.H., Franssen, H., and Wokke, J.H.J. (1995a). Improvement of multifocal motor neuropathy during long-term weekly treatment with human immunoglobulin. *Neurology* **45**: 987–988.

Van den Berg, L.H., Kerkhof, H., Oey, P.L., Franssen, H., Mollee, I., Vermeulen, M., Jennekens, F.G.I., and Wokke, J.H.J. (1995b). Treatment of multifocal motor neuropathy with high dose intravenous immunoglobulins: a double blind, placebo controlled study. *J. Neurol. Neurosurg. Psychiatry* **59**: 248–252.

Waxman, S.G. (1980). Determinants of conduction velocity in myelinated nerve fibers. *Muscle Nerve* **3**: 141–150.

Waxman, S.G. and Foster, R.E. (1980). Ionic channel distribution and heterogeneity of the axon membrane in myelinated fibers. *Brain Res. Rev.* **2**: 205–240.

6 Immunopathological studies in immune-mediated neuropathies

M. Corbo and A.P. Hays

Introduction

The aim of immunopathological evaluation of nerve is to characterize the cellular and humoral features of the immune system in disease states as it is expressed in tissue sections. The information provides insight into the pathogenesis of tissue injury at the cellular level, and it can be used to classify diseases for diagnostic purposes. The main effectors of cell injury include the T cells, B cells, macrophages, immunoglobulins, complement system, and cytokines. The chief function of the immune system is to respond to foreign antigen in a highly specific way to eliminate pathogenic agents, but the immunological reaction can injure tissue or the immune system can act abnormally to attack a self antigen and produce an autoimmune disease. Historically, Guillain-Barré syndrome (GBS) was first thought to be an autoimmune disorder mediated by lymphocytes and macrophages, in part because it resembles an animal model, experimental allergic neuropathy. This disorder can be induced by immunization of experimental animals by nerve tissue (or myelin antigen), and it can be produced by transfer of T cells (but not immunoglobulins) into a naive animal (Arnason and Soliven 1993). However, the animal model may not be analogous to the human disease based on recent immunological and immunopathological studies of GBS (see below).

Progress in the immunopathology of human disease was slow until about 1980 and later when conceptual and methodological advances emerged. Studies of GBS have provided increasing evidence that autoreactive antibodies to peripheral nerve antigens are important in the pathogenesis of the disease. At about the same time, Latov et al. (1980) discovered that the IgM paraprotein of some of the patients with chronic demyelinating neuropathy recognized a peripheral myelin antigen. These observations focused interest on the humoral immune system as a possible cause of autoimmune disorders of nerve. This idea prompted numerous immunohistochemical studies using antibodies as reagents to identify components of the immune system in peripheral nerve. During the last 15 years, new reagents of increased specificity using affinity-purified immunoglobulins or F(ab′)2 fragments and monoclonal antibodies have become commercially available for more definitive histochemical studies.

The results of the early histochemical studies of

peripheral nerve have been modified by later work. For example, the first available probes for identified human complement proteins were limited in number and specificity. In potential autoimmune neuropathies, antibodies to C3 or C3b recognized only diffuse protein in the endoneurium, a non-specific finding, but they usually did not react with complement components as part of an immune complex with immunoglobulin on myelin sheaths (Takatsu et al. 1985). Later, when antibodies to C3d, a split fragment of C3b, became available commercially, the reagent could demonstrate the complement component in truncated form at the same site as the IgM (Hays et al. 1988). This new antibody reagent provided important evidence that autoantibodies are pathogenic in several disorders of nerve including GBS (Hafer-Macko et al. 1996a,b). Nerve biopsies that contain immune complexes of IgM or IgG and C3d on nerve fibers help distinguish immune-mediated disorders from others for diagnostic purposes.

Methodology

Nerve biopsy studies are important both for research and diagnostic purposes. Routinely, the nerve is submitted for routine histology (paraffin sections) and resin histology (semi-thin sections of plastic sections, about 1 μm thick) for diagnosis of vasculitic neuropathy, amyloidosis and other disorders. The neuropathy is classified as an axonopathy or a myelinopathy based on semi-thin sections, and if necessary, examination of teased nerve fibers or electron microscopic evaluation of the nerve. Immunohistochemical stains are best performed using cryosections of snap-frozen, unfixed tissue for analysis of immunoglobulins and complement proteins although some investigators prefer paraffin sections of formalin fixed tissue (Brandtzaeg 1981). Normally, the endoneurium contains abundant IgG with less IgA and little or no detectable IgM. To remove loosely bound immunoglobulins from the tissue, freshly cut sections are first washed in phosphate buffered saline, pH 7.4, for 5–10 minutes before they are fixed with acetone or ethanol. The sections are then immunostained with fluorescein-conjugated rabbit antibodies that recognize the heavy chain of IgG, IgA, and IgM and epitopes of C3d (Takatsu et al. 1985). Some prefer to immunostain fibrinogen as a marker for a protein that has broken through from the circulation into extravascular sites as an artifact of the surgical procedure or of a delay in freezing or fixing the tissue to help to interpret deposits of immunoglobulins and complement proteins. The conjugated antibodies are diluted 1:20 except for those specific for IgG, which is diluted 1:100. This technique is designated as the *direct method* and is distinguished from the *indirect method* where the antibody reagent is unconjugated and is subsequently localized using a second or third antibody conjugate of fluorochrome, texas red, peroxidase, or another molecule for indirectly visualizing the antigen. Routinely, we perform immunostaining for C5b-9 (membrane attack complex) using a monoclonal antibody in the indirect method. This recognizes a neoantigen of the complex, an epitope that is only expressed after the terminal components of complement have been activated. Immunoperoxidase stains of immunoglobulins and complement proteins yield similar results, and the method has the advantage of providing a permanent preparation. The immunofluorescence method can be used for high resolution confocal microscopy (Corbo et al. 1992; Santoro et al. 1992), and it can be easily employed for double or paired labeling of two different antigens in the same section, for example, IgM and C3d (Hays et al. 1988).

Other histochemical stains are performed as indicated by the pathological findings. If mononuclear inflammatory cells are present, B cells can be distinguished from T cells as a first step to identifying a B cell lymphoma or an inflammatory disorder (Thomas et al. 1990b). If immune complexes are found in the nerve, they can be stained for lambda and kappa light chains to determine whether the immunoglobulin is limited to one type, a finding that suggests monoclonality (Takatsu et al. 1985). In amyloidosis, the light chain form of amyloid in primary amyloidosis can be distinguished from that of the protein, transthyretin, in familial amyloidotic neuropathy by immunohistochemical stains using antibodies of an appropriate specificity (Ii et al. 1992). Other examples are described in the following sections.

The indirect immunofluorescence method can also be used to determine whether an autoantibody binds to potential target antigens that are expressed in the central or peripheral nervous system. Cryosections of normal tissue are prepared in a similar fashion or are unfixed, but then are exposed to the serum of the patient in serial dilutions ranging from 1:20 to 1:1000 or higher for 1 hour. The bound immunoglobulin is detected with a conjugated antibody to one or more human immunoglobulin isotypes, usually human IgG and IgM (Takatsu et al. 1985; Corbo et al. 1992). The patient's serum is omitted or replaced by serum of a normal individual as a control. Serum from normal individuals contain low titer autoantibodies to neural tissue, particularly to neurofilament protein of axons. Therefore, only antibodies that bind to neural structures at high titers of 1: 100 or greater are considered to be potentially pathogenic. In paraneoplastic neuropathy, for example, high titer IgG binds to nuclei of nerve cells of the dorsal root ganglion and the central nervous system in patients with a small cell carcinoma of the lung and anti-Hu antibodies (Graus et al. 1985).

Neuropathy associated with monoclonal gammopathy

Waldenström's macroglobulinemia and IgM monoclonal gammopathy of undetermined significance (MGUS)

Neuropathies associated with IgM monoclonal gammopathy were described initially in patients with Waldenström's macroglobulinemia, and infiltration of nerve by malignant B cells was thought to be a possible mechanism of nerve damage (Logothetis et al. 1960). Most nerve biopsies do not show neoplastic infiltration, however, and the first observation of monoclonal IgM (M-protein, paraprotein) deposits in sural nerve suggested that the immunoglobulin is a pathogenic autoantibody (Iwashita et al. 1974; Propp et al. 1975). In some patients with either MGUS or malignant IgM gammopathies, the monoclonal IgM reacts with peripheral nerve myelin antigens (Latov et al. 1980; Latov & Steck 1995), first identified as myelin-associated glycoprotein (MAG) (Braun et al. 1982). In morphological studies, the affected sural nerves in patients with anti-MAG monoclonal gammopathy typically present the characteristic features of a chronic demyelinating neuropathy (Propp et al. 1975; Nemni et al. 1983; Smith et al. 1983; Mendell et al. 1985), consistent with the myelin specificity of the autoantibodies. In both MGUS (Smith et al. 1983; Mendell et al. 1985; van den Berg et al. 1996) and Waldenström's macroglobulinemia (Propp et al. 1975; Vital et al. 1975). Electron microscopic examination shows widening of myelin lamellae at the minor dense line, typically located in the outer half of the myelin sheath. This myelin morphological alteration is considered to be relatively specific for these IgM neuropathies, although it has been described in other conditions (King and Thomas 1984; Vital et al. 1986). Lymphocytes are usually not encountered; but sparse histiocytes are found, and they rarely penetrate the surface of myelin sheaths and seem to strip off layers of myelin (Vital et al. 1991), a typical feature of GBS and chronic inflammatory demyelinating polyneuropathy. Unmyelinated axons are frequently spared, and only in the more severe cases are there abnormalities of the corresponding Schwann cell processes.

Direct immunohistochemical studies of the sural nerve or other nerves from patients with anti-MAG M-proteins demonstrate IgM deposits on myelin sheaths (Figure 6.1a) (Mendell et al. 1985; Takatsu et al. 1985). The IgM in the deposits are limited to one immunoglobulin light chain, usually a kappa type, the same light chain type as the corresponding circulating paraprotein (Propp et al. 1975; Mendell et al. 1985; Takatsu et al. 1985). The monoclonal IgM in the deposits and the serum also have the same idiotypic determinant (Takatsu et al. 1985). The IgM is localized to the periphery of nerve fibers, and it corresponds to zones of widened myelin lamellae (Mendell et al. 1985). Less often, the paraprotein is found in a periaxonal location. Complement components, such as C1q, C3d, and C5, colocalize with the monoclonal IgM on myelin sheaths (Figure 6.1b), suggesting a complement-mediated form of demyelination (Hays et al. 1988; Monaco et al. 1990); however, no C5b-9 (membrane attack complex) is found in nerve in most cases (Kissel et al. 1986; A.P. Hays and G. Rosoklija, unpublished data). The finding of immune complexes of monoclonal IgM and C3d on myelin sheaths of sural nerve is a useful diagnostic feature of these neuropathies although the abnormality is not completely specific. Also, a minority of the

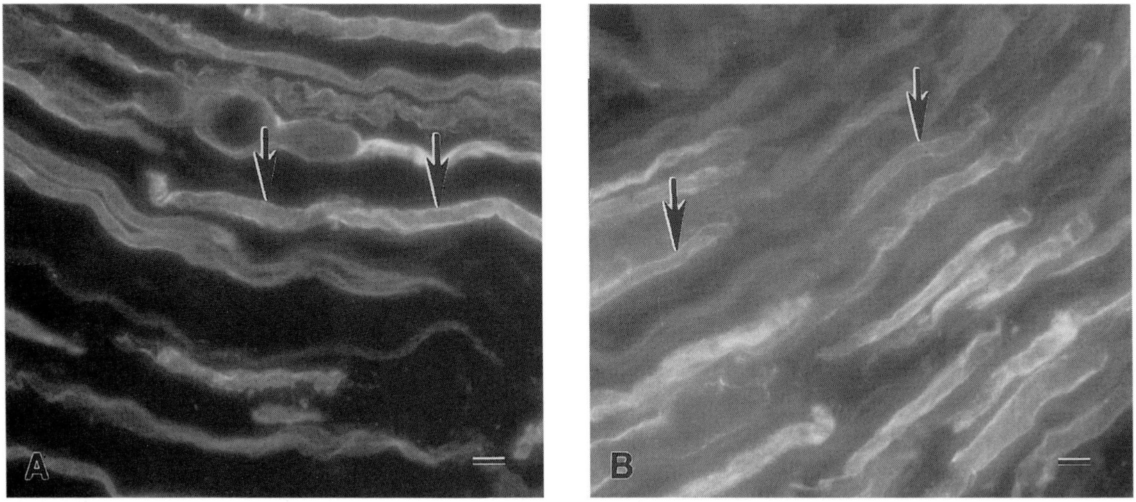

Figure 6.1 *Longitudinal cryosections of a sural nerve biospy specimen in a patient with neuropathy and an IgM paraprotein reactive to myelin-associated glycoprotein. The sections are stained by the direct immunofluorescence method using fluorescein-conjugated antibodies that recognize human IgM (A) and C3d (B). Myelin sheaths exhibit strongly immunoreactive IgM and C3d (arrows). The staining is chiefly located along the edge of myelin sheaths when observed in transverse sections (not shown). Less intense immunostaining of C3d is present in the endoneurium. The fluorescein-conjugated antibodies to C3d also react with whole C3, and this complement component is located in endoneurium in normal nerve. Bars: 10 μm.*

patients have no detectable IgM or C3d (or both) in the nerve biopsy.

The compact portions of myelin sheaths are not immunostained for IgM by the direct immunofluorescence method, but the compact myelin is bound by the IgM when the human anti-MAG antibodies are applied to normal human peripheral nerve using the indirect immunohistochemical method (Abrams et al. 1982; Smith et al. 1983; Nobile-Orazio et al. 1984; Takatsu et al. 1985; van den Berg et al. 1996). This is in contrast to the known periaxonal localization of MAG, which is not expressed in compact myelin (Trapp and Quarles 1984). The differences between the direct and indirect immunofluorescence methods can be explained by the observation that the IgM monoclonal antibodies bind to a carbohydrate epitope that is shared by MAG and by several other glycoproteins and glycolipids in peripheral nerve (Latov & Steck 1995). These antigens include Po glycoprotein, PMP22 and two sulfated glucuronyl glycolipids, and they are expressed in the compact portion of myelin sheaths of peripheral nerve. In an immunohistochemical study using sera from 20 patients with this form of neuropathy, the intensity of bound IgM to myelin sheaths correlated better with the titers of antibodies against MAG than those against the crossreactive glycolipid sulfoglucuronyl paragloboside (SGPG) (van den Berg et al. 1996).

In some cases, the monoclonal IgM disclosed specificities other than anti-MAG (Dellagi et al. 1982; Ilyas et al. 1985) even though demyelination seemed to be the chief mechanism of nerve injury. Some of these monoclonal IgM paraproteins react with GM1 ganglioside, disialosyl gangliosides or sulfatide (see below). When monoclonal IgM reacts with chondroitin sulfate C, a constituent of axons and connective tissue, the sural nerve biopsy shows the morphological features of an axonal neuropathy, and the axon rather than myelin is considered to be the chief site of nerve damage (Nemni et al. 1983; Sherman et al. 1983; Mamoli et al. 1992). Nemni et al. (1983) demonstrated electron-opaque amorphous material in the extracellular space of the endoneurium. The material is probably composed of the monoclonal IgM based on the direct immunofluorescence pattern of immunoreactive IgM heavy chains and light chains in the same nerves (Sherman et al. 1983). It also contains strongly immunoreactive C3d

(A.P. Hays, unpublished data), a finding that suggests that the IgM autoantibody reacts with antigen. These extracellular components are presumably localized in the connective tissue of the endoneurium as indicated by binding of the paraprotein to endoneurium using the indirect immunofluorescence method (Freddo et al. 1985). The monoclonal IgM anti-chondroitin sulfate C can bind also to the Schmidt-Lanterman incisures (Quattrini et al. 1991).

IgG and IgA monoclonal gammopathies of undetermined significance

IgG and IgA paraproteins in patients with neuropathy are less common than those with IgM paraproteins, and the reported pathological nerve findings are heterogeneous. Nerve biopsies from patients with IgG monoclonal gammopathy and neuropathy have shown signs of either demyelination or axonal degeneration (Read et al. 1978; Ohnishi and Hirano 1981; Sewell et al. 1981). The sural nerve of two patients had deposits of immunoreactive IgG on myelin sheaths (Sewell et al. 1981; Bosch et al. 1982). Three other patients with an axonal neuropathy had an IgG paraprotein that reacted with the low molecular weight subunit of neurofilament protein (68 kDa). Direct immunohistochemical studies of nerve showed deposits of IgG limited to one light chain type in the axons (Nemni et al. 1990; Fazio et al. 1992). Moorhouse et al. (1992) described localization of immunotactoid-like structures within the axons of myelinated and unmyelinated nerve fibers in the sural nerve of a patient with an IgG paraprotein and axonal neuropathy.

In patients with IgA monoclonal gammopathies a variable pathological picture of demyelinating, axonal, or mixed neuropathies have been reported (Nemni et al. 1991; Simmons et al. 1993). Another patient had amyotrophic lateral sclerosis, breast carcinoma and an IgA paraprotein that bound to the high molecular weight subunit of neurofilament protein (200 kDa) and a surface membrane antigen of unknown identity (Hays et al. 1990). At autopsy, the axons and motor nerve cell bodies contained strongly immunostained IgA of the same subtype as the circulating paraprotein.

Multiple myeloma and osteosclerotic myeloma

Peripheral neuropathy in multiple myeloma is uncommon (Kelly et al. 1981). Although tumor infiltration of the nerve can occur (Barron et al. 1960; Hesselvik 1969), it is usually not found even with extensive postmortem examination of the peripheral nervous system (Victor et al. 1958). More commonly, amyloid infiltrates nerves in multiple myeloma (see below); however, the neuropathy in most cases are not associated with either amyloidosis or tumor infiltration (Kelly et al. 1981). The neuropathy is clinically heterogeneous but most often exhibits progressive sensorimotor dysfunction. The nerves show axonal degeneration with loss of myelinated and unmyelinated fibers, and signs of axonal regeneration (Walsh 1971; Asbury and Johnson 1978; Ohi et al. 1985). Evidence of axonal atrophy as a primary process with secondary demyelination has been obtained in the nerve biopsy (Ohi et al. 1985). Infrequently, the pathological changes in nerve of myelomatous polyneuropathy suggest a demyelinating process (Victor et al. 1958; Asbury and Johnson 1978; Delauche et al. 1981). Immunohistochemical stains of biopsied nerve demonstrate greater staining of IgG and one of the light chains in the endoneurium (A.P. Hays, unpublished data), but the immunoglobulin and the C3 component of complement is not selectively concentrated at the periphery of nerve fibers as in anti-MAG neuropathy.

Osteosclerotic myeloma is an uncommon variant of myeloma in the USA, but is more common in Japan. Over half of the patients develop peripheral neuropathy (Kelly et al. 1981). Some of them also have the disorder as part of the POEMS syndrome (Nakanishi et al. 1984) consisting of polyneuropathy, organomegaly, endocrinopathy, an M-protein and skin changes. The biopsy of sural nerve often discloses axonal degeneration, demyelination and remyelination associated with small perivascular infiltrates of mononuclear inflammatory cells in the epineurium (Kelly et al. 1981, 1983; Nakanishi et al. 1984). An IgA monoclonal protein is frequently detected in the serum of patients, less commonly an IgG paraprotein. The immunoglobulin usually has a lambda light chain, in contrast, to that of multiple myeloma where kappa light chains predominate. Deposition of IgG was found in the perineurium of one patient (Lavenstein et al. 1979), but whether the immunoglobulins are important in the pathogenesis of the neuropathy is unclear. Amyloid deposition is generally absent.

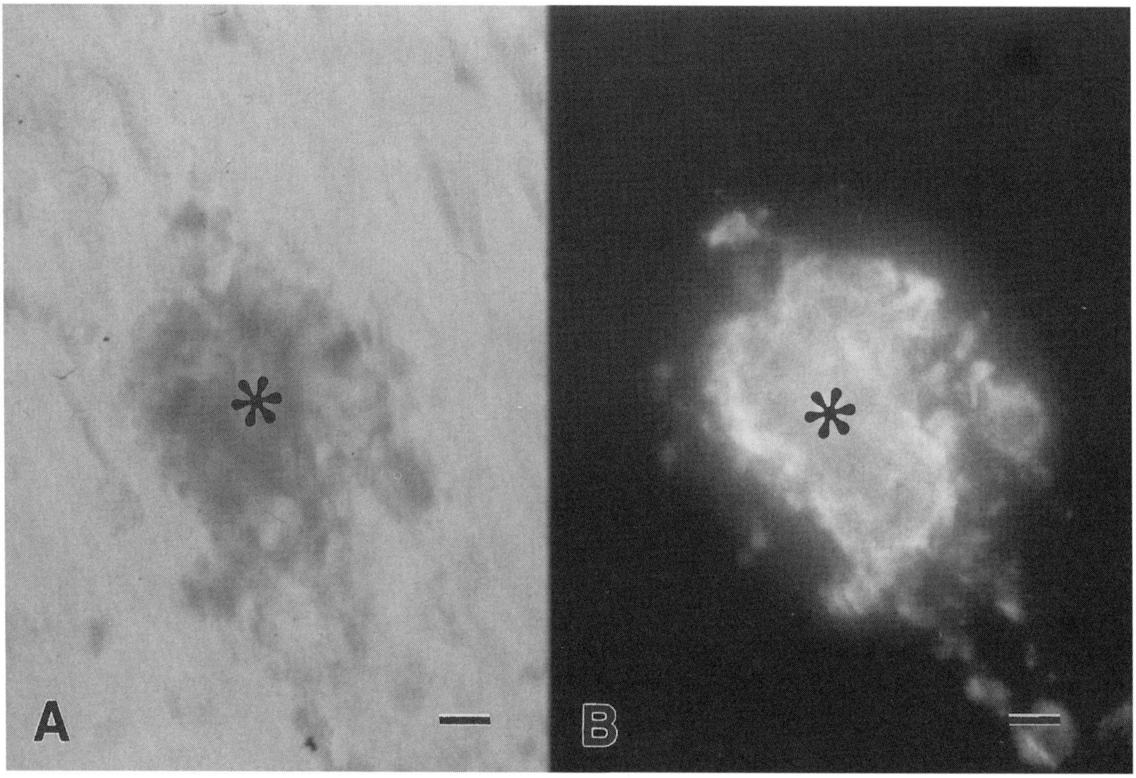

Figure 6.2 *Cryosections of sural nerve in a patient with primary amyloidosis. (A) The endoneurium of nerve shows a mass of amyloid (asterisk) stained by Congo red. (B) The same deposit of amyloid (asterisk) is strongly immunoreactive for C5b-9 (membrane attack complex). (C) In a different section of the nerve, deposits of amyloid in the endoneurium are strongly immunostained for kappa light chains (asterisk). The intensity of staining of lambda light chains in the amyloid does not exceed that of the endoneurium (not shown). The findings provide presumptive evidence of amyloid derived from a monoclonal kappa immunoglobulin light chain. Bars: 10 μm.*

Neuropathy associated with primary amyloidosis

Primary amyloidosis and amyloidosis of multiple myeloma are caused by extracellular accumulation of amyloid, and it is derived from a monoclonal light chain immunoglobulin (Dalakas and Cunningham 1986; Ii et al. 1992). Amyloid is a generic term as many different proteins give rise to the formation of this pathogenic substance. In any one case of amyloidosis, the substance originates from a single major protein and is usually composed of a polypeptide fragment rather than the whole molecule (Glenner 1980). The amyloid of familial amyloidotic neuropathy differs from the amyloid of primary amyloidosis because it is derived from a different protein, usually transthyretin. Histologically, all forms of amyloid are homogeneous, hyaline, and metachromatic with crystal violet or methyl violet. The material is congophilic (Figure 6.2a), and it has a green birefringence when viewed using polarized light (Glenner 1980; Elghetany and Saleem 1988). All types of amyloid contain amyloid P component, a glycoprotein that is a useful immunohistochemical marker of the substance (Shirahama et al. 1981). Ultrastructurally, amyloid is identified by a characteristic fine structure consisting of 7.5–10 nm linear, non-branching, aggregated fibrils (Glenner 1980). Electron microscopy may rarely show amyloid fibrils when tinctorial stains are negative (Kyle and Greipp 1983).

The neuropathy in primary amyloidosis, myelomatous amyloidosis and familial amyloidotic neuropathy

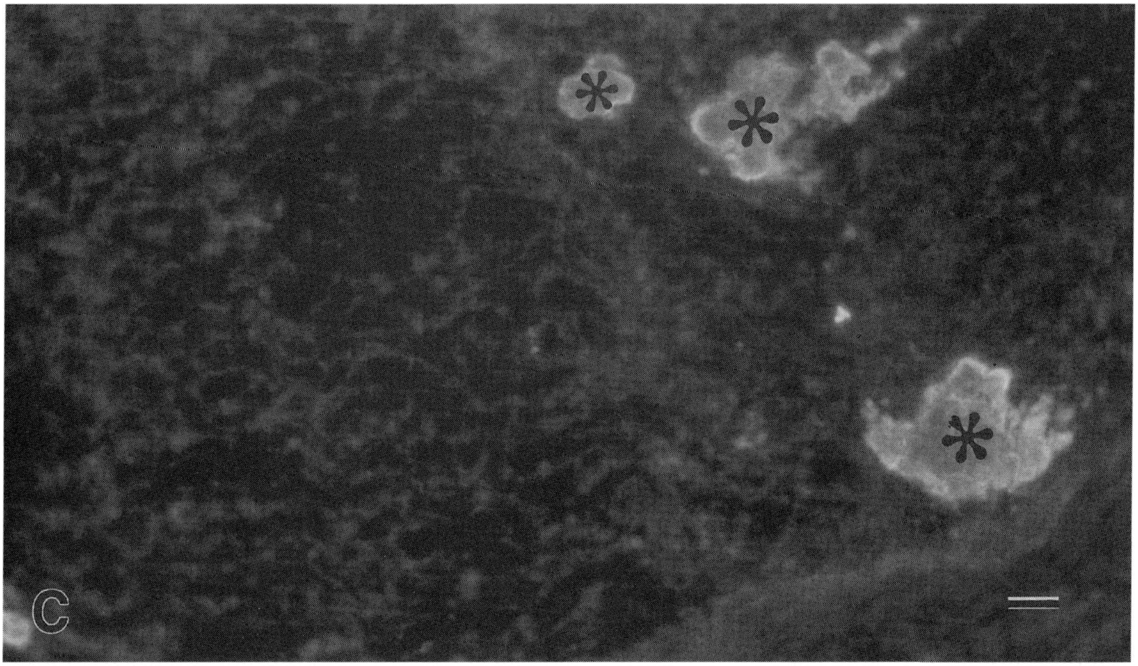

Figure 6.2 (*cont.*)

have similar clinical and pathological features (Kelly et al. 1981; Dalakas and Cunningham 1986; Ii et al. 1992). The patients have a slowly progressive sensorimotor neuropathy, often beginning with paresthesias or lancinating pain or both (Ii et al. 1992). Motor and autonomic dysfunction usually develop later. Semi-thin peripheral nerve sections show active axonal degeneration and marked loss of myelinated fibers, especially the small myelinated ones. Unmyelinated fibers are frequently involved and decreased in number. Teased fiber studies show features of predominantly axonal degeneration (Thomas and King 1974; Kelly et al. 1979). The epineurial and endoneurial connective tissues are infiltrated by amyloid, in globular or in diffuse form (Thomas and King 1974; Asbury and Johnson 1978; Kelly et al. 1979). The walls of the vasa nervorum may be thickened by the presence of amyloid deposition (Thomas and King 1974; Kelly et al. 1979; Verghese et al. 1983). Post-mortem studies of patients with amyloid polyneuropathy and autonomic symptoms, show amyloid infiltration of peripheral nerves, dorsal roots, dorsal root ganglia and sympathetic ganglia with loss of ganglion cells (Davies-Jones & Esiri 1971; Nordborg et al. 1973; Verghese et al. 1983).

Immunohistochemical stains of nerve help to distinguish the light chain type of amyloid of multiple myeloma or primary amyloidosis from the amyloid composed of transthyretin in familial amyloidotic polyneuropathy (Dalakas and Cunningham 1986; Ii et al. 1992). In primary amyloidosis, amyloid deposits react with antisera to either kappa or lambda light chains (Figure 6.2c) (Dalakas and Cunningham 1986; Sommer and Schroder 1989; Ii et al. 1992) but not with antibodies specific for transthyretin. In familial amyloidotic neuropathy, the deposits are negative for light chains but contain immunoreactive transthyretin. Rarely, amyloid is composed of some other protein.

How amyloid produces injury of nerve fibers is not well understood. Nerve can be compressed in some instances when deposits of amyloid are localized in the perineurium or surrounding connective tissue causing the carpal tunnel syndrome (Asbury and Johnson 1978). Also, amyloid deposits in the endoneurium may compress and distort cytons and nerve fibers in the ganglia and peripheral nerves, respectively, explaining the pathological aspect of 'dying back' axonopathy and Wallerian degeneration. Vessel lumens may be narrowed and, sometimes, this can cause infarcts of nerve (Asbury and Johnson 1978). Compression or ischemic injury of nerve

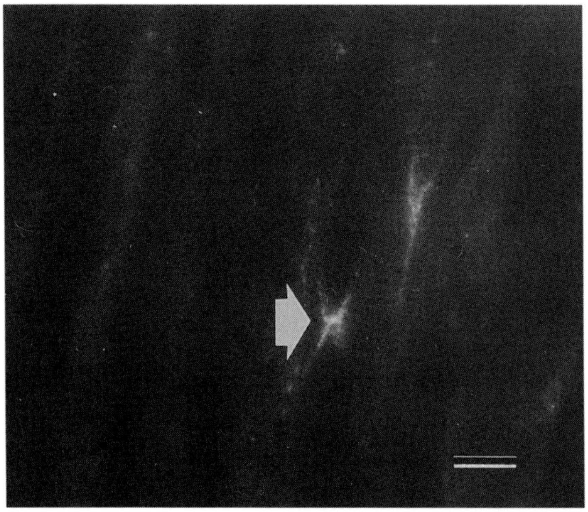

Figure 6.3 *Longitudinal cryosection of sural nerve in a patient with multifocal motor conduction block and elevated titer of anti-GM1 ganglioside antibodies. The section is stained by the direct immunofluorescence method using fluorescein-conjugated antibodies specific for human IgM. Strongly immunoreactive IgM is demonstrated at a node of Ranvier (arrow). The IgM is concentrated in the nodal gap but extends over the surface of the paranodal myelin. Another deposit of IgM is present on paranodal myelin of only one internode because the adjacent internode is not included in the plane of the section. Bar: 10 μm. (Permission to use this photograph and the caption in modified form was granted by Raven Press. This material includes Figure 4 and caption of Chapter 33, p. 394 in* Advances in Neurology, *vol. 56,* Amyotrophic Lateral Sclerosis and Other Motor Neuron Diseases, *edited by L.P. Rowland, published 1991).*

fibers does not explain well the preferential involvement of small diameter myelinated fibers and unmyelinated fibers. Alternatively, amyloid may have a selective toxic effect on nerve fibers (Trotter et al. 1977; Verghese et al. 1983). Immunohistochemical stains of nerve show that amyloid contains abundant complement proteins including membrane attack complex (C5b-9) (Figure 5.2b) in both primary amyloidosis and familial amyloidotic neuropathy (Zanusso et al. 1992; Isozaki et al. 1993). The mechanism of localized activation of the complement system in amyloid is not known, but complement proteins, particularly membrane attack complex, could injure nerve fibers and cause axonal degeneration.

Neuropathies associated with autoantibodies to GM1 ganglioside and other glycoconjugates

Motor neuron disease and chronic motor neuropathies

IgM monoclonal or polyclonal autoantibodies with anti-GM1 ganglioside activity have been associated with lower motor neuron disease or slowly progressive motor neuropathy with or without conduction block. To date, however, few pathological studies have been reported in these conditions. Human anti-GM1 antibodies bind to GM1 at the surface of motor neurons (Thomas et al. 1990a; Corbo et al. 1992), and both GM1 and crossreactive glycoproteins are present at the nodes of Ranvier in peripheral nerve (Corbo et al. 1993b; Apostolski et al. 1994). In one patient with anti-GM1 antibodies and multifocal motor conduction block, sural nerve biopsy demonstrated IgM deposits at the nodes of Ranvier by direct immunofluorescence (Figure 6.3) (Santoro et al. 1990), and the serum caused demyelination and conduction block when injected into rat sciatic nerve (Santoro et al. 1992). Post-mortem pathological studies were performed in two patients with slowly progressive motor neuropathy (Rowland et al. 1982; Adams et al. 1993), one of whom had multifocal conduction block and elevated anti-GM1 antibodies. The histology of the nervous system in both patients showed axonal degeneration in the anterior roots and central chromatolysis of spinal motor neurons. Loss of up to 60% motor neurons was found in spinal cord in one of the cases. Biopsy of the right ulnar nerve in a third patient, who had symptoms of motor neuron disease, revealed a neuropathy with onion bulb formations (Auer et al. 1989). A fourth patient had multifocal motor neuropathy and increased anti-GM1 antibody titer, and a nerve biopsy specimen from a region of conduction block showed focal demyelination (Kaji et al. 1993). In this case, no immunohistochemical studies were performed. Sural nerve biopsy in patients with motor neuropathy is usually normal, but some patients have mild changes of demyelination (Krarup et al. 1990), perivascular inflammatory infiltrates (van den Bergh et al. 1989; Krarup et al. 1990), or loss of myelinated axons (Parry and Clarke 1988; Pestronk et al. 1988; Krarup et al. 1990).

The pathological separation of motor neuron disease from purely motor neuropathy is problematic, although the demonstration of a marked loss of motor neurons by autopsy is definitive in amyotrophic lateral sclerosis (Hays 1991). We have recently studied the pathological abnormalities in biopsies of the motor branch of the obturator nerve to the gracilis muscle in patients with motor disorders (Corbo et al. 1997). Six patients had motor neuropathy, as defined by electrophysiological findings, either multifocal motor conduction block or motor conduction slowing or both. Three of them had evidence of a demyelinating neuropathy with small onion bulb formations, and three showed evidence of a chronic axonopathy. All six patients had a significantly higher density of regenerative clusters of small myelinated fibers in comparison with motor nerves of patients with motor neuron disease. This morphological finding in these biopsies helped to distinguish motor neuropathy from motor neuron disease in our series of patients. The six patients with motor neuropathy had no simple relation between conduction block (three patients), titers of anti-GM1 antibodies (four patients) and demyelination or axonal degeneration in the motor nerve. Abnormal deposits of immunoglobulin and complement were not found in the motor nerve of any of these patients.

Acute and chronic inflammatory neuropathies

Acute inflammatory neuropathy (GBS) is typically a demyelinating neuropathy associated with infiltration of endoneurium by mononuclear inflammatory cells, chiefly lymphocytes and monocytes or macrophages (Arnason and Soliven 1993). Demyelination occurs diffusely, but tends to be more severe around venules and capillaries (Asbury and Johnson 1978). Electron microscopic examination demonstrates macrophages that penetrate the basal lamina and invade the outer portion of otherwise intact myelin sheaths. These macrophages seem to strip away a layer of the myelin sheath (Prineas 1972). This pattern is in contrast to lymphocytes which do not seem to make contact with nerve fibers. Immunohistochemical studies of nerve have shown deposition of C3d on the surface of myelinated nerve fibers in the early stage of the disease before they are attacked by macrophages (Hafer-Macko et al. 1996a,b).

More recently, an axonal form of GBS has been reported (Feasby et al. 1986), and some of the patients have a syndrome of acute motor axonal neuropathy (Griffin et al. 1996). The nerve is infiltrated by mononuclear inflammatory cells, but monocytes and macrophages predominate with only sparse lymphocytes. Axonal degeneration is found pathologically with little or no demyelination. Ultrastructurally, macrophages are located in the periaxonal space between the myelin sheath and axolemma and rarely within axons (Griffin et al. 1996). Immunohistochemical stains show deposition of C3d at nodes of Ranvier (Hafer-Macko et al. 1996a) in the early stage of the disease. GBS had been linked to *Campylobacter jejuni* infection and high-titer serum antibodies to GM1 gangliosides and other glycolipids as potential target antigens of immune-mediated injury of myelin and axons (Yuki et al. 1990, van den Berg et al. 1992; Griffin et al. 1996). Serum IgG from a patient with acute motor neuropathy and anti-GM1 antibodies bound to nodes of Ranvier of teased myelinated fibers of cauda equina using an indirect immunohistochemical method (Gregson et al. 1991). The immunopathological findings in nerve supports the concept that autoantibodies are important in the pathogenesis of GBS.

Chronic inflammatory demyelinating polyneuropathy (CIDP) has a slowly progressive or relapsing pattern of disease, and the disorder is thought to be a autoimmune disorder resembling GBS. The nerve has pathological features of a chronic demyelinating disorder, sometime with small onion bulbs (Asbury and Johnson 1978). Mononuclear inflammatory cells infiltrate the endoneurium, but about half of the cases lack lymphocytes. Immunohistochemical stains are usually negative for immune complexes, but C3d deposits can be found on the surface of myelin sheaths during a relapse (Hays, unpublished data). Patients with motor neuropathy and multifocal motor conduction block (see above) may represent a form of CIDP (Parry 1993).

Neuropathies associated with anti-sulfatide antibodies

Monoclonal or polyclonal IgM anti-sulfatide antibodies have been reported in association with predominantly sensory neuropathy (Li et al. 1991). Nerve

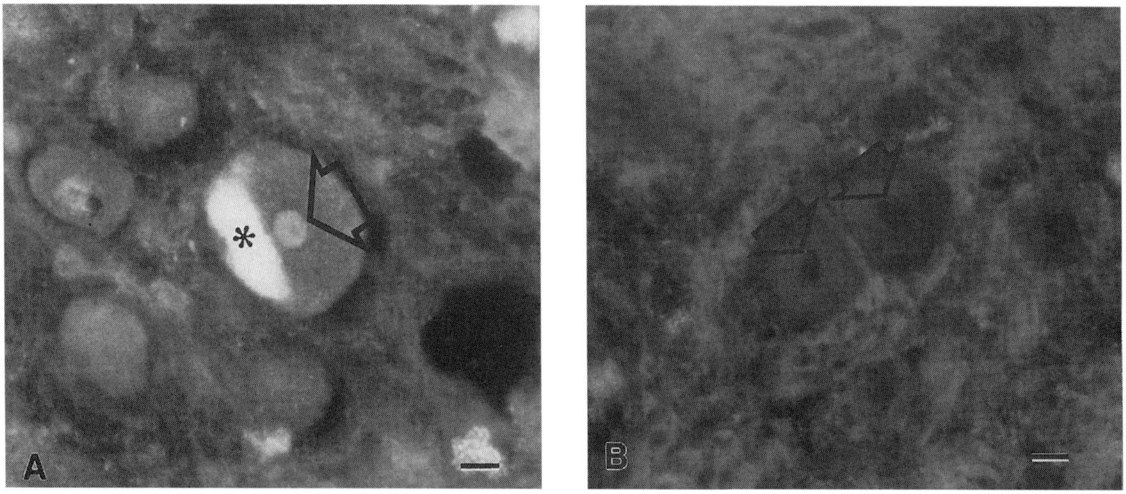

Figure 6.4 *Cryosections of normal dorsal root ganglion stained by an indirect immunofluorescence method. (A) The cryosection was exposed to a 1:400 dilution of serum from a patient with a small cell carcinoma of the lung and high titer anti-Hu antibodies. After 1 hour of incubation, the section was washed in buffer and stained with fluorescein-conjugated antibodies to human IgG. Immunoreactive IgG is bound to a nucleus of a dorsal root ganglion cell (arrow) and, to a lesser degree, to the cytoplasm. The bright (white) mass in the cytoplasm (asterisk) is normal autofluorescent lipofuscin. Immunostained IgG is present diffusely in the connective tissue, and it largely reflects endogenous, extracellular IgG which is found in normal tissue. (B) The cryosection is exposed to serum of a normal subject and subsequently immunostained for human IgG. No IgG is bound to nuclei of two ganglion cells (arrows), but diffuse immunoreactive IgG is present in the connective tissue. Bars: 20 μm.*

biopsy showed a normal nerve or chronic axonal degeneration although one specimen had signs of a chronic myelinopathy (Quattrini et al. 1992; Nemni et al. 1993). Immunocytochemical studies revealed that the anti-sulfatide antibodies bound to unfixed human neuroblastoma cells and the surface of unfixed rat dorsal root ganglia neurons, and to ethanol-fixed sections of central and peripheral myelin of human tissue (Quattrini et al. 1992). Direct immunostaining of sural nerve for immunoglobulins was normal except for two patients with serum antibodies against both sulfatide and chondroitin sulfate C. These two nerves had increased staining of IgM in the endoneurium, resembling the pattern in patients with anti-chondroitin sulfate C antibodies (see above) (Nemni et al. 1993).

Paraneoplastic neuropathies

Peripheral neuropathies may be associated with neoplasms, but without direct infiltration of nerves by neoplastic cells (McLeod 1993). These paraneoplastic neuropathies are clinically and pathologically heterogeneous, but most of them are sensorimotor neuropathies caused by degeneration of axons or the whole nerve cell. The best defined syndrome is the neuropathy associated with a small cell carcinoma of the lung and anti-Hu autoantibodies (Posner 1995). The patients have a subacute, sensory neuropathy or more frequently an encephalomyelitis with or without a sensory neuropathy and motor neuropathy. At post-mortem, loss of nerve cells and mononuclear inflammatory infiltration are found in the central nervous system and dorsal root ganglia. Nerve biopsies show active axonal degeneration and loss of myelinated fibers in the absence of regenerative clusters of small myelinated nerve fibers. In most cases, inflammatory cells are absent, but they may show perivascular mononuclear inflammatory cells in the epineurium or microvasculitis (Younger et al. 1994). The anti-Hu IgG antibodies bind to nuclei of nerve cells of the dorsal root ganglia (Figure 6.4) and CNS using the indirect immunohistochemical method (Graus et al.

1985). At a high serum dilution of over 1:100, the immunostaining of nerve cells is nearly specific for the syndrome. The diagnosis is confirmed by Western blot analysis of the serum which demonstrates binding of the IgG to a group of proteins of 35–40 kDa (Posner 1995).

Vasculitic neuropathies

Necrotizing vasculitis may be limited to the PNS clinically or be part of a systemic disorder, usually a collagen vascular disease. The histological diagnosis of necrotizing vasculitis requires inflammatory cell infiltration and necrosis of blood vessel walls. The necrosis is usually fibrinoid in type. In peripheral nerve, the epineurial arterioles or venules are typically involved by the vasculitic process. The size of the affected vessels is generally large, but hypersensitivity vasculitis or microvasculitis and non-systemic vasculitis of nerve involve small diameter vessels (Dyck et al. 1987). Inflammatory lesions of vasa nervorum may be widespread and numerous, but may be sparse and require examination of many different levels of the tissue block to find diagnostic features of vasculitis. According to Said et al. (1988), the combination of nerve and muscle sampling increases the chance of visualizing the lesions in vasculitic neuropathy. Histological clues of necrotizing vasculitis in the epineurium include hemorrhage, thrombosis or recanalization of epineurial vessels, and perivascular inflammatory cell infiltrates with or without hemosiderin-laden macrophages; however, these findings are considered to be circumstantial evidence of nerve vasculitis and are not sufficient for diagnosis. Active destructive lesions are marked by necrosis of vessel wall associated with intramural infiltration of polymophonuclear leukocytes or mononuclear inflammatory cells or both. Active necrotizing vasculitis with eosinophilic infiltration was described in Churg–Strauss syndrome (Oh et al. 1986). Thickening of the intima, large discontinuities of the internal elastic lamina and focal scarring of the media sometimes with perivascular infiltrates of chronic inflammatory cells is characteristic of an older, repaired vascular lesion.

In the active lesion, the mononuclear cells consist of predominantly T lymphocytes, mostly CD8 cytotoxic/suppressor cells, and macrophages (Kissel et al. 1989). Many T lymphocytes express Ia antigen, suggesting that they are activated. In the nerve biopsy from other patients, Panegyres et al. (1990) observed a significant number of B lymphocytes in mononuclear cell infiltrates, whereas CD4 and CD8 T cells were present in roughly equal proportion. In our series of nerve biopsies in vasculitic neuropathy both CD4 and CD8-positive cells were found in the inflammatory infiltrates, but CD4 expressing cells predominated as a rule.

In addition, immunocytochemical analysis of endothelial adhesion molecules reveal that intercellular adhesion molecule-1 (ICAM-1) is strongly expressed on the surface of the intima of large and medium sized vessels of the epineurium, and in most cases on endothelium of endoneurial capillaries, suggesting an active role in the pathogenesis of vasculitic neuropathy (Corbo et al. 1993a). Endothelial leukocyte adhesion molecule-1 (ELAM-1) and vascular cell adhesion molecule-1 (VCAM-1) show a less intense expression in some cases. Deposits of immunoglobulin and complement proteins including membrane attack complex in the walls of vascular lesions or of uninflamed vessels have been described (Conn et al. 1972; Nemni et al. 1988; Kissel et al. 1989; Panegyres et al. 1990; Hawke et al. 1991).

Signs of Wallerian degeneration and loss of myelinated fibers represent the usual pathological picture observed in the affected nerves. Some nerve fascicles may be more severely involved than others. Nerve fiber loss that predominated in the center of the nerve fascicle is thought to be a characteristic consequence of ischemic insult. Teased fiber preparations show axonal degeneration. Ultrastructural study documents the degeneration of unmyelinated fibers (Vital and Vital 1985).

Conclusions

Immunopathological studies of the PNS have begun to provide important information about the pathogenesis of autoimmune neuropathies during the last 15 years. Selective deposition of immunoglobulins and complement components, particularly C3d, on myelinated nerve fibers supports the concept of autoantibody-mediated disease in several disorders including the polyneuropathy in patients with an anti-MAG IgM paraprotein, chronic progressive motor neuropathy with or without multifocal motor conduction block and GBS. The finding of immune complexes in sural nerve are largely limited to the anti-MAG neuropathy for diagnostic purposes, but the yield could be extended potentially with biopsy of motor nerves and technological advances. Similarly, immunohistochemical evaluation of B cells, T cells, monocytes/macrophages and cytokines in human nerves have been limited chiefly to research studies of neuropathies. Among these disorders are diabetic neuropathy which has an inflammatory disorder of nerve in some instances suggesting a possible autoimmune disorder (Younger et al. 1996). The eventual goal is to apply the methods of immunopathology, and use the information for diagnosis and clinical management of patients.

References

Abrams, G.M., Latov, N., Hays, A.P., Sherman, W., and Zimmerman, E.A. (1982). Immunocytochemical studies of human peripheral nerve with serum from patients with polyneuropathy and paraproteinemia. *Neurology* (NY) **32**: 821–826.

Adams, D., Kuntzer, T., Steck, A.J., Lobrinus, A., Janzer, R.C., and Regli, F. (1993). Motor conduction block and high titres of anti-GM1 ganglioside antibodies: pathological evidence of a motor neuropathy in a patient with lower motor neuron syndrome. *J. Neurol. Neurosurg. Psychiatry* **56**: 982–987.

Apostolski, S., Sadiq, S.A., Hays, A., Corbo, M., Suturkova-Milosevic, L., Chaliff, P., Stefansson, K., LeBaron, R.G., Ruoslant, E., and Hays, A.P. (1994). Identification of Gal(β1-3)GalNAc bearing glycoproteins at the nodes of Ranvier in peripheral nerve. *J. Neurosci. Res.* **38**: 134–141.

Arnason, B.G.W. and Soliven, B. (1993). Acute inflammatory demyelinating polyradiculoneuropathy. In *Peripheral Neuropathy*, 3rd edn, ed. P.J. Dyck, P.K. Thomas, J.W. Griffin, P.A. Low and J.F. Poduslo, pp. 1437–1497. Philadelphia: W.B. Saunders Company.

Asbury, A.K. and Johnson, P.C. (1978). *Pathology of Peripheral Nerve: Major Problems in Pathology*, vol 7, pp. 148–155. Philadelphia: W.B. Saunders.

Auer, R.N., Bell, R.B., and Lee, M.A. (1989). Neuropathy with onion bulb formations and pure motor manifestations. *Can. J. Neurol. Sci.* **16**: 194–197.

Barron, K.D., Rowland, L.P., and Zimmerman, H.M. (1960). Neuropathy with malignant tumor metastases. *J. Neurol. Ment. Dis.* **131**: 10–31.

Bosch, E.P., Ansbacher, L.E., Goeken, J.A., and Cancilla, P.A. (1982). Peripheral neuropathy associated with monoclonal gammopathy studies of intraneural injections of monoclonal immunoglobulin sera. *J. Neuropathol. Exp. Neurol.* **41**: 446–459.

Brandtzaeg, P. (1981). Prolonged incubation time in immunohistochemistry: effects on fluorescence staining of immunoglobulins and epithelial components in ethanol – and formaldehyde – lixed paraffin-embedded tissues. *J. Histochem. Cytochem.* **29**: 1302–1315.

Braun, P.E., Frail, D.E., and Latov, N. (1982). Myelin-associated glycoprotein is the antigen for a monoclonal IgM in polyneuropathy. *J. Neurochem.* **32**: 1261–1265.

Conn, D.L., McDuffie, F.C., and Dyck, P.J. (1972). Immunopathologic study of sural nerves in rheumatoid arthritis. *Arthritis Rheum.* **15**: 135–143.

Corbo, M., Nemni, R., Previtali, S., Innaccone, S., Zocchi, M., and Canal, N. (1993a). Immunocytochemical analysis of the intercellular adhesion molecules in the vasculitic neuropathy. *Can. J. Neurol. Sci.* **20** (suppl. 4): 76 (abstract).

Corbo, M., Quattrini, A., Latov, N., and Hays, A.P. (1993b). Localization of GM1 and Gal(β1-3)GalNAc antigenic determinants in peripheral nerve. *Neurology* **43**: 809–814.

Corbo, M., Quattrini, A., Lugaresi, A., Santoro, M., Latov, N., and Hays, A.P. (1992). Patterns of reactivity of human anti-GM1 antibodies with spinal cord and motor neurons. *Ann. Neurol.* **32**: 487–493.

Corbo, M., Abouzahr, M.K., Latov, N., Iannaccone, S., Quattrini, A., Nenni, R., Canal, N., and Hays, A.P. (1997). Motor nerve biopsy structures in motor neuropathy and motorneuron disease. *Muscle Nerve* **20**: 15–21.

Dalakas, M.C. and Cunningham, G. (1986). Characterization of amyloid deposits in biopsies of 15 patients with 'sporadic' (non-familial or plasma cell dyscrasic) amyloid polyneuropathy. *Acta Neuropathol. (Berl.)* **69**: 66–72.

Davies-Jones, G.A.B. and Esiri, M.M. (1971). Neuropathy due to amyloid in myelomatosis. *Br. Med. J.* **2**: 444.

Delauche, M.C., Clauve, J.P., and Seligmann, M. (1981). Peripheral neuropathy and plasma cell neoplasias: a report of 10 cases. *Br. J. Haematol.* **48**: 383–392.

Dellagi, K., Brouet, J.C., Perreau, J., and Paulin, D. (1982). Human monoclonal IgM with autoantibody activity against intermediate filaments. *Proc. Natl. Acad. Sci. USA* **79**: 446–450.

Dyck, P.J., Benstead, T.J., Conn, D.L., et al. (1987). Non-systemic vasculitic neuropathy. *Brain* **110**: 843–854.

Elghetany, M.T. and Saleem, A. (1988). Methods for staining amyloid in tissues: a review. *Stain Technol.* **63**: 201–212.

Fazio, R., Nemni, R., Quattrini, A., Lorenzetti, I., and Canal, N. (1992). IgG monoclonal proteins from patients with axonal peripheral neuropathies bind to different epitopes of the 68 kDa neurofilament protein. *J. Neuroimmunol.* **36**: 97–104.

Feasby, T.E., Gilbert, J.J., Brown, W.F., Bolton, C.F., Hahn, A.F., Koopman, W.F., and Zochodne, D.W. (1986). An acute axonal form of Guillain-Barré polyneuropathy. *Brain* **109**: 1115–1126.

Freddo, L., Hays, A.P., Sherman, W.H., and Latov, N. (1985). Axonal neuropathy in a patient with IgM M-protein reactive with nerve endoneurium. *Neurology* **35**: 1321–1325.

Glenner, G.G. (1980). Amyloid deposits and amyloidosis: the B-fibrilloses. *N. Engl. J. Med.* **302**: 1283–1292.

Graus, F., Cordon-Cardo, C., and Posner, J.B. (1985). Neuronal antinuclear antibody in sensory neuronopathy from lung cancer. *Neurology* **35**: 538–543.

Gregson, N.A., Jones, D., Thomas, P.K., and Willison, H.J. (1991). Acute motor neuropathy with antibodies to GM1 ganglioside. *J. Neurol.* **238**: 447–451.

Griffin, J., Li, C.Y., Ho, T.W., Tian, M., Gao, C.Y., Xue, P., Mishu, B., Cornblath, D.R., Macko, C., McKhann, G.M., and Astbury, A.K. (1996). Pathology of motor-sensory axonal Guillain-Barré syndrome. *Ann. Neurol.* **39**: 17–28.

Hafer-Macko, C.E., Hsieh, S.T., Li, C.Y., Ho, T.W., Sheikh, K., Cornblath, D.R., McKhann, G.M., Asbury, A.K., and Griffin, J.W. (1996a). Acute motor axonal neuropathy: an antibody-mediated attack on axolemma. *Ann. Neurol.* **40**: 635–644.

Hafer-Macko, C.E., Sheikh, K.A., Li, C.Y., Ho, T.W., Cornblath, D.R., McKhann, G.M., Asbury, A.K., and Griffin, J.W. (1996b). Immune attack on the Schwann cell surface in acute inflammatory demyelinating polyneuropathy. *Ann Neurol.* **39**: 625–635.

Hawke, S.B., Davies, L., Pamphlett, R., Guo, Y.P., Pollard, J.D., and McLeod, J.G. (1991). Vasculitic neuropathy. A clinical and pathological study. *Brain* **114**: 2175–2190.

Hays, A.P. (1991). Separation of motor neuron diseases from pure motor neuropathies: pathology. In *Amyotrophic Lateral Sclerosis and Other Motor Neuron Diseases, Advances in Neurology*, vol. 56, ed. L.P. Rowland, pp. 385–398. New York: Raven Press.

Hays, A.P., Lee, S.S.L., and Latov, N. (1988). Immune reactive C3d on the surface of myelin sheaths in neuropathy. *J. Neuroimmunol.* **18**: 231–244.

Hays, A.P., Roxas, A., Sadiq, S.A., Vallejos, H., D'Agati, V., Thomas, F.P., Torres, R., Sherman, W.H., Bailey-Braxton, D., Hays, A.G., Rowland, L.P., and Latov, N. (1990). A monoclonal IgA in a patient with motor neuron disease reacts with neurofilaments and surface antigen on neuroblastoma cells. *J. Neuropath. Exp. Neurol.* **49**: 383–398.

Hesselvik, M. (1969). Neuropathological studies on myelomatosis. *Acta Neurol. Scand.* **45**: 95–108.

Ii, K., Kyle, R.A., and Dyck, P.J. (1992). Immunohistochemical characterization of amyloid proteins in sural nerves and clinical associations in amyloid neuropathy. *Am. J. Pathol.* **141**: 217–226.

Ilyas, A.A., Quarles, R.H., Dalakas, M.C., Fishman, P.H., and Brady, R.O. (1985). Monoclonal IgM in a patient with paraproteinaemic polyneuropathy binds to gangliosides containing disialosyl groups. *Ann. Neurol.* **18**: 655–659.

Isozaki, E., Rosoklija, G., Neri, D., Herbert, J., and Hays, A.P. (1993). Two different forms of amyloid in polyneuropathy activate the classical complement pathway. *Neurology* **43** (suppl.): A232.

Iwashita, H., Argyrakis, A., Lowitsch, K., and Spaar, F.W. (1974). Polyneuropathy in Waldenström's macroglobulinemia. *J. Neurol. Sci.* **21**: 341–354.

Kaji, R., Oka, N., Tsuji, T., Mezaki, T., Nishio, T., Akiguchi, I., and Kimura, J. (1993). Pathological findings at the site of conduction block in multifocal motor neuropathy. *Ann. Neurol.* **33**: 152–158.

Kelly, J.J., Kyle, R.A., Miles, J.M., and Dyck, P.J. (1981). The spectrum of peripheral neuropathy in myeloma. *Neurology (NY)* **31**: 24–31.

Kelly, J.J., Kyle, R.A., Miles, J.M., and Dyck, P.J. (1983). Osteosclerotic myleloma and peripheral neuropathy. *Neurology (Minneap.)* **33**: 202–210.

Kelly, J.J., Kyle, R.A., O'Brien, P.C., and Dyck, P.J. (1979). The natural history of peripheral neuropathy in primary systemic amyloidosis. *Ann. Neurol.* **6**: 1–7.

King, R.H.M. and Thomas, P.K. (1984). The occurrence and significance of myelin with unusually large periodicity. *Acta Neuropathol. (Berl)* **63**: 319–329.

Kissel, J.T., Rammohan, K.W., and Mendell, J.R. (1986). Absence of complement membrane attack complex in nerves from patients with polyneuropathy and a monoclonal anti-MAG IgM gammopathy. *Neurology* **36** (suppl.): 79.

Kissel, J.T., Riethman, J.L., Omerza, J., Rammohan, K.W., and Mendell, J.R. (1989). Peripheral nerve vasculitis: immune characterization of the vascular lesions. *Ann. Neurol.* **25**: 291–297.

Krarup, C., Stewart, J.D., Sumner, A.J., Pestronk, A., and Lipton, S.A. (1990). A syndrome of asymmetric limb weakness with motor conduction block. *Neurology* **40**: 118–127.

Kyle, R.A. and Greipp, P.R. (1983). Amyloidosis (AL): clinical and laboratory features of 229 cases. *Mayo Clin. Proc.* **58**: 665–683.

Latov, N., Hays, A.P., and Sherman, W.H. (1988). Peripheral neuropathy and anti-MAG antibodies (review). *Crit. Rev. Neurobiol.* **3**: 301–332.

Latov, N., Sherman, W.H., Nemni, R., Galassi, G., Shyong, J.S., Penn, A.S., Chess, L., and Osserman, E.F. (1980). Plasma cell dyscrasia and peripheral neuropathy with a monoclonal antibody to peripheral nerve myelin. *N. Engl. J. Med.* **303**: 618–621.

Latov, N. and Steck, A.J. (1995). Neuropathies associated with anti-glycoconjugate antibodies and IgM monoclonal gammopathies. In *Peripheral Nerve Disorders*, 2nd edn, ed. A. Asbury and P.K. Thomas, pp. 153–174. Oxford: Butterworth/Heinemann.

Lavenstein, B., Dalakas, M., and Engel, W.K. (1979). Polyneuropathy in 'nonsecretory' osteosclerotic multiple myeloma with immunoglobulin deposition in peripheral nerve tissue. *Neurology (Minneap.)* **29**: 611.

Li, F., Pestronk, A., Griffin, J., Feldman, E.L., Cornblath, D., Trotter, J., Zhu, S., Yee, W.C., Phillips, D., Peeples, D.M., and Winslow, B. (1991). Polyneuropathy syndromes associated with serum antibodies to sulfatide and myelin associated glycoprotein. *Neurology* **41**: 357–362.

Logothetis, J., Silverstein, P., and Coe, J. (1960). Neurological aspects of Waldenström's macroglobulinemia. *Arch. Neurol.* **3**: 564–573.

Mamoli, A., Nemni, R., Camerlingo, M., Quattrini, A., Castro, L., Lorenzetti, L., and Canal, N. (1992). A clinical, electrophysiological, morphological and immunological study of chronic sensory neuropathy with ataxia and paraesthesia. *Acta Neurol. Scand.* **85**: 110–115.

McLeod, J.G. (1993). Paraneoplastic neuropathies. In *Peripheral Neuropathy*, 3rd edn, ed. P.J. Dyck, P.K. Thomas, J.W. Griffin, P.A. Low and J.F. Poduslo, pp. 1583–1590. Philadelphia: W.B. Saunders Company.

Mendell, J.R., Zahenk, Z., Whitaker, J.N., Trapp, B.D., Yates, A.J., Griggs, R.C., and Quarles, R.H. (1985). Polyneuropathy and IgM monoclonal gammopathy, studies on the pathogenic role of anti-myelin associated glycoprotein antibody. *Ann. Neurol.* **17**: 243–254.

Monaco, S., Bonetti, B., Ferrari, S., et al. (1990). Complement dependent demyelination in patients with IgM monoclonal gammopathy and polyneuropathy. *N. Engl. J. Med.* **322**: 649–652.

Moorhouse, D.F., Fox, R.I., and Powell, H.C. (1992). Immunotactoid-like endoneurial deposits in a patient with monoclonal gammopathy of undetermined significance and neuropathy. *Acta Neuropathol.* **84**: 484–494.

Nakanishi, T., Sobue, I., Toyokura, Y., Hishitani, H., Kuroiwa, Y., Satoyoshi, E., Tsubacki, T., Igata, A., and Ozaki, Y. (1984). The Crow-Fukase syndrome, a study of 102 cases in Japan. *Neurology* **34**: 712–720.

Nemni, R., Corbo, M., Fazio, R., Qualtrini, A., Comi, G., and Canal, N. (1988). Cryoglobulinaemic neuropathy. A clinical, morphological and immunocytochemical study of 8 cases. *Brain* **111**: 541–552.

Nemni, R., Fazio, R., Quattrini, A., Lorenzetti, I., Mamoli, D., and Canal, N. (1993). Antibodies to sulfatide and to chondroitin sulfate C in patients with chronic sensory neuropathy. *J. Neuroimmunol.* **43**: 79–86.

Nemni, R., Feltri, M.L., Fazio, R., Quattrini, A., Lorenzetti, I., Corbo, M., and Canal, N. (1990). Axonal neuropathy with monoclonal IgG kappa that binds to a neurofilament protein. *Ann. Neurol.* **28**: 361–364.

Nemni, R., Galassi, G., Latov, N., Sherman, W.H., Olarte, M.R., and Hays, A.P. (1983). Polyneuropathy in nonmalignant IgM plasma cell dyscrasia: a morphological study. *Ann. Neurol.* **14**: 43–54.

Nemni, R., Mamoli, A., Fazio, R., Camerlingo, M., Quattrini, A., Lorenzetti, I., Comola, M., Galardi, M., and Canal, N. (1991). Polyneuropathy associated with IgA monoclonal gammopathy: a hypothesis of its pathogenesis. *Acta Neuropathol.* **81**: 371–376.

Nobile-Orazio, E., Hays, A.P., Latov, N., Perman, G., Golier, J., Shy, M.E., and Freddo, L. (1984). Specificity of mouse and human monoclonal antibodies to myelin-associated glycoprotein. *Neurology (Cleveland)* **34**: 1336–1342.

Nordborg, C., Kristensson, K., Olsson, Y., and Sourander, P. (1973). Involvement of the autonomic nervous system in primary and secondary amyloidosis. *Acta Neurol. Scand.* **49**: 31–38.

Oh, S.J., Herrara, G.A., and Spalding, D.M. (1986). Eosinophilic vasculitic neuropathy in the Churg–Strauss syndrome. *Arthritis Rheum.* **29**: 1173–1175.

Ohi, T., Kyle, R.A., and Dyck, P.J. (1985). Axonal attenuation and secondary segmental demyelination in myeloma neuropathies. *Ann. Neurol.* **17**: 255–261.

Ohnishi, A. and Hirano, A. (1981). Uncompacted myelin lamellae in dysglobulinemic neuropathy. *J. Neurol. Sci.* **51**: 131–140.

Panegyres, P.K., Blumbergs, P.C., Leong, A.S-Y., and Bourne, A.J. (1990). Vasculitis of peripheral nerve and skeletal muscle: clinicopathological correlation and immunopathic mechanisms. *J. Neurol. Sci.* **100**: 193–202.

Parry, G.J. (1993). Motor neuropathy with multifocal conduction block. In *Peripheral Neuropathy*, 3rd edn, ed. P.J. Dyck, P.K. Thomas, J.W. Griffin, P.A. Low and J.F. Poduslo, pp. 1518–1524. Philadelphia: W.B. Saunders Company.

Parry, G.J. and Clarke, S. (1988). Multifocal acquired demyelinating neuropathy masquerading as motor neuron disease. *Muscle Nerve* **11**: 103–107.

Pestronk, A., Cornblath, D.R., Ilyas, A.A., Baba, H., Quarles, R.H., and Griffin, J.W. (1988). A treatable multifocal motor neuropathy with antibodies to GM1 ganglioside. *Ann. Neurol.* **24**: 73–78.

Posner, J.B. (1995). Anti-Hu autoantibody associated sensory neuropathy/ encephalomyelitis: a model of paraneoplastic syndrome. *Perspect. Biol. Med.* **38**: 167–181.

Prineas, J.W. (1972). Acute idiopathic polyneuritis. An electron microscopic study. *Lab. Invest.* **26**: 133–147.

Propp, R.P., Means, E., Deibel, R., Sherer, G., and Barron, K. (1975). Waldenström's macroglobulinemia and neuropathy. *Neurology* **25**: 980–988.

Quattrini, A., Corbo, M., Dhaliwal, S.K., Sadiq, S.A., Lugaresi, A., Oliveira, A., Uncini, A., and Latov, N. (1992). Anti-sulfatide antibodies in neurological disease: binding to rat dorsal root ganglia neurons. *J. Neurol. Sci.* **112**: 152–159.

Quattrini, A., Nemni, R., Fazio, R., Iannaccone, S., Lorenzetti, I., Grassi, F., and Canal, N. (1991). Axonal neuropathy in a patient with monoclonal IgM kappa reactive with Schmidt–Lanterman incisures. *J. Neuroimmunol.* **33**: 73–79.

Read, D.J., Banhegan, R.I., and Matthews, W.B. (1978). Peripheral neuropathy and benign IgG paraproteinemia. *J. Neurol. Neurosurg. Psychiatry* **41**: 215–219.

Rowland, L.P., Defendini, R., Sherman, W., Hirano, A., Olarte, M.R., Latov, N., Lovelace, R.E., Inoue, K., and Osserman, E.F. (1982). Macroglobulinemia with peripheral neuropathy simulating motor neuron disease. *Ann. Neurol.* **11**: 532–536.

Said, G., Lacroix-Ciaudo, C., Fujimura, H., Blas, C., and Faux, N. (1988). The peripheral neuropathy of necrotizing arteritis: a clinicopathological study. *Ann. Neurol.* **23**: 461–465.

Santoro, M., Thomas, F.P., Fink, M.E., Lange, D.F., Uncini, A., Wadia, N.H., Latov, N., and Hays, A.P. (1990). IgM deposits at nodes of Ranvier in a patient with amyotrophic lateral sclerosis, anti-GM1 antibodies, and multifocal motor conduction block. *Ann. Neurol.* **28**: 373–377.

Santoro, M., Uncini, A., Corbo, M., Staugaitis, S.M., Thomas, F.P., Hays, A.P., and Latov, N. (1992). Experimental conduction block induced by serum from a patient with anti-GM1 antibodies. *Ann. Neurol.* **31**: 385–390.

Sewell, H.F., Matthews, J.B., Gooch, E., Millac, P., Willox, A., Stern, M.A. and Walker, F. (1981). Autoantibody to nerve tissue in a patient with peripheral neuropathy and IgG paraprotein. *J. Clin. Pathol.* **34**: 1163–1166.

Sherman, W.H., Latov, N., Hays, A.P., Takatsu, M., Nemni, R., Galassi, G., and Ossermau, E.F. (1983). Monoclonal IgM_k antibody precipitating with chondroitin sulfate C from patients with axonal polyneuropathy and epidermolysis. *Neurology* **33**: 192–201.

Shirahama, T., Skinner, M., and Cohen, A.S. (1981). Immunocytochemical identification of amyloid in formalin-fixed paraffin sections. *Histochemistry* **72**: 161–171.

Simmons, Z., Bromberg, M.B., Feldman, E.L., and Blaivas, M. (1993). Polyneuropathy associated with IgA monoclonal gammopathy of undetermined significance. *Muscle Nerve* **16**: 77–83.

Smith, I.S., Kahn, S.N., Lacey, B.W., King, R.H., Eames, R.A., Whybrew, D.J., and Thomas, P.K. (1983). Chronic demyelinating neuropathy associated with benign IgM paraproteinaemia. *Brain* **106**: 169–195.

Sommer, C. and Schroder, J.M. (1989). Amyloid neuropathy: immunocytochemical localization of intra- and extracellular immunoglobulin light chains. *Acta Neuropathol.* **79**: 190–199.

Takatsu, M., Hays, A.P., Latov, N., Abrams, G.M., Nemni, R., Sherman, W.H., Nobile-Orazio, E., Saito, T., and Freddo, L. (1985). Immunofluorescence studies of patients with neuropathy and IgM M-proteins. *Ann. Neurol.* **181**: 173–181.

Thomas, P.K. and King, R.H.M. (1974). Peripheral nerve changes in amyloid neuropathy. *Brain* **97**: 395–406.

Thomas, F.P., Thomas, J.E., Sadiq, S.A., van den Berg, L.H., Latov, N., and Hays, A.P. (1990a). Human monoclonal anti-Gal(β1-3)GalNAc autoantibodies bind to the surface of bovine spinal motoneurons. *J. Neuropathol. Exp. Neurol.* **49**: 89–95.

Thomas, F.P., Vallejos, V., Foiti, D.R., Miller, J.R., Barrett, R., Fetell, M.R., Knowles, D.M., Latov, N., and Hays, A.P. (1990b). B cell small lymphocytic lymphoma and chronic lymphocytic leukemia with peripheral neuropathy, two cases with neuro pathologic findings and lymphocyte marker analysis. *Acta Neuropathol.* **80**: 197–202.

Trapp, B.D. and Quarles, R.H. (1984). Immunocytochemical localization of the myelin-associated glycoprotein. *J. Neuroimmunol.* **6**: 231–249.

Trotter, J.L., Engel, W.K., and Ignoczak, T.F. (1977). Amyloidosis with plasma cell dyscrasia: an overlooked cause of adult onset sensorimotor neuropathy. *Arch. Neurol.* **34**: 209–214.

Van den Berg, L.H., Marrink, J., de Jager, A.E.J., de Joug, H.J., van Imhoff, G.W., Latov, N., and Sadiq, S.A. (1992). Anti-GM_1 antibodies in patients with Guillaiu-Barré syndrome. *J. Neurol. Neurosurg. Psychiatry* **55**: 8–11.

Van den Berg, L.H., Hays, A.P., Nobile-Orazio, E., et al. (1996) Anti-MAG and anti-SGPG antibodies in neuropathy. *Muscle Nerve* **19**: 637–643.

Van den Bergh, P., Logigian, E.L., and Kelly, J.J. (1989). Motor neuropathy with multifocal conduction blocks. *Muscle Nerve* **11**: 26–31.

Van den Berg, L.H., Marrink, J., de Jager, A.E.J., de Jong, H.J., van Imholt, G.W., Latov, N., and Sadiq, S.A. (1992). Anti-GM_1 antibodies in patients with Guillain–Barré syndrome. *J. Neurol. Neurosurg. Psychiatry* **55**, 8–11.

Verghese, J.P., Bradley, W.B., Nemni, R., and McAdam, P.W.J. (1983). Amyloid neuropathy in multiple myeloma and other plasma cell dyscrasias: a hypothesis of the pathogenesis of amyloid neuropathies. *J. Neurol. Sci.* **59**: 237–246.

Victor, M., Banker, B.Q., and Adams, R.D. (1958). The neuropathy of multiple myeloma. *J. Neurol. Neurosurg. Psychiatry* **21**: 73–88.

Vital, C., Dumas, P., Latinville, D., Dib, M., Vital, A., and Bechenmacher, C. (1986). Relapsing inflammatory demyelinating polyneuropathy in a diabetic patient. *Acta Neuropathol. (Berl)* **71**: 94–99.

Vital, C., Henry, P., Loiseau, P., Julien, J., Vallat, J.M., Tignol, J., Bonnad, E., and Hedreville-Talon, M.A. (1975). Les neuropathies peripheriques de la maladie de Waldenström's: etude histologique et ultrastructurale de cinq cas. *Ann. Anat. Pathol.* **20**: 93–108.

Vital, A., Latinville, D., Aupy, M., et al. (1991). Inflammatory demyelinating lesions in two patients with IgM monoclonal gammopathy and polyneuropathy. *Neuropathol. Appl. Neurobiol.* **17**: 415–420.

Vital, A. and Vital, C. (1985). Polyarteritis nodosa and peripheral neuropathy: ultrastructural study of 13 cases. *Acta Neuropathol. (Berl.)* **67**: 136–141.

Walsh, J.C. (1971). The neuropathy of multiple myeloma. *Arch. Neurol.* **25**: 404–414.

Younger, D.S., Dalmau, J., Inghirami, G., Sherman, W.H., and Hays, A.P. (1994). Anti-Hu-associated peripheral nerve and muscle microvasculitis. *Neurology* **44**: 181–183.

Younger, D.S., Rosoklija, G., Hays, A.P., Trojaborg, W., and Latov, N. (1996). Diabetic peripheral neuropathy: a clinicopathologic and immunohistochemical analysis of sural nerve biopsies. *Muscle Nerve* **19**: 722–727.

Yuki, N., Yoshino, H., Sato, S., and Miyatake, T. (1990). Acute axonal polyneuropathy associated with anti-GM1 antibodies following *Campylobacter jejuni* enteritis. *Neurology* **40**: 1900–1902.

Zanusso, G.L., Moretto, G., Bonetti, B., Monaco, S., and Rizzuto, N. (1992). Complement neoantigen and vitronectin are components of plaques in amyloid AL neuropathy. *Ital. J. Neurol. Sci.* **13**: 493–499.

PART III Immune-mediated neuropathies

7 Guillain-Barré syndrome and variants

F.G.A. van der Meché

Introduction

The Guillain-Barré features of subacute symmetrical ascending paralysis of the Guillain-Barré syndrome (GBS) have been first described by Landry in 1859. In 1916 Guillain-Barré and Strohl added the characteristic cerebrospinal fluid (CSF) findings of a raised protein content with a near normal cell count. Haymaker and Kernohan described in 1949 for a group of 50 patients the inflammatory changes in the peripheral nervous system. The development of the experimental allergic neuritis (EAN) in 1955 by Waksman and Adams initiated subsequently immunological research in this field. From this time onward clinical, epidemiological, neurophysiological and immunological studies have shed new light on the syndrome and resulted in clinical trials evaluating specific treatment in the 1980s. In 1978 and reassessed in 1990 by Asbury and Cornblath diagnostic criteria for GBS have been developed. They are predominantly based upon clinical criteria: more or less symmetrical paresis with reduction and finally disappearance of reflexes with a progressive phase of maximally 4 weeks. CSF analysis and electromyography (EMG) characteristics add further support. Important is the exclusion of any specific cause. Within the limits of these criteria a large variability of clinical features exists. The classical form may be further characterized by distal, global or more proximal weakness and the absence or presence of sensory signs (van der Meché et al. 1988; Visser et al. 1995). Furthermore, cranial nerve variants such as the Miller Fisher syndrome and a lower bulbar variant do exist. In addition to these clinical characteristics EMG and pathology may both add information concerning the extent of axonal involvement and the latter method also about the nature of the inflammatory lesions (van der Meché et al. 1988; Honavar et al. 1991). Microbiological studies may reveal specific infections such as *Campylobacter jejuni*, cytomegalovirus, Epstein–Barr virus, *Mycoplasma pneumoniae* and HIV. Immunological studies may give evidence for immune activation or more specifically for autoantibodies, e.g. directed against the gangliosides GM1 or GQ1b. Finally, epidemiological circumstances may be important such as the late summer occurrence of a paralytic syndrome in children and young adults in China (McKhann et al. 1993).

At present consensus exists to define GBS in the first place clinically and to add subsequently to these

Table 7.1 *Guillain-Barré syndrome*

Clinically defined by
– more or less symmetrical weakness
– disappearing myotatic reflexes
– nadir within 4 weeks, usually within 2 weeks
– no other identifiable cause

Further characterization of clinically defined GBS

Neurological examination
Classically ascending
– sensorimotor
– pure motor
– severe sensory/autonomic
– distal, proximal, global weakness
– hyperacute with severe prognosis
Cranial nerve variant
– Miller Fisher syndrome
– lower bulbar variant
Epidemiology
– late summer outbreak, in children in China
– vaccination programs, e.g. rabies
Electrodiagnostic studies
– demyelination versus axonal
– diffuse conduction block
Pathological studies
– demyelination versus axonal
– inflammatory characteristics
Microbiological studies
– *C. jejuni*
– CMV, EBV, HIV
– *Mycoplasma pneumoniae*
Immunological studies
– activation markers
– autoantibodies

Notes:
CMV: cytomegalovirus; EBV: Epstein–Barr virus, GBS: Guillain-Barré syndrome; HIV: human immunodeficiency virus.

clinically defined cases of GBS further characteristics (Table 7.1) (Ad Hoc Committee WHO 1993; van der Meché and van Doorn 1995). In the future it may be that subgroups may be identified with a specific pathogenesis and clinical picture that may respond to a particular therapy. At present two effective therapies are known: plasma exchange (PE) and high-dose immunoglobulins intravenously given (IgIV). There is a further indication that pure motor GBS is associated with *C. jejuni* infection and high titers of anti-GM1 IgG antibodies and that these patients respond better to IgIV than to PE (Visser et al. 1995).

Clinical description

Classically ascending Guillain-Barré syndrome

The main clinical characteristics have already been discussed above. By definition the nadir has been reached within 4 weeks, but about 70% of patients do so within 2 weeks. It has been argued that in fact the distinction between GBS and chronic inflammatory demyelinating polyneuropathy (CIDP) is rather arbitrarily (van der Meché 1994). In CIDP by definition the nadir is reached beyond 2 months. But also an intermediate group has been described (Honavar et al. 1991). In fact it may therefore be suggested that a continuum exists with regard to the time of the nadir with a sharp peak during the first few weeks and the long tail of patients who have a much longer and usually less fulminating course (van der Meché and van Doorn 1995).

About 80% of the patients will present or will develop sensory symptoms and signs. In a literature review of the clinical features of 924 cases, summarized by Hughes and Winer (1984), 85% had involvement of arms and legs on admission. Fourteen percent had weakness limited to the legs and only 1% had arm weakness alone. In patients with tetraparesis, however, arm weakness may be more pronounced in a small proportion. Half of the patients will present with cranial nerve involvement, most frequently facial weakness.

For some reason distribution of weakness in the individual extremities has generally been held to be more proximal than distal. In the literature the proximal predominance varies from 4% in the arms to 58% in the legs (van der Meché 1994). In our own series of 147 patients proximal predominance was present in a quarter; in another quarter deficit was more distally and in the remaining half global (Visser et al. 1995). A distal predilection is easily explained, either by random demyelination, or vulnerability of the longer axons (van der Meché et al. 1988). A predilection of shorter motor fibers is not easily understood and even more complex since sensory signs are not more extensive proximally in patients with proximal motor deficit.

A pure motor form has been described in 3% of the large series of Ropper (1994). Visser et al. (1995) found in a series of 147 patients a pure motor form in 17%. Furthermore, they demonstrated that these patients, in contrast to patients with sensory involvement, nearly always had predominantly distal motor deficit, rarely cranial nerve involvement, and presumably due to the sparing of proximal muscles, relatively less need for artificial ventilation. Also reflexes may be spared until more severe paresis develops due to an intact afferent pathway (van der Meché et al. 1988). Furthermore, an association was found with high titers of anti-GM1 IgG antibodies and somewhat more patients had a preceding *C. jejuni* infection. The majority of these patients did not fulfil the electrophysiological criteria for the demyelination as suggested by Asbury and Cornblath (1990). Interestingly, it was found that a differential effect of treatment was observed in this group. Patients treated with IgIV fared better compared with the patients treated with PE. In the IgIV group (n=16), 13% was not able to walk independently 6 months after onset of the disease and 55% in the PE group (n=11; p=0.02). This difference was even more pronounced in the pure motor group with proven *C. jejuni* infection (p=0.002). This preliminary finding may suggest that IgIV is able to prevent severe axonal degeneration in at least a number of cases. Further studies should clarify this.

A special variant of the pure motor GBS is the paralytic syndrome observed in China. A clinical analysis of 514 cases of this syndrome has been reported by Zhang and Li (1979). Over the last few years more clinical details have become available (McKhann et al. 1993). It concerns children or sometimes young adults, usually from rural areas, who develop paralytic disease in the late summer. Reflexes are lost in weak muscles and no sensory signs are found. At the nadir 30% need artificial respiration. Recovery may be partial but is often complete. CSF shows no pleiocytosis but increased protein content is present in 60% of the cases. The electrophysiology, however, lacks the typical characteristics of demyelination. Indeed in a preliminary communication it has now been indicated that in many of these patients axonal changes predominate (Asbury et al. 1993).

A more controversial subject is the existence of a primary axonal variant in Western countries. In general, axonal damage has been interpreted as a bystander effect of severe immune-mediated demyelination. The possibility of a primary axonal neuropathy was initially suggested by Feasby et al. in 1986, based on five extremely severely afflicted patients. These patients had inexcitable motor nerves, denervation potentials and poor recovery in three out of four survivors. The one patient who died showed at post-mortem in only 5% of the nerve fibers demyelination, but in over 30% axonal degeneration. Two later autopsy studies with similar clinical and electrophysiological characteristics suggested that demyelination might have been the primary pathological process (Fuller et al. 1992; Berciano et al. 1993).

In a longitudinally electrophysiological study of eight patients who developed severe axonal damage, according to clinical and electrophysiological criteria, it was demonstrated that in the majority conduction block, the hall-mark of demyelination, was found before the development of the electrophysiological characteristics of axonal damage (van der Meché et al. 1991a). Also Brown et al. (1993) demonstrated conduction block very distally in the motor nerves. They argue, however, that the conduction block observed might be attributed to the wave of Wallerian degeneration from the more proximal localized axonal lesion to the periphery. As long as the terminal end has not yet degenerated, it still is possible to stimulate the nerve distally. In contrast, more proximally the nerve is inexcitable due to the fact that axonal degeneration has already taken place at that level. Based on the still lose criteria for axonal GBS Yuki (1994) has suggested a pathogenesis of severe GBS with axonal involvement. *C. jejuni* may induce either GM1 or GD1a IgG antibodies that might damage the axons. The evidence is however based upon anecdotal studies.

The state of the art may be summarized as follows:

1. Severe axonal degeneration exists and results in poor recovery. A primary axonopathic mechanism may well exist, but is as yet unproven and may be difficult to prove considering the following:

2. Electrophysiologically it is difficult to distinguish the different causes of low distal amplitude and inexcitable nerves. Demyelination may be more exaggerated distally, where also the reduced safety factor at the transition of myelinated to unmyelinated nerve ending renders conduction more vulnerable, all resulting in a low CMAP due to demyelination. On the other hand axonal degeneration may take place over a long distance of the nerve fibre or a mere loss of contact of terminal nerve branches may occur; both yield similar electrophysiological results despite of course an important prognostic difference. Furthermore, transient conduction block may not necessarily be attributed to demyelination, but may be explained by a bypassing wave of Wallerian degeneration. Only persistent or resolving conduction block is with certainty caused by demyelination (van der Meché et al. 1991a).
3. Pathologically, axonal changes may predominate, even in case of a severe primary demyelinating attack. Severe primary demyelination may occur without severe cellular infiltration (Honavar et al. 1991). Focal, severe demyelination resulting in axonal damage will finally be seen at all lower segments of the nerve as Wallerian axonal degeneration, thereby increasing the chance of finding axonal degeneration many fold over the finding the local spot of demyelination;
4. In EAN dose dependently a demyelinating or an axonal form of the experimental neuropathy may be elicited (Hartung et al. 1988). This indicates that it may be a matter of severity of the same pathogenic process;
5. The proof of an association between severe GBS with axonal involvement and *C. jejuni* infection plus GM1 of GD1a IgG antibodies is as yet preliminary and considering the arguments above premature with respect to a primary axonal disease.

The discussion of a possible axonal form of GBS stresses the importance of the concept given in the Introduction. As long as the hyperacute severe form of GBS is studied within the concept of clinically defined GBS further studies of larger groups of patients may solve the issue.

Autonomic and sensory variants do occur either apart or in combination. These are however rare diseases (for a review see van der Meché 1994).

Cranial nerve syndromes

Two clinical variants may be distinguished: one in which initially the oculomotor nerves are involved, the Miller Fisher syndrome, and another in which lower bulbar muscles are the first to be involved. Both forms tend to develop facial weakness and a descending paresis of the extremities, especially of the proximal muscles. Due to this, patients may need intubation to prevent obstructive apnea or artificial ventilation due to diaphragmatic weakness. In addition to these more severe examples, very mild forms may occur.

The Miller Fisher syndrome consists of ophthalmoplegia, ataxia and areflexia. The variability in 52 cases described in the literature has been surveyed by Schum and Geysel (1975). There has been a long dispute whether the Miller Fisher syndrome has a peripheral or a central cause, but it is now generally believed to be of peripheral nature, although it may be difficult to exclude some central involvement (Ropper 1994).

The lower bulbar variant, also called the pharyngeal cervical brachial variant by Ropper (1994), is characterized by difficulties in swallowing, speech, facial weakness and descending weakness starting in the shoulders.

In 26 patients with the onset of the disease in cranial nerves we identified an ophthalmoplegic group ($n=17$) and a lower cranial nerve variant ($n=9$), based on the early signs. Later in the disease, however, considerable overlap occurs. At the nadir of the disease 72% of the patients above 50 years of age and 12% of the patients below 50 years needed artificial respiration. The prognosis was generally good, some deficit occurred after 6 months in the older age group, but this was of minor functional importance (Ter Bruggen et al. 1991).

Diagnosis and prognosis

The diagnosis is mainly based on the clinical criteria discussed. Other diseases may sometimes be considered such as acute brainstem or spinal disorders, poliomyelitis, tick bite paralysis, botulism, acute myopathy or hypo- or hyperkalemia. Other neuropathies that may need to be considered are toxic neuropathies caused by alcohol, heavy metals, insecticides, solvents and drugs including cytotoxic agents such as vincristin. Acute or subacute neuropathies may also be due to vitamin B1 deficiency, porphyria, the neuropathy of critical illness, lymphomatose infiltration, vasculitis, Lyme borreliosis and poliomyelitis. In the last two conditions increased cell counts in CSF are usually present and confirmatory tests available. The cranial nerve syndromes may be confused with brainstem encephalitis, Wernicke encephalopathy, myasthenia gravis and botulism.

The diagnosis may be further supported by the characteristic findings in the CSF. Classically the protein content is raised with a normal cell count. In the first week of the disease the increase of protein content is still limited. In our experience in over 100 patients, 50% will then have a raised protein content, whereas the proportion increases to 80% in the second week. Only about 10% of the patients will have a cell count above 3 mm^{-3}. If the cell count is raised above normal with in other respects the usual form of GBS it is important to consider HIV infection as the triggering mechanism and as an alternative Lyme borreliosis. Since the total protein raise is due to leakage through the damaged blood–brain barrier, oligoclonal banding or the IgG index is of no diagnostic value. In general CSF studies are not very valuable in the typical case as usually the a priori chance of the diagnosis is very high and a negative test does not exclude the diagnosis of GBS.

Electrophysiological studies may show the characteristics of demyelination: slowing of conduction, conduction block, i.e. abnormal decrease of the compound muscle action potential after more proximal stimulation compared with distal stimulation, abnormal dispersion either after distal stimulation or after more proximal stimulation. Note that reduction of the compound muscle action potential (CMAP) after more proximal stimulation may be due to conduction block and to abnormal dispersion. As both are due to demyelination there is no need to differentiate between the two for diagnostic purposes. Previously we suggested the more descriptive term: length dependent amplitude reduction (van der Meché et al. 1988). In a group of 135 GBS patients the sensitivity of the EMG to detect signs of polyneuropathy was 85% at the end of the first week, but the sensitivity to detect demyelination was lower; the specificity was 100% (Meulstee 1994).

The EMG has been implicated as a prognostic factor. As discussed above severe axonal degeneration results in a low CMAP. It may therefore be expected that a low CMAP is related to a more severe clinical course. This has indeed been demonstrated in several studies (van der Meché 1994). We confirmed that the distal CMAP is significantly related to the outcome criterion of independent locomotion 6 months after the disease (Meulstee 1994; van der Meché 1994). In a longitudinal study of 135 patients it was found that only about 10% of the variability in duration until independent locomotion was explained by the size of the CMAP at the nadir. Therefore the CMAP is an unreliable clinical prognostic factor if considered alone.

Other factors found to be of prognostic value are the speed of deterioration, deficit at the nadir, the need of artificial respiration, the duration of the plateau phase and treatment. In the North American plasma exchange trial patients who were slowly deteriorating and randomized after the first week, who were under 30 years of age and who did not need artificial respiration, received plasma exchange and had CMAPs above 20% of normal were independently ambulant at 6 months. In contrast, if the patients were over 60 years of age and had all other factors in the negative direction, the proportion of patients independently ambulant at 6 months was only 19% (McKhann et al. 1988).

At present as discussed above it is not clear how biological factors such as *C. jejuni* infection and anti-GM1 antibodies are related to prognosis. In a preliminary study we found that patients above 50 years who had a *C. jejuni* infection and anti-GM1 antibodies had only a chance of 10% to be able to walk 2 months after onset, whereas younger patients without these factors had a 75% chance (van der Meché et al. 1993).

Pathogenesis

In considering pathogenic factors one should keep in mind that the GBS is very variable and also that

Table 7.2 *Relations between Guillain-Barré subpattern,* C. jejuni *and anti-ganglioside antibodies*

	Antiganglioside antibody	*C. jejuni* association	Ganglioside-like structures present on *C. jejuni*	Crossreaction demonstrated
Classical Guillain-Barré syndrome (often pure motor)	GM1	+	+	+
Chinese paralytic syndrome	GM1	+	Not investigated	Not investigated
Miller Fisher syndrome	GQ1b	+	+	+
Lower bulbar variant	GT1a/GD1a?	Not investigated	Not investigated	Not investigated
Sensory variant	GD1b?	Not investigated	Not investigated	Not investigated

in more typical cases pathological and electrophysiological studies have shown a large variability (van der Meché et al. 1988; Honavar et al. 1991). GBS is however generally assumed to be an immune-mediated polyneuropathy. In about 70% the disease is preceded by an infectious disease (Table 7.1). The histology shows perivascular infiltrates and macrophages involved in myelin destruction. Furthermore a variety of immunological studies have shown activation of the immune system. T and B cells become activated at the onset of the disease as evidenced by an increase of the activation markers in serum (for a review see Hartung et al. 1993; van der Meché and van Doorn 1995). In short, IL-6, a promotor of immune globulin synthesis was found to be increased both in serum and CSF of GBS patients. The soluble IL-2 receptor and IL-2 itself are increased in serum. Other interleukines that are variably increased in serum or CSF include interferon gamma and TNFα, which has a toxic effect on myelin and Schwann cells. IL-2 and TNFα have been shown to correlate with the clinical course in longitudinal studies. Furthermore, for TNFα a correlation with disease severity has been suggested. Also the number of activated T lymphocytes expressing the activation markers HLA-DR, the transferrin receptor and the membrane bound IL-2 receptor is increased. Macrophages, suggested to be the chief antigen-presenting cells in inflammatory foci, are activated as suggested by increased serum levels of the secretory product neopterin and by enhanced in vitro production of oxygen free radicals. The involvement of complement has been substantiated by the finding of increased concentrations of the soluble terminal complement in serum and CSF and increased concentrations of the low molecular weight product C3a and C5a in CSF alone.

In contrast to the indirect approach summarized above, a more direct way to study the immune pathogenesis has been developed over the last few years. In the following, the association of an antecedent *C. jejuni* infection with different patterns of GBS will be discussed, together with the possible role of this infection in the initiation of the production of the anti-ganglioside antibodies and the present evidence of the pathogenic significance of these auto-antibodies (Table 7.2).

Kaldor and Speed (1984) described for the first time in a large series of classical ascending GBS patients the significance of *C. jejuni* infection as a preceding event in GBS. The incidence of 38% has been repeated by others (Kuroki et al. 1991; van der Meché et al. 1992, 1993; Enders et al. 1993; Vriesendorp et al. 1993). A relation with a more severe disease has been suggested by a number of studies (Kaldor and Speed 1984; Winer et al.1988; Yuki et al. 1991; van der Meché et al. 1992, 1993; Vriesendorp et al. 1993, Jacobs et al. 1996), but not in all (Enders et al. 1993). In any case the association is not absolute as many patients with a *C. jejuni* infection have a benign course (van der Meché et al. 1991b). The study of anti-gangliosides antibodies in GBS parallelled the study of *C. jejuni.* These antibodies may recognize different epitopes on individual gangliosides; some of these epitopes are shared between different gangliosides and therefore crossreactivity between gangliosides does occur. Alternatively, patients may have several antibodies reacting with different epitopes. Anti-GM1 antibodies are most extensively investigated. They are, however, not specific for GBS as they are also found in patients with for example CIDP, lower motor neuron disease and multifocal motor neuropathy (Pestronk et al. 1990; Chaudhry et al. 1993). High titer IgG anti-GM1 antibodies has been associated with predominantly motor GBS (Kornberg et al. 1994; Visser et al. 1995). The presence of these antibodies have been related to a more severe clinical course (Yuki et al. 1991; Ilyas et al. 1992; Simone et al. 1993; Van der Meché et al. 1993), but this was not confirmed in all studies (Enders et al., 1993; Vriesendorp et al., 1993). This discrepancy may be due to the limited number of patients in some studies, the methodology of follow-up and the technique of antibody testing, but also the influence of other prognostic factors, such as age and *C. jejuni*, has to be taken into account. Furthermore, the immune globulin isotype may be important as it has been suggested above that especially IgG antibodies may be related to more severe axonal loss. Subsequently it was shown that *C. jejuni* infection and anti-GM1 antibodies regularly occur together in individual patients. In a group of 129 patients this association was significant (van der Meché et al. 1992), which led to the hypothesis that *C. jejuni* may contain a GM1-like structure,that induces anti-GM1 antibodies. It has now been shown that *C. jejuni* isolated from GBS patients does contain GM1-like structures (Moran et al. 1991; Yuki et al. 1993a). An other important step has been that Oomes et al. (1995) demonstrated that indeed anti-GM1 antibodies from GBS sera could be absorbed by *C. jejuni* bacteria, but not by *E. coli*; this confirmed with patient material that the concept of molecular mimicry may play a role in the pathogenesis. The next prerequisite is of course whether GM1 epitopes are present in the right places on the peripheral nervous system and whether they do play a pathogenic role. GM1 indeed is present at the nodal and paranodal level, and in addition at the nerve terminals (Corbo et al. 1993). A preliminary report of two GBS patients suggests that anti-GM1 containing plasma raises the stimulus threshold of the phrenic nerve in a nerve-diaphragm preparation and blocks up to 30% of the fibres (Vincent et al. 1994).

In the Chinese paralytic syndrome in children an association was also found with *C. jejuni* infection and with anti-GM1 antibodies (McKhann et al. 1993; Kornberg et al. 1994). Further information whether *C. jejuni* cultured from these patients may be able to absorb the anti-GM1 antibodies has not yet been obtained.

The findings in the Chinese syndrome so far, however, fit well in with the findings in the pure motor variant of GBS (Visser et al. 1995). It is best summarized as a strong relation between IgG anti-GM1 antibodies with a pure motor neuropathy with little electrophysiological evidence for demyelination. Although axonal changes may predominate, the clinical course in both the pure motor GBS as well as in the Chinese paralytical syndrome often have a benign course; therefore it should be anticipated that the major changes are at the level of the nerve endings. Any damage at that level may be followed by fast recovery. This concept is also in agreement with our findings that the classical electrophysiological signs of denervation do not predict a poor outcome (Meulstee 1994).

The Miller Fisher syndrome is strongly related to anti-GQ1b antibodies; in four studies these antibodies were found in 23 of 26 patients tested (Chiba et al. 1992; Willison et al. 1993; Yuki et al. 1993b; Jacobs et al. 1995). A preceding *C. jejuni* infection has been documented in the study of three patients by Jacobs et al. (1995). Furthermore, in this study it was shown that three strains of bacteria isolated from the Miller Fisher patients were able to absorb the anti-GQ1b antibodies, whereas control strains of *C. jejuni* were not. The strains isolated from Miller Fisher patients were on the other hand not able to absorb anti-GM1 antibodies of a classical GBS patient. The antibodies therefore recognized epitopes on *C. jejuni* bacteria in a strain-specific manner. This is supported by the findings of Yuki (1994) who demonstrated GQ1b-like structures on *C. jejuni* strains cultured from Miller Fisher patients. That molecular mimicry may also play a role in Miller Fisher syndrome is further supported by the finding of the preferential localization of GQ1b in the oculomotor nerves (Chiba et al. 1993) and the pathophysiological effect of anti-GQ1b antibodies containing sera. Roberts et al. (1994) demonstrated that three such sera were able to block miniature endplate potentials and completely block the electrically evoked muscle potentials in the mouse phrenic nerve-diaphragm preparation.

Anecdotal information suggests that the lower bulbar variant may be related to anti-GT1a and GD1a antibodies (Mizoguchi et al. 1994) and sensory neuropathy with anti-GD1b antibodies; from the latter ganglioside it is known that it is mainly localized in dorsal root ganglia (for a review see van der Meché and van Doorn 1995).

If these antiganglioside antibodies do indeed play a significant pathogenic role it may follow that more complex clinical patterns are constructed for the contribution of several antibody-mediated mechanisms. In our series it is shown that high titer anti-GM1 antibodies do occur also in mixed sensorymotor GBS; anti-GM1 antibodies may nevertheless be responsible for the motor part of the clinical deficit. Furthermore, anti-GQ1b antibodies do occur in classical GBS, usually only if clear ocular involvement is present (B.C. Jacobs and L.H. Visser, unpublished observation).

Treatment

Supportive treatment is still of primary importance, despite the fact that specific immune modulating therapy is now available. Respiratory insufficiency and cardiovascular instability do often occur and these functions should be carefully monitored. More rarely paralytic ileus may develop. Thromboembolic complications, compression neuropathies, decubitus, contractures and urinary infections are all largely preventable. Pain may be burdensome and often difficult to treat. Optimal positioning on special mattresses is usually of great help. Neuropathic pain medication like tricyclic antidepressant or carbamazepine may have some additional effect (see Chapter 26), but is often disappointing. Epidural morphine infusion is in use in several centers.

Monitoring of patients in an intensive care unit is necessary in any patient with fast progression or who is already severely paralysed. Progressive weakness of the respiratory muscles and muscles involved in swallowing especially should be monitored with great care. Aspiration in a patient with respiratory weakness may result in acute respiratory distress. Decreasing respiratory force is paralleled by a decreasing vital capacity. Elective intubation is indicated in patients who are still deteriorating if the vital capacity is about 15 ml kg^{-1} or just above 1 litre in a 70 kg person (Ropper 1992). In addition to the vital capacity, an increasing respiratory rate and subjective increased effort of breathing are indicators of impending respiratory failure. Paradoxical movements of thorax and abdomen are a late feature. Blood gas analysis may not be very informative; pCO_2 and pO_2 may remain within normal limits until respiratory failure occurs. If atelectasis or respiratory infection occurs, however, these complications may result in shunting and lowering of the pO_2 with increased respiratory effort. By monitoring the vital capacity, respiratory rate and the subjective breathing load such complications may, however, be prevented by physical therapy and elective intubation.

Cardiovascular dysautonomia should be treated only when really necessary, as the response to medication may be unpredictable. Hypotension may best be treated by an increase of fluid infusions.

Specific treatment

PE and more recently intravenous immunoglobulin (IgIV) have been shown to be effective, corticosteroids are still under study, others like liquorpheresis are experimental. The efficacy of PE has been demonstrated in two large clinical trials including 245 patients in the North American trial and 220 patients in the French trial, respectively (Guillain-Barré Syndrome Study Group 1985; French Cooperative Group on PE in GBS 1987). In the North American trial a total of 200–250 ml kg^{-1} of plasma was exchanged in 7–14 days, in 40–50 ml kg^{-1} exchanges on three to five occasions. In the French study, two plasma volumes were exchanged on 4 alternate days. In the PE group of both studies improvement started earlier and artificial respiration was significantly decreased compared with the control group. Moreover, the median time until independent locomotion was decreased by 32 and 41 days, respectively, compared with the control group in the two studies. In the North American trial there was still a significant improvement at 6 months in the walking ability of patients who had received PE. These findings indicate not only a considerable decrease in morbidity, but also a considerable degree of economic savings as a result of PE.

The main drawbacks of PE treatment are contra-indications and treatment failures during the PE course. Moreover, PE facilities are not available everywhere or immediately applicable in acute situations. Furthermore, it is usually a burden for the patient. An alternative to PE is IgIV which has been shown to be effective in a variety of immune-mediated diseases (Dwyer 1992). A multicentre study has been conducted in the Netherlands comparing IgIV with PE in 150 patients (van der Meché et al. 1992). A dose of 0.4 g kg^{-1} bodyweight was given over 5 consecutive days. The predefined aim of the study was to show equal efficacy; such a study is called 'a conservative trial'. The main outcome criterion was functional improvement 4 weeks after entry. In fact, significantly more patients in the IgIV group improved over the first 4 weeks (53% versus 34% in the PE group, 95% confidence interval of the difference 3–34%, $p=0.024$). Also secondary outcome criteria favoured IgIV, namely the time until functional improvement ($p=0.05$), the fraction of patients with multiple complications ($p<0.01$) and the fraction of patients needing artificial ventilation in the second week ($p<0.05$). Based on the main aim of this conservative trial we concluded that indeed IgIV is at least as effective as PE, but may be superior. Some discussion was initiated by Ropper (1992) concerning a better outcome of the NA-trial PE group, compared with the Dutch PE group. Differences in referral pattern, entry criteria and method of analysis explain this difference (van der Meché 1994).

The Dutch and French trials, that had similar pre-entry disease duration, and that were both analysed according to the intention to treat paradigm, had a similar outcome in the PE groups. The French study, therefore, validates the Dutch results. A recently finished intercontinental study coordinated by Professor Hughes in London, compared IgIV, PE and a combination. It appeared that IvIg was as effective as PE whereas the combination was not superior (Plasma Exchange/Sandoglobin Guillain-Barré Trial Group 1997).

After treatment the patients may improve, stabilize or further deteriorate. In the individual case it is impossible to determine whether therapy actually caused improvement or the improvement had occurred spontaneous. On the other hand, patients who continue to deteriorate may have had a worse outcome without therapy. The only sure way to conclude that an individual patient responds to therapy is when after initial stabilization or improvement for 1 or a few weeks, secondary deterioration occurs. Such 'treatment-related clinical fluctuations' occur in about 10% after IgIV or PE and may be taken as additional evidence for biological efficacy (Kleyweg and van der Meché 1991). In general it seems unnecessary to change or extend therapy if patients do not start to improve during therapy. In the Dutch trial only about one-quarter made some functional recovery either with IgIV or PE in the first 2 weeks after randomization. One-quarter and one-third designated in the IgIV group and PE group, respectively, deteriorated in this period. This is consistent with the experiences in CIDP; here also the onset of improvement may take 1 week or more. Furthermore, after a treatment course, either IgIV or PE, the patient usually is in his third week of the disease. At that time treatment has very limited effect upon the clinical course (GBS Study Group 1985).

GBS may also follow a severe course in children (Kleyweg et al 1989) so that specific treatment is indicated. No formal trials have been performed in children alone, but comparison with historical controls has suggested a similar benefit from PE in children to that in adults (Lamont et al. 1991). It is therefore advisable to treat children with GBS with IgIV.

Recently, there has been renewed interest in corticosteroid therapy. Haass et al. (1988) described 11 patients of whom eight started to improve within 48 hours after the first dose of 1000 mg methylprednisolone. No relapses occurred if the dose was tapered in 5-day steps. The mean time to be at least independently ambulant was 49 days. Recently, the GBS Steroid Trial Group (1993) reported negative results following treatment for 5 days with 500 mg of methylprednisolone. In this study, however, PE was permitted if required and the increased application of PE in the placebo group may have masked some positive effects of methylprednisolone.

Stimulated by a report of synergistic action between IgIV and high dose methylprednisolone in idiopathic thrombocytopenic purpura, the Dutch GBS study group has performed a pilot study of combined treatment in 25 GBS patients, the results of which have been compared with the 74 IgIV treated patients in the previous trial. After 4 weeks 76% in the methylprednisolone/IgIV group functionally improved, whereas 53% improved in the IgIV group in the previous study ($p=0.04$) (Dutch Guillain-Barré Study Group 1994). The results stimulated a large scale randomized trial that is now in progress.

Future developments

Two major factors may influence developments in the near future: subgroups of the syndrome may be split off as distinct disease entities, and further treatment programmes may be developed in relation to different subgroups. At present it is still appropriate to include all patients who fulfil the major clinical syndrome criteria in the category of GBS and name them 'GBS clinically defined'. Subgroups can further be characterized according to epidemiological, clinical, electrodiagnostic, microbiological and immunological findings.

Specific treatment may develop from monotherapy with IgIV or PE to multimodal therapy. In particular, IgIV may easily be combined with other immune-modulating drugs. Interleukines or substances antagonizing interleukines like TNF-α are also future candidates to be tested in GBS. Furthermore, drugs that modify the final common path of tissue destruction like oxygen free radical scavengers or drugs promoting nerve regeneration (e.g. nerve growth factors) may potentially be of use.

Conclusions

The clinical variability of GBS in relation to a variety of epidemiological and laboratory findings has led to some confusion about subtyping different forms of GBS. At present the data do not allow a specific distinction of subgroups. In the individual patient a diagnosis of 'GBS clinically defined' may be made and further characterized by epidemiological, electrophysiological, pathological, microbiological and immunological findings. This may be finally the best way to identify in large groups of patients trends in specific pathogenic mechanisms possibly amenable for individualized treatment. Pathogenetically, more and more evidence is accumulating favoring molecular mimicry between microorganisms and peripheral nerve constituents as a major mechanism. Different strains from *C. jejuni* have been implicated to give rise to anti-GM1 antibodies in classical GBS and to anti-GQ1b antibodies in case of MillerFisher syndrome.

Therapy is both supportive and specific. Plasma exchange was the first specific treatment shown to be effective. Now high dose immunoglobulins are shown to be at least as effective.This form of treatment is more easily applicable and has therefore replaced plasma exchange in many centers. The combination of immunoglobulins with either high dose steroids and plasma exchange are currently being evaluated in two independent clinical trials. Future treatment studies may implicate new immune modulating drugs, drugs that protect the nerves against the final common path of tissue destruction such as free oxygen radical scavengers and finally drugs that promote neural growth.

References

Ad Hoc Committee WHO AIREN. (1993). Acute onset flaccid paralysis. World Health Organization, Geneva.

Asbury, A.K. and Cornblath, D.R. (1990). Assessment of current diagnostic criteria for Guillain-Barré syndrome. *Ann. Neurol.* **27**(suppl.): S21–S24.

Asbury, A.K., Li, C.Y., Ho, T., Macko, C., Xue, P., Stadlan, E.M., Ramos-Alvarez, M., Valenciano, L., Gao, C.Y., Cornblath, D.R., McKhann, G.M., and Griffin, J.W. (1993). Clinicopathological features of Guillain-Barré syndrome in China and elsewhere. *J. Neurol.* **241**(suppl.): S32.

Berciano, J., Coria, F., Montón, M., Calleja, J., Figols, J., and Lafarga, M. (1993). Axonal form of Guillain-Barré syndrome: evidence for macrophage-associated demyelination. *Muscle Nerve* **16**: 744–751.

Brown, W.F., Feasby, Th.E., and Hahn, A.F. (1993). Electrophysiological changes in the acute 'axonal' form of Guillain-Barré syndrome. *Muscle Nerve.* **16**: 200–205.

Chaudhry, V., Corse, A.M., and Cornblath, D.R. (1993). Multifocal motor neuropathy: response to human immune globulin. *Ann. Neurol.* **33**: 237–242.

Chiba, A., Kusunoki, S., Shimizu, T., and Kanazawa, I. (1992). Serum IgG antibody to ganglioside GQ1b is a possible marker of Miller Fisher syndrome. *Ann. Neurol.* **31**: 677–679.

Chiba, A., Kusunoki, S., Obata, H., Machinami, R., and Kanazawa, I. (1993). Serum anti-GQ1b IgG antibody is associated with ophthalmoplegia in Miller Fisher syndrome and Guillain-Barré syndrome: clinical and immunohistochemical studies. *Neurology* **43**: 1911–1917.

Corbo, M., Quattrini, A., Latov, N., and Hays, A.P. (1993). Localization of GM1 and Gal(β1–3)GalNAc antigenic determinants in peripheral nerve. *Neurology* **43**: 809–814.

Dutch Guillain-Barré Study Group. (1994). Treatment of Guillain-Barré syndrome with high-dose immune globulins combined with methylprednisolone: a pilot study. *Ann. Neurol.* **35**: 749–752.

Dwyer, M.D. (1992). Manipulating the immune system with immune globulin. *N. Eng. J. Med.* **326**: 107–116.

Enders, U., Karch, H., Toyka, K.V., Michels, M., Zielasek, J., Pette, M., Heesemann, J., and Hartung, H.P. (1993). The spectrum of immune responses to *Campylobacter jejuni* and glycoconjugates in Guillain-Barré syndrome and in other neuroimmunological disorders. *Ann. Neurol.* **34**: 136–144.

Feasby, T.E., Gilbert, J.J., Brown, W.F., Bolton, C.F., Hahn, A.F., Koopman, W.F., and Zochodne, D.W. (1986). An acute axonal form of Guillain-Barré polyneuropathy. *Brain* **109**: 1115–1126.

French Cooperative Group on Plasma Exchange in Guillain-Barré Syndrome. (1987). Efficiency of plasma exchange in Guillain-Barré syndrome: role of replacement fluids. *Ann. Neurol.* **22**: 753–761.

Fuller, G.N., Jacobs, J.M., Leweis, P.D., and Lane, R.J.M. (1992). Pseudoaxonal Guillain- Barré syndrome: severe demyelination mimicking axonopathy. A case with pupillary involvement. *J. Neurol. Neurosurg. Psychiatry* **55**: 1079–1083.

Guillain, G., Barré, J.A., and Strohl, A. (1916). Sur un syndrome de radiculo-nevrite avec hyperalbuminose du liquide cephalo-rachidien sans reaction cellulaire. Remarques sur les caracteres cliniques et graphiques des reflexes tendineux. *Bulletin et memories de la society medicale des hopitaux de Paris. Masson et Cie* **40**: 1462–1470.

Guillain-Barré Syndrome Steroid Trial Group. (1993). Double-blind trial of intravenous methylprednisolone in Guillain-Barré syndrome. *Lancet* **341**: 586–590.

Guillain-Barré Syndrome Study Group. (1985). Plasmapheresis and acute Guillain Barré syndrome. *Neurology* **35**: 1096–1104.

Haass, A., Trabert, W., Gressnich, N., and Schimrigk, K. (1988). High-dose steroid therapy in Guillain-Barré syndrome. *J. Neuroimmunol.* **20**: 305–308.

Hartung, H.-P., Heininger, K., Schafer, B., Fierz, W., and Toyka, K.V. (1988). Immune mechanisms in inflammatory polyneuropathy: advances in neuroimmunology. *Ann. N.Y. Acad. Sci.* **540**: 122–161.

Hartung, H.-P., Stoll, G., and Toyka, K.V. (1993). Immune reactions in the peripheral nervous system. In *Peripheral Neuropathy*, 3rd edn, ed. P.J. Dyck and P.K. Thomas, pp. 418–444. Philadelphia: Saunders.

Haymaker, W. and Kernohan, J.W. (1949). The Landry-Guillain-Barré syndrome: Clinicopathologic report of fifty fatal cases and a critique of the literature. *Medicine.* **25**: 59–141.

Honavar, M., Tharakan, J.K.J., Hughes, R.A.C., Leibowitz, S., and Winer J.B. (1991). A clinicopathological study of the Guillain-Barré syndrome. Nine cases and literature review. *Brain* **114**: 1245–1269.

Hughes, R.A.C., and Winer, J.B. (1984). Guillain-Barré syndrome. In *Recent Advances in Cinical Neurology*, 4th edn, ed. W.B. Matthews and G.H. Glaser, pp. 19–49. Edinburgh: Churchill Livingstone.

Ilyas, A.A., Mithen, F.A., Dalakas, M.C., Chen, Z.W., and Cook, S.D. (1992). Antibodies to acidic glycolipids in Guillain-Barré syndrome and chronic inflammatory demyelinating polyneuropathy. *J. Neurol. Sci.* **107**: 111–121.

Jacobs, B.C., Endtz, H.Ph., van der Meché, F.G.A., Hazenberg, M., Achtereekte, H.A.M., and van Doorn, P.A. (1995). Serum anti-GQ1b IgG antibodies recognize surface epitopes on *Campylobacter jejuni* from patients with Miller Fisher syndrome. *Ann. Neurol.* **37**: 260–254.

Jacobs, B.C., van Doorn, P.A., Schmitz, P.I.M. et al. (1996). *Campylobacter jejuni* infections and anti-GM1 antibodies in Guillain-Barré syndrome. *Ann. Neurol.* **40**: 181–187.

Kaldor, J. and Speed, B.R. (1984). Guillain-Barré syndrome and *Campylobacter jejuni*: a serological study. *Br. Med. J.* **288**: 1867–1870.

Kleyweg, R.P. and van der Meché, F.G.A. (1991). Treatment related fluctuations in Guillain-Barré syndrome after high-dose immunoglobulins or plasma-exchange. *J. Neurol. Neurosurg. Psychiatry* **54**: 957–960.

Kleyweg, R.P., van der Meché, F.G.A., Loonen, M.C.B., de Jonge, J., and Knip, B. (1989). The natural history of the Guillain-Barré syndrome in 18 children and 50 adults. *J. Neurol. Neurosurg. Psychiatry* **52**: 853–856.

Kornberg, A.J., Pestronk, A., Bieser, K., Ho, T.W., McKhann, G.M., Wu, H.S., and Jiang, Z. (1994). The clinical correlates of high-titer IgG anti-GM1 antibodies. *Ann. Neurol.* **35**: 234–237.

Kuroki, S., Haruta, T., Yoshioka, M., Kobayashi, Y., Nukina, M., and Nakanishi, H. (1991). Guillain-Barré syndrome associated with *Campylobacter* infection. *Pediatr. Infect. Dis. J.* **10**: 149–151.

Lamont, P.J., Johnston, H.M., and Berdoukas, V.A. (1991). Plasmapheresis in children with Guillain-Barré syndrome. *Neurology* **41**: 1928–1931.

Landry, O. (1859). Note sur la paralysie ascendante aigue. *Gazette Hebdomadaire* **6**: 474–476.

McKhann, G.M., Cornblath, D.R., and Griffin, J.W. (1993). Acute axonal neuropathy: a frequent cause of flaccid paralysis in China. *Ann. Neurol.* **33**: 333–342.

McKhann, G.M., Griffin, J.W., Cornblath, D.R., Mellits, E.D., Fisher, R.S., Quaskey, S.A., and the Guillain-Barré Syndrome Study Group. (1988). Plasmapheresis and Guillain-Barré syndrome: analysis of prognostic factors and the effect of plasmapheresis. *Ann. Neurol.* **23**: 347–353.

Meulstee, J. (1994). *Electrodiagnostic studies in Guillain-Barré syndrome.* Thesis Erasmus University Rotterdam.

Mizoguchi, K., Hase, A., Obi, T., Matsuoka, H., Takatsu, M., Nishimura, Y., Irie, F., Seyama, Y., and Hirabayashi, Y. (1994). Two species of antiganglioside antibodies in a patient with a pharyngeal-cervical-brachial variant of Guillain-Barré syndrome. *J. Neurol. Neurosurg. Psychiatry* **57**: 1121–1123.

Moran, A.P., Rietschel, E.T., Kosunen, T.U., and Z Ähringer, U. (1991). Chemical characterization of *Campylobacter jejuni* lipopolysaccharides containing N-acetylneuraminic acid and 2,3-diamino-2,3-dideoxy-*d*-glucose. *J. Bacteriol.* **173**: 618–626.

Oomes, P.G., Jacobs, B.C., Hazenberg, M.P.H., Bänffer, J.R.J., and van der Meché, F.G.A. (1995). Anti-GM1 IgG antibodies and *Campylobacter* bacteria in Guillain-Barré syndrome: evidence of molecular mimicry. *Ann. Neurol.* **38**: 170–175.

Pestronk, A., Chaudhry, V., Feldman, E.L., Griffin, J.W., Cornblath, D.R., Denys, E.H., Glasberg, M., Kuncl, R.W., Olney, R.K., and Yee, W.C. (1990). Lower motor neuron syndromes defined by patterns of weakness, nerve conduction abnormalities and high titers of antiglycolipid antibodies. *Ann. Neurol.* **27**: 316–326.

Plasma Exchange/Sandoglobulin Guillain-Barré Trial Group. (1997). Randomised trial of plasma exchange, intravenous immunoglobulin, and combined treatments in Guillain-Barré syndrome. *Lancet* **349**: 225–230.

Roberts, M., Willison, H., Vincent, A., and Newsom-Davis, J. (1994). Serum factor in Miller Fisher variant of Guillain-Barré syndrome and neurotransmitter release. *Lancet* **343**: 454–455.

Ropper, A.H. (1992). The Guillain-Barré Syndrome. *N. Engl. J. Med.* **326**: 1130–1136.

Ropper, A.H. (1994). Miller Fisher syndrome and other acute variants of Guillain-Barré syndrome. In *Baillière's Clinical Neurology*, vol. 2, no. 1, pp. 95–106.

Schumm, F. and Geysel, A. (1975). Das Fischer-syndrom, eine Sonderform des Landry-Guillain-Barré-Syndroms. *Nervenarzt* **46**: 678–687.

Simone, I.L., Annunziata, P., Maimone, D., Liguori, M., Leante, R., and Livrea, P. (1993). Serum and CSF anti-GM1 antibodies in patients with Guillain-Barré syndrome and chronic inflammatory demyelinating polyneuropathy. *J. Neurol. Sci.* **114**: 49–55.

Ter Bruggen, J.P., van der Meché, F.G.A., de Jager, A.E.J., Polman, C.H., and Wokke, J.H.J. (1991). Upside Guillain-Barré syndrome. *Clin. Neurol. Neurosurg.* **93**: 177.

Van der Meché, F.G.A. (1994). The Guillain-Barré syndrome. In *Baillière's Clinical Neurology*, vol. 2, no. 1, pp. 73–94.

Van der Meché, F.G.A., Meulstee, J., and Vermeulen, M., and Kievit, A. (1988). Patterns of conduction failure in the Guillain-Barré syndrome. *Brain* **111**: 405–416.

Van der Meché, F.G.A., Meulstee, J., Kleyweg, R.P. (1991a). Axonal damage in Guillain-Barré syndrome. *Muscle Nerve* **14**: 997–1002.

Van der Meché, F.G.A., Oomes, P.G., Kleyweg, R.P., Bänffer, J.R.J, and Meulstee, J. (1991b). Axonal Guillain-Barré. *Neurology* **41**: 1530–1531.

Van der Meché, F.G.A., Schmitz, P.I.M., and Dutch Guillain-Barré Study Group. (1992). A randomized trial comparing intravenous immune globulin and plasma exchange in Guillain-Barré syndrome. *N. Engl. J. Med.* **326**: 1123–1129.

Van der Meché, F.G.A., Oomes, P.G., and Schmitz, P.I.M. (1993). The clinical significance of biological prognostic factors including anti-GM1 antibodies in Guillain-Barré syndrome. In *Guillain-Barré Syndrome*, ed. C.J. Gibbs Jr and G.M. McKhann, pp. 251–255: Stuttgart: Thieme.

Van der Meché, F.G.A., and van Doorn, P.A. (1995). Guillain-Barré syndrome and chronic inflammatory demyelinating polyneuropathy: immune mechanisms and update on current therapies. *Ann. Neurol.* **37** (suppl. 1): S14–S31.

Vincent, A., Roberts, M., Willison, H., and Newsom-Davis, J. (1994). Plasma from patient with raised anti-GM1 antibodies passively transfer conduction block. *J. Neuroimmunol.* **54**: 204.

Visser, L.H., van der Meché, F.G.A., van Doorn, P.A., Jacobs, B.C., Kleyweg, R.P., Oomes, and the Dutch Guillain-Barré Study Group. (1995). Guillain-Barré syndrome without sensory loss (acute motor neuropathy): a subgroup with specific clinical, electrodiagnostic and laboratory features. *Brain* **118**: 841–847.

Vriesendorp, F.J., Mishu, B., Blaser, M.J., and Koski, C.L. (1993). Serum antibodies to GM1, GD1b, peripheral nerve myelin and *Campylobacter jejuni* in patients with Guillain-Barré syndrome and controls: correlation and prognosis. *Ann. Neurol.* **34**: 130–135.

Waksman, B.H. and Adams, R.D. (1955). Allergic neuritis: an experimental disease of rabbits induced by the injection of peripheral nervous tissue and adjuvants. *J. Exp. Med.* **102**: 213–235.

Willison, H.J., Veitch, J., Paterson, G., and Kennedy, P.G.E. (1993). Miller Fisher syndrome is associated with serum antibodies to GQ1b ganglioside. *J. Neurol. Neurosurg. Psychiatry* **56**: 204–206.

Winer, J.B., Hughes, R.A.C., Anderson, M.J., Jones, D.M., Kangro, H., and Watkins, R.P.F. (1988). A prospective study of acute idiopathic neuropathy. II. Antecedent events. *J. Neurol. Neurosurg. Psychiatry* **51**: 613–618.

Yuki, N. (1994). Pathogenesis of axonal Guillain-Barré syndrome: hypothesis. *Muscle Nerve.* **17**: 680–682.

Yuki, N., Sato, S., Itoh, T., and Miyatake, T. (1991). HLA-B35 and acute axonal polyneuropathy following *Campylobacter* infection. *Neurology* **41**: 1561–1563.

Yuki, N., Sato, S., Tsuji, S., Ohsawa, T., and Miyatake, T. (1993b). Frequent presence of anti-GQ1b antibody in Fisher's syndrome. *Neurology* **43**: 414–417.

Yuki, N., Taki, T., Inagaki, F., Kasama, T., Takahashi, M., Saito, K., Handa, S., and Miyatake, T. (1993a). A bacterium lipopolysaccharide that elicits Guillain-Barré syndrome has a GM1 ganglioside-like structure. *J. Exp. Med.* **178**: 1771–1775.

Yuki, N., Taki, T., Takahashi, T., Saito, K., Inagaki, F., Kasama, T., Yoshirol, H., Handa, S., and Miyatake, T. (1994). Molecular mimicry between gangliosides and *Campylobacter jejuni* isolated from Guillain-Barré syndrome and Fisher syndrome. *Muscle Nerve* (suppl.) **1**: S222.

Zhang, Z.L. and Li, T.N. (1979). Acute polyradiculoneuritis: clinical analysis of 514 cases. *Chin. J. Neurol. Psychiatry* **12**: 17–21.

8 Chronic inflammatory demyelinating polyneuropathy

M. Vermeulen

History and definition

At the beginning of this century my colleagues at the University Hospital of Amsterdam recognized a disorder which we now refer to as chronic inflammatory demyelinating polyneuropathy (CIDP). This was evident from a book published in 1911 on neuromuscular diseases written by one of them, Wertheim Salomonson (1911). In this book he described a disorder named polyneuritis idiopathica subacuta. The following is a summary of his description of this disorder.

This neuropathy, polyneuritis idiopathica subacuta, is characterized by a prodromal phase, deterioration of neurological functions and death or spontaneous improvement. In the prodromal phase patients may have gastrointestinal disturbances, fatigue, fever, pain or paresthesiae. This is followed by muscle weakness which may lead to generalized paralysis. There are usually sensory signs and symptoms, but weakness predominates. The neurological signs and symptoms are often rather symmetrical. Muscle atrophy and cranial nerve involvement may occur. Cardiac and respiratory complications may lead to death. Weakness usually starts in the legs, with arms being involved later. Weakness is sometimes restricted to the legs. Initially weakness is often confined to muscles innervated by one nerve, for instance the peroneal or tibial nerve in the legs or the median or ulnar nerve in the arms. Of the cranial nerves the facial nerve is most frequently affected. Bladder or bowel dysfunction is rare. The reflexes usually disappear. He goes on with a description of delirium which may occur in these patients followed by a description of different types of recovery. Some patients recover within 2 months, most patients take 6 months to recover and recovery may even occur after 1 year.

For this chapter on chronic inflammatory demyelinating polyneuropathy (CIDP) it is important that he observed cases which develop more slowly and that remissions and exacerbations may occur. Without references he mentioned that similar patients with recurrences were seen by Grocco, Déjerine, Eichhorst, Targowla, Sorgo, Schlier, Thomas and Oppenheim. In 1958 Austin in his landmark publication on recurrent polyneuropathies discussed reports of these neurologists mentioned by Wertheim Salomonson. Austin thought that a number of older reports could not be accepted as examples of recurrent polyneuropathy. He did not accept the case described by Grocco because of the presence of abdominal pains, vomiting, aphonia and sphincter disturbances. The descriptions by Eichhorst and Sherwood had too little clinical information, the case of Sorgo was probably a neuropathy caused by obliterative vascular (collagen) disease and that of Schlier was related to other diseases. This clearly demonstrates that since the first reports the diagnosis of these recurrent neuropathies were the subject of discussion. From the description by Wertheim Salomonson it is clear that he considered what we now have named the Guillain-Barré syndrome (GBS) and CIDP, as one and the same disorder. The only difference is the course that is the rate of progression of weakness and the occurrence of relapses.

In the previously mentioned paper by Austin emphasis is laid on recurrent neuropathies. He reviewed 32 cases of recurrent polyneuropathy and nine cases of acute symmetrical polyneuropathy with recurrences after withdrawal of corticosteroid treatment. He described a patient whom he had treated with adrenocorticotrophic hormone (ACTH) therapy. Repeated exacerbations and remissions over a 5 year period were clearly related to the waxing and waning of this treatment. Thomas et al described five patients with either recurrences or a more protracted initial course. All were treated with corticosteroids (Thomas et al. 1969). In 1975 Dyck et al. described chronic and relapsing patients and suggested that these patients should be separated from the acute syndrome. These authors emphasized that the acute monophasic inflammatory polyradiculoneuropathy usually reaches its maximum deficit in 3 weeks and begins to improve before 6 months. The patients with the acute syndrome also had a better prognosis since after an average follow-up period of 7.5 years only 4% of the chronic and recurrent cases had completely recovered. Although the course and the prognosis of the acute syndrome is different from the chronic and recurrent cases, many similarities could be detected. Weakness, sensory disturbances, cranial nerve involvement, cerebrospinal fluid (CSF) protein elevations, electrophysiological findings and pathological features save for hypertrophic changes, were not different between acute and chronic patients.

In 1976 Prineas and McLeod emphasized that the chronic and relapsing forms are related disorders. They concluded that chronic and relapsing neuropathies differ from the acute syndrome chiefly in regard to the rate of evolution and the severity of the initial episode of the neuropathy. In a review on the idiopathic polyradiculoneuropathies, Horowitz (1989) discussed the separation of chronic and recurrent forms from the acute disorders. He concluded that cases intermediate in their characteristics between the two conditions could conceivably indicate the presence of a spectrum in the temporal evolution of a single disorder. Horowitz questioned whether the actual incidence of a history of preceding infections is different between patients with the acute and chronic forms. He refers to a study by McCombe et al in patients with CIDP which showed that 32% of patients had a preceding illness or a vaccination (McCombe et al. 1987). This high incidence is not very much different from that observed in GBS. The difference in the frequency of assisted ventilation between the acute and chronic forms was also questioned by Horowitz. He stressed that most patients with GBS recover without respiratory difficulties and that a substantial number of patients with the chronic form develop respiratory insufficiency. Horowitz concluded that those who divide the acute and chronic syndromes treat a semiological complex as a nosologic entity.

Several committees have tried to define the acute and chronic syndromes. In 1978 GBS was arbitrarily defined by an ad hoc committee of the National Institute of Neurological Disorders and Stroke as an acute polyradiculoneuropathy in which symptoms usually reach their worst within 4 weeks (Asbury et al. 1978). In 1991 a panel of neurologists for the American Academy of Neurology Task Force on Acquired Immunodeficiency Syndrome stipulated the minimum progressive phase of CIDP as greater than 2 months (Ad Hoc subcommittee 1991). These definitions leave an intermediate group which has been named subacute idiopathic demyelinating polyradiculoneuropathy (SIDP). In 1992 Hughes proposed a classification into GBS with a progressive phase up to 4 weeks, SIDP with a progressive phase from 4 to 12 weeks and CIDP with a progressive phase greater than 12 weeks (Hughes et al. 1992).

In recent years it became increasingly evident that GBS is no longer a simple concept. The same may be true for CIDP. GBS may involve more than one type of pathological process. Feasby et al. (1986) showed that some patients had an acute axonal neuropathy, rather than a demyelinating disorder. Therefore the name 'acute inflammatory demyelinating polyneuropathy' is not appropriate for all patients with GBS. Even in the group with clear demyelinating features the pathogenesis may be different. In some patients demyelination is mediated predominantly by lymphocytes, in others it is primarily antibody mediated. Similarly, Julien et al. (1989) described patients with a chronic relapsing polyneuropathy, who had primary axonal lesions. Apart from a distinction between acute and chronic forms, there may be differences in pathogenesis within these groups.

The distinction between acute and chronic forms is not only an academic exercise as it determines the choice of treatment. A beneficial effect of steroids could not be demonstrated in GBS in contrast to patients with CIDP. Whether treatment response is different in the pathogenetic subgroups of patients with GBS or CIDP discussed above remains to be seen. In the criteria for the diagnosis CIDP, electrophysiological features considered consistent with demyelination are still required, indicating that pure axonal forms are not accepted.

Clinical features

In typical cases there is weakness with sensory impairments in arms and legs, both distally and proximally with slight asymmetries. The reflexes of arms and legs disappear. The onset is insidious. There may be a progressive deterioration or a course with remissions and exacerbations. All the clinical features reported in patients with GBS have been seen in CIDP, including cranial nerve involvement, respiratory failure and autonomic disturbances (Prineas and McLeod 1976; McCombe et al. 1987).

Pure motor (Donaghy 1994) and pure sensory forms have been described (Jay and Oh 1988). Weakness usually starts in the legs but may begin in the arms. Cranial nerve impairment may be the first sign (Donaghy and Earl 1985). Some reflexes may remain present even in severely affected patients. Initially when the signs and symptoms are mild and very slowly progressive this neuropathy is often not recognized by general physicians. Usually, these patients are advised to take things easier because the symptoms are attributed to 'stress'.

When there are remissions and exacerbations the diagnosis is not difficult. In contrast to patients with a chronic progressive form, the distinction from other chronic neuropathies may not be easy. Very important in the distinction from other neuropathies is the distribution of weakness which in CIDP is rarely confined to the distal muscles of the legs. The probability of CIDP is very low in patients who present with moderate to severe weakness of the legs without weakness of arm muscles. Similarly, in patients with a peripheral neuropathy and preserved arm reflexes, the diagnosis CIDP is unlikely (van Doorn et al. 1991). Tremor is not rare in CIDP. It usually increases with action. There is no relation between severity of the neuropathy and tremor. Tremor may occur in the presence of slight weakness and may begin when the patient is improving. Several drugs can be given to treat this often disabling tremor. Primidone is often effective when other treatments fail.

Laboratory analysis

Blood

Routine blood examination is usually normal in CIDP patients. As CIDP may be associated with systemic diseases, abnormalities consistent with these disorders can be found. CIDP has been observed in patients with thyrotoxicosis (McCombe et al. 1987), inflammatory bowel disease, hepatitis and after infections with cytomegalovirus and human immunodeficiency virus (Barohn et al. 1989).

Usually, patients with monoclonal gammopathy are excluded from studies on patients with CIDP. There is no doubt this is the right decision in patients with IgM monoclonal proteins, but patients over 50 years of age with IgG gammopathy of undetermined significance and the typical signs and symptoms of CIDP can probably best be treated as patients with CIDP in the absence of gammopathy.

Many different assays have been described to demonstrate antibodies against nervous tissue. A mixed hemagglutination test to demonstrate anti-human peripheral nerve antibodies has been shown to be positive in 50% of CIDP patients and in only 3% of patients with other neuropathies (Van Doorn et al. 1987). Similar results were reported for a complement fixation assay which measured C3b. In this study 50% of CIDP patients had positive results compared with 13% of patients with other neuropathies (Hays et al. 1988). Of the tests against cultured cells, an immune fluorescence assay to detect antibodies against hybrid mouse neuroblastoma/rat glioma NBL cell line 108 cc showed the best results; 43% of CIDP patients had these antibodies compared with 7% of patients with other neuropathies (van Doorn et al. 1988).

In other tests to detect antibodies the percentage of positive results in CIDP patients was low or was not much different from that in patients with other neuropathies, or patients with other neuropathies.

Recently, it was concluded that selective high titer serum IgG and IgM binding to B-tubulin has specificity for CIDP, that these antobodies occur in 50–60% of CIDP patients and that they may serve as a marker of the disease (Kornberg and Pestronk 1993). Van Schaik et al. (1994) using Western blot techniques could not confirm the high occurrence of these antibodies in CIDP.

Cerebrospinal fluid

Cerebrospinal fluid (CSF) protein is usually elevated; in four series the occurrence ranged from 87 to 95% (Dyck et al. 1975; Prineas and McLeod 1976; McCombe et al. 1987; Barohn et al. 1989). The level is often above 1 g l^{-1}. If a value of more than 1 g l^{-1} is found in a patient with a chronic peripheral neuropathy, the likelihood of CIDP increases. A normal value considerably decreases the probability of CIDP. In a series of patients with the clinical diagnosis CIDP who had improved after intravenous immunoglobulin treatment, the mean CSF protein value was 1.08 g l^{-1} (range 0.35–3.41g l^{-1}). The mean number of cells was 5×10^6/l, ranging from 0 to 20×10^6/l (van Doorn et al. 1991b). Others have also reported slight increases in cell number in 3%–13% of patients (Dyck et al. 1975; Prineas and McLeod 1976; McCombe et al. 1987; Barohn et al. 1989). An increased number of cells should alert to the presence of infections like HIV and *Borrelia burgdorferi*. If the signs and symptoms are not typical for CIDP the presence of cells should raise the suspicion of neoplastic meningitis.

Electrophysiology

In 1958 Austin in his review on recurrent polyneuropathy mentioned conduction block as an important feature of the disease. In 1969 Thomas et al. concluded that reduced nerve conduction velocity is useful diagnostically, indicating the presence of segmental demyelination. In 1975 Dyck et al. in their review came to the conclusion that there is a diffusely slow conduction velocity and that the most marked slowing is often very proximal (Dyck et al. 1975). Recently, several sets of criteria have been proposed for electrodiagnostic identification of patients with CIDP. In the evaluation of these criteria it is important to realize that physicians wish to distinguish patients with CIDP early in the course of the disease from patients with other disorders resembling CIDP. The problem is never how to distinguish a healthy nurse from a patient who very obviously is suffering from CIDP. Therefore, the proposed criteria should be tested by comparing electrophysiologic data of CIDP patients obtained at the time of their initial evaluation with that of patients with other neurological disorders, relevant in the differential diagnosis. One such comparison has been published (Bromberg 1991). Bromberg investigated the sensitivity and specificity of three sets of electrodiagnostic criteria shown in Table 8.1. Electrophysiological data were obtained from three groups of patients. One group consisted of 70 patients who were actively followed and who fulfilled clinical criteria for CIDP. Criteria included a progressive, relapsing or stepwise course with weakness and sensory disturbance, CSF cytoalbuminic dissociation in most patients, response to corticosteroids and plasma exchange, and exclusion of other diagnoses such as associated monoclonal gammopathy, multifocal motor neuropathy or systemic dysimmune disorders. The electrophysiological data were obtained at the time of their initial evaluation. The two control groups consisted of patients with diabetes mellitus and clinically evident polyneuropathy of mild to moderate severity and patients who fulfilled criteria for motor neuron disease. Sensitivity (true positive rate) of each of the three criteria were 50% for set I,

Table 8.1. *Three sets of electrophysiologic criteria for chronic inflammatory demyelinating polyneuropathy (CIDP)*

Set I

Must demonstrate three of the following abnormalities in motor nerves.

1. Reduced conduction velocity in two or more nerves: <75% of LLN.
2. Partial conduction block or abnormal temporal dispersion in one or more nerves: <70% P/D ratio.
3. Prolonged distal latency in two or more nerves: >130% of ULN
4. Prolonged F wave latency in one or more nerves: >130% of ULN

Set II

Must demonstrate three of the following abnormalities in motor nerves.

1. Reduction in conduction velocity in two or more nerves:
   <80% of LLN if CMAP amplitude >80% of LLN, or
   <70% of LLN if CMAP amplitude <80% of LLN.
2. Partial conduction block or abnormal temporal dispersion in one or more nerves (median, ulnar, peroneal):
   (a) partial conduction block: <80% P/D ratio if duration of negative peak of proximal CMAP is <115% of distal duration.
   (b) abnormal temporal dispersion and possible conduction block: <80% P/D ratio if duration of negative peak of proximal CMAP is >115% of distal CMAP duration.
3. Prolonged distal latency in two or more nerves:
   >125% of ULN in CMAP amplitude >80% of LLN, or
   >150% of ULN if CMAP amplitude <80% of LLN.
4. Prolonged F-wave latency in two or more nerves:
   >120% of ULN if CMAP amplitude is >80% LLN, or
   >150% of ULN if CMAP amplitude is <80% LLN, or absent F wave after 10 to 15 trials.

Set III

Must demonstrate the following abnormality in motor nerves.

1. Reduction in conduction velocity in two or more nerves:
   <70% of LLN.

Notes:
LLN: lower limit of normal; P/D: proximal to distal compound muscle action potential (CMAP) amplitude ratio; ULN: upper limit of normal.

46% for set II and 43% for III. (For I, II and III see Table 8.1.)

Specificity (true negative rate) was 100% for the three sets. Sensitivity could be increased by excluding patients in whom not every testable motor nerve was evaluated. This resulted in sensitivities of 64% for set I, 60% for II and 48% for III. When the same was carried out for the control groups, one patient with diabetes fulfilled set III. Many combinations were tried to see what the maximum sensitivity is without reduction of specificity. A sensitivity of 66% appeared to be the highest limit. Above this level there is a sharp decline of the specificity. A sensitivity of 66% can be achieved by the modified set I and III. Modified set I is the same as set I of Table 8.1 except that reduction in conduction velocity and prolonged distal latency need be present in only one nerve to be counted as one of the three abnormalities. Similarly, modified set III is the same as set III shown in Table 7.1 except that reduction of velocity needs be present in one nerve. Modified set I has several advantages over III. This set requires greater numbers of abnormalities which increases diagnostic confidence by excluding hereditary neuropathies and focal entrapment neuropathies. Hereditary motor sensory neuropathy type I can be distinguished from the acquired demyelinating disorders by the absence of conduction block or abnormal temporal dispersion. Slowing of conduction is more uniform over the nerves in patients with hereditary neuropathy. A disadvantage of criteria based on nerve conduction only is that it underestimates the presence of an acquired demyelinating process. This can be improved by testing for conduction block or abnormal temporal dispersion in several nerves.

There is considerable debate about the best method to define conduction block or temporal dispersion. Oh et al. (1994) showed that the reduction of CMAP amplitude with proximal stimulation ranges from 25 to 41% of the distal CMAP in normal subjects. An important finding was that there is a significant difference between CMAP elicited from the posterior tibial nerve and other nerves. For the median, ulnar and peroneal nerves the normal limit was 25% when amplitudes were measured from peak to peak and 30% for negative peak measurements. The values were 36% and 41%, respectively, for the tibial nerve. This means that if the modified set I discussed above is chosen as the best set of tests to diagnose CIDP, the definition of partial conduction block or abnormal dispersion can be used for all nerves except for the tibial nerve for which the negative peak amplitude reduction should be more than 40% in case of abnormality. Oh et al. (1994) compared different methods of measuring conduction block such as measurements of peak to peak amplitudes, negative peak amplitude, negative peak area and total area. Of these, total area measurements appeared to be the most sensitive but specificity in relevant controls was not investigated. When different methods of temporal dispersion were compared the measurement of negative peak duration was the most sensitive measure, but again specificity is not known.

In conclusion, the modified set I appears to be the most useful set of tests to diagnose CIDP. Care should be taken in the interpretation of results obtained from the posterior tibial nerve as for that nerve criteria of conduction block are different from other nerves.

Nerve biopsy

There is much controversy over the value of nerve biopsy in CIDP. Pollard (1993) concluded that nerve biopsy is a valuable adjunct in the diagnosis of CIDP whereas Bahron et al. (1989) were less enthousiastic. According to Pollard the quintescential pathological feature of CIDP is inflammatory demyelination. In his series of biopsies these were present in four of five biopsies from adults, but in only one of four biopsies from children. Bahron et al. found inflammation in only 11% of 56 biopsies. The difference may be explained by selection because Bahron et al. performed biopsy in nearly all their patients with CIDP whereas Pollard selected his patients. Pollard did first electrophysiological studies and when sensory nerve action potentials were absent and the motor responses were of very low amplitude, biopsy was performed. The reason for biopsy was that in these patients demyelination was difficult to prove with electrophysiological techniques. The presence of inflammatory changes in half of the nerve biopsies found by Pollard was similar in that of a series of biopsies described by Dyck et al. (1975). It is therefore likely that the sensitivity of nerve biopsies is approximately 50% in selected cases in whom the diagnosis remains in doubt after clinical, CSF and electrophysiological studies. Usually the probability of CIDP is either very low or very high in suspected cases after clinical, blood, CSF and electrophysiologic studies have all been performed. In these cases it is very unlikely that nerve biopsy will considerably change the diagnostic pretest probability.

Pathogenesis

The pathogenesis of GBS and CIDP is probably the same but once the disease has been induced GBS is in contrast to CIDP a short lasting disorder. Patients with GBS may be severely disabled for many months but this is not caused by a continuous immune-mediated attack on the peripheral nerves. The immune-mediated attack probably lasts not more than 1–2 weeks but it usually takes much longer for nerves to recover depending on the extent of axonal damage. In CIDP the immune-mediated attack may continue for many years but even after 10 years this process may stop. Therefore, immunosuppressive or modulating treatment late in the course of GBS is not effective whereas in CIDP marked improvements may be seen even several years after the first symptoms. For a better understanding of the disease process in CIDP we not only need to know how the immune systems attacks peripheral nerves as in GBS, but also why this process may continue.

The animal model of GBS, experimental allergic neuritis (EAN), is regarded as relevant to some aspects of the human disorder. A similar model for CIDP may help us learn why in GBS the immune attack is short lasting and self-limited in contrast to CIDP. Harvey and coworkers showed that a chronic relapsing or progressive disease can be induced in adult outbred New Zealand white rabbits inoculated with a single dose of purified bovine peripheral nerve myelin and Freund's adjuvant (Harvey et al. 1987).

This chronic model in certain mouse strains appears to be linked to immune response genes in the region of H-2. In addition to genetic susceptibility other factors play a role. The age of the animals at the onset of disease induction is an important factor (Harvey et al. 1987). The antigen plays a role as induction with crude polyantigenic myelin emulsions results more often in chronic disease than after induction with myelin basic protein. The presence of a persisting antigen depot at the injection site has also been stressed as an important factor. In the study of Pollard's group chronic disease was induced by purified myelin administered in an amount ten times greater than that necessary to induce the acute disease.

Which of these factors play a role in the human disorder? Are immunogenetic factors related to CIDP? Several studies investigated the association between HLA antigens and CIDP. Increased frequency of HLA-A3, A30/31, B7, B8 and DR2 have been reported. In our own series of patients we found an association with B5, B16 and CW2 (van Doorn et al. 1991a). Nevertheless, we are not convinced that there is an association between CIDP and these genetic factors as when *p* values are corrected for the number of antigens that are tested in the different HLA loci, the results are no longer significant.

There are no differences in age at which CIDP or GBS develops as was shown in the animal model. Differences in antecedent infections between CIDP and GBS may exist which would support the suggestion from animal studies that the antigen which induces the disease is different; however, there are no well designed studies comparing the antecedent events in GBS and CIDP. There is no evidence that there is persisting antigenic stimulating in CIDP and it is unlikely that there is a difference in the dose of the antigen which induces CIDP or GBS. Therefore, the question how to explain the induction of acute or chronic disease is far from resolved. Similarly, in other autoimmune disorders like idiopathic thrombocytopenia it is unknown why some develop acute and others chronic forms of the disease.

Variants of CIDP

Focal neuropathy preceding CIDP

Verma et al. (1990) described three patients with mononeuropathic limb weakness 2, 11 and 23 years, respectively, before a fullblown CIDP developed. The first patient initially had left hand weakness. This weakness waxed and waned for almost 2 years. Following a febrile episode this patient noted weakness of the left leg. The symptoms progressed over the next 5–6 years. Eight years after the first symptoms he also developed weakness of the right leg. Nine years after the first symptoms this patient had mild atrophy in the left forearm and left thigh muscles, weakness of the proximal and distal muscles in the left upper limb, right upper limb and all muscles in the lower limbs. Reflexes were absent and plantar reflexes were flexor. There was impairment of light touch and pinprick sensations over the left thumb and the index, middle and ring fingers. Vibration was decreased distally in both feet.

The second patient first noted paresthesiae on the dorsum of the right foot followed by foot drop. Improvement began a month later and he was asymptomatic 6 months later. The right foot drop recurred 4, 7 an 11 years later. When the latter footdrop recurred he also developed weakness of the left lower extremity and weakness of both hands.

Neurological findings 11 years after the first symptoms included atrophy of muscles in both hands and in the right anterior tibial compartment. Weakness was more pronounced distally in upper and lower limbs. Reflexes were diminished in the upper limbs and absent in the lower limbs. Light touch and pinprick sensations were impaired distally in all limbs with a distal-proximal gradient and were absent on the dorsum of the right foot.

The third patient had at the age of 5 years a 2-month episode of focal weakness of the right leg which resolved spontaneously. At the age of 28 years she had a recurrence of weakness in the right leg followed a year later by weakness in the other three limbs. In addition to weakness she developed areflexia and minimal sensory impairment distally.

Other diagnoses than CIDP were considered in these patients but were rejected. Relapsing and progressive mononeuropathy multiplex occurs also in vasculitis but the patients described by Verma et al. had no evidence of vasculitis. Other causes of focal neuropathy like trauma, entrapment, neurofibromatosis, acromegaly, hypothyroidism, amyloidosis, sarcoidosis and leprosy were excluded or extremely unlikely. Three patients had electrophysiological signs of conduction block and histologically there was evidence of focal demyelination-remyelination. Cell infiltration was demonstrated in two of the three patients. These patients resemble three patients described by Donaghy and Earl (1985) in whom ocular palsies preceded CIDP.

Multifocal demyelinating neuropathy with persistent conduction block.

Lewis et al. (1982) described patients with subacute onset of sensorimotor symptoms of one or two nerves in the arms. Progression was slow and relentless as distinct new nerve lesions became apparent. Arms were always more affected than legs. Reflexes generally were absent in the arms but preserved in the legs. All sensory modalities were impaired in severely involved nerves. Electrophysiological studies demonstrated conduction block. Distal motor latencies were normal and many segments of the nerve had normal or nearly normal conduction velocities. Some patients were treated with steroids and improved. These patients resemble those described by Pestronk et al. (1988). The main difference is the absence of sensory disturbances in the patients described by Pestronk et al. and the poor response to steroids. This poor response to steroids and even deterioration has also been reported in patients with pure motor forms of CIDP (Donaghy et al. 1994).

The only difference between CIDP, multifocal demyelinating neuropathy and multifocal motor neuropathy may be the number of focal demyelinating lesions. If only a few are present large nerve segments including distal segments may remain free from conduction blocks. If these few lesions are restricted to motor nerves the clinical signs of multifocal motor neuropathy develop and if a few lesions are present in sensory and motornerves the clinical signs of multifocal demyelinating neuropathy will emerge. If the lesions develop rapidly in many nerves distally and proximally in both legs and arms, patients will have the typical signs of CIDP; however, patients with pure motor signs may have a different disorder as treatment response to steroids is different.

CIDP and central lesions

There are several reports of the coexistence of central and peripheral nervous system lesions in patients with CIDP. Feasby et al. (1990) divided these reports into several categories; cases of CIDP where 'multiple sclerosis (MS) lesions' have been demonstrated clinically, pathologically, or by diagnostic techniques, cases of MS where peripheral nerve abnormalities have been detected pathologically or electrophysiologically and cases where central and peripheral lesions have developed simultaneously. A review of these reports suggests a greater than chance occurrence of the two conditions MS and CIDP.

The study of Feasby et al. shows that most patients with CIDP do not have evidence of MS and that the concurrence of these two diseases is uncommon. In the study of Feasby et al. six of 19 patients with CIDP had magnetic resonance imaging (MRI) evidence of small subcortical lesions. Five of these six patients were over 55 years of age. These authors applied the following criteria to these results; they required two of the following three criteria: at least one lesion > 6 mm, a lesion abutting the ventricular bodies and an infratentorial lesion. Applying these criteria none of the five patients over age 55 years could be classified as having MS lesions. The lesions seen in the sixth patient who was 38 years old were not typical of MS.

Differential diagnosis

Table 8.2 lists the diagnoses in patients who were referred to our department with a diagnosis of CIDP but in whom the diagnosis had to be changed.

Chronic idiopathic axonal neuropathy

This is a slowly progressive neuropathy which may resemble CIDP because it is a chronic neuropathy

Table 8.2 *Final diagnosis in patients referred with diagnosis CIDP in whom diagnosis had to be changed*

Chronic idiopathic axonal polyneuropathy
Hereditary motor and sensory neuropathy type I
X-linked hereditary motor and sensory neuropathy
Hereditary liability to pressure neuropathy
POEMS syndrome
X adrenoleucodystrophy
Amiodarone polyneuropathy
Diabetic plexopathy
Radiation plexopathy
Motor neuron disease
Hypothyroidism and polyneuropathy
Non-systemic vasculitic neuropathy
Tumor of the filum terminale

and because of the loss of fast conducting axons in the legs which may result in considerable slow nerve conduction velocities of the leg nerves. (Notermans et al. 1993). The distinction from CIDP should not be difficult as clinical signs, electrophysiological tests and CSF examinations are different. Weakness in chronic idiopathic axonal neuropathy is usually restricted to distal leg muscles. In CIDP weakness is usually present in distal and proximal muscles and there usually is not much difference between weakness in the legs and arms in CIDP (van Doorn et al. 1991b). Loss of fast conducting axons in the legs may result in slowed nerve conduction velocities in the leg nerves in patients with axonal neuropathies but slow nerve conduction velocities in the arm nerves is not a feature of chronic idiopathic axonal neuropathy.

Hereditary motor and sensory neuropathy Type I (HMSN-I)

This neuropathy is not difficult to distinguish from CIDP when patients present with the typical features of HMSN-I and a family history. In typical cases the first symptoms develop during the first two decades of life. The clinical course in adults is stationary over long periods of time and when there is progression this is extremely slow. This neuropathy does not usually lead to major disability. This is in contrast to CIDP in which there is rapid progression of deterioration, often leading to major disability. Electrophysiological tests usually may help to distinguish between HMSN-I and CIDP. In HMSN-I there is diffuse slowing of all nerves whereas in CIDP there may be much difference in conduction velocities of two nerves in the same arm. The diffuse slowing in HMSN-I does usually not result in conduction block, a feature which is typical for the acquired demyelinating disorders. CSF protein is usually not elevated to levels over 1 gl^{-1} in HMSN. Exceptions have been described; some HMSN patients have CSF protein levels of more than 1 gl^{-1} and there is one report of large CMAP amplitude reduction on proximal versus distal stimulation of the median nerve in a patient with HSMN-I (Hoogendijk et al. 1992). If there remains doubt, testing for the presence of the DNA duplication in chromosome 17p 11.2 may be helpful. If a patient with slowed nerve conduction velocities and with family members with a similar neuropathy clearly deteriorates, two possibilities should be considered; first X-linked HMSN which will be discussed in the next paragraph and second the development of CIDP in a patient with HMSN-I. Prednisone responsiveness in patients with HMSN-I has been reported. Patients with HMSN-I may be extra vulnerable to CIDP.

X-linked HMSN

In contrast to patients with HMSN-I, males with X-linked HMSN may have rapidly progressive deterioration after the first two decades of life, which may lead to major disability. The suspicion of X-linked HMSN should be raised if in a family with hereditary neuropathy the males are severely affected whereas the females have mild or subclinical disease. In X-linked HMSN the onset is in early childhood. In most of the males gait becomes severely impaired. Intrinsic hand muscles become involved in the early teens. Total areflexia is uncommon.

POEMS syndrome

If patients present with a demyelinating polyneuropathy and all the features of the POEMS syndrome (polyneuropathy, organomegaly, endocrinopathy, monoclonal gammopathy and skin changes) it is unlikely that these patients will be diagnosed and treated as CIDP. The POEMS syndrome, however, is a variant of osteosclerotic myeloma in which only one or two of the features of the POEMS syndrome may be present (Miralles et al. 1992). The diagnosis of

Table 8.3 *Features that raise the suspicion of osteosclerotic myeloma in patients with a demyelinating polyneuropathy*

Polycythemia
Anemia
Leukocytosis
Thrombocytosis
Elevated erythrocyte sedimentation rate
Hyperpigmentation
Hypertrichosis
Thickened skin
Raynaud's phenomenon
Peripheral edema
Lymphadenopathy
Hepatomegaly
Splenomegaly
Ascites
Pleural effusions
M protein
Hypothyroidism

osteosclerotic myeloma should be considered in patients with a demyelinating polyneuropathy who in addition have one of the features listed in Table 8.3. If none of these features is present a search for osteosclerotic bone lesions in patients with a demyelinating polyneuropathy is not recommended.

X adrenoleucodystrophy

This disorder may mimic a chronic neuropathy when weakness and sensory disturbances develop in the variant referred to as adrenomyeloneuropathy. Distinction from CIDP is usually not difficult as there are signs of a spastic paraparesis. In a recent series of patients described by van Geel et al. (1994) adrenomyeloneuropathy occurred more frequently than the variant with progressive cerebral impairment (Mori et al. 1981). The same group also found that electrophysiological tests do not fulfil the criteria of a demyelinating peripheral nerve disorder. The diagnostic assay for this disorder is the detection of the C26/C22 fatty acid ratio.

Amiodarone polyneuropathy

Amiodarone is an anti-ventricular arrhythmia agent which may cause, even after standard dosages, a distal symmetric sensorimotor polyneuropathy, often accompanied by tremor. Electrophysiological studies showed marked decreased conduction velocities and nerve biopsy revealed predominant symmetrical demyelination. The skin may show a bluish discoloration.

Plexopathy

Diabetic amyotrophy may present with progressive asymmetrical proximal weakness in the legs. The knee jerks are depressed or absent. The anterolateral muscle group in the lower legs may be affected simultaneously. Distinction from CIDP is usually not difficult as the signs are in most patients restricted to the legs.

Radiation-induced lumbosacral plexopathies may develop slowly and progressively over many years and may therefore resemble a chronic polyneuropathy. The absence of abnormalities in the arms and the absence of electrophysiological signs consistent with demyelination soon point to a diagnosis other than CIDP.

Motor neuron disease

CIDP may be predominantly motor. In these patients distinction between CIDP and motor neuron disease may be difficult (Parry and Clarke 1988). Careful electrophysiological studies aimed at the demonstration of conduction block and velocity slowing will differentiate the two disorders. Loss of fast conducting fibers in motor neuron disease may mimic slowed nerve conduction by demyelination. In these patients with motor neuron disease and slowed nerve conduction velocities the distal action potentials are usually very small.

Hypothyroidism

Electrophysiological studies in patients with symmetrical polyneuropathy and hypothyroidism may be consistent with a demyelinating neuropathy. Symmetrical polyneuropathy in these patients usually starts in the legs and within a few months the hands are also affected. Reflexes are usually absent in the legs and depressed in the arms. Muscle cramps are frequent and creatine kinase concentrations may be elevated. In patients with signs and symptoms of CIDP, serum thyroxine levels are usually determined to exclude this neuropathy. If hypothyroidism is found in patients with a demyelinating neuropathy, the diagnosis osteosclerotic myeloma should be considered.

Non-systemic vasculitic neuropathy

In this neuropathy, clinically only the nerves are affected. There are no or few constitutional symptoms or serological abnormalities. The clinical pattern may be that of multiple mononeuropathy, asymmetrical neuropathy, distal neuropathy and sensory polyneuropathy. Electrophysiological studies will show signs of axonal neuropathy.

Tumor of the filum terminale

These patients may have progressive weakness and sensory disturbances suggesting a chronic peripheral neuropathy. Bourque and Dyck (1990) described a patient who was initially referred with the diagnosis of a polyneuropathy (Charcot-Marie-Tooth) who turned out to have an ependymoma of the filum terminale, as was the case in a patient referred to us with the diagnosis CIDP. Bourque and Dyck emphasized that in patients with greater weakness in plantar flexors than in dorsiflexors, intraspinal disease should be suspected rather than periperal neuropathy.

Treatment

Whether the results of studies on the effectiveness of treatment are relevant for clinical practice depends on the choice of outcome measures. In the early experimental phase, the aim of most studies is to investigate if there is any effect at all of the treatment on the disease process. Studies like these increase our knowledge of the disease and of the biological effect of treatment. To investigate effects on the disease process we need the most sensitive measures. In these studies measures of impairment which assess disturbed function of peripheral nerves are the best outcome measures. Examples are electrophysiological parameters and dynamometric analysis of muscle weakness. If these studies demonstrate that the compound muscle action potentials increase, that the nerve conduction velocities are less slow or that muscle strength measured with a dynamometer improves, it remains to be shown that these changes are relevant for the patient. Clinically relevant information is usually provided by disability measures. Disability, which refers to functional performance can be expressed for instance in the ability to walk. Studies with these disability measures can be used for clinical decisions. Treatment recommendations can only be based on trials which used measures of disability. It is confusing that in the field of peripheral nerve disorders a neurological disability score (Molenaar et al. 1995) is used which in fact does not measure disability but impairment. This scale measures cranial nerve function, reflexes, muscle strength and sensory disturbances, which all reflect impairment. Especially in studies on patients with CIDP, these clinically less relevant impairment scores were used. In contrast, studies in patients with GBS usually had disability scales as the main outcome measure. Measures of impairment are often recommended because they are considered to be more objective measures, but these may be less valuable than the so-called 'soft clinical measures', provided that these clinical scales have been investigated. In physics accuracy and precision are important in measurement. Similarly, in clinical measurements comparable characteristics of measures such as reliability and validity should tested.

In the following paragraphs treatments will only be discussed that were tested in clinical trials.

Prednisone

Some patients fulfil all the criteria for CIDP but are hardly disabled. In these patients treatment can be postponed until deterioration occurs. At present there is no evidence that the course of the disease in the long-term is favourably influenced when treatment is started as early as possible.

Prednisone has in many centers for a long time been the standard treatment in CIDP; however, this treatment is based on rather weak evidence. Several uncontrolled series of patients treated with steroids have been reported and only one clinical trial (Dyck et al. 1982). In this controlled trial patients were treated with prednisone or no treatment. The neurologist who did the assessments had probably knowledge of the treatment as the method section did not describe how this was avoided. The method of randomization was unacceptable. The first patient in each 'age-duration-sex' group was randomly assigned to prednisone or no treatment. The second patient received the alternative therapy followed by random assignment to the third patient and so on. This is unacceptable as the second, fourth and so on treatment can be predicted which might influence the decision to include patients in the trial. The main outcome assessment was carried out with the already discussed neurological disability score which as explained before is not a disability score but an impairment scale.

The median change after 3 months was −1.5 for the controls and 10.0 for the treatment group (p=0.016). The number of patients in the control group with improvement of 10 or more points was three of 14 and in the treatment group eight of 14 which is not statistically different. Moreover, five patients treated with prednisone were excluded from the final analysis. One of these five patients died, according to the authors, from cardiac arrhythmia possibly related to hyperglycemia. Another patient was excluded because he could not return for follow-up but the reason was that he remained respirator bound at another hospital. The authors rightly conclude that their study provide no answer to the value of prednisone usage for longer than 3 months, especially when benefit is balanced against the risk of hyperglycemic hyperosmolar coma, cataracts of the eye, infection and aseptic necrosis of the hips.

The beneficial effects of steroids can therefore hardly be based on this trial, but is based on uncontrolled experience of many different centers. In a large series of CIDP patients 65% improved after treatment with steroids (Barohn et al. 1989). There are no prospective studies on the disadvantages of treatment with steroids in CIDP patients.

Many different prednisone treatment schedules have been described. Dalakas et al. (1981) advised starting with 100 mg prednisone in a single dose daily for 3–4 weeks. This is reduced to 100 mg on even days and 10 mg on uneven days in 9 weeks by reducing the dose by 10 mg every week on uneven days. In two weeks the dose on uneven days is reduced to zero. The 100 mg dose on alternate days is continued for 1–3 months after which the dose is reduced by 5 mg every 3–4 weeks until 80 mg is reached. Thereafter the dose is reduced by 2.5 mg every 3–4 weeks until 50 mg is reached. The scheme continues with a reduction of 2.5 mg every month until 20 mg. Further reduction is by 1 mg every 1–2 months. Others have advocated a much lower initial dose. Donaghy (1993) recommended an initial daily dose of 60 mg, falling to 45 mg daily after 2 weeks and converting to 45 mg on alternate days over the next 2–3 months.

The question is whether the dose of prednisone can be lowered by adding azathioprine. This question has not been investigated in a clinical trial, although there has been a trial in which prednisone was compared with prednisone in combination with azathioprine (Dyck et al. 1985). The aim of this trial was not to compare the effectiveness of treatment with steroids with that of a much lower dose of steroids combined with azathioprine. What this trial did investigate was if the combination of azathioprine and prednisone resulted in more improvement than prednisone alone. No difference could be detected.

Plasma exchange

There are two double-blind clinical trials in which plasma exchange was compared with sham exchange. In the first study the analysis included 15 patients treated with plasma exchange and 14 with sham exchange (Dyck et al. 1986). Outcome was assessed at 3 weeks. Patients were asked whether their neurological status had improved, worsened or remained the same. There was no difference in responses between the groups. In the plasma exchange group seven of 15 had improved on the neurological disability score compared with nine of 14 in the sham exchange group. There were some differences but whether these were clinically relevant is doubtful. Five patients in the plasma exchange group improved more than any patient in the sham exchange group and the differences in electrophysiological parameters were in favor of the plasma exchange group.

In the second study 18 patients with CIDP were randomized to plasma exchange or sham plasma exchange (Hahn et al. 1996a). After a wash-out period patients were crossed over to the alternate treatments. Several outcome measures were used of which a functional clinical assessment was the most relevant. Of the 15 patients who completed the study 12 improved by 1–5 (median 3) points on an 11 point scale.

Intravenous immunoglobulin

After it had been shown that patients with CIDP may improve after infusion with plasma from blood bank donors, a beneficial effect of immunoglobulin infusion was demonstrated in eight of nine patients treated with intravenous immunoglobulin (IVIG) (Vermeulen et al. 1985). Similar uncontrolled results were reported by others. In a cross-over study in patients with CIDP who had responded to treatment with IVIG it was shown that these patients did respond to IVIG as discontinuation was followed by deterioration and improvement followed after IVIG administration (van Doorn et al. 1990). After infusion of albumin which could not be distinguished from IVIG by patient or physician, no improvement was seen. This study shows that CIDP patients may improve after IVIG administration. It does not answer the question whether IVIG is the preferred treatment in CIDP. In a double-blind placebo-controlled trial in newly diagnosed patients with CIDP the results of treatment with IVIG were disappointing (Vermeulen et al. 1993). Four of 15 patients in the IVIG group responded to treatment and three of 13 patients in the placebo group. Improvement was measured using a disability scale. Similarly, there were no differences between the groups either on the MRC weakness score of 12 muscle groups or in neurophysiological parameters. A clear beneficial effect of IVIG was demonstrated in a study from Canada (Hahn et al. 1996b). A two-group analysis of the first trial period of this cross-over study showed that 16 patients had been assigned to IVIG and 14 to placebo. On average the placebo group had worsened slightly, whereas the IVIG group on average improved 1–3 points on a non-linear 11 point functional scale. Recently IVIG was compared with plasma exchange. No differences were found between the groups (Dyck et al. 1995).

Conclusions

Despite little progress in knowledge of the pathogenesis of CIDP, patients with this disorder are better off than they were 30 years ago. This has resulted from better recognition of this neuropathy and by the spreading awareness that most of these patients have a treatable disorder. The understanding of this disease at the molecular level is scanty. We do not know against which molecules the immune attack is directed and when this attack has been initiated, we do not know why some patients have a self-limited disorder and others do not.

Many different treatments have been tested. It is difficult to base firm guidelines for treatment on the published studies. Patients may improve after treatment with steroids, but at the price of severe side-effects. Improvement can be achieved with IVIG but the costs of this treatment are very high. The question is whether the side-effects of steroids can be reduced by a regimen with pulse doses of steroids followed by a low maintenance dose or whether rapid improvement can be induced by short-lasting treatment with IVIG followed by low dose treatment with steroids to prevent relapse. To answer these questions we need clinical studies with appropriate outcome measures. Electrophysiological measures are not suitable for this purpose. Instead, disability measures should be used with acceptable reliability and validity.

References

Ad hoc subcommittee of the American Academy of Neurology AIDS Task Force. (1991). Research criteria for diagnosis of chronic inflammatory demyelinating polyneuropathy (CIDP). Neurology **41**: 617–618.

Asbury, A.K., Arnason, B.G.W., Karp, H.R., and McFarlin, D.F. (1978). Criteria for diagnosis of Guillain-Barré syndrome. *Ann. Neurol.* **3**: 565–566.

Austin, J.H. (1958). Recurrent polyneuropathies and their corticosteroid treatment. With five-year observations of a placebo controlled case treated with corticotrophin, cortisone, and prednisone. *Brain* **81**: 157–192.

Barohn, R.J., Kissel, J.T., Warmolts, J.R., and Mendell, J.R. (1989). Chronic inflammatory demyelinating polyneuropathy, clinical characteristics, course and recommendations for diagnostic criteria. *Arch. Neurol.* **14**: 878–884.

Bourque, P.R., and Dyck, P.J. (1990). Selective calf weakness suggests intraspinal pathology, not peripheral neuropathy. *Arch. Neurol.* **47**: 79–80.

Bromberg, M.B. (1991). Comparison of electrodiagnostic criteria for primary demyelination in chronic polyneuropathy. *Muscle Nerve* **14**: 968–976.

Dalakas, M.C. and Engel, W.K. (1981). Chronic relapsing (dysimmune) polyneuropathy: pathogenesis and treatment. *Ann. Neurol.* **9**: 134–145.

Donaghy, M. (1993). Disorders of peripheral nerves. In *Brain's Disease of the Nervous System*, ed. J. Walton, 10th edn, p. 605. Oxford: Oxford Medical Publications.

Donaghy, M. and Earl, C.J. (1985). Ocular palsy preciding chronic relapsing polyneuropathy by several weeks. *Ann. Neurol.* **17**: 49–50.

Donaghy, M., Mills, K.R., and Boniface, S.J. (1994). Pure motor demyelinating neuropathy: deterioration after steroid treatment and improvement with intravenous immunoglobulin. *J. Neurol. Neurosurg. Psychiatry* **57**: 778–783.

Dyck, P.J., Lais, A.C., Ohta, M., Bastron, J.A., Okazaki, H., and Groover, R.V. (1975). Chronic inflammatory polyradiculoneuropathy. *Mayo Clin. Proc.* **50**: 621–637.

Dyck, P.J., O'Brien, P.C., and Oviatt, K.F. (1982). Prednisone improves chronic inflammatory demyelinating polyradiculoneuropathy more than no treatment. *Ann. Neurol.* **11**: 136–141.

Dyck, P.J., O'Brien, P., Swanson, C., Low, P., and Daube, J. (1985). Combined azathioprine and prednisone in chronic inflammatory demyelinating polyneuropathy. *Neurology* **35**: 1173–1176.

Dyck, P.J., Daube, J., O'Brien, P., Pineda, A., Low, P.A., and Windebank, A.J. (1986). Plasma exchange in chronic inflammatory demyelinating polyneuropathy. *N. Engl. J. Med.* **31**: 314–461–465.

Dyck, P.J., Litchy, W.J., Kratz, K.M., and Suarez, G.A. (1995). A plasma exchange versus immune globulin infusion trial in chronic inflammatory demyelinating polyradiculoneuropathy. *Ann. Neurol.* **36**: 838–845.

Feasby, T.E., Gilbert, J.J., Brown, W.F., Bolton, C.F., Hahn, A.F., Koopman, W.F., and Zochodne, D.W. (1986). An acute axonal form of Guillain-Barré polyneuropathy. *Brain* **109**: 1115–1126.

Feasby, T.E., Hahn, A.F., Koopman, W.J., and Lee, D.H. (1990). Central lesions in chronic inflammatory demyelinating polyneuropathy. An MRI study. *Neurology* **40**: 476–478.

Hahn, A.F., Bolton, C.F., Pillay, N., Chalk, C., Benstead, T., Bril, V., Shumak, K., Vandervoort, M.K., and Feasby, T.E. (1996a). Plasma-exchange therapy in chronic inflammatory demyelinating polyneuropathy. A double-blind, sham-controlled, cross-over study. *Brain* **119**: 1055–1066.

Hahn, A.F., Bolton, C.F., Zochodne, D., and Feasby, T.E. (1996b). Intravenous immunoglobulin treatment in chronic inflammatory demyelinating polyneuropathy. A double-blind, placebo controlled, cross-over study. *Brain* **119**: 1067–1077.

Harvey, G.K., Pollard, J.D., Schindhelm, K., and Antony, J. (1987). Chronic experimental allergic neuritis. An electrophysiological and histological study in the rabbit. *J. Neurol. Sci.* **81**: 215–225.

Hays, A.P., Lee, S.S., and Latov, N. (1988). Immune reactive C3d on the surface of myelin sheaths in neuropathy. *J. Neuroimmunol.* **18**: 231–244.

Hoogendijk, J.E., De Visser, M., Bour, L.J., Jennekens, F.G.I., and Ongerboer de Visser, B.W. (1992). Conduction block in hereditary motor and sensory neuropathy type I. *Muscle Nerve* **15**: 520–521.

Horowitz, S.H. (1989). The idiopathic polyneuradiculoneuropathies: a historical guide to an understanding of the clinical syndromes. *Acta Neurol. Scand.* **80**: 369–386.

Hughes, R., Sanders, E., Hall, S., Atkinson, P., Colchester, A., and Payan, P. (1992). Subacute idiopathic demyelinating polyradiculoneuropathy. *Arch. Neurol.* **49**: 612–616.

Jay, J.L. and Oh, S.J. (1988). Sensory neuropathy as a variant of chronic inflammatory demyelinating neuropathy (CIDN). *Neurology* **38**(Suppl.): 189.

Julien, J., Vital, C., Lagueny, A., Ferrer, X., and Brechenmacher, C. (1989). Chronic relapsing idiopathic polyneuropathy with primary axonal lesions. *J. Neurol. Neurosurg. Psychiatry* **52**: 871–875.

Kornberg, A.J. and Pestronk, A. (1993). Immune-mediated neuropathies. *Cur. Opin. Neurol.* **6**: 681–687.

Lewis, R.A., Sumner, A.J., Brown, M.J., and Asbury, A.K. (1982). Multifocal demyelinating neuropathy with persistent conduction block. *Neurology* **32**: 958–964.

McCombe, P.A., Pollard, J.D., and McLeod, J.G. (1987). Chronic inflammatory demyelinating polyradiculoneuropathy. A clinical and electrophysiological study of 92 cases. *Brain* **110**: 1617–1630.

Miralles, G.D., O'Fallon, J.R., and Talley, N.J. (1992). Plasma-cell dyscrasia with polyneuropathy. The spectrum of POEMS syndrome. *N. Engl. J. Med.* **327**: 1919–1923.

Molenaar, D.S.M., de Haan, R., and Vermeulen, M. (1995). Impairment, disability, or handicap in peripheral neuropathy: analysis of the use of outcome measures in clinical trials in patients with peripheral neuropathies. *J. Neurol. Neurosurg. Psychiatry* **59**: 165–169.

Notermans, N.C., Wokke, J.H.J., Franssen, H., Van der Graaf, Y., Vermeulen, M., Van den Berg, L.H., Bär, P.R., and Jennekens, F.G.I. (1993). Chronic idiopathic polyneuropathy presenting in middle or old age: a clinical and electrophysiological study of 75 patients. *J. Neurol. Neurosurg. Psychiatry* **56**: 1066–1071.

Oh, S.J., Kim, D.E., and Kurwoglu, H.R. (1994). What is the best diagnostic index of conduction block and temporal dispersion? *Muscle Nerve* **17**: 489–493.

Parry, G.J. and Clarke, S. (1988). Multifocal acquired demyelinating neuropathy masquerading as motor neuron diseases. *Muscle Nerve* **11**: 103–107.

Pestronk, A., Cornblath, D.R., Ilyas, A.A., Baba, H., Quarles, R.H., Griffin, J.W., Alderson, K., and Adams, R.M. (1988). A treatable multifocal motor neuropathy with antibodies to GM1 gangliosides. *Ann. Neurol.* **23**: 73–78.

Pollard, J.D. (1993). Chronic inflammatory demyelinating polyradiculopathy. In *Guillain-Barré Syndrome*, ed. G.J. Parry, pp. 175–179. New York: Thieme.

Prineas, J.W. and McLeod, J.G. (1976). Chronic relapsing polyneuritis. *J. Neurol. Sci.* **27**: 427–458.

Thomas, P.K., Lascelles, R.G., Hallpike, J.F., and Hewer, R.L. (1969). Recurrent and chronic relapsing Guillain-Barré polyneuritis. *Brain* **92**: 589–606.

Van Doorn, P.A., Brand, A., and Vermeulen, M. (1987). Clinical significance of antibodies against peripheral nerve tissue in inflammatory polyneuropathy. *Neurology* **37**: 1798–1803.

Van Doorn, P.A., Brand, A., Strengers, P.F.W., Meulstee, J., and Vermeulen, M. (1990). High-dose intravenous immunoglobulin treatment in chronic inflammatory demyelinating polyneuropathy: a double-blind placebo-controlled cross over study. *Neurology* **40**: 209–212.

Van Doorn, P.A., Brand, A., and Vermeulen, M. (1988). Anti-neuroblastoma cell line antibodies in inflammatory demyelinating polyneuropathy; inhibition in vitro and in vivo by IV immunoglobulin. *Neurology* **38**: 1592–1596.

Van Doorn, P.A., Schreuder, G.M.Th., Vermeulen, M., d'Amaro, J., and Brand, A. (1991a). HLA antigens in patients with chronic inflammatory demyelinating polyneuropathy. *J. Neuroimmunol.* **32**: 133–139.

Van Doorn, P.A., Vermeulen, M., Brand, A., Mulder, P.G.M., and Busch, H.F.M. (1991b). Intravenous immunoglobulin treatment in patients with chronic inflammotory demyelinating polyneuropathy. Clinical and laboratory characteristics associated with improvement. *Arch. Neurol.* **48**: 217–20.

Van Geel, B.M., Assies, J., Weverling, G.J., and Barth, P.G. (1994). Predominance of the adrenomyeloneuropathy phenotype of X-linked adrenoleucodystrophy in The Netherlands. A survey of 30 kindreds. *Neurology* **44**: 2343–2346.

Van Schaik, I.N., Vermeulen, M., Van Doorn, P.A., and Brand, A. (1994). Anti-β-tubulin antibodies in patients with chronic inflammatory demyelinating polyneuropathy. *J. Neurol.* **242**: 599–603.

Verma, A., Tandon, R., Adesina, A.M., Pendlebury, W.W., Fries, T.J., and Bradley, W.G. (1990). Focal neuropathy preceding chronic inflammatory demyelinating polyneuropathy by several years. *Acta Neurol. Scand.* **81**: 516–521.

Vermeulen, M., Van Doorn, P.A., Brand, A., Strengers, P.F.W., Jennekens, F.G.I., and Busch, H.F.M. (1993). Intravenous immunoglobulin treatment in patient with chronic inflammatory demyelinating polyneuropathy: a double blind, placebo controlled study. *J. Neurol. Neurosurg. Psychiatry* **56**: 36–39

Vermeulen, M., Van der Meché, F.G.A., Speelman, J.D., Weber, A., and Busch, H.F.M. (1985). Plasma and gamma-globulin infusion in chronic inflammatory polyneuropathy. *J. Neurol. Sci.* **70**: 317–326.

Wertheim Salomonson, J.K.A. (1911). *Pathologie en therapie der neuritis, myositis, zenuwgezwellen, neuralgie en myalgie.* Amsterdam: Scheltema en Holkema.

9 Acute and chronic sensory neuronopathy

G. Sobue

Introduction and historical review

At the time of Romberg, more than a century ago, tabes dorsalis was the most common cause of sensory ataxia (Romberg 1851 cited in Smith et al. 1994); diphtheritic neuropathy and arsenic neuropathy were the major differential diagnoses for tabes dorsalis. With the decrease in prevalence of these disorders, diseases affecting the primary sensory neurons have become less common. In 1948, Denny-Brown described two patients with primary sensory neuropathy associated with carcinoma (Denny-Brown 1948), which was characterized by subacute and progressive course of the disease with evidence of polymyositis, in addition to that which he called degeneration of the dorsal root ganglia. Subsequently, similar cases have been reported using many nosological eponyms (Henson et al. 1954; Horwich et al. 1977). Certain patients with similar subacute or sometimes chronic sensory neuropathy, which predominantly affected proprioceptive sensation and presented as sensory ataxia with good preservation of motor nerve functions, however, had no evidence of malignancy (Charron et al. 1980; Kaufman et al. 1981; Mitsumoto et al. 1985; Dalakas 1986; Sobue et al. 1979, 1987, 1988, 1993). Similar chronic sensory neuropathies manifesting as a sensory ataxia were also thought to be caused by megavitaminosis of pyridoxine(vitamin B6)(Schaumburg et al. 1983), and by intoxication with cisplatin, an anti-cancer drug (Hadley et al. 1979). Among these sensory neuropathies, particularly those affecting kinesthetic sensation, cases with evidence of Sjögren's syndrome and Sicca syndrome had accumulated (Kaltreider and Talal 1969; Hull et al. 1984; Kennett and Harding 1986; Malinow et al. 1986; Graus et al. 1988; Mellgren et al. 1989; Griffin et al. 1990; Kumazawa et al. 1993; Sobue et al. 1993; Grant et al. 1997). Most of these cases showed a chronic progressive course but some were subacute or acute in onset. The pathological hallmark is sensory (Mallinow et al. 1986; Griffin et al. 1990; Smith et al. 1994) and there may also be sympathetic and ciliary ganglionitis (Kumazawa et al. 1993) with T cell invasion, designated ganglionitis or ganglioneuronopathy.

On the other hand, sensory neuronopathy with acute onset and frequently accompanied by a prodromal febrile episode and a long-standing sensory deficit, as well as a well-preserved motor function, has been identified. Dyck and coworkers(1968) briefly described two cases of acute sensory neuropathy with multifocal radicular sensory loss, suggesting the dorsal root ganglia as the locus of the disease. Sterman and colleagues (1980) subsequently reported three patients who presented with acute severe paresthesia, sensory ataxia and loss of sensation following a preceding febrile illness, who exhibited well-preserved motor function and poor recovery from sensory ataxia, which suggests the dorsal root ganglia may be the major lesion (Sterman et al. 1980). Windebank et al. (1990) reviewed the clinical, electrophysiological and pathological features of clinically pure sensory neuropathy, which was acute in onset, and suggested an immune-mediated process at the level of the posterior root or dorsal root ganglion. Acute sensory ganglionitis associated with severe autonomic involvement frequently associated with a prodromal febrile episode has also been recognized as one spectrum of sensory neuronopathy (Colan et al. 1980). In those cases, albumino-cytologic dissociation and well-preserved motor functions were common. Dorsal root ganglionitis and an almost normal ventral root, accompanied by severe dysautonomia, has also been reported (Hodson et al. 1984; Fagius et al. 1983; Tohgi et al. 1989). In these conditions, the ganglionitis resulting in severe axonal degenerations was the major and likely the primary process in the pathology. There was a fairly good recovery of autonomic function in spite the sensory deficit which is generally long-standing(Yasuda et al. 1995). These cases would also be related to the Guillain-Barré syndrome (GBS), particularly the axonal form of the motor nerve counterpart (Feasby et al. 1986). In practice such cases are sometimes difficult to distinguish from acute sensory demyelinating neuropathy, a pure sensory variant of GBS which mostly exhibits sensory ataxia (Dawson et al. 1988; Miralles et al. 1992).

In this chapter, I focus on the non-malignant sensory neuronopathy primarily affecting the dorsal root ganglia with an underlying immune-mediated inflammatory mechanism, which often exhibits autonomic nerve involvement. Motor functions are electrophysiologically, pathologically and clinically well preserved. These conditions are divided into two categories in their clinical course and mode of onset: acute and chronic variations. Similar conditions associated with malignant diseases are described in a separate chapter.

Chronic sensory neuronopathy

Clinical features

This disorder is characterized by a chronic insidious onset of sensory neuronopathy, which is initially a multiple mononeuritis or frequently trigeminal mononeuritis and later develops to involve the entire body including the trunk and extremities, although motor nerve functions are completely preserved. Pathologically the dorsal root ganglion neurons are primarily involved in the immune-mediated mechanism. This disorder is associated with autonomic dysfunction of various degrees. Two conditions are included in this category: those associated with Sjögren's or sicca syndrome and the idiopathic cases, except for cases with malignancy. The two conditions share common clinical, electrophysiological and pathological features, although some features are characteristic of each condition.

Chronic sensory neuronopathy associated with Sjögren's syndrome or sicca syndrome

Case presentation

A 76-year-old woman noticed numbness and dysesthesia on the right side of her face when she was 64 years old. The dysesthesis progressed over the following 4 years to involve the ulnar side of the right arm, radial side of the left arm, and lateral side of the lower legs. Beginning at age 71 years, she developed unsteadiness of gait and pseudoathetoid movement of the fingers on both sides. Xerostomia and Adie's pupils were present at this time. Loss of light touch and pain were observed in the dermatomes of the spinal segment (C5 to T5 and below T9 on the right, C4 to T4 and below T10 on the left), in the trunk, and in the extremities, as well as on the right side of her face. There was profound loss of vibratory and joint sense in the four extremities. All tendon reflexes were absent. There was no Babinski's sign. Her gait was ataxic and Romberg's sign was markedly positive. There was no apparent muscular wasting. She showed severe postural hypotension with 70 mmHg systolic and 40 mmHg diastolic pressure, but heart rate increased with the postural blood pressure change. Heart rate variation (R-R interval) in response to deep breathing was significantly diminished. Minor's iodine-starch test in an artificial climate chamber showed distinct anhidrotic areas in the dermatomes of the spinal segments at C4 to T5 on the right side and below T5 on the left side of the trunk as well as the four extremities. Sensory nerve action potentials were absent in the median, tibial and sural nerves, and motor nerve conduction velocity and the amplitude of the maximum compound action potentials were normal in the median and tibial nerves. Somatosensory evoked potentials(SEPs) with right median nerve stimulation at the wrist did not elicite any response in the cervical and cortical record and Erb's point. Protein content and the number of cells in CSF were normal. Xerostomia was confirmed by the salivary secretion test following the citrus stimulation test, but Schirmer's and Rose bengal test were negative. Antibody titers to Ro(SS-A) and microsomes were significantly elevated, but other autoantibodies, including those to La(SS-B), were not. Minor salivary gland biopsy revealed destruction of acinar cells and extensive periacinar lymphocytic infiltrations. Sural nerve biopsy revealed a loss of large myelinated fibers and fiber sprouting. Lymphocyte infiltration in the tunica intima and media of the small artery, indicating the presence of chronic phase of the angitis, was present.

The diagnostic criteria for Sjögren's syndrome (Fox et al. 1986) were fulfilled, which included sicca syndrome of xerostomia and xerophthalmia, pathological abnormality of mononuclear cell infiltration and the destruction of the acinar cells in the salivary gland seen on biopsy or keratoconjunctivitis and confirmed by Rose bengal or Schirmer's test. Autoantibodies to Ro(SS-A) or La(SS-B) were positive. Polyclonal or monoclonal elevation of the serum gamma globulin was frequently seen. The female preponderance(more than 80%) is characteristic particularly compared with idiopathic cases (Griffin et al. 1990; Sobue et al. 1993), and generally occurs in the middle-aged or elderly. The common initial symptom is paresthesia localized in the very distal portion of the extremities or frequently in the area of the trigeminal nerve branch (Kaltreider and Talal 1969; Hull et al. 1984; Kennett and Harding 1986; Griffin et al. 1990; Sobue et al. 1993; Grant et al. 1997), as is demonstrated in the present case. In the most patients, progression of sensory symptoms is asymmetrical and multifocal, similar to those of multiple mononeuritis. Each episode of focal sensory neuropathy is acute or subacute, but the overall clinical progression is generally chronic. The expression of sensory symptoms is not temporally synchronized in most patients, as one extremity is initially involved and then other extremities are involved. In the advanced stage, the sensory impairment involves the trunk, frequently segmental or asymmetrical, but more prominent sensory involvement is commonly seen in the distal portions of the extremities and the distal portions of the trigeminal (middle face) and the truncal nerves (anterior abdominal wall). Kinesthetic and position sense of the joints are severely involved in the proximal extremity joints (shoulder, hip and knee joints) as well as in the distal extremity joints (Sobue et al. 1993). Vibratory sense is also severely involved in a similar pattern of distribution to that of joint sense, but involvement is also noted in the trunk and face. Kinesthetic proprioceptive sense is more prominently involved than is superficial sensation, but this difference is not distinctive in many cases. Most patients exhibit sensory ataxia in the limbs, pseudoathetotic movement and sensory ataxic gait; the advanced case is bound to the wheel chair and requires help in the activities of daily life. Some cases become static in clinical severity. Motor strength remains essentially normal, and muscle atrophy is not generally present. Deep tendon reflexes are generally diminished or absent. As for the autonomic signs, Adie's tonic pupils are frequently present (Hull et al. 1984; Kennett and Harding 1986; Mellgren et al. 1989; Griffin et al. 1990; Watershoot et al. 1991; Kumazawa et al. 1993; Sobue et al. 1993). Orthostatic hypotension and fluctuating blood pressure are common (Griffin et al. 1990; Kumazawa et al. 1993; Sobue et al. 1993). Segmental anhidrosis along the spinal dermatomes as was seen in the present case is frequently seen (Kumazawa et al. 1993) Raynaud's phenomenon is also seen (Sobue et al. 1993). These autonomic signs are likely to be more prominent in cases with Sjögren's syndrome than in idiopathic cases.

The clinical course and distribution of the sensory and autonomic involvement is variable among cases as a consequence of the multifocal distribution of the lesions. Cases only exhibiting cranial neuropathy, such as trigeminal neuropathy, or cases with multiple cranial neuropathy involving the trigeminal, acoustic and glossopharyngeal nerves and Adie's pupil also could be included in the same category. Some cases with Adie's pupils and segmental anhidrosis designated as Ross's syndrome (1958) may also be included in this disorder (Kumazawa et al. 1993). In the early stage, cases with multiple mononeuritis showing a temporary migrating pattern restricted to sensory impairment of paresthesia simulates 'migrant sensory neuropathy' described by Wartenberg (1958), but at this early stage most of the cases do not fulfil the diagnostic criteria for Sjögren's syndrome. In our experience, some of the cases showing 'non-systemic vasculitic neuropathy' (Dyck et al. 1987) come to show more generalized sensory deficits over several years of follow-up and exhibit sensory ataxic neuropathy without the criteria of Sjögren's syndrome(Sobue et al. 1989, 1993). Some cases were also reported as sensorimotor neuropathy which involves motor nerves as well (Alexander et al. 1982, 1992; Mellgren et al. 1989;). The underlying pathological process which involves the motor nerves is not well understood, but may be related to the non-systemic vasculitis which is occasionally seen in the nerves of patients with Sjögren's syndrome (Kaltreider and Talal 1969; Peyronnard J-M et al. 1982; Said et al. 1988; Mellgren et al. 1989; Kumazawa et al. 1993).

Idiopathic chronic sensory neuronopathy

The clinical, electrophysiological and pathological features of sensory neuronopathy are similar to those of cases associated with Sjögren's syndrome (Kaufman et al. 1981; Dalakas 1986; Mellgren et al. 1989; Sobue et al. 1988, 1993), but autonomic dysfunction as in Raynaud's phenomenon, orthostatic hypotension and Adie's pupils are less common in this condition. The male/female ratio is much higher than in Sjögren's syndrome (Griffin et al. 1990; Sobue et al. 1993). Laboratory data for sicca syndrome characteristic for Sjögren's syndrome is of course less common in this condition. Diagnosis for Sjögren's syndrome in chronic sensory neuronopathy is frequently established when the neuropathy develops during long-term follow-up (Kennett and Harding 1986; Graus et al. 1988; Kumazawa et al. 1993; Sobue et al. 1993), so that patients categorized as idiopathic occasionally are diagnosed as having Sjögren's syndrome in the later phase. Whether Sjögren's syndrome observed in chronic sensory neuronopathy is essentially the same as in cases primarily diagnosed as Sjögren's syndrome without neuropathy is the issue to be established in some cases. Sensory neuronopathy is frequently associated with autonomic dysfunction which may eventually result in diminished salivation and lacrimation independent of the primary immune-mediated destruction of the salivary or lacrimal glands. In such cases, the precise diagnosis based on minor salivary gland biopsy and autoantibodies for the diagnostic criteria for Sjögren's syndrome (Fox et al. 1986) is essential.

Laboratory features

Electrophysiological features

Routine peripheral motor nerve conduction velocities and amplitudes of compound muscle action potentials are generally normal, while sensory action potentials are not detectable in many cases, or their amplitude is markedly diminished (Dalakas et al. 1986; Kennett and Harding 1986; Mallinow et al. 1986; Laloux et al. 1988; Mellgren et al. 1989; Griffin et al. 1990; Sobue et al. 1979, 1987, 1988, 1993). The neurogenic pattern in needle EMG is not obtained in most cases. SEP could be elicited in focally involved cases (Laloux et al. 1988), but cortical and cervical somatosensory evoked potentials and evoked potentials from Erb's point are barely recorded by median nerve stimulation at the wrist (Mallinow et al. 1986; Kachi et al. 1994). When the median nerve is stimulated at more proximal points, clear potentials are recorded from Erb's point, but cortical SEPs are still hardly elicited. SEP study indicates that the sensory nerves are centrally and peripherally involved in this condition, and the involvement is more prominent in the distal portion in the peripheral nerve, which is concordant with the pathological conditions of sensory ganglionitis and central-peripheral distal axonopathy (Kachi et al. 1994).

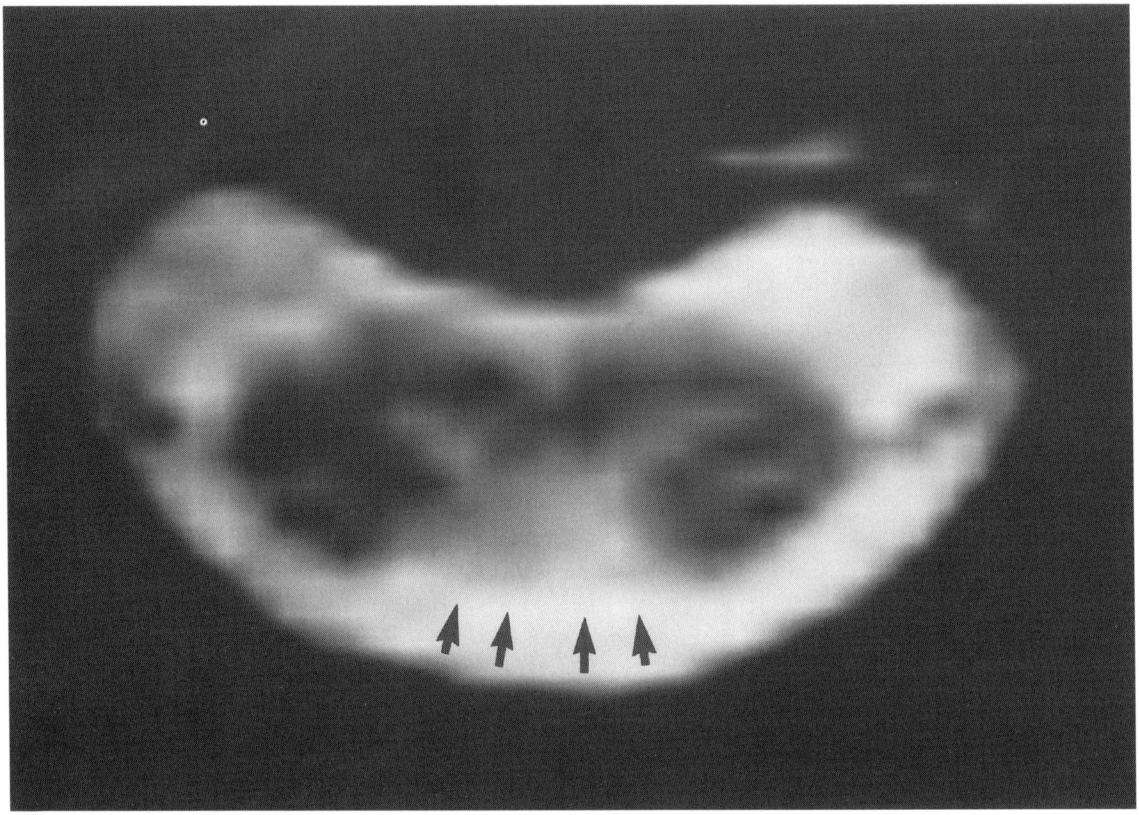

Figure 9.1 *Axial T2*-weighted gradient echo-images of the cervical spinal cord at the C4–5 segment on the patients with Sjögren's syndrome-associated neuropathy. A high-intensity signal is present in the posterior column (arrows). Reproduced from Sobue et al.,* Neurology *(**45**: 592–593, 1995), by permission).*

MRI study

The T2*-weighted images of the spinal cord occasionally demonstrate the high-intensity area in the posterior column, which is consistent with the view that the sensory ganglion neurons are primarily and extensively involved, and is also consistent with SEP findings (Sobue et al, 1995) (Figure 9.1). In cases in which the sensory loss extends to the arms, legs and trunk, the T2*-weighted high-intensity area is present in both the fasciculus cuneatus and fasciculus gracilis, consistent with the distribution of sensory loss (Sobue et al. 1995).

Laboratory study

The CSF protein level is generally normal, and pleocytosis is not present, but the elevated gamma globulin concentration or a single monoclonal gamma globulin(IgAk, IgMk) band may be detected (Dalakas 1986). Polyclonal elevation of serum IgG or IgA is observed in most patients. In cases with Sjögren's syndrome, the autoantibody of anti-Ro(SS-A) antigen is frequently positive, but anti-La(SS-B) is positive in only a few patients. The antinuclear antibody is also frequently positive in many patients. Antineuronal antibodies (anti-Hu) were evaluated in sensory neuronopathy and also in those with Sjögren's syndrome (Griffin et al. 1990; Chalk et al. 1993), and were negative in the patients without small-cell lung cancer (Chalk et al. 1993). These authors state that the anti-Hu antibody is a marker of a patient's immune response to a small-cell lung cancer. However, another group (Moll et al. 1993) reported that antineuronal antibodies were detectable in about half of the patients with Sjögren's syndrome-associated sensory neuronopathy, while they were not positive in patients with Sjögren's syndrome without neuropathy (Chalk et al. 1993).

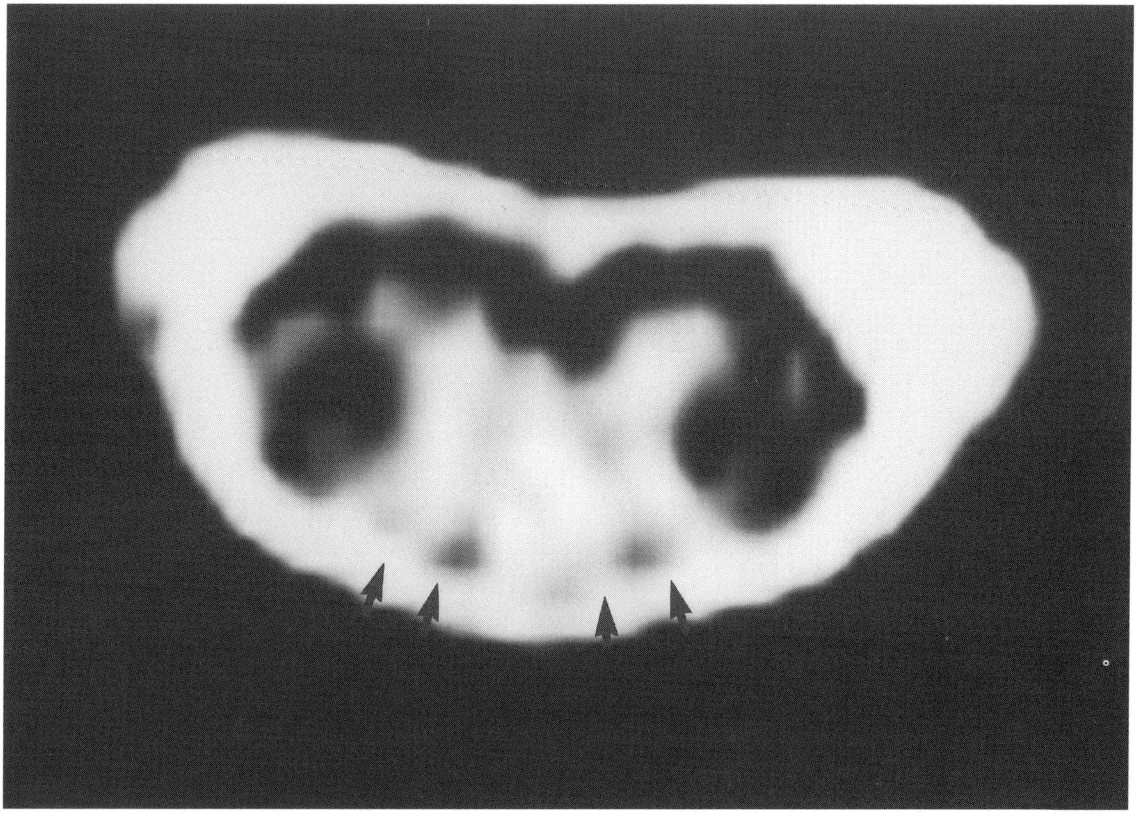

Figure 9.2 *Axial T2*-weighted gradient echo-images of the cervical spinal cord at the C4–5 segment on the patient with acute autonomic and sensory neuronopathy. A high-intensity signal is present in the posterior column (arrows).*

Pathological findings

Major pathological changes exist in the dorsal root ganglion with lymphocytic infiltration, neuronal degeneration and loss, and residual satellite cell nodules (Mallinow et al. 1986; Griffin et al. 1990). These features are common in both conditions with Sjögren's syndrome associated and idiopathic cases (Okajima et al. 1983; Sobue et al. 1988), and also resemble those described in sensory neuronopathy with carcinoma (Denny-Brown 1948; Henson et al. 1954; Horwich et al. 1977). The lymphocytes in the dorsal root ganglia in cases of Sjögren's syndrome are mainly T cells, predominantly of the cytotoxic/suppressor type (Griffin et al. 1990), while the helper/inducer cells are mainly found in lymphoid infiltrates in Sjögren's syndrome (Adamson et al. 1983). Large myelinated fibers corresponding to the primary sensory neurons are diminished in the peripheral nerves, while unmyelinated fibers are fairly well preserved (Kaufman et al. 1981; Hankey and Gubbay 1987; Dalakas 1986; Graus et al. 1988; Laloux et al. 1988; Sobue et al. 1988, 1993; Mellgren et al. 1989; Griffin et al. 1990). Active axonal degeneration in the teased fiber preparation is observed in patients with a shorter duration of illness (Mellgren et al. 1989; Sobue et al. 1993). Hypertrophic neuropathy with onion bulb formation in the sural nerve was exceptionally reported in a Sjögren's syndrome-associated case (Marbini et al. 1982). In the central rami of the primary sensory neurons, extensive axon loss is also present (Okajima et al. 1983; Sobue et al. 1988). The myelinated fibers in the dorsal column of the spinal cord are also severely depleted, which is confirmed in the high intensity area by T2*-weighted magnetic resonance imaging (MRI) (Sobue et al. 1995) (Figure 9.1). These pathologies of the central and peripheral rami of the sensory neurons are also similar in both Sjögren's syndrome-associated and idiopathic cases. Small epineurial arterioles with intimal proliferation and mural and perivascular mononuclear cell infiltration, indicating chronic necrotizing angiopathy, is occasionally seen in Sjögren's syndrome (Kaltreides 1969; Moilina et al. 1985; Said et al. 1988; Mellgren et al. 1989; Kumazawa et al. 1993), which suggests that the angiopathic process plays a role in the development of peripheral neuropathy, particularly in motor nerve involvement and the distally accentuated manner of peripheral nerve damage in Sjögren's syndrome-associated cases (Mellgren et al. 1989; Sobue et al. 1993; Kachi et al. 1994). Sympathetic and ciliary ganglia would also be involved corresponding to the clinical manifestations of the Adie's pupils, segmental anhidrosis and segmental distribution of the sensory loss (Kumazawa et al. 1993). The dorsal root ganglion, sympathetic and parasympathetic ganglion and peripheral nerve involvement is multifocal, inducing multifocal expression of sensory and autonomic symptoms.

Systemic infiltrations of lymphocytes in the visceral organs, including the liver, lung, thyroid, kidney, intestine, and other lymphoid tissues, are frequent (Sobue et al. 1988), but symptoms consequent to this lymphoid infiltration are rarely manifested.

Prognosis and treatment

Initial paresthesia and localized sensory deficit is frequently low, and some cases have been reported to be substantially improved by corticosteroid therapy (Griffin et al. 1990; Sobue et al. 1993). Compensation and learning for deafferentation may also promote gradual functional improvement. Corticosteroid therapy or plasmapheresis may be efficient in the early stage of the disease (Griffin et al. 1990); however, when sensory disturbances are fully developed, and sensory loss, particularly sensory ataxia is predominant, and the sensory deficit becomes long-standing, the resistance to immune-suppression therapy probably results from sensory ganglion neuron loss (Kaufman et al. 1981; Dalakas 1986; Kennett and Harding 1986; Mallinow et al. 1986; Sobue et al. 1987, 1988, 1993; Laloux et al. 1988).

Acute sensory neuronopathy

Clinical features

This entity is characterized by acute onset of sensory loss, predominantly of sensory ataxia, areflexia and well preserved motor power. Autonomic dysfunction may be present, but cases with prominent involvement of autonomic function as well as sensory neuronopathy may be categorized as acute autonomic and sensory neuronopathy. Acute sensory neuronopathy has been seen in association with cancer, particularly small-cell carcinoma of the lung (Horwich et al. 1977), but in this chapter, idiopathic cases are described.

Acute sensory neuronopathy

In 1980, Sterman et al. presented three cases. In all cases, the febrile illness was followed by antibiotic treatment, particularly penicillin or its derivatives. These patients suddenly experienced numbness and pain over the face and entire body including the trunks and extremities. Signs appeared rapidly with sensory ataxia, generalized areflexia, and widespread sensory loss in all modalities, but predominantly in proprioceptive sensibility. Sensory action potentials were extremely diminished or unobtainable, whereas motor power was preserved intact. There were no denervation potentials and motor nerve conduction as well as distal latency and compound muscle action potentials were completely preserved. The protein levels in the CSF were elevated without pleocytosis. Sensory disturbance was maximal within 1 week of onset, subsequently remained static and all cases developed a severe static residual sensory deficit including sensory ataxia during the 5-year follow-up. No evidence of neoplastic disease or immunological disorder was found. No autonomic sign was described in these cases, but autonomic dysfunction would not be the major symptom compared with the sensory deficit.

The clinical symptoms with limitation to the sensory system, entire body involvement including face, trunk and extremities and long-standing sensory deficit suggest that ganglionopathy is the primary process in this condition. Low-amplitude or unobtainable sensory potentials are consistent with secondary breakdown of the peripheral axons associated with degeneration of the dorsal root ganglion neurons. The underlying mechanism is not known but some immune-mediated process might be involved in the pathogenesis. The blood–brain barrier may be incomplete in the dorsal root ganglia and may permit penetration by immune agents, which would explain why the dorsal root ganglion cell is selectively involved (Sterman et al. 1980). Subsequently, similar cases were sporadically reported (Mori et al. 1981; Sahashi et al. 1985; Knazam et al. 1990; Taly et al. 1991), but most of these were associated to some extent with autonomic dysfunction, so that some have been described as sensory autonomic or autonomic sensory neuronopathy. Windebank et al. (1990) reviewed 42 cases with sensory neuronopathy selected by the criteria of acute pure sensory neuropathy. Electrophysiological testing typically showed the absence of sensory potentials, and CSF was usually acellular with normal protein levels, in contrast to Stermann's report (1980). Sural nerve biopsy showed axonal degeneration and axonal atrophy without inflammation. These pathological, electrophysiological and clinical features also suggested ganglioneuronitis possibly mediated by some immune mechanism. As the demyelinating nature was not generally present, these cases were not confirmed as a sensory variant of acute inflammatory demyelinating polyradiculoneuropathy (AIDP).

Acute autonomic and sensory neuronopathy

Colan et al. reported in 1980 an unusual case of acute neuropathy of autonomic and sensory dysfunction with completely well-preserved motor power which they called acute autonomic and sensory neuropathy. This disease is characterized by dorsal root ganglioneuronopathy and extensive involvement of the autonomic ganglion neurons (Fujii et al. 1982; Fagius et al. 1983; Hodson et al. 1984; Tohgi et al. 1989; Kanda et al. 1990; Yasuda et al. 1994, 1995). It may be essentially similar to acute sensory neuronopathy except for the severe involvement of the sympathetic and parasympathetic ganglion neurons and clinically severe autonomic dysfunction. In this chapter, I will refer to this condition as acute autonomic and sensory neuronopathy. This condition must also be distinguished from acute pandysautonomia (Young et al. 1969; Appenzeller and Kornfeld 1973), and the autonomic and sensory form of GBS (Dawson et al. 1988; Miralles et al. 1992).

Case presentation

A 27-year-old woman experienced abdominal pain and diarrhea about 10 days after suffering from a flu-like upper respiratory infection. She also complained of nausea, vomiting, and general fatigue. She then developed constipation with abdominal distention, and was admitted to the gastroenterology department of the hospital with a diagnosis of paralytic ileus of unknown origin. On the tenth day of hospitalization, she complained of numbness in her arms and legs and exhibited a gait disturbance. She was then referred to the department of neurology. On neurological examination, the pupils were irregularly shaped and unreactive to light. Corneal reflexes were absent. There was a complete loss of sensation in all modalities over the entire body as well as in the area of the second and third branches of the bilateral trigeminal nerves. There was a deficit in severe deep sensation in all extremities leading to sensory ataxia and pseudoathetosis. Orthostatic hypotension with syncope, urinary retention, paralytic ileus, and anhidrosis were present. Muscle volume and strength were generally well preserved. Deep tendon reflexes were generally absent. Electrophysiologically, there were well-preserved motor action potentials whereas there were no sensory action potentials on nerve conduction studies, SEPs and blink reflexes in affected portions. CSF examination showed albumino-cytological dissociation. The autonomic dysfunctions, anhidrosis, gastrointestinal dysfunction, and orthostatic hypotension improved 1 year after the onset. The sensory symptoms remained in static residual deficit and she was not able to walk unaided even after 5 years of onset due to severe sensory ataxia. She also complained of productive cough and suffering from spontaneously occurring severe tingling deep pain.

Most patients had experienced antecedent febrile illness, especially respiratory tract infection. The acute onset of an abdominal disorder can be the first presenting symptom and subsequent somatosensory neurological symptoms then lead to the appropriate diagnosis in some cases. A patient with this symptom treated by laparotomy (Colan et al. 1980) has been reported. Orthostatic hypotension, impairment of sweating and urinary disturbance are common. Coefficient of variation in R-R intervals in the lying position was reduced. The pupils responded to conjunctival instillation of 0.1% epinephrine, but not to cocaine. Pharmacologically, hypersensitivity of the pupils and the lack of sweating following local application of pilocarpine indicate postganglionic denervation in autonomic dysfunction. Appreciable recovery of autonomic dysfunction tends to occur; however, orthostatic hypotension with syncope remained unchanged in some cases for more than 2 years after onset (Fujii et al. 1982; Fagius et al. 1983; Tohgi et al. 1989). The most common distribution pattern of sensory loss is the entire body including the face. Sensation was severely impaired for all modalities, especially of proprioception and vibration sense, so that patients were unable to walk due to sensory ataxia. All sensory modalities were severely impaired or lost and occasionally there was a patchy improvement of sensation over the body, but long-standing severe residual sensory deficits impairing daily activity are commonly seen in most patients. Generalized areflexia is common but CNS involvement is not present.

Pathological and laboratory features

There have been no reports of autopsied cases of pure sensory neuronopathy, but the pathological features of sensory neuronopathy in the condition described here would share features with those of acute autonomic and sensory neuronopathy, three cases of which have been described (Fagius et al. 1983; Hodson et al. 1984; Tohgi et al. 1989). The primary sensory neurons and their axons are severely involved. The nerve cell bodies of the dorsal root ganglion have often disappeared, with or without lymphoid cell infiltration. Biopsy specimen of the sural nerve, the most distal portion of the primary sensory neurons, exhibits severe loss of large and small myelinated and unmyelinated fibers, but inflammatory cell invasions are not generally present. The dorsal columns of the spinal cord and dorsal roots exhibit an extensive loss of myelinated fibers. The ventral horn motor neurons are on the contrary well preserved. The nerve cell bodies in the thoracic sympathetic ganglion, celiac ganglion and Auerbach's plexus were largely destroyed in those with acute autonomic and sensory neuronopathy(Fagius et al. 1983; Tohgi et al. 1989).

Well-preserved motor action potentials and normal motor conduction with no sensory action potentials on nerve conduction studies are characteristic. SEPs and blink reflexes were not elicited in affected portions. CSF examination may show albumino-cytological dissociation.

Axial MRI in the posterior column of the cervical, thoracic and lumbar spinal cord may demonstrate lesions in some patients (Yasuda et al. 1994) (Figure 8.2). The T2*-weighted high-intensity area in the posterior column of the spinal cord at all levels can be detected, which is consistent with the pathological findings reported from autopsy cases. These lines of evidence suggest that the main lesion responsible for the sensory deficit in this disease is the dorsal root ganglion neurons (ganglioneuronopathy) with secondary degeneration of the posterior column in the spinal cord and the peripheral rami in the nerve trunks.

Prognosis and treatment

Sensory deficits are generally severe and longstanding. The major residual sensory deficit is sensory ataxia due to profound impairment of proprioceptive sensibility (Sterman et al. 1980; Mori et al. 1981; Fagius et al. 1983; Hodson et al. 1984; Sahashi et al. 1985; Tohgi et al. 1989; Yasuda et al. 1994, 1995). On the contrary, the autonomic dysfunction in cases with autonomic and sensory neuronopathy shows a favorable recovery at 1 year follow-up in many cases (Yasuda et al. 1995). Some patients were treated empirically by immune suppression with corticosteroids or plasmapheresis, but consistent favorable effects have not been obtained. L-threo-2,3,-dihydroxyphenyl-serine(L-DOPS) may be effective for the improvement of orthostatic hypotension (Kanda et al. 1990).

Pathogenetic considerations

Antecedent febrile illness is frequently followed by days of silence and the acute onset of sensory deficit mostly extending over the entire body. Poor recovery is probably due to the destruction of the dorsal root ganglion cells in the underlying process. Albumino-cytological dissociation is frequently seen. These characteristics suggest an immune mechanism directly attacking the dorsal root ganglion cells or the sympathetic and parasympathetic ganglion cells, an etiology similar to that of the GBS, although the nature of the demyelinating neuropathy is not known. The causative agent for the antecedent febrile illness has not been elucidated, but Epstein-Barr virus antibody titres were pathologically elevated in the serum of some cases (Fujii et al. 1982; Kanda et al. 1990). The cases reported by Windebank et al.(1990) may be somewhat different in pathoetiology from those described by Sterman et al.(1980) and others (Mori et al. 1981; Yasuda et al. 1995). In their series, CSF protein elevation was rare and antecedent illness was not common although not precisely described.

Differential diagnosis of the acute and chronic sensory neuronopathy

Acute or chronic sensory symptoms without motor nerve involvement, even if autonomic symptoms are present, is the most important feature for a differential diagnosis. Cases of acute sensory GBS or acute ataxic GBS would exhibit a sensory deficit (Dawson et al. 1988; Miralles et al. 1992); occasionally the sensory ataxia is permanently present as a residual sign (Sobue et al. 1983). There may be evidence of demyelinating features such as conduction block, slow conduction and temporal dispersion in the compound muscle action potentials. In most cases, motor function involvement is shown electrophysiologically and clinically, suggesting the pathological process is not restricted to the sensory system. Malignant sensory neuronopathy is indistinguishable from cases without malignancy only by the clinical manifestations (Denny-Brown 1948; Henson et al. 1954). The autoantibody against neuronal antigen, anti-Hu antibody, would be helpful (Chalk et al. 1993), and an extensive survey for small-cell bronchial carcinoma would assist in making the diagnosis. Toxic neuropathies due to cisplatin (Hadley and Herr 1979), mercury (Jacobs et al. 1977), adriamycin (Spencer and Schaumburg 1978), pyridoxine (Schaumburg et al. 1983), and podophyllin (O'Mahony et al. 1990; Chang et al. 1992) are the major causative agents of chronic sensory neuronopathy, as they attack the dorsal root ganglion neurons. Particularly, cisplatin and pyridoxine megavitaminosis would present profound sensory ataxia. The history of exposure to these toxic substances is an essential clue to establish the diagnosis. Hereditary sensory and autonomic neuropathy (Dyck 1993), familial amyloidotic neuropathy (Sobue et al. 1990) and Friedreich's ataxia (Dyck 1993) would also exhibit the symptoms corresponding to involvement of the sensory ganglion neurons. In these conditions, a familial history of the disease with young age of onset would be a diagnostic clue and characteristic associated signs such as insensitivity to pain, persistent trophic change of the extremities, severe persistent autonomic symptoms, as well as motor power deficiency, cerebellar signs and deformity of the feet, may help make the diagnosis. In familial amyloidosis, ganglionopathy preferentially occurs in small diameter sensory neurons (Sobue et al. 1990). DNA analysis for the responsible gene has become available to make the final diagnosis in some of these hereditary diseases. Chronic biliary cirrhosis is rarely associated with chronic sensory neuronopathy (Charron et al. 1980); however, this neuronopathy is indistinguishable from that associated with Sjögren's syndrome or the idiopathic condition because biliary cirrhosis is one of the manifestations of Sjögren's syndrome and the related lymphocyte invasion is a result of immune mechanism directed against the biliary duct (Fox et al. 1986; Sobue et al. 1988).

References

Adamson, T., Fox, R., Frisman. D., and Howell, F. (1983). Immunohistologic analysis of lymphoid infiltrates in primary Sjögren's syndrome using monoclonal antibodies. *J. Immunol.* **130**: 203–208.

Alexander, E.L. (1992). Central nervous system disease in Sjögren's syndrome. *Rheum. Dis. Clin. N. Am.* **18**: 637–672.

Alexander, E.L., Provost, T.T., Stevens, M.B., and Alexander, G.E. (1982). Neurologic complications of primary Sjögren's syndrome. *Medicine* **61**: 247–257.

Appenzeller, O. and Kornfeld, M. (1973). Acute pandysautonomia. *Arch. Neurol.* **29**: 510–519.

Chalk, C.H., Lennon, V.A., Stevens, J.C., and Windebank, A.J. (1993). Seronegativity for type 1 antineuronal nuclear antibodies ('anti-Hu')in subacute sensory neuropathy patients without cancer. *Neurology* **43**: 2209–2211.

Chang, M.H., Lin, K.P., Wu, Z.A., and Liao, K.K. (1992). Acute ataxic sensory neuronopathy resulting from podophyllin intoxication. *Muscle Nerve* **15**: 513–514.

Charron, L., Peyronnard, J.M., and Marchand, L. (1980). Sensory neuropathy associated with primary biliary cirrhosis. *Arch. Neurol.* **37**: 84–87.

Colan, R.V., Snead, O.C., Oh, S.J., and Kashlan, M.B. (1980). Acute autonomic and sensory neuropathy. *Ann. Neurol.* **8**: 441–444

Dalakas, M.C. (1986). Chronic idiopathic ataxic neuropathy. *Ann. Neurol.* **19**: 545–554.

Dawson, D.M., Samuels, M.A., and Morris, J. (1988). Sensory form of acute polyneuritis. *Neurology* **38**: 1728–1731.

Denny-Brown, D. (1948). Hereditary sensory neuropathy with muscular changes associated with carcinoma. *J. Neurol. Neurosurg. Psychiatry* **11**: 73–87.

Dyck, P.J. (1993). Neuronal atrophy and degeneration predominantly affecting peripheral sensory and autonomic neurons. *In Peripheral Neuropathy*, 3rd edn, vol. 2, ed. P.J. Dyck et al., pp. 1065–1093. Philadelphia: W.B. Saunders.

Dyck, P.J., Benstead, T.J., Conn, B.D., Stevens, J.C., Windebank, A.J., and Low, P.A. (1987). Non-systemic vasculitic neuropathy. *Brain* **110**: 843–854.

Dyck, P.J., Gutrecht, J.A., Bastron, J.A. et al. (1968). Histologic and teased fiber measurements of sural nerve in disorders of lower motor and primary sensory neurons. *Mayo Clin. Proc.* **43**: 81–123.

Feasby, T.E., Gilbert, J.J., Brown, W.F. et al. (1986). An acute axonal form of Guillain-Barré polyneuropathy. *Brain* **109**: 1115–1126.

Fagius, J., Westerberg, C.E., and Olsson, Y. (1983). Acute pandysautonomia and sensory deficit with poor recovery. A clinical, neurophysiological and pathological case study. *J. Neurol. Neurosurg. Psychiatry* **46**: 725–733.

Fox, R., Robinson, C.A., Curd, J.G., Kozin, F., and Howell, F.V. (1986). Sjögren's syndrome: proposed criteria for classification. *Arthritis Rheum.* **29**: 577–585.

Fujii, N., Tabira, T., Shibazaki, H., Kuroiwa, Y., Ohnishi, A., and Nagaki, J. (1982). Acute autonomic and sensory neuropathy associated with elevated Epstein–Barr virus antibody. *J. Neurol. Neurosurg. Psychiatry* **45**: 656–665.

Grant, I.A., Hundes, G.E., Homberger, H.A., and Dyck, P.J. (1997). Peripheral neuropathy associated with sicca complex. *Neurology* **48**: 855–862.

Graus, F., Pou, A., Kanterewicz, E., and Anderson, N.E. (1988). Sensory neuronopathy and Sjögren's syndrome: clinical and immunologic study of two patients. *Neurology* **38**: 1637–1639.

Griffin, J.W., Cornblath, D.R., Alexander, E., Campbell, J., Low, P.A., Bird, S., and Feldman, E.L. (1990). Ataxic sensory neuropathy and dorsal root ganglionitis associated with Sjögren's syndrome. *Ann. Neurol.* **27**: 304–315.

Hadley, D. and Herr, H.W. (1979). Peripheral neuropathy associated with cisdichlor diamminoplatinum (II). *Cancer* **44**: 2026–2032.

Hankey, G. and Gubbay, S. (1987). Peripheral neuropathy associated with sicca syndrome. *J. Neurol. Neurosurg. Psychiatry* **50**: 1085–1086.

Henson, R.A., Russell, D.S., and Wilkinson, M. (1954). Carcinomatous neuropathy and myopathy: a clinical and pathological study. *Brain* **77**: 82–121.

Hodson, A,K., Hurwitz, B.J., and Albrecht, R. (1984). Dysautonomia in Guillain-Barré syndrome with dorrsal root ganglioneuropathy, Wallerian degeneration, and fatal myocarditis. *Ann. Neurol.* **15**: 88–95.

Horwich, M.S., Cho, L., Porro, R.S., and Posner, J.B. (1977). Subacute sensory neuropathy: a remote effect of carcinoma. *Ann. Neurol.* **2**: 7–19.

Hull, R.G., Morgan, S.H., Harding, A.E., and Hughes, G.R.V. (1984). Sjögren's syndrome presenting as a severe sensory neuropathy including involvement of the trigeminal nerve. *Br. J. Rheumatol.* **23**: 301–303.

Jacobs, J.M., Carmichael, N., and Cavanagh, J.B. (1977). Ultrastructural changes in the nervous sytem of rabbits poisoned with methyl mercury. *Toxicol. Appl. Pharmacol.* **39**: 249–261.

Kachi, T., Sobue, G., Yamamoto, M., and Igata, A. (1994). Sensory conduction study in chronic sensory ataxic neuropathy. *J Neurol. Neurosurg. Psychiatry* **57**: 941–944.

Kaltreides, H.B. and Talal, N. (1969). The neuropathy of Sjögren's syndrome: trigeminal nerve involvement. *Ann. Intern. Med.* **70**: 751–762.

Kanda, F., Uchida, T., Jinnai, K., Tada, K., Shiozawa, S., Fujita, T., and Ohnishi, A. (1990). Acute autonomic and sensory neuropathy: a case report. *J. Neurol.* **237**: 442–447.

Kaufman, M.D., Hopkins, L.C., and Hurwitz, B.J. (1981). Progressive sensory neuropathy in patients without carcinoma: a disorder with distinctive clinical and electrophysiological findings. *Ann. Neurol.* **9**: 237–242.

Kennett, R.P. and Harding, A.E. (1986). Peripheral neuropathy associated with the sicca syndrome. *J. Neurol. Neurosurg. Psychiatry* **49**: 90–92.

Knazan, M., Bohlega, S., Berry, K., and Eisen, A. (1990). Acute sensory neuropathy with preserved SEPs and long-latency reflexes. *Muscle Nerve* **13**: 381–384.

Kumazawa, K., Sobue, G., Yamamoto, K., and Mitsuma, T. (1993a). Segmental anhidrosis in the spinal dermatomes in Sjögren's syndrome-associated neuropathy. *Neurology* **43**: 1820–1823.

Kumazawa, K., Sobue, G., Yamamoto, K., Shimada, N., and Mitsuma, T. (1993b). Autonomic dysfunction in sensory ataxic neuropathy with Sjögren's syndrome. *Clin. Neurol.(Tokyo)* **33**: 1059–1065.

Laloux, P., Brucher, J.M., Sindic, C.J.M., and Laterre, E. C. (1988). Subacute sensory neuronopathy associated with Sjögren's sicca syndrome. *J. Neurol.* **235**: 352–354.

Mallinow, K., Yannakakis, G.D., Glusman, S.M., Edlow, D.W., Griffin, J., Pestronk, A., Powell, D.L., Ramsey-Goldman, R. Eidelman, B.H., Medsger, T.A. Jr, Alexander, E.L. (1986). Subacute sensory neuronopathy secondary to dorsal root ganglionatis in primary Sjögren's syndrome. *Ann. Neurol.* **20**: 535–537.

Marbini, A., Gemignani, F., Manganelli, P., Govoni, E., Bragaglia, M.M., and Ambanelli, U. (1982). Hypertrophic neuropathy in Sjögren's syndrome. *Acta Neuropathol.* (Berl.) **57**: 309–312.

Mellgren, S., Conn, D.L., Stevens, J.C., and Dyck, P.J. (1989). Peripheral neuropathy in primary Sjögren's syndrome. *Neurology* **39**: 390–304.

Miralles, F., Montero, J., and Matos, J.M. (1992). Pure sensory Guillain-Barré syndrome. *J. Neurol. Neurosurg. Psychiatry* **55**: 414–415.

Mitsumoto, H., Wilbourn, A.J., and Massarweh, W. (1985). Acquired 'pure' sensory polyneuropathy (APSP): unique clinical features in 30 patients. *Neurology* **35** (suppl. 1): 295–371.

Molina, R., Provost, T.T., and Alexander, E.L. (1985). Peripheral inflammatory vascular disease in Sjögren's syndrome. *Arthritis Rheum.* **28**: 1341–1347.

Moll, J. W.B., Markusse, H.M., Vecht, Ch.J., and Henzen-Logmans, S.C. (1993). Antineuronal antibodies in patients with neurologic complications of primary Sjögren's syndrome. *Neurology* **43**: 2574–2581.

Mori, K., Ide, Y., Mori, M., et al. (1981). A case of acute inflammatory polyradiculoneuropathy with anesthesis over the entire body. *Clin. Neurol.(Tokyo)* **21**: 392–395.

O'Mahony, S., Keohane C., Jacobs, J., O'Riordain, D., and Whelton, M. (1990). Neuropathy due to podophyllin intoxication. *J. Neurol.* **237**: 110–112.

Okajima, T., Yamamura, S., Hamada, K., et al. (1983). Chronic sensory and autonomic neuropathy. *Neurology* **33**: 1061–104.

Peyronnard, J.M., Charron, L., Beaudet, F., and Couture, F. (1982). Vasculitic neuropathy in rheumatoid disease and Sjögren syndrome. *Neurology* **32**: 839–845.

Romberg, M.H. (1851). Lehrbuch der Nerven-Krankheiten des Menschen. Alexander Duncker, Berlin. Japanese translation by Takahashi, A., et al. (1994). *Neurol. Med. (Tokyo)* 110–113.

Ross, A.T. (1958). Progressive selective sudomotor denervation: a case with coexisting Adie's syndrome. *Neurology* **8**: 809–817.

Sahashi, K., Takahashi, A., Ibi, T., Gotoh, S., Matsui, T. (1985). Acute predominantly sensory neuropathy. *Klin. Wochenschr.* **63**: 319–324.

Said, G., Lacroix-Ciaudo, C., Fujimura, H., Blas, C., and Faux, N. (1988). The peripheral neuropathy of necrotizing arteritis: a clinicopathological study. *Ann. Neurol.* **23**: 461–46.

Schaumburg, H., Kaplan, J., Windebank, A., Vick, N., Rasmus, S., Pleasure, D., and Brown, M.J. (1983). Sensory neuropathy from pyridoxine abuse: a new megavitamin syndrome. *N. Engl. J. Med.* **309**: 445–448.

Smith, B.E., Windebank, A.J., and Dyck, P.J. (1994). Nonmalignant inflammatory sensory polyganglionopathy. In *Peripheral Neuropathy*, ed. P.J. Dyck, P.K. Thomas et al., pp.1525–1531. Philadelphia: W.B. Saunders.

Sobue, G. and Yanagi, T. (1979). Chronic ataxic polyneuritis with polyclonal hypergammaglobulinemia. *Neurol. Med. (Tokyo)* **11**: 380–382.

Sobue, G., Nakao, N., Kumazawa, K., and Mitsuma, T. (1989). Migrating multiple mononeuritis and non-systemic angitis. *Clin. Neurol. (Tokyo)* **29**: 1210–1215.

Sobue, G., Nakao, N., Murakami, K., et al. (1990). Type 1 familial amyloid polyneuropathy, a pathological study of the periphral nervous system. *Brain* **113**: 903–922.

Sobue, G., Senda, Y., Matsuoka, Y., and Sobue, I. (1983). Sensory ataxia: a residual disability of Guillain-Barré syndrome. *Arch. Neurol.* **40**: 86–89.

Sobue, G., Yanagi, T., and Hashizume, Y. (1988). Chronic progressive sensory ataxic neuropathy with polyclonal gammopathy and disseminated focal perivascular cellular infiltrations. *Neurology* **38**: 463–467.

Sobue, G., Yasuda, T., Kachi, T., Mizuno, K., and Yanagi, T. (1987). Clinico-pathological characteristics of idiopathic chronic progressive sensory-ataxic polyneuropathy. *Clin. Neurol.(Tokyo)* **27**: 745–755.

Sobue, G., Yasuda, T., Kachi, T., Sakakibara, T., and Mitsuma, T. (1993). Chronic progressive sensory ataxic neuropathy: clinicopathological features of idiopathic and Sjögren's syndrome-associated cases. *J. Neurol.* **240**: 1–7.

Sobue, G., Yasuda, T., Kumazawa, K., Yamamoto, K., and Mitsuma, T. (1995). MR demonstrates dorsal column involvement of the spinal cord in Sjögren's syndrome-associated neuropathy. *Neurology* **45**: 592–593.

Spencer, P.S. and Schaumburg, H.H. (1978). Pathobiology of neurotoxic axonal degeneration. In *Physiology and Pathobiology of Axons*, ed. S.G. Waxman, pp. 265–282. New York: Raven Press.

Sterman, A.B., Schaumburg, H.H., and Asbury, A.K. (1980). The acute sensory neuronopathy syndrome: a distinct clinical entity. *Ann. Neurol.* **7**: 354–358.

Taly, A.B., Prasad, A., Vasanth, S.K., and Nagaraja, D. (1991). Acute ataxic neuropathy: a clinical, electrophysiological and morphological study. *Acta Neurol. Scand.* **84**: 398–402.

Thomas, P.K. (1992) The Guillain-Barré syndrome: no longer a simple concept. *J. Neurol.* **239**: 361–2.

Tohgi, H., Sano, M., Sasaki, K., Suzuki, H., Sato, T., Iwasaki, T., and Satodate, R. (1989). Acute autonomic and sensory neuropathy: report of an autopsy case. *Acta Neuropathol.(Berl.)* **77**: 659–663.

Wartenberg, R. (1958). Migrant sensory neuritis. In *Neuritis, Sensory Neuritis and Neuralgia*, ed. R. Wartenberg, pp. 233–247. Oxford: Oxford University Press.

Watershoot, M.P., Guerit, J.M., Lambert, M., and deBarsy, T. (1991). Bilateral tonic pupils and polyneuropathy in Sjögren's syndrome: a common pathophysiological mechanism? *Eur. Neurol.* **31**: 114–116.

Windebank, A.J., Blexrud, M.D., Dyck, P.J., Daube, J.R., and Karnes, J.L. (1990). The syndrome of acute sensory neuropathy: clinical features and electrophysiologic and pathologic changes. *Neurology* **40**: 584–591.

Yasuda, T., Sobue, G., Hirose, Y., Mimura, M., and Yanagi, T. (1994). MR of acute autonomic and sensory neuropathy. *Am. J. Neuroradiol.* **15**: 114–115.

Yasuda, T., Sobue, G., Mokuno, K., Hakusui, S., Ito, T., Hirose, Y., and Yanagi, T. (1995). Clinico-pathophysiological features of acute autonomic and sensory neuropathy: a long-term follow-up study. *J. Neurol.* **242**: 623–628.

Young, R.R., Asbury, A.K., and Corbett, J.L. (1969). Pure pandysautonomia with recovery. *Trans. Am. Neurol. Assoc.* **94**: 355–357.

10 Acute and chronic autonomic neuropathies

G.A. Suarez and P.A. Low

Introduction

The diagnosis of a patient with an autonomic neuropathy is challenging to many neurologists because autonomic fibers innervate many organs producing protean clinical manifestations. The difficulties include long lists of possible causes, an extensive laboratory survey of all potential etiologies, complexity of electrophysiological studies, and relatively limited information on pathogenesis and treatment; however, this picture is rapidly changing for several reasons. With the recent advent of non-invasive objective tests for the assessment of autonomic function, it is now possible to characterize and quantitate autonomic function in the neuropathies using standardized, comprehensive, sensitive, and specific tests.

Evaluation and quantitation of autonomic indices is important because: (1) autonomic indices reflect small myelinated and unmyelinated fiber function, (2) in certain neuropathies, the presence of autonomic failure is associated with poor prognosis, i.e. diabetes and amyloidosis, and (3) autonomic indices are used to objectively evaluate the response to treatment, i.e. idiopathic autonomic neuropathy.

In this chapter, we will describe: (1) the clinical evaluation of autonomic function with emphasis on the autonomic neuropathies, (2) laboratory and diagnostic tests used in the evaluation of autonomic neuropathies, and (3) classification and description of the acute and chronic autonomic neuropathies.

Clinical evaluation

The clinical evaluation of a patient with a suspected autonomic neuropathy begins with a detailed neurological and autonomic history. In taking the autonomic history, particular attention should be directed to assess orthostatic, sudomotor, secretomotor, gastrointestinal, genitourinary, and ocular symptoms.

Orthostatic hypotension (OH) may be manifested as dizziness, orthostatic lightheadedness, near syncope, or syncope after standing. There are some patients in whom orthostatic symptoms only occur after certain conditions, such as a hot bath, exercise, or prolonged standing. Symptoms may be worse or only present postprandially or after alcohol ingestion. Patients with postural orthostatic tachycardia syndrome

(POTS) have orthostatic dizziness but usually associated with palpitations and tremulousness.

Sudomotor symptoms are investigated by asking patients whether they sweat on a hot summer day, after a hot shower, or after exercise. Some patients complain of heat intolerance. The patient may feel dizzy, hot, or flushed after exercise or a hot shower but after careful questioning, they would not sweat globally or in specific areas of their body. Secretomotor symptoms are sought by asking about dry eyes or dry mouth. Gastrointestinal symptoms, such as anorexia, early satiety, bloating, nausea, or vomiting are common among patients with gastrointestinal dysfunction secondary to an autonomic neuropathy. Weight loss is a frequent symptom and sign in patients with gastroparesis. Diarrhea may alternate with constipation. Urinary retention occasionally preceded by frequent micturition are the symptoms associated with parasympathetic failure affecting the urinary bladder. Ocular symptoms relate to difficulties in accommodation. Patients may complain of photophobia in bright sunlight or may have poor night vision.

Erectile failure is a prominent symptom in men with sexual dysfunction secondary to autonomic neuropathy. Patients may initially have partial erectile failure, followed by complete impotence. Symptoms of ejaculatory dysfunction are more difficult to elicit. Retrograde ejaculation may indicate sympathetic dysfunction. Patients should be asked whether the urine looked turbid after sexual intercourse. Spermatozoa may be seen in the urine if there is retrograde ejaculation.

Autonomic examination

Patients with a suspected autonomic neuropathy should undergo a complete neurological examination. In addition, the physical examination ought to be focused or directed to the following areas.

Blood pressure and heart rate

Blood pressure (BP) and heart rate (HR) are measured after 5–10 minutes of rest in both the supine position and after standing for 1 minute. If OH is suspected but not detected, the patient is asked to do a light exercise, such as ten squats, before rechecking the BP. For this review, OH is defined as a reduction in systolic BP of ≥30 mm Hg, a drop in diastolic BP of ≥30 mm Hg, or a mean arterial BP drop of ≥20 mm Hg. Ideally, BP recording should be performed in duplicate. In patients with generalized sympathetic (adrenergic failure), OH is present and not associated with reflex tachycardia. If reflex tachycardia is present, OH may be secondary to hypovolemia or deconditioning.

Sudomotor function

Dryness of the skin, whether globally or regionally, should be assessed during the examination. This is usually accomplished by gently stroking the skin with the examiner's finger pads. A qualitative test to assess sudomotor function by running a heavy spoon over the skin has been described (Tsementzis and Hitchcock 1985).

Pupils

Pupillary shape, size, and response to light and accommodation are assessed. The presence of a tonic pupil is sought by maintaining a light stimulus for 1 minute to the apparently unreactive pupil.

Vasomotor and trophic functions

In patients with distal sympathetic neuropathies or toxic neuropathies, particular attention should be paid to acral vasomotor and trophic changes. The presence of cyanosis, pallor, or mottling should be noted. Hyperalgesia (painful stimulus perceived more painful) or allodynia (perception of pain from a non-painful stimulus) are assessed by palpating the skin. Nail changes, such as excessive fragility, discoloration, thickening, and Mee's lines may be seen in the arsenical and toxic neuropathies. Alopecia or hypertrichosis may also be a prominent sign in some of the toxic neuropathies.

After the office or bedside evaluation, the clinician needs to recognize the presence or absence of autonomic dysfunction and try to recognize patterns of autonomic failure that define specific syndromes. The clinician needs to decide if further studies are necessary. If the physician recognizes that symptoms do not require extensive evaluation because the cause is apparent or the disorder is benign, no further tests are needed. In many of the autonomic neuropathies, however, laboratory evaluation not only complements

Table 10.1 *Autonomic reflex screen*

1. QSART distribution
2. Orthostatic blood pressure (BP) and heart rate (HR) response to tilt
3. Heart rate response to deep breathing (HR_{DB})
4. Valsalva ratio (VR)
5. Beat-to-beat BP (BP_{BB}) top Valsalva maneuver, tilt and deep breathing

the autonomic history and examination, but also provides helpful information to determine the presence of autonomic failure, the level of the lesion (pre- or postganglionic), the autonomic system involved, and the severity of autonomic failure.

Tests to assess autonomic function in autonomic neuropathies

Non-invasive studies measure effector function of complicated autonomic reflexes. Because they provide indirect information, the use of a single test is probably inadequate. It is necessary to carry out a battery of comprehensive autonomic tests that would allow the clinician to determine the presence, extent, and severity of a suspected autonomic lesion. The tests should be carried out using quantitative, non-invasive, and reliable tests of known sensitivity and specificity. At the Mayo Autonomic Reflex Laboratory, we use a battery of tests (autonomic reflex screen) that fulfills the requirements described above (Table 10.1).

Preparation of patients for autonomic tests is important to minimize confounding variables. Prior to testing, patients must avoid the following:

- food, caffeine-containing drinks, and tobacco products for 3 hours
- alcohol for 12–24 hours
- cold and antiallergic over-the-counter medications, antidepressants, antihistamines, diuretics, and α- and β-agonists for 48 hours
- calcium channel blockers and α- and β-antagonists for 24 hours (if medically permissible). Diabetic patients should have no evidence of hypoglycemia
- excessive cold and heat exposure for 30 minutes
- patients in severe pain should postpone testing.

When an autonomic neuropathy is suspected, it is important to characterize and quantitate autonomic indices to determine the presence or absence of autonomic failure, distribution, level of the lesion (pre- or postganglionic), system involved (adrenergic, cardiovagal, sudomotor), and severity of autonomic deficits. The assessment of autonomic indices is also helpful to monitor the progress and response to treatment.

Sudomotor function tests

The eccrine sweat glands are innervated by nerve fibers that are sympathetic and cholinergic in origin. In the autonomic neuropathies, involvement of sympathetic sudomotor fibers is commonly seen. A complete lesion may produce anhidrosis, while a partial lesion may initially elicit excessive sweating. Distal anhidrosis is quite common in many autonomic and somatic neuropathies. The mechanism is due to postganglionic denervation. In other neuropathies, such as amyloid, the mechanism is probably due to a combination of pre- and postganglionic denervation.

When evaluating a patient with a suspected autonomic neuropathy, we assess sudomotor function with the quantitative sudomotor axon reflex test (QSART) and the thermoregulatory sweat test (TST). The principle of the QSART is shown in Figure 10.1. The neural substrate consists of an axon reflex mediated by postganglionic sympathetic sudomotor fibers (Low et al. 1983a). Acetylcholine (ACh) is iontophoresed and stimulates nicotinic receptors of one population of eccrine sweat glands. This evokes a nerve impulse that travels antidromically to a branch point, and then orthodromically to release acetylcholine from the nerve terminal. Acetylcholine traverses the neuroglandular junction and binds to M3 muscarinic receptors on a second population of sweat glands and evokes a sweat response (Torres et al. 1991). The sweat response terminates when ACh is inactivated and cleaved into acetate and choline by acetylcholinesterase present in subcutaneous tissues.

The test is performed as follows. Acetylcholine is iontophoresed using a constant current generator in a multicompartmental sweat cell, which is applied to the skin. The same cell is used to measure the sweat

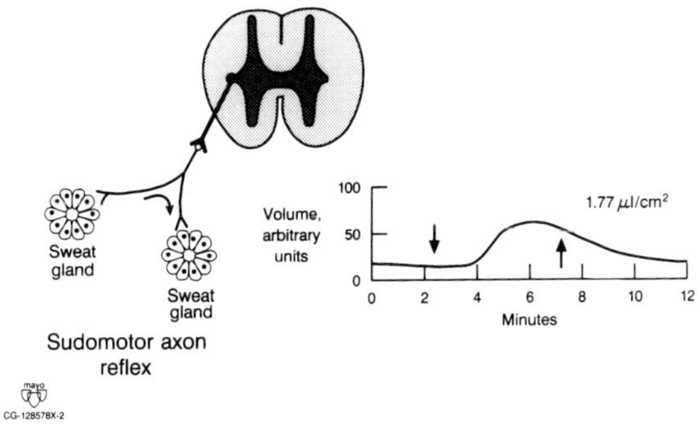

Figure 10.1 *Left: the neural pathway for the axon-reflex sweat response. Right: a representative QSART response. Reproduced with permission from Low PA, Opfer-Gehrking TL, Kihara M: In vivo studies on receptor pharmacology of the human eccrine sweat gland.* Clin. Auton. Res. *2: 29–34, 1992.*

response, which is quantitated using a sudometer. Output from the sudometer is displayed and analysed on a computer. Standard QSART recordings are made from the following four sites: medial forearm, proximal leg, distal leg, and proximal foot. The recordings are symmetric but, for practical purposes, we routinely record from the left side; however, when clinically necessary, we will record from the right side, i.e. after a left sural nerve biopsy. The normal QSART response has a latency of 1–2 minutes with a rapid rise time and a sweat volume. The relatively prolonged latency is mainly due to the iontophoresis of ACh. The response returns to baseline (Figure 9.1) within 5 minutes after the stimulus is over. The test is sensitive, specific, and reproducible in controls and in patients with neuropathy (Low et al. 1986). A normal QSART indicates integrity of the postganglionic sympathetic sudomotor axon. The response may be normal or abnormal provided iontophoresis is successful and eccrine sweat glands are present. Abnormal patterns are: (1) reduced, (2) absent, (3) excessive, or (4) persistent. Patterns 3 or 4 may be seen in painful distal small fiber neuropathy (Stewart et al. 1992). QSART recordings have been performed in many neuropathies (Low et al. 1986; Stewart et al. 1992; Suarez et al. 1994). In patients with idiopathic autonomic neuropathy, abnormalities of QSART correlate well with severity of autonomic failure and with other tests of autonomic function (Suarez et al. 1994).

The TST is a test of efferent sympathetic sudomotor pathways. The efferent pathways begin in the hypothalamus, descending via multisynaptic pathway in the spinal cord, and synapsing with preganglionic neurons located in the intermediolateral column. Preganglionic neurons connect with postganglionic neurons located in the pre- and paravertebral autonomic ganglia. The test requires the application of topical powders (alizarine red mixed with sodium carbonate and cornstarch) to the entire body and observation of the sweat pattern. The powder is light orange when dry and purple when wet. The stimulus is an elevation in core temperature which activates thermal receptors in the anterior hypothalamus and, to a lesser degree, receptors in the skin and spinal cord. Fealey (1993) suggested using an elevation in oral temperature of 1°C, provided the patient is not dehydrated or hypothermic. It is important to emphasize that the patient should avoid anticholinergic medications, including common cold over-the-counter drugs, for at least 48 hours prior to testing. A sweat cabinet is the method of choice for heat stimulus, with adequate control of ambient temperature and humidity. Alternatively, elevation of ambient temperature or an infrared heat source could be used as a heat stimulus. If the head is omitted, the latency to thermoregulatory sweating is delayed. A semi-quantitative approach to measure the percentage of anhidrosis was recently introduced by Fealey et al. (1989). An abnormal sweat response may be due to a lesion anywhere along the sympathetic sudomotor pathways. Several patterns are recognized: (1) normal, (2) distal, (3) focal, (4) global (more than 80% anhidrosis), (5) regional (large areas of anhidrosis but less than 80%), and (6) mixed patterns. The percentage of body anhidrosis correlates well with the severity of autonomic failure in patients with idiopathic autonomic neuropathy (Suarez et al. 1994). The TST, used in combination with QSART, is helpful in differentiating a pre- from a postganglionic sudomotor lesion. When anhidrosis is recorded on TST but sweating is normal with QSART, the lesion is preganglionic. If anhidrosis is present with both TST and QSART, the lesion is postganglionic.

A sweat imprint method was described by Kennedy and Navarro (1993) as a quantitative measure of sudomotor function. The sweat imprint depends on the direct stimulation of sweat glands with iontophoresis of 1% pilocarpine for 5 minutes. A silastic impression material is used over the stimulated surface, and upon hardening, each sweat droplet leaves an imprint which is measured and quantitated. Kennedy and Sakuta (1984) have described studies of sweat droplet morphometry in human diabetic neuropathy using the sweat imprint. A good correlation was established between sweat histogram abnormalities and perception of pain thresholds in patients with diabetic neuropathy (Kennedy and Sakuta 1984; Navarro et al. 1989). Navarro et al. (1989) used the silastic method in patients with diabetic neuropathy and found that sudomotor abnormalities correlated well with measures of thermal sensation but had a low concordance with nerve conduction studies, which suggests that small fiber function may be separately affected from large fiber function in diabetic neuropathy.

Cardiovagal function

Heart rate response to deep breathing

This is probably the most reliable and frequently used method to assess baroreflex function (Low 1993a). Both major afferent and efferent pathways are vagal. There are several factors that influence the heart rate deep breathing (HR_{DB}): age, rate of breathing, position of subject, hypocapnia, depth of breathing, medication, and different methods of analysis (Low and Pfeifer 1993). A review of the factors affecting HR_{DB} has recently been published (Ewing 1993; Low and Pfeifer 1993). There are several methods for evaluation of HR_{DB}: the E:I ratio, HR range, and the mean circular resultant. The E:I ratio is derived by dividing the R–R maximum by the R–R minimum. This method is affected by ectopic beats, drifting HR, and suppressed by resting tachycardia. The HR range, which is the difference between maximum and minimum HR is also affected by ectopic beats and is insensitive to the mean HR. The mean circular resultant is a measure of the synchronization between the HR variation and respiration. One of the drawbacks is that it needs a long recording period, but it is generally unaffected by ectopic beats and shifting mean HR. In most laboratories, the E:I ratio or HR range are the preferred methods. We used the HR range with only eight respiratory cycles to avoid hypocapnia. Ectopic beats and artefacts are relatively easy to detect and exclude from the analysis. Each autonomic laboratory should establish their own control values. There is extensive experience with the use of this test in the detection and characterization of cardiovagal dysfunction in the peripheral neuropathy, especially diabetic neuropathy (Low and McLeod 1993).

The Valsalva ratio

The Valsalva ratio (VR) is a ratio of the maximal to the minimal HR in response to the Valsalva maneuver. The maneuver is performed as follows. The patient, in the supine position, is asked to maintain a column of mercury at 40 mm Hg for 10–15 seconds via a bugle with an air leak (to ensure an open glottis). The maneuver is repeated until two reproducible responses are obtained. The mechanisms of the different phases of the Valsalva maneuver are shown in Table 10.2. Although VR mainly reflects cardiovagal function, it is also dependent on BP alterations and cardiac sympathetic function. The true stimuli of the VR is the reduction in BP in phase II and BP overshoot in phase IV. If beat-to-beat BP recordings are not available during the Valsalva maneuver, the true stimuli is not observed.

Several variables may affect the VR including: age, position, volume status, expiratory pressure, and duration of the effort. These are described in detail elsewhere (Low 1993a). We use an expiratory pressure of 40 mm Hg (Benarroch et al. 1991). Pressures below 20 mm Hg are inadequate (Korner et al. 1976), and pressure above 60 mm Hg are difficult to reproduce.

Adrenergic function

Orthostatic blood pressure recording

Orthostatic BP recording in response to standing or upright tilt are recorded simultaneously using a sphygmomanometer cuff over the upper arm and with beat-to-beat BP recording with a continuous non-invasive BP monitor (Finapres monitor). Manual recordings are performed in duplicate, ensuring that the arm is at

Table 10.2 *Mechanisms of phases of the Valsalva maneuver*

Phase	Event	Major mechanism
I	Brief (1–3 s) increase in BP	Mechanical compression of aorta
II_e	Small reduction in MAP; larger reduction in PP	Reduction in venous return; counteracted by vagal release
II_l	Rise in BP in second half of phase II	Activation of vasomotor and cardiac sympathetics; continued effects of vagal release
III	Brief (1–3 s) fall in BP	Release of mechanical compression of the aorta
IV	Sustained BP overshoot	Maintained vasomotor sympathetic activation and normalization of cardiac output

Note:
MAP: mean arterial pressure; PP: pulse pressure; BP: blood pressure.

heart level (Webster et al. 1984). BP is measured in the supine position after 5 or 10 minutes of rest. The subject is then tilted to an angle of 80° for 5 or more minutes. Cuff recordings are generally obtained at minute intervals. The Finapres device is a photoplethysmographic technique that permits non-invasive continuous measurements of beat-to-beat BP. It generates an arterial waveform similar to that of peripheral arterial waveform. The Finapres-recorded pressures have shown good correlation with intra-arterial pressures (Imholtz et al. 1988). Some investigators have reported poor correlation between Finapres and intra-arterial recordings (Nijboer et al. 1988). We have observed that to obtain good concordance between Finapres and brachial cuff recordings, particular attention to detail of finger cuff application and maintenance of a warm hand are of utmost importance.

Beat-to-beat blood pressure recordings during the Valsalva maneuver (VM)

Using non-invasive BP recording, four phases of the VM are recognized. Phases I and III are mechanically induced by compression and decompression of the aorta. Phase II is divided into early phase II (II_e) and late phase II (II_l). Early phase II is due to a reduction in venous return causing a fall in cardiac output, which is partially counteracted by vagal release with concomitant tachycardia. Late phase II is due to an increase peripheral resistance secondary to an increase in efferent sympathetic traffic to muscle (resistance and capacitance beds). In normal subjects within 4–5 seconds, the falling BP is arrested. In phase IV, preload (venous return) and cardiac output have normalized, while there is still significant peripheral vasoconstriction, causing the classical BP overshoot seen in phase IV with concomitant baroreflex response of transient bradycardia (Sandroni et al. 1991). In patients with adrenergic failure, there is a progressive decline in BP during phase II_e, without recovery of BP during phase II_l and absent blood pressure overshoot (phase IV). In some patients, presyncope or syncope may occur during the VM. A method of quantitation of adrenergic failure based on the severity of the changes of the VM has been recently published (Low 1993b).

Classification of autonomic neuropathies

The classification of autonomic neuropathy has been expanded in the last decade, in part due to the development of objective and non-invasive tests of autonomic function and also because of an improved understanding of basic mechanisms of autonomic failure and the development of new therapies. In some neuropathies, the brunt of the neuropathic process affects the parasympathetic and sympathetic system producing widespread autonomic dysfunction that dominates the clinical picture. Amyloidosis and idiopathic autonomic neuropathy (IAN) are typical examples. On the other hand, in many neuropathies that affect small fiber function or a combination of large and small fiber involvement, the degree of autonomic dysfunction may go unnoticed, unless sensitive tests are performed. These abnormalities may not dominate the overall clinical picture but may predispose to certain complications, i.e. cardiac arrhythmias in the setting of Guillain-Barré syndrome (GBS). This classification is modified from a previous review of autonomic neuropathies (Table 10.3) (Low and McLeod 1993).

The acute autonomic neuropathies

There is a spectrum of acute autonomic neuropathies. There is significant overlap among the disorders in this group. Some degree of autonomic

Table 10.3 *Classification of autonomic neuropathies*

I. Acute autonomic neuropathies

A. Idiopathic autonomic neuropathy (pandysautonomia)
B. Acute paraneoplastic autonomic neuropathy
C. Acute cholinergic neuropathy
D. Guillain-Barré syndrome
E. Botulism
F. Porphyria
G. Drug-induced acute autonomic neuropathies
  1. Cis-platinum
  2. Vincristine
  3. Vacor
  4. Amiodarone
  5. Perhexiline
H. Toxic acute autonomic neuropathies
  1. Heavy metals
  2. Organic solvents
  3. Acrylamide

II. Chronic peripheral autonomic neuropathies

A. Distal sympathetic neuropathies
  1. Distal small fiber neuropathy
  2. Peripheral neuropathies
B. Pure cholinergic neuropathies
  1. LEMS
  2. Chronic idiopathic anhidrosis
  3. Adie's syndrome
  4. Chagas' disease
C. Pure adrenergic neuropathy
D. Combined sympathetic and parasympathetic failure
  Autonomic dysfunction clinically *important*
  1. Amyloid
    a. Sporadic systemic amyloid neuropathy
    b. Multiple myeloma associated amyloid neuropathy
    c. Familial amyloidotic polyneuropathy (FAP)
  2. Diabetic autonomic neuropathy
  3. Chronic idiopathic autonomic neuropathy
  4. Chronic paraneoplastic autonomic including panautonomic neuropathy
  5. Sensory neuronopathy with autonomic failure
  6. Pure autonomic failure
  7. Familial dysautonomia (Riley–Day syndrome)
E. Combined sympathetic and parasympathetic failure
  Autonomic dysfunction usually clinically *unimportant*
  1. Hereditary neuropathies
    a. Hereditary motor and sensory neuropathies
    b. Friedreich's ataxia
    c. Hereditary sensory neuropathy
    d. Adrenomyeloneuropathy
    e. Fabry's disease
  2. Connective tissue disease
    a. Rheumatoid arthritis
    b. Systemic lupus erythematosus and mixed connective tissue diseases
  3. Infectious
    a. Leprosy
    b. AIDS
  4. Immune-mediated
  Chronic inflammatory demyelinating polyradiculoneuropathy (CIDP)
  5. Metabolic: uremia
  6. Nutritional deficiencies
    a. Subacute combined degeneration
    b. Alcoholic neuropathy
  7. Dysautonomia of old age
  8. Amyotrophic lateral sclerosis
F. Disorders of reduced orthostatic tolerance
  1. Postural orthostatic tachycardia syndrome (POTS)

Note:
LEMS: Lambert–Eaton myasthenic syndrome.

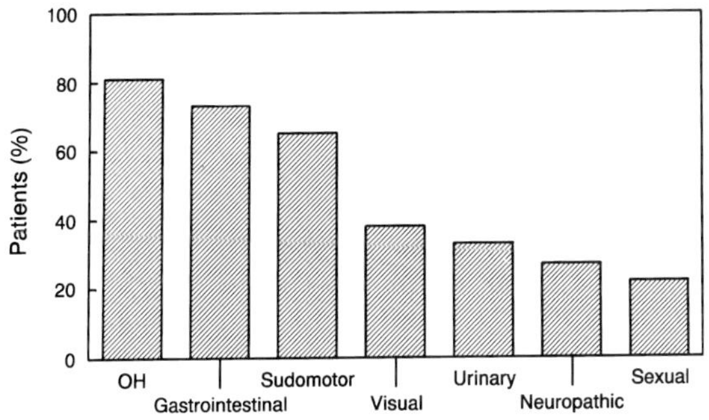

Figure 10.2 *Mean percentage of patients with symptoms of autonomic dysfunction by category and somatic neuropathic involvement at onset in 27 patients with IAN (actue pandysautonomia). OH: orthostatic symptoms. Reproduced with permission from Suarez GA, Fealey RD, Camilleri M, Low PA: Idiopathic autonomic neuropathy: clinical, neurophysiologic, and follow-up studies on 27 patients.* Neurology *44: 1675–1682, 1994.*

dysfunction occurs in patients with GBS. There is also some degree, albeit mild, of somatic involvement in the acute idiopathic autonomic neuropathy. Idiopathic autonomic neuropathy is at one end of the spectrum, with widespread and severe parasympathetic and sympathetic dysfunction. GBS is at the other end, as the brunt of the disorder affects the somatic nervous system.

There is also evidence suggesting that there are restricted forms of autonomic neuropathies with selective involvement of autonomic systems (Suarez et al. 1994). Some cases affect the cholinergic system, other cases are manifested as neurogenic motility disorders (Camilleri et al. 1993), and still other cases are postviral and manifest with excessive orthostatic tachycardia with restricted adrenergic and sudomotor deficits (POTS).

In some autonomic neuropathies such as IAN, there are several reasons to suspect that the pathogenesis is immune-mediated. The following is a description of individual autonomic neuropathies.

Idiopathic autonomic neuropathy (pandysautonomia)

The syndrome of acute IAN (acute pandysautonomia) is relatively uncommon but highly characteristic (Suarez et al. 1994), and the distinctive features are: (1) acute or subacute onset and monoplasic course, (2) frequent history of preceding infection, (3) spectrum of autonomic involvement ranging from panautonomic failure to restricted forms, and (4) relative or complete sparing of somatic fibers.

Characteristically, the disease occurs in a previously healthy subject with the acute or subacute onset of sympathetic and parasympathetic failure. Widespread sympathetic failure is manifested as OH and anhidrosis. Parasympathetic failure is manifested as severe constipation or diarrhea, dry eyes, dry mouth, and disturbance of bladder function. Gastrointestinal symptoms are common and include early satiety, bloating, nausea, vomiting, and weight loss. There may be an antecedent viral infection, such as herpes (Neville and Sladen 1984), infectious mononucleosis (Yahr and Frontera 1975), and Coxsackie virus (Pavesi et al. 1992). In a recent review of the Mayo experience based on 27 patients (Suarez et al. 1994). a presumed antecedent viral infection occurred in 16 of 27 patients (59%). A flu-like illness or upper respiratory infection was the most frequent antecedent infection, occurring in 11 patients.

Young et al. (1969, 1975) described the original case of acute pandysautonomia. This report was remarkable for the relative purity of autonomic involvement and the patient's complete recovery. Subsequent reports (Appenzeller and Kornfeld 1973; Yahr and Frontera 1975; Colan et al. 1980; Fagius et al. 1983; Low et al. 1983b; Neville and Sladen 1984; Taubner and Salonova 1984; Hart and Kanter 1990; Feldman et al. 1991; Stoll et al. 1991; Pavesi et al. 1992; Suarez et al. 1994) have usually been limited to single case reports and characterized by heterogeneity of onset, autonomic failure, and different degrees of recovery.

In our recent review of 27 patients with IAN, after follow-up for a mean duration of 32 months, 81% of the patients had an acute or subacute onset that was followed by a monophasic course. Orthostatic, gastrointestinal, and sudomotor were the most frequent type of symptoms occurring in more than 50% of patients (Figure 10.2). Orthostatic symptoms, such as dizziness, orthostatic lightheadedness, or syncope upon standing, occur in 21 patients (78%). Gastrointestinal symptoms were reported by 19 patients (70%) and consisted of various combinations of nausea, vomiting, diarrhea, and constipation with intestinal ileus. Seven patients (26%) had somatic sensory symptoms 'tingling' and 'numbness' in the distal extremities. Somatic neuropathic symptoms were typically associated with normal nerve conduction studies.

Neurological examination confirms the presence of OH, fixed HR, and tonic pupils. Muscle strength, deep tendon reflexes, and sensation are generally normal, although minor distal sensory deficits may occur. In our group of patients, neuropathic deficits were quantitated using the neuropathic disability score (NDS) (Schondorf and Low 1993). The mean total NDS score was 6.5. Seven patients had mild distal neuropathic sensory deficits.

Laboratory investigations

Nerve conduction studies are generally normal, although minor abnormalities may be occasionally seen. The ARS and TST are markedly abnormal. The TST shows widespread anhidrosis (Figure 10.3). The results of the QSART are diffusely abnormal indicating postganglionic sudomotor sympathetic failure. Orthostatic hypotension, as a sign of widespread adrenergic failure, is commonly present with a fixed HR and a reduction in phase II of the VM that exceeds 40 mm Hg. Salivation and tear secretion are reduced. Gastrointestinal motility is abnormal (Camilleri et al. 1993). We characterized and quantitated the autonomic deficits using the composite autonomic scoring scale (CASS; Figure 10.4) (Suarez et al. 1994). The spectrum of autonomic involvement varied from selective cholinergic failure to different degrees of parasympathetic and sympathetic dysfunction. Adrenergic and sudomotor systems were most frequently involved. At initial presentation, 63% of the patients had severe autonomic failure and 11 had moderate autonomic dysfunction. Supine plasma norepinephrine may be normal or reduced when compared to controls but fails to rise upon standing.

The sural nerve biopsy findings have been recently described (Suarez et al. 1994). The biopsy may be normal or may reveal different degrees of axonal degeneration and myelin remodeling. In our series of cases, small mononuclear cell infiltrates surrounding an epineurial vessel were found in one patient.

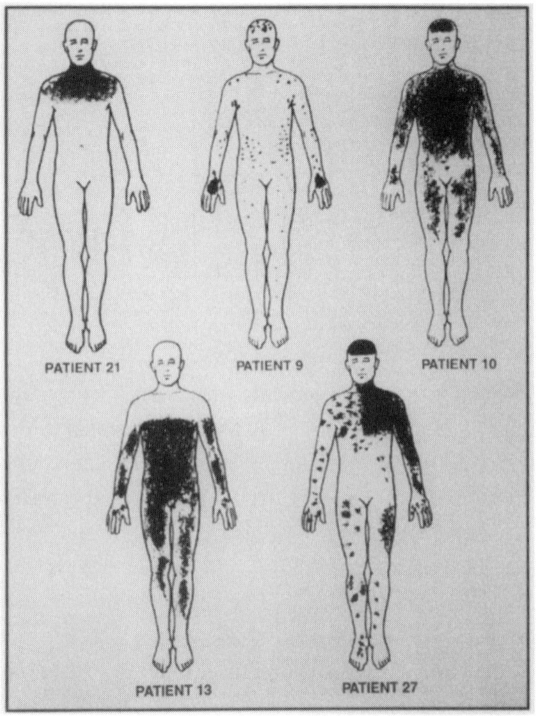

Figure 10.3 *Representative thermoregulatory sweating abnormalities in idiopathic autonomic neuropathy. Distributions of involvement were distal (patient 10, patient 13, extremities), global with tiny 'islands' of preserved sweating (patients 9 and 27), segmental (patient 13, upper body). Striking preserved segmental sweating occurred (patient 27). Sweating in black shaded areas. Reproduced with permission from Suarez GA, Fealey RD, Camilleri M, Low PA: Idiopathic autonomic neuropathy: clinical, neurophysiologic, and follow-up studies on 27 patients.* Neurology *44: 1675–1682, 1994.*

Differential diagnosis

The main differential diagnoses are paraneoplastic autonomic neuropathy, acute cholinergic neuropathy, and GBS. Idiopathic autonomic neuropathy may be indistinguishable from paraneoplastic autonomic neuropathy until a cancer is found, usually a small-cell carcinoma of the lung. In those patients, ANNA-1 (anti-Hu) antibodies may be positive. The

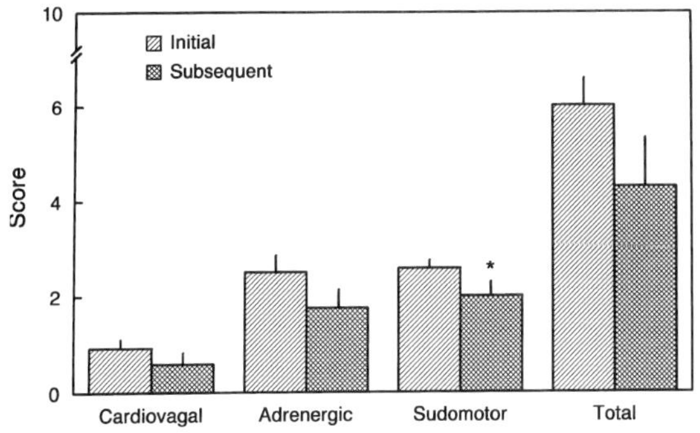

Figure 10.4 *Mean scores (±SEM) on the composite autonomic scoring scale at initial evaluation and subsequent follow-up of patients with autonomic deficits.* *p=0.05. *Reproduced with permission from Suarez GA, Fealey RD, Camilleri M, Low PA: Idiopathic autonomic neuropathy: clinical, neurophysiologic, and follow-up studies on 27 patients.* Neurology *44: 1675–1682, 1994.*

acute cholinergic neuropathies do not involve the adrenergic system and, therefore, do not present significant OH. In GBS, the brunt of the pathological process affects the somatic nervous system producing diffuse muscle weakness and areflexia that dominates the clinical picture, providing a clear distinction from IAN. The temporal profile separates the acute autonomic neuropathy from the chronic autonomic neuropathies. Occasionally, the clinician may be confronted with a case of IAN with a chronic course. In such cases, amyloidosis may be included in the differential diagnosis and is usually excluded by the appropriate pathological studies.

Mechanism

The underlying pathogenesis of IAN is likely immune-mediated. The evidence for this is based on the following: (1) an acute or subacute onset and antecedent presumed viral infection, (2) relative selectivity of autonomic fiber, (3) monophasic course, (4) absence of an associated disease, and (5) inflammatory infiltrates on sural nerve biopsies.

Course and prognosis

The course of IAN is variable. From our series of patients, a distinct pattern emerged. The majority of patients had a monophasic course with a progressive phase followed by a plateau and remission, or a prolonged stable deficit without remission and no recurrences. We used the CASS to monitor the degree of recovery and the progression of the disease. Although there was a trend toward recovery of function after 32 months, it was not complete (Figure 10.4) at follow-up. Mean CASS had improved by 28%, but only six patients (22%) had marked improvement of autonomic deficits.

Management

As there is suggestive evidence of an immune-mediated process, it may be reasonable to consider plasma exchange, intravenous gamma globulin or prednisone as an early therapeutic intervention in patients with progressive disability. Some patients seem to show improvement on these treatments, although there is no conclusive evidence of efficacy of these approaches. If immune therapy is undertaken, it is important to quantitate neurological and autonomic status before and after treatment to document whether these treatments are efficacious. Prednisone may be used at a dosage of 60 mg daily for 4 weeks, then taper the dosage over the following weeks. Supportive treatment for the management of OH and bowel and bladder symptoms are also important. Our approach for the management of orthostatic symptoms is the combination of non-pharmacological and pharmacological approaches. This subject has been recently reviewed (Low 1993c). Briefly, patients should expand their plasma volume by hydration and increasing salt intake. The patients should drink a minimum of five glasses of fluid per day and should take 10–20 g of salt in the diet. Patients should also try sleeping with the head of the bed elevated 11–22 cm, to minimize nocturia and salt depletion. Pharmacological treatment is an important part of the overall therapeutic regimen. The first-line therapeutic agents are listed in Table 10.4.

Postural orthostatic tachycardia syndrome

POTS refers to a syndrome characterized by orthostatic tachycardia associated with lightheadedness,

Table 10.4 *First-line treatment of orthostatic hypotension*

High-salt diet (10–12 g/day)
Large-volume fluid intake (≥600 ml/day)
Fludrocortisone 0.1–0.6 mg/day
Ibuprofen (400 mg three times daily)
Phenylpropanolamine (25 mg three times daily)

palpitations, tremulousness, anxiety, and nausea. POTS is another manifestation of a restricted autonomic neuropathy (Schondorf and Low 1993). The disorder typically occurs in young women, between the ages of 20 and 50 years (Hoeldtke and Davis 1991; Schondorf and Low 1993). Patients may be supersensitive to β-agonists, such as isoproterenol. Autonomic deficits are present in approximately two-thirds of patients. These patients have distal sudomotor failure on the QSART and TST. The HR_{DB} is usually normal but often excessively large. Beat-to-beat BP to the VM are abnormal with an exaggerated phase II_e and reduced or absent phase II_l. Phase IV may be normal or may be excessively large. The HR to tilt is abnormal with an excessive tachycardia from 120 to 170 beats/minute on tilt-up. Patients with excessive venous pooling have a reduction in pulse pressure. Some patients have a hypertensive response. The management of POTS has been recently reviewed (Low et al. 1995).

Acute cholinergic neuropathy

Patients with a restricted cholinergic neuropathy have alacrima, blurred vision, xerostomia, anhidrosis, constipation, and urinary retention but do not have orthostatic hypotension. Gastrointestinal symptoms are quite common, presenting with abdominal pain and ileus during the early stages, followed by gastroparesis and constipation during the chronic phase. In some patients, gastrointestinal motility abnormalities may dominate the clinical picture. Acute cholinergic neuropathy is likely a restricted form of the idiopathic autonomic neuropathy, with abnormalities limited to the postganglionic cholinergic neuron.

Guillain-Barré syndrome (acute inflammatory demyelinating polyradiculoneuropathy)

Autonomic involvement is not uncommon in GBS but is not a requirement for diagnosis. The major diagnostic features are the acute onset of an ascending, predominantly motor, polyradiculoneuropathy. Patients may have tachycardia, associated with wide fluctuations in BP with alternating hypertension and hypotension (Low and McLeod 1993). Bladder and bowel dysfunction may be present but usually does not dominate the overall clinical picture (Kogan et al. 1981; Wheeler et al. 1984; Truax 1984). Life-threatening dysautonomia may occur in some patients with GBS. It usually occurs in the acute phase of the disease and tends to correlate with the severity of somatic involvement. It may be more frequent in patients with respiratory failure, but this association is not always present (Lichtenfeld 1971; Tuck and McLeod 1981). Sinus tachycardia and orthostatic hypotension alternating with hypertensive crisis, may be seen. Less frequent autonomic symptoms include constipation, gastroparesis, sexual impairment, and rectal incontinence.

Tests of autonomic function are often abnormal and include impaired cardiovagal (Persson and Solders 1983), sudomotor (Tuck and McLeod 1981), vasomotor (Appenzeller and Marshall 1963; Tuck and McLeod 1981), and adrenergic (Harati and Low 1990; Low and McLeod 1993) function. Sinus tachycardia, bradyarrhythmias, heart block, and even asystole have been described. Sinus arrest may occur after strong vagal stimulation, i.e. tracheal suction (Truax 1984).

The management of patients with GBS and autonomic instability requires close supervision in the intensive care unit (ICU) with monitoring of HR and BP (Ropper 1993). In patients with transient paroxysmal hypertension alternating with hypotension, the use of antihypertensive medication is not recommended because the patient may be supersensitive to these agents. If the patient develops sustained hypertension, then the use of a combined α- and β-adrenergic blocker has been suggested. In addition to careful monitoring of HR and BP in the ICU setting, the management and prevention of autonomic failure is of utmost importance. It is important to maintain an adequate blood volume as the denervated vascular bed may be extremely sensitive to volume depletion. To prevent deconditioning, the patient should be mobilized as soon as possible to avoid the orthostatic intolerance of prolonged bed rest.

Botulism

The main features are the acute development of cholinergic neuropathy, ptosis, blurred vision, extra-ocular muscle weakness and bulbar weakness, which may progress to generalized neuromuscular paralysis. The typical syndrome begins 12–36 hours after the ingestion of contaminated foods. Autonomic symptoms are those of a severe cholinergic neuropathy, with anhidrosis, dry eyes and mouth, paralytic ileus, and urinary retention (Nix et al. 1985). Orthostatic hypotension is not common but has been reported (Vita et al. 1987). The type of botulinum toxin may relate to the frequency, severity, and duration of autonomic failure. Botulism type B appears to be more frequently associated with cholinergic neuropathy.

Laboratory studies have shown abnormal cardiovagal tests and orthostatic hypotension (Vita et al. 1987). Esophageal manometric studies are abnormal (Nix et al. 1985). Electrophysiological studies showed reduced compound muscle action potential amplitude with facilitation with rapid repetitive stimulation. Single fiber electromyography (EMG) may show a neuromuscular transmission defect with blocking and increased jitter. Autonomic deficits improve before the resolution of the neuromuscular blockade. Adrenergic function with orthostatic hypotension recovers before parasympathetic function.

Botulism is a clinical diagnosis, confirmed by the identification of the toxin in the food or the patient's serum (Pickett 1988). The treatment is mainly supportive with ventilatory assistance in patients with respiratory failure. Antitoxins are used, but their efficacy is unknown. Guanidine has been used in some cases with mixed results (Cherington and Ryan 1970; Faich et al. 1971; Jenzer et al. 1975).

Porphyria

The hepatic porphyrias are autosomal-dominant disorders of the heme biosynthesis. The main clinical features of the group of hepatic porphyrias are peripheral neuropathy with autonomic involvement, skin symptoms, and central nervous system manifestations. Acute or subacute onset of a predominantly peripheral motor neuropathy dominates the clinical picture in acute intermittent porphyria. Autonomic dysfunction is frequent in acute intermittent porphyria, and autonomic hyperactivity predominates over autonomic failure. Dysautonomia may also occur in variegate porphyria. Persistent tachycardia may be an early feature of an attack and may also precede the onset of somatic neuropathy. Other clinical features of autonomic neuropathy include abdominal pain, nausea and vomiting, severe constipation, diarrhea, bladder distension, and sweating abnormalities (hyper- and hypohidrosis). Painless vomiting may occur, associated with hypertension and tachycardia. Sudden death during an acute porphyric attack has been attributed to cardiac arrhythmias.

Autonomic studies have shown abnormal sympathetic and parasympathetic function (Stewart and Hensley 1981; Fagius 1993). Pathologic studies have shown involvement of the vagus nerve and sympathetic ganglia. Prevention of the ingestion of porphyrogenic drugs is critical. The therapy of the acute attack consists of a combination of supportive measures, such as hydration, nutrition, pain control, and intravenous administration of heme (Windebank and Bonkovsky 1993).

Autonomic neuropathies associated with drugs, industrial agents, and heavy metals

Cis-*platinum*

Cis-platinum is an antineoplastic drug used frequently for the treatment of lung, gynecological, and other malignancies. Its side-effects include peripheral neuropathy, ototoxicity, and retrobulbar neuritis. Neuropathy may be present in patients who have received a cumulative dose of 200–800 mg m^{-2}, usually corresponding to four courses of therapy (Rosenfeld and Broder 1984). Autonomic symptoms with orthostatic hypotension and secretomotor failure have been reported in patients receiving *cis*-platinum (Rosenfeld and Broder 1984).

Vincristine

Vincristine is a cytotoxic agent used in the treatment of lymphoma, leukemia, and other malignancies. The mechanism of action of vincristine is not completely known but appears to disrupt the microtubules and interferes with axonal transport. It is neurotoxic, and peripheral neuropathy is a limiting factor in its use. Its neurotoxicity is dose related and cumulative with repeated dosing. Vincristine usually needs to be stopped after a cumulative dose of 30–50 mg (Legha 1986). Orthostatic hypotension, constipation, abdominal pain, ileus and urinary retention have been reported in association with vincristine (Legha 1986; Hancock and Naysmith 1975). Abnormal cardiovascular responses have been described (Hancock and Naysmith 1975).

Amiodarone

Amiodarone is an antiarrhythmic agent that causes a sensory motor peripheral neuropathy in approximately 10% of the patients (Martinez-Arizala et al. 1983; Santoro et al. 1992). Pathological studies of sural nerves have shown characteristic lamellated lysosomal inclusions (Pellissier et al. 1984; Jacobs and Costa-Jussà 1985). Autonomic failure with orthostatic hypotension has been reported (Manolis et al. 1987). When the drug is discontinued, slow improvement of the neuropathy occurs.

Perhexiline maleate

Perhexilene maleate is used for the treatment of angina pectoris (Fraser et al. 1977). Fraser et al. (1977) reported three patients who developed an autonomic neuropathy characterized by orthostatic hypotension and abnormal Valsalva ratio following perhexiline maleate treatment.

Vacor

Vacor is a rodenticide that antagonizes nicotinamide metabolism. Ingestion is usually accidental or deliberate (suicidal or homicidal). It causes acute hypoglycemic ketoacidosis associated with a somatic and autonomic neuropathy. Autonomic symptoms include postural hypotension and gastrointestinal dysfunction (Johnson et al. 1980; LeWitt 1980). Nicotinamide may be beneficial if administered during the early stages of intoxication (Johnson et al. 1980).

Toxic autonomic neuropathies

Heavy metals

Autonomic symptoms may be present to a certain extent in the different intoxications, but no systematic evaluation of autonomic function in heavy metal intoxication has been reported. In thallium poisoning, tachycardia and hypertension may be present, usually associated with peripheral neuropathy (Bank et al. 1972). In arsenic poisoning, distal hyper- or hypohidrosis have been described (LeQuesne and McLeod 1977). Inorganic mercury poisoning occurs mainly in children, and its clinical manifestations include tachycardia, hypertension, acrodynia, and excessive sweating (Warkany and Hubbard 1948).

Organic solvents

Prolonged occupational exposure (mean of 16 years) to a variety of organic solvents including aliphatic, aromatic, and other hydrocarbons has been associated with abnormalities of cardiovascular autonomic function (HR_{DB}) (Matikainen and Juntunen 1985). Peripheral neuropathy was also present in those patients.

Intentional inhalation of *n*-hexane and methyl-*n*-butyl-ketone may result in a rapidly progressive polyneuropathy associated with distal sudomotor failure, vasomotor instability, postural hypotension, and erectile failure.

Acrylamide

The soluble monomeric form of acrylamide is toxic and occurs mainly in the industrial setting. It causes a sensory neuropathy with distal hyperhidrosis and signs of exfoliative dermatitis. In experimental studies, there is degeneration of sympathetic and parasympathetic fibers.

Distal small fiber neuropathy

Clinical features

Distal small fiber neuropathy (DSFN) is characterized by distal dysesthesias and postganglionic sympathetic dysfunction occurring in the absence of significant somatic neuropathy. Symptoms include superficial burning and a deeper aching pain. The pain is most common in the sole and toe-pads with latter involvement of the dorsum. Troublesome allodynia, where light touch and firm pressure, as with weight bearing, causes pain, is common. Sympathetic dysfunction is manifest as vasomotor changes, with pallor, sometimes alternating with rubor (with accentuation of pain – erythromelalgia), cyanosis and mottling, are common. Sudomotor dysfunction, manifest as excessive sweating or as anhidrosis is also common.

Distal small fiber neuropathy may be a manifestation of neuropathies such as diabetes, inherited, immune-mediated, or related to AIDS. The majority of cases of distal small fiber neuropathy are idiopathic and run a benign course. The neurologic examination in idiopathic DSFN is usually unremarkable. Strength is normal. Sensation may be mildly impaired, especially for sharp-dull discrimination and temperature perception, or it is normal. Reflexes are usually normal. EMG and nerve conduction studies are normal or unremarkable. The most sensitive diagnostic test is QSART or TST showing distal anhidrosis (Stewart et al. 1992).

Investigations

The majority of patients with distal small fiber neuropathy will have abnormalities of QSART in the distal lower extremities (Stewart et al. 1992). The diagnostic yield is enhanced if multiple recording sites are used. QSART shows normal sweat volume in the forearm and anhidrosis in the lower extremities, maximal distally. Computer-assisted sensory examination for small fiber function may be helpful (Jamal et al. 1987). Jamal found abnormalities in sensory testing in 25 of 25 patients; however, the actual sensitivity is uncertain as these patients were selected into the study on the basis of impaired sensory examinations.

Pure cholinergic neuropathies

Chronic idiopathic anhidrosis

Clinical features

The core features are acquired widespread anhidrosis in the absence or generalized adrenergic and cardiovagal failure. These patients have total or subtotal anhidrosis and are heat intolerant, becoming hot, flushed, dizzy, dyspneic, and weak, when the ambient temperature is high or when they exercise. Distal vasomotor changes may be present, but orthostatic hypotension, or other evidence of generalized adrenergic failure, or symptomatic somatic neuropathy, are absent. Pupillary abnormalities may be present. It is important to recognize, as it is relatively common and often confused with the more malignant autonomic disorders, such as multiple system atrophy, pure autonomic failure, and the autonomic neuropathies. Chronic idiopathic anhidrosis probably comprises a heterogenous group of disorders with restricted autonomic failure. Segmental anhidrosis with Adies pupil (Ross syndrome) is well recognized (Ross 1958) and is often one type of chronic idiopathic anhidrosis, although rare cases of Ross syndrome are associated with more widespread autonomic failure. The prognosis appears to be distinctly better than the progressive autonomic disorders. The sweating deficit may remain stable, progress, or, infrequently, regress. The great majority of patients do not subsequently develop adrenergic failure.

Investigations

These patients have widespread anhidrosis on thermoregulatory sweat test. The majority of cases are associated with postganglionic impairment (Low et al. 1986). Orthostatic hypotension is absent, and cardiovascular heart rate tests, supine and standing plasma norepinephrine, and beat-to-beat BP responses to tilt and the Valsalva maneuver show no evidence of autonomic failure.

Treatment

Treatment is focused on the avoidance of heat stress. These patients should live in an air-conditioned environment. Some patients seem to have an altered comfort zone, setting their home thermostats to relatively lower temperatures (often in the low 60s). They should avoid vigorous exercise in a hot environment as they are more prone to heat injury, including heat exhaustion and heat stroke.

Adie's syndrome

The typical tonic pupil is a large pupil that does not react to direct light. It is due to a postganglionic parasympathetic lesion. Because of denervation supersensitivity, it pupilloconstricts to subthreshold concentrations of parasympathomimetic agents, such as pilocarpine 0.125% or methacholine 2.5%, whereas the normal pupil would be unaffected. The pupillary abnormality may be unilateral or bilateral and may occur in isolation or in association with more widespread neurological or autonomical abnormalities. Adie's syndrome refers to the combination of a tonic pupil with areflexia (Markus 1906; Weber 1933; Johnson and Spalding 1974). Widespread sympathetic failure is uncommon but is well documented (Johnson and Spalding 1974). Another combination is tonic pupil and segmental anhidrosis, sometimes referred to as Ross syndrome (Ross 1958). This syndrome is important to recognize as the widespread anhidrosis does not indicate a progressive autonomic disorder (Low et al. 1986). Yet another combination is tonic pupil(s) with chronic inflammatory demyelinating polyradiculoneuropathy (CIDP). Another combination is tonic pupil(s) with a sensory neuronopathy as part of Sjögren's syndrome. These patients have widespread autonomic failure with anhidrosis, orthostatic hypotension, impairment of cardiovagal function and keratoconjunctivitis sicca and xerostomia (Griffin et al. 1990). Adie's pupil may also occur as part of the autonomic paraneoplastic neuropathy. The site of the lesion is likely in the ciliary ganglion and degenerative changes have been described in autopsy tissue (Harriman and Garland 1968).

Chagas' disease

Chagas' disease is caused by *Trypanosoma cruzi*, an intracellular protozoan. *T. cruzi* is found in the Americas from the southern USA to southern Argentina. Acute Chagas' disease is rare in the USA and chronic Chagas', which develops years to decades after primary infection, is seen in increasing numbers in South American immigrants, especially from Central America. The most commonly affected organs are the heart, resulting in biventricular cardiomegaly and conduction defects, and the gastrointestinal tract (Koberle 1968). Autonomic syndromes are manifest as a chronic cholinergic neuropathy. The dysautonomia has been briefly reviewed (Johnson and Spalding 1974; Harati and Low 1990). Patients develop megaduodenum and megacolon and complain of increasing dysphagia and constipation. Other parts of the gastrointestinal and urinary tracts, gall bladder, and salivary glands may be affected (Ferreira-Santos 1961; Koberle 1963).

Autonomic function tests may be abnormal. There may be orthostatic hypotension, baroreflex abnormalities, impaired heart rate response to standing and Valsalva maneuver (Amorim et al. 1968, 1982; Manco et al. 1969; Gallo et al. 1975; Palmero et al. 1981). Plasma norepinephrine may be reduced (Iosa et al. 1989). Cardiac nerves undergo degeneration (Amorim et al. 1968; Manco et al. 1969). Multifocal inflammatory lesions associated with demyelination are present in the peripheral nervous system in humans and in the murine experimental model (Said et al. 1985). There is evidence that the destruction of the peripheral and sympathetic nervous systems has an autoimmune basis, T lymphocytes and possibly humoral factors being responsible for an attack on neural elements. Antigenic determinants may be shared by the parasite and host. A recent placebo-controlled clinical trial of mixed gangliosides has demonstrated improved BP control with treatment possibly due to an indirect neurotropic effect (Iosa et al. 1991). The disease may be transmitted in endemic areas in South America by the bite of a reduviid bug. Transmission may also occur via blood transfusions, a more likely mode of infection within the USA. The diagnosis of chronic Chagas' disease is made by detecting antibodies to *T. cruzi* using complement fixation, immunofluorescence or ELISA assay. False positive test may occur with leishmaniasis. When one test is positive, the test is usually confirmed by two additional tests (Kirchoff 1991).

Amyloid neuropathy

Amyloid neuropathies could be subdivided into sporadic primary amyloid and familial amyloid polyneuropathy (FAP). Amyloid is a fibrillar protein with a β-pleated sheet configuration that has a typical apple-green birefringence when viewed under the polarizing microscope. Immunohistochemical tests permit a classification based on the type of amyloid. The AL type is associated with primary amyloidosis. The AF type with transthyretin (prealbumin) as the main protein component is associated with inherited amyloidosis.

Sporadic primary amyloid neuropathy (Kyle and Dyck 1993)

A disabling and relentlessly progressive polyneuropathy is found in patients with primary amyloidosis. It has a typical clinical picture characterized by: (1) systemic features, (2) cardiovascular involvement, (3) renal disease, and (4) peripheral neuropathy with prominent autonomic failure.

It tends to affect middle-aged men, and initial neuropathic symptoms are 'numbness' and 'loss of pain' affecting the distal extremities. There is a predominant loss of unmyelinated and small myelinated fibers in the peripheral nerve, but large fiber involvement is also generally present. Autonomic symptoms are prominent and dominate the clinical picture. Peripheral vasomotor and sudomotor control are markedly impaired. Postural hypotension with syncope is an early symptom. The pattern of anhidrosis suggests a preganglionic sympathetic component, in addition to a postganglionic sympathetic failure. Gastrointestinal symptoms with alternating constipation and diarrhea are common. The deposition of amyloid fibrils in the esophagus causes dysphagia. Impotence is common in men. Weight loss and macroglossia are helpful clinical clues to the diagnosis. Renal insufficiency with proteinuria and cardiac conduction abnormalities and ventricular arrhythmias are the leading causes of death (Olofsson et al. 1983).

Electrophysiological studies show evidence of an axonal polyneuropathy. Autonomic tests show evidence of severe adrenergic, sudomotor, and cardiovagal failure. Thermoregulatory sweat test and QSART show also prominent anhidrosis.

The diagnosis is confirmed by the presence of amyloid deposits in different tissues. Sural nerve, subcutaneous fat aspirate, and rectal biopsies are the tissues most frequently obtained. Primary amyloid neuropathy carries an ominous prognosis. In one large series of 229 patients with primary systemic amyloidosis (Kyle and Greipp 1983), median survival from the time of diagnosis of peripheral neuropathy and orthostatic hypotension was 60 and 9.5 months, respectively. Poor prognostic indices were weight loss, cardiac failure, and light chains in the urine.

Familial amyloid polyneuropathy (FAP)

All forms of FAP are dominantly inherited. There are several clinical phenotypes, but the clinical features and course have been best studied for familial autonomic polyneuropathy type I. They have in common peripheral neuropathy with prominent autonomic symptoms. They differ in age of onset, genetic abnormality, clinical phenotype, and other tissue involvement. The first to be described was the Portuguese variety originally recognized by Andrade in 1952. The amyloid is derived from abnormal transthyretin (TTR), formally known as prealbumin. The first mutation reported was a methionine for valine substitution at position 30 in the molecule. Since then, other point mutations of the TTR gene have been described.

FAP type I

FAP type I was originally described by Andrade in northern Portugal. It is the most common form of FAP and has also been described elsewhere. Neuropathic symptoms begin in the third or fourth decade but may occur later in life. The initial symptoms are pain and paresthesias affecting the feet and legs first and later in the hands. This is often associated with pain and temperature sensory loss, producing a syndrome masquerading lumbosacral syringomyelia. Other sensory modalities are affected later. Autonomic symptoms are present since the onset and sometimes dominate the entire clinical picture. These include postural hypotension, anhidrosis, impotence, difficulty in voiding urinary and urinary retention, and constipation alternating with diarrhea. Pupillary abnormalities with escalloped margins may be present.

The loss of pain and temperature sensation may lead to the occurrence of inadvertent skin burns and persistent ulcers in the feet. Neuropathic joint degeneration also occurs. Muscle weakness and areflexia appear as the disease advances. The amyloid deposits are found in peripheral nerve, within sensory and autonomic ganglia and other organs such as the kidneys and heart. The disease runs a progressive course, with renal failure and cardiac complications as the leading cause of death.

The mechanism of the neuropathy is unknown. Electrophysiological studies show an axonal distal sensory polyneuropathy with significant autonomic failure.

Sural nerve biopsies have shown reduction in small myelinated and non-myelinated fibers with widespread amyloid deposits throughout. Immunochistochemical studies of the amyloid deposits are helpful in providing evidence for hereditary amyloidosis. Inherited amyloidosis specifically reacts with antiserum against TTR.

Treatment is mainly supportive and symptomatic. Preliminary reports of liver transplantation in a small number of cases are encouraging, but no definitive results are available.

FAP type II (Rukavina or Indiana form)

In FAP II, symptoms begin in early mid-life with carpal tunnel syndrome, related to amyloid deposition in the flexor retinaculum. A more generalized predominantly sensory and autonomic neuropathy occurs later, but the outlook is not as severe as FAP I. Amyloid infiltration of the vitreous resulting in vitreous opacities is common. Different point mutations at position 58 and 84 in the TTR gene have been demonstrated. Asymptomatic carriers could be identified using recombinant DNA techniques.

Treatment is mainly symptomatic. Treatment of carpal tunnel syndrome by surgical decompression usually produces relief of symptoms.

FAP type III (van Allen or Iowa form)

In FAP III, the clinical features resemble those of type I FAP, but autonomic involvement is not as conspicuous. There is an increased incidence of duodenal ulcers, as well as early renal involvement. The amyloid fibrils consist of a variant of apolipoprotein A1.

FAP type IV

FAP IV is characterized by ocular manifestations. The presence of lattice corneal dystrophy, corneal opacities due to amyloid infiltration, is a cardinal clinical feature. A slowly progressive facial palsy with facial skin changes may occur later. A mild generalized somatic neuropathy without major autonomic features supervenes later.

Diabetic autonomic neuropathy

Diabetic autonomic neuropathy has recently been reviewed in detail (Suarez and Low 1994).

References

Amorim, D.S., Godoy, R.A., Manco, J.C., Tanaka, A., and Gallo Jr, L. (1968). Effects of acute elevation in blood pressure and of atropine on heart rate in Chagas' disease. A preliminary report. *Circulation* **38**: 289–294.

Amorim, D.S., Manco, J.C., Gallo Jr, L., and Marin-Neto, J.A. (1982). Chagas heart disease as an experimental model for studies of cardiac autonomic function in man. *Mayo Clin. Proc.* **57** (suppl.): 46–60.

Appenzeller, O. and Kornfeld, M. (1973). Acute pandysautonomia. Clinical and morphologic study. *Arch. Neurol.* **29**: 334–339.

Appenzeller, O. and Marshall, J. (1963). Vasomotor disturbance in Landry-Guillain-Barré syndrome. *Arch. Neurol.* **9**: 368–372.

Bank, W.J., Pleasure, D.E., Suzuki, K., Nigro, M., and Katz, R. (1972). Thallium poisoning. *Arch. Neurol.* **26**: 456–464.

Benarroch, E.E., Opfer-Gehrking, T.L., and Low, P.A. (1991). Use of the photoplethysmographic technique to analyse the Valsalva maneuver in normal man. *Muscle Nerve* **14**: 1165–1172.

Camilleri, M., Balm, R.K., and Low, P.A. (1993). Autonomic dysfunction in patients with chronic intestinal pseudo-obstruction. *Clin. Auton. Res.* **3**: 95–100.

Cherington, M. and Ryan, D.W. (1970). Treatment of botulism and guanidine. *N. Engl. J. Med.* **282**: 195–197.

Colan, R.V., Snead III, O.C., Oh, S.J., and Kashlan, M.B. (1980). Acute autonomic and sensory neuropathy. *Ann. Neurol.* **8**: 441–444.

Ewing, D.J. (1993). Noninvasive evaluation of heart rate: the time domain. In *Clinical Autonomic Disorders: Evaluation and Management*, ed. P.A. Low, pp. 297–314. Boston: Little, Brown and Company.

Fagius, J., Westerberg, C.E., and Olsson, Y. (1983). Acute pandysautonomia and severe sensory deficit with poor recovery. A clinical, neurophysiological and pathological case study. *J. Neurol. Neurosurg. Psychiatry* **46**: 725–733.

Fagius, J. (1993). Syndromes of autonomic overactivity: clinical presentation, assessment, and management. In *Clinical Autonomic Disorders: Evaluation and Management*, ed. P.A. Low, pp. 197–208. Boston: Little, Brown and Company.

Faich, G.A., Graebner, R.W., and Sato, S. (1971). Failure of guanidine therapy in botulism A. *N. Engl. J. Med.* **285**: 773–776.

Fealey, R.D. (1993). The thermoregulatory sweat test. In *Clinical Autonomic Disorders: Evaluation and Management*, ed. P.A. Low, pp. 217–229. Boston: Little, Brown and Company.

Fealey, R.D., Low, P.A., and Thomas, J.E. (1989). Thermoregulatory sweating abnormalities in diabetes mellitus. *Mayo Clin. Proc.* **64**: 617–628.

Feldman, E.L., Bromberg, M.B., Blaivas, M., and Junck, L. (1991). Acute pandysautonomic neuropathy. *Neurology* **41**: 746–748.

Ferreira-Santos, R. (1961). Megacolon and megarectum in Chagas' disease. *Proc. R. Soc. Med.* **54**: 1047–1053.

Fraser, D.M., Campbell, I.W., and Miller, H.C. (1977). Peripheral and autonomic neuropathy after treatment with perhexiline maleate. *Br. Med. J.* **2**: 675–676.

Gallo Jr, L., Marin-Neto, J.A., Manco, J.C., Rassi, A., and Amorim, D.S. (1975). Abnormal heart rate responses during exercise in patients with Chagas disease. *Cardiology* **60**: 147–162.

Griffin, J.W., Cornblath, D.R., Alexander, E., Campbell, J., Low, P.A., Bird, S., and Feldman, E.L. (1990). Ataxic sensory neuropathy and dorsal root ganglionitis associated with Sjögren's syndrome. *Ann. Neurol.* **27**: 304–315.

Hancock, B.W. and Naysmith, A. (1975). Vincristine-induced autonomic neuropathy. *Br. Med. J.* **3**: 207.

Harati, Y. and Low, P.A. (1990). Autonomic peripheral neuropathies: diagnosis and clinical presentation. In *Current Neurology*, ed S.H. Appel, pp. 105–176. Yearbook Medical Publishers.

Harriman, D.G.F. and Garland, H.G. (1968). The pathology of Adie's syndrome. *Brain* **91**: 401–418.

Hart, R.G. and Kanter, M.C. (1990). Acute autonomic neuropathy. Two cases and a clinical review. *Arch. Intern. Med.* **150**: 2373–2376.

Hoeldtke, R.D. and Davis, K.M. (1991). The orthostatic tachycardia syndrome: evaluation of autonomic function and treatment with octreotide and ergot alkaloids. *J. Clin. Endocrinol. Metab.* **73**: 132–139.

Imholtz, B.P.M., van Montfans, G.A., Settels, J.J., van der Hoeven, G.M.A., Karemaker, J.M. and Wieling, W. (1988). Continuous noninvasive blood pressure monitoring: reliability of Finapres device during Valsalva manoeuvre. *Cardiovasc. Res.* **22**: 390–397.

Iosa, D., DeQuattro, V., Lee, D.D., Elkayam, U., and Palmero, H. (1989). Plasma norepinephrine in Chagas cardioneuromyopathy: a marker of progressive dysautonomia. *Am. Heart J.* **117**: 882–887.

Iosa, D., Massari, D.C., and Dorsey, F.C. (1991). Chagas' cardioneuropathy: effect of ganglioside treatment in chronic dysautonomic patients – a randomized double-blind parallel placebo-controlled study. *Am. Heart J.* **122**: 775–785.

Jacobs, J.M. and Costa-Jussa, F.R. (1985). The pathology of amiodarone neurotoxicity. II. Peripheral neuropathy in man. *Brain* **108**: 753–769.

Jamal, G.A., Hansen, S., Weir, A.I. and Ballantyne, J.P. (1987). The neurophysiologic investigation of small fiber neuropathies. *Muscle Nerve* **10**: 537–545.

Jenzer, G., Mumenthaler, M., Ludin, H.P., and Robert, F. (1975). Autonomic dysfunction in botulism B: a clinical report. *Neurology* **25**: 150–153.

Johnson, D., Kubic, P., and Levitt, C. (1980). Accidental ingestion of Vacor rodenticide: the systems and sequelae in a 25-month-old child. *Am. J. Dis. Child.* **134**: 161–164.

Johnson, R.H. and Spalding, J.M.K. (1974). *Disorders of the Autonomic Nervous System.* Philadelphia: F.A. Davis Company.

Kennedy, W.R. and Navarro, X. (1993). Evaluation of sudomotor function by sweat imprint methods. In *Clinical Autonomic Disorders: Evaluation and Management*, ed. P.A. Low, pp. 253–261. Boston: Little, Brown and Company.

Kennedy, W.R. and Sakuta, M. (1984). Collateral reinnervation of sweat glands. *Ann. Neurol.* **15**: 73–78.

Kirchoff, L.V. (1991). Trypanosomiasis. In *Harrison's Principles of Internal Medicine*, ed. J. Wilson et al., New York: McGraw Hill.

Koberle, F. (1963). Enteromegaly and cardiomegaly in Chagas' disease. *Gut* **4**: 399–405.

Koberle, F. (1968). Chagas disease and Chagas syndromes. *Adv. Parasitol.* **6**: 63–116.

Kogan, B.A., Solomon, M.H., and Diokno, A.C. (1981). Urinary retention secondary to Landry-Guillain-Barré syndrome. *J. Urol.* **126**: 643–644.

Korner, P.I., Tonkin, A.M., and Uther, J.B. (1976). Reflex and mechanical circulatory effects of graded Valsalva maneuvers in normal man. *J. Appl. Physiol.* **40**: 434–440.

Kyle, R.A. and Dyck, P.J. (1993). Amyloidosis and neuropathy. In *Peripheral Neuropathy*, 3rd edn, ed. P.J. Dyck, P.K. Thomas, J.W. Griffin, P.A. Low and J.F. Poduslo, pp. 1294–1309. Philadelphia: W.B. Saunders.

Kyle, R.A. and Greipp, P.R. (1983). Amyloidosis: clinical and laboratory features in 229 cases. *Mayo Clin. Proc.* **58**: 665–683.

Legha, S.S. (1986). Vincristine neurotoxicity. Pathophysiology and management. *Med. Toxicol.* **1**: 421–427.

LeQuesne, P.M. and McLeod, J.G. (1977). Peripheral neuropathy following a single exposure to arsenic. *J. Neurol. Sci.* **32**: 437–451.

LeWitt, P.A. (1980). Neurotoxicity of the rat poison Vacor. A clinical study of 12 cases. *N. Engl. J. Med.* **302**: 73–77.

Lichtenfeld, P. (1971). Autonomic dysfunction in the Guillain-Barré syndrome. *Am. J. Med.* **50**: 772–780.

Low, P.A., Caskey, P.E., Tuck, R.R., Fealey, R.D., and Dyck, P.J. (1983a). Quantitative sudomotor axon reflex test in normal and neuropathic subjects. *Ann. Neurol.* **14**: 573–580.

Low, P.A., Dyck, P.J., Lambert, E.H., Brimijoin, W.S., Trautmann, J.C., Malagelada, J.R., Fealey, R.D., and Barrett, D.M. (1983b). Acute panautonomic neuropathy. *Ann. Neurol.* **13**: 412–417.

Low, P.A., Zimmerman, B.R., and Dyck, P.J. (1986). Comparison of distal sympathetic with vagal function in diabetic neuropathy. *Muscle Nerve* **9**: 592–596.

Low, P.A. (1993a). Laboratory evaluation of autonomic failure. In *Clinical Autonomic Disorders: Evaluation and Management*, ed. P.A. Low, pp. 169–195. Boston: Little, Brown and Company.

Low, P.A. (1993b). Composite autonomic scoring scale for laboratory quantification of generalized autonomic failure. *Mayo Clin. Proc.* **68**: 748–752.

Low, P.A. (1993c). Neurogenic orthostatic hypotension. In *Current Therapy in Neurologic Disease*, 4th edn, ed. R.T. Johnson and J.W. Griffin, pp. 21–26. St. Louis: Mosby Year Book.

Low, P.A., Opfer-Gehrking, T.L., Textor, S.C., Benarroch, E.E., Shen, W.-K., Schondorf, R., Suarez, G.A., and Rummans, T.A. (1995). Postural tachycardia syndrome (POTS). *Neurology* **45** (suppl. 5): S19–S25.

Low, P.A. and McLeod, J.G. (1993). The autonomic neuropathies. In *Clinical Autonomic Disorders: Evaluation and Management*, ed. P.A. Low, pp. 395–421. Boston: Little, Brown and Company.

Low, P.A. and Pfeifer, M.A. (1993). Standardization of clinical tests for practice and clinical trials. In *Clinical Autonomic Disorders: Evaluation and Management*, ed. P.A. Low, pp. 287–296. Boston: Little, Brown and Company.

Manco, J.C., Gallo Jr, L., Godoy, R.A., Fernandes, R.G., and Amorim, D.S. (1969). Degeneration of the cardiac nerves in Chagas' disease. *Circulation* **40**: 879–885.

Manolis, A.S., Tordjman, T., Mack, K.D., and Estes III, N.A. (1987). Atypical pulmonary and neurologic complications of amiodarone in the same patient. Report of a case and review of the literature. *Arch. Intern. Med.* **147**: 1805–1809.

Markus, C. (1906). Notes on a peculiar pupil phenomenon in cases of partial iridoplegia. *Trans. Ophthalmol. Soc. U.K.* **26**: 50–56.

Martinez-Arizala, A., Sobol, S.M., McCarty, G.E., Nichols, B.R., and Rakita, L. (1983). Amiodarone neuropathy. *Neurology* **33**: 643–645.

Matikainen, E. and Juntunen, J. (1985). Autonomic nervous system dysfunction in workers exposed to organic solvents. *J. Neurol. Neurosurg. Psychiatry* **48**: 1021–1024.

Navarro, X., Kennedy, W.R., and Fries, T.J. (1989). Small nerve fiber dysfunction in diabetic neuropathy. *Muscle Nerve* **12**: 498–507.

Neville, B.G. and Salden, G.E. (1984). Acute autonomic neuropathy following primary herpes simplex infection. *J. Neurol. Neurosurg. Psychiatry* **47**: 648–650.

Nijboer, J.A., Dorlas, J.C., and Lubbers, J. (1988). The difference in blood pressure between upper arm and finger during physical exercise. *Clin. Physiol.* **8**: 501–510.

Nix, W.A., Eckardt, V.F., and Kramer, G. (1985). Reversible esophageal motor dysfunction in botulism. *Muscle Nerve* **8**: 791–795.

Olofsson, B.-O., Ericksson, P., and Ericksson, A. (1983). The sick sinus syndrome in familial amyloidosis with polyneuropathy. *Int. J. Cardiol.* **4**: 71–73.

Palmero, H.A., Caeiro, T.F., and Iosa, D. (1981). Prevalence of slow heart rates in chronic Chagas' disease. *Am. J. Trop. Med. Hyg.* **30**: 1179–1182.

Pavesi, G., Gemignani, F., Macaluso, G.M., Ventura, P., Magnani, G., Fiocchi, A., Medici, D., Marbini, A., and Mancia, D. (1992). Acute sensory and autonomic neuropathy: possible association with Coxsackie B virus infection. *J. Neurol. Neurosurg. Psychiatry* **55**: 613–615.

Pellissier, J.F., Pouget, J., Cros, D., de Victor, B., Serratrice, G., and Toga, M. (1984). Peripheral neuropathy induced by amiodarone chlorhydrate. A clinicopathological study. *J. Neurol. Sci.* **63**: 251–266.

Persson, A. and Solders, G. (1983). R–R variations in Guillain-Barré syndrome: a test of autonomic dysfunction. *Acta Neurol. Scand.* **67**: 294–300.

Pickett, J.B. (1988). AAEE case report no. 16: botulism. *Muscle Nerve* **11**: 1201–1205.

Ropper, A.H. (1993). Acute autonomic emergencies and autonomic storm. In *Clinical Autonomic Disorders: Evaluation and Management*, ed. P.A. Low, pp. 747–760. Boston: Little, Brown and Company.

Rosenfeld, C.S. and Broder, L.E. (1984). Cisplatin-induced autonomic neuropathy. *Canc. Treat. Rep.* **68**: 659–660.

Ross, A.T. (1958). Progressive selective sudomotor denervation: a case with co-existing Adie's syndrome. *Neurology* **8**: 809–817.

Said, G., Joskowicz, M., Barreira, A.A., and Eisen, H. (1985). Neuropathy associated with experimental Chagas' disease. *Ann. Neurol.* **18**: 676–683.

Sandroni, P., Benarroch, E.E., and Low, P.A. (1991). Pharmacological dissection of components of the Valsalva maneuver in adrenergic failure. *J. Appl. Physiol.* **71**: 1563–1567.

Santoro, L., Barbieri, F., Nucciotti, R., Battaglia, F., Crispi, F., Ragno, M., Greco, P., and Caruso, G. (1992). Amiodarone-induced experimental acute neuropathy in rats. *Muscle Nerve* **15**: 788–795.

Schondorf, R. and Low, P.A. (1993). Idiopathic postural orthostatic tachycardia syndrome: an attentuated form of acute pandysautonomia? *Neurology* **43**: 132–137.

Stewart, J.D., Low, P.A., and Fealey, R.D. (1992). Distal small fiber neuropathy: results of tests of sweating and autonomic cardiovascular reflexes. *Muscle Nerve* **15**: 661–665.

Stewart, P.M. and Hensley, W.J. (1981). An acute attack of variegate porphyria complicated by severe autonomic neuropathy. *Aust. N. Z. J. Med.* **11**: 82–83.

Stoll, G., Thomas, C., Reiners, K., Schober, R., and Hartung, H.P. (1991). Encephalo-myelo-radiculo-ganglionitis presenting as pandysautonomia. *Neurology* **41**: 723–726.

Suarez, G.A., Fealey, R.D., Camilleri, M., and Low, P.A. (1994). Idiopathic autonomic neuropathy: clinical, neurophysiologic, and follow-up studies on 27 patients. *Neurology* **44**: 1675–1682.

Suarez, G.A. and Low, P.A. (1994). Peripheral nervous system complications of diabetes mellitus or hypoglycemia. In *Handbook of Clinical Neurology*, ed. P.J. Vinken, G.W. Bruyn and H.L. Klawans. Amsterdam: Elsevier (in press).

Taubner, R.W. and Salanova, V. (1984). Acute dysautonomia and polyneuropathy. *Arch. Neurol.* **41**: 1100–1101.

Torres, N.E., Zollman, P.J., and Low, P.A. (1991). Characterization of muscarinic receptor subtype of rat eccrine sweat gland by autoradiography. *Brain Res.* **550**: 129–132.

Truax, B.T. (1984). Autonomic disturbances in Guillain-Barré syndrome. *Neurology* **4**: 462–468.

Tsementzis, S.A. and Hitchcock, E.R. (1985). The spoon test: a simple bedside test for assessing sudomotor autonomic failure. *J. Neurol. Neurosurg. Psychiatry* **48**: 378–380.

Tuck, R.R. and McLeod, J.G. (1981). Autonomic dysfunction in Guillain-Barré syndrome. *J. Neurol. Neurosurg. Psychiatry* **44**: 983–990.

Vita, G., Girlanda, P., Puglisi, R.M., Marabello, L., and Messina, C. (1987). Cardiovascular-reflex testing and single-fiber electromyography on botulism. A longitudinal study. *Arch. Neurol.* **44**: 202–206.

Warkany, J. and Hubbard, D.M. (1948). Mercury in urine of children with acrodynia. *Lancet* **1**: 829–830.

Weber, F.P. (1933). Dr. Markus's original case of Markus's syndrome ('myotonic pupil' with absence of patellar and achilles reflexes) shown twenty-seven and a half years ago. *Proc. R. Soc. Med.* **26**: 530–531.

Webster, J., Newnham, D., Petrie, J.C., and Lovell, H.G. (1984). Influence of arm position on measurement of blood pressure. *Br. Med. J.* **288**: 1574–1575.

Wheeler Jr, J.S., Siroky, M.B., Pavlakis, A., and Krane, R.J. (1984). The urodynamic aspects of the Guillain-Barré syndrome. *J. Urol.* **131**: 917–919.

Windebank, A.J. and Bonkovsky, H.L. (1993). Porphyric neuropathy. In *Peripheral Neuropathy*, 3rd edn, ed. P.J. Dyck, P.K. Thomas, J.W. Griffin, P.A. Low and J.F. Poduslo, pp. 1161–1168. Philadelphia: W.B. Saunders.

Yahr, M.D. and Frontera, A.T. (1975). Acute autonomic neuropathy. Its ocurrence in infectious mononucleosis. *Arch. Neurol.* **32**: 132–133.

Young, R.R., Asbury, A.K., Adams, R.D., and Corbett, J.L. (1969). Pure pan-dysautonomia with recovery. *Trans. Am. Neurol. Assoc.* **94**: 355–357.

Young, R.R., Asbury, A.K., Corbett, J.L., and Adams, R.D. (1975). Pure pan-dysautonomia with recovery. Description and discussion of diagnostic criteria. *Brain* **98**: 613–636.

11 Vasculitic neuropathies

G. Said

Introduction

Vasculitis is a common and treatable cause of neuropathy. The neuropathy often occurs in the context of a multisystem disorder but in a substantial proportion of patients, especially among those seen by neurologists, the neuropathy is the first and only manifestation of vasculitis. In most cases, necrotizing arteritis of the type observed in polyarteritis nodosa is responsible for the lesions, but classification of vasculitis is still uncertain. In contrast, the mechanism of the nerve lesions associated with vasculitis is rather uniform, with nerve ischemia as the common consequence of the occlusion of blood vessels in necrotizing arteritis.

Vasculitis and the peripheral nervous system

The vasculitides are often classified according to the size of vessels predominantly affected (Winkelmann 1980), but overlaps are common and the nomenclature of the systemic vasculitides remains enigmatic (Lie 1994) (Table 11.1). Recent attempts to classify systemic vasculitides (Jennette et al. 1994) did not bring much clarification. The large vessel vasculitis which includes giant cell arteritis and Takayasu's arteritis are seldom associated with peripheral neuropathy. In the medium-sized vessel vasculitis, which includes polyarteritis nodosa and Kawasaki disease, neuropathy occurs only in patients with polyarteritis nodosa.

Using this recent classification, the group of small vessel vasculitis includes Wegener's granulomatosis, the Churg–Strauss syndrome, and what is called microscopic polyangiitis with involvement of capillaries which is sometimes associated with polyarteritis nodosa. Actually the group of microscopic polyangiitis does not represent a clear entity because overlaps with polyarteritis nodosa is very common, with involvement of capillaries occurring in a number of patients with otherwise typical polyarteritis nodosa. In addition, the Churg–Strauss syndrome which associates asthma and eosinophilia with eosinophil-rich and granulomatous inflammation involving the respiratory tract, and necrotizing vasculitis affecting small to medium-sized vessels is often difficult to differentiate from classical polyarteritis nodosa. Essential cryoglobulinemia vasculitis is included in microscopic polyangiitis but in our experience cryoglobulinemia may be associated with

Table 11.1 *A revised, practical classification of vasculitis*

Primary vasculitides affecting large, medium, and small-sized blood vessels
Takayasu arteritis
Giant cell (temporal) arteritis
Isolated angiitis of the central nervous system
Affecting predominantly medium and small-sized blood vessels
Polyarteritis nodosa
Churg–Strauss syndrome
Wegener's granulomatosis
Affecting predominantly small-sized blood vessels
Microscopic polyangiitis
Schönlein-Henoch syndrome
Cutaneous leukocytoclastic angiitis
Miscellaneous conditions
Bürger's disease
Cogan syndrome
Kawasaki disease

Note:
Reproduced from Lie (1994).

small vessel involvement as well as with typical polyarteritis nodosa. Thus, no classification of systemic vasculitis is fully satisfactory as underlined by Lie (1994). From a neurological point of view, the lesions observed in vasculitic neuropathy are ischemic lesions resulting from occlusion of the vasa nervorum, mainly in the course of polyarteritis nodosa.

Necrotizing arteritis affects blood vessels of the size of those located in the epineurium; because of that, necrotizing arteritis is commonly associated with symptomatic or subclinical peripheral nerve involvement through a mechanism of nerve ischemia (Kussmaul and Maier 1866; Lovshin and Kernohan 1948; Asbury and Johnson 1978). Clinical neuropathy occurs in 50–75% of the patients with systemic vasculitis of the polyarteritis nodosa group (Godeau and Guillevin 1982; Moore and Cupps 1983), but subclinical lesions are even more common. The same pattern of lesions of blood vessels occurs in allergic angiitis. Peripheral neuropathy also occurs in the context of Wegener's granulomatosis (Stern et al. 1965) but less often as the presenting manifestation of the disease than in polyarteritis nodosa.

We have recently reviewed the clinical and pathological data of 200 patients in whom we found necrotizing vasculitis in nerve and/or in muscle biopsy specimens and much of the data used in this chapter comes from this study (G. Said, unpublished observations).

Peripheral neuropathy of necrotizing arteritis

Clinical aspects

Focal and multifocal neuropathy are the most common patterns of vasculitic neuropathy, but distal symmetrical sensory or sensorimotor neuropathy also occurs in this context. In our series of patients, focal neuropathy (mononeuritis) affected 16.5% of patients with demonstrated necrotizing arteritis (NA), and multifocal neuropathy (mononeuritis multiplex) in 56.5% of them. Distal symmetrical sensory or sensorimotor neuropathy was present in 50 patients (25%). Any peripheral nerve can be affected but in the vast majority of our patients the peroneal nerve was involved. This nerve was affected unilaterally in 62.5% of the patients, and bilaterally affected in one-third of patients. Unilateral involvement of the popliteal nerve was present in 27.5% of patients, both popliteal nerves were affected in 5% of them. Unilateral involvement of the ulnar nerve occurred in 25.5% of patients, bilateral involvement in 8%. The median nerve was affected on one side in 21.5% of patients, and on both sides in 3%. Unilateral involvement of the radial nerve was present in 8% of patients, and in 2% on both sides. Unilateral involvement of the femoral nerve was observed in 6% of the patients. Proximal sciatic nerve or sciatic root involvement was observed in 2% of patients. Involvement of the fifth and seventh cranial nerves was observed only once. Signs of central nervous system (CNS) involvement were present in 3% of our patients, but systematic magnetic resonance imaging (MRI) of the brain would probably detect many more patients with silent involvement of the CNS. CNS manifestations were present in 20–40% of patients in other series (Godeau and Guillevin 1982; Moore and Cupps 1983). CNS involvement seems to be more common in very severe forms of polyarteritis nodosa, and also occurs later in the course of the disease (Frohnert and Sheps

1967). Early treatment with corticosteroids may have modified the occurrence of CNS complications.

Weakness, numbness and pain are common in the affected territory, but general muscle weakness and myalgia are also often noted. The onset of the neuropathy is typically abrupt and the deficit severe. In many cases, however, the deficit is partial, affecting only part of a nerve territory. Also the course of the neuropathy may be slowly progressive in some cases, especially in the elderly. The cerebrospinal fluid (CSF) is usually normal, but a mild elevation of the protein content occurs. Recovery from motor deficit due to ischemic neuropathy takes months because the nerve lesions are axonal. Residual pains are common and may be difficult to differentiate from relapses of the neuropathy.

Electrophysiological aspects

The electrophysiological studies show an axonal neuropathy in all cases. Some authors have suggested using electrophysiological data to orientate the site of the nerve biopsy (Wees et al. 1981). Occasionally, an early ischemic conduction block has been observed (Ropert and Metral 1990; Cornblath and Sumner, 1991), but conduction block is more suggestive of nerve entrapment or of acute focal demyelination, as observed in Guillain-Barré syndrome (GBS) or in other forms of acquired demyelinative neuropathy, than of an ischemic nerve lesion. Needle electromyography will reveal signs of denervation with spontaneous activity seen as fibrillation potentials and positive sharp waves. Early in the course of ischemic neuropathy, the motor unit morphology may remain relatively normal.

Morphological aspects

Demonstration of necrotizing asteritis in biopsy specimens

The diagnosis of NA needs histological confirmation, which can be easily achieved through a biopsy of a specific skin lesion; otherwise, nerve and/or muscle biopsies are advised in the search for characteristic lesions of muscular or epineurial arteries (Maxeiner et al. 1952; Parry et al. 1981; Wees et al. 1981; Pages et al. 1984; Davies 1994). Biopsy of the kidney is less frequently diagnostic, even in patients with nephropathy. It is impossible to tell how often the diagnosis of necrotizing arteritis is not achieved histologically, and it must be remembered that a negative biopsy does not rule out the diagnosis of NA; however, in our experience repetition of the biopsies is seldom helpful.

The yield of nerve biopsy is obviously improved by careful selection of the nerve to be biopsied and by examination of serial sections. Healing of a nerve biopsy site in the lower limbs is especially slow in patients with vasculitis who receive corticosteroids. These patients should not be allowed to walk before complete healing of the biopsy site.

In patients with vasculitic neuropathy due to necrotizing arteritis, vasculitis can be demonstrated in the muscle or nerve specimen, or in both. In our recent evaluation, in 27% of our patients with vasculitic neuropathy, the specific vascular lesion was found in the muscle specimen only, in 35% in the nerve specimen only, and in 27% of patients in both the nerve and muscle specimens. It is thus wiser to sample both the nerve and the muscle during the same procedure (Bonnin et al. 1948; Said et al. 1988; Panegyres et al. 1990), especially when the peroneal nerve is affected. In such cases, we biopsy the superficial peroneal nerve and the peroneus brevis muscle during the same procedure, under local anesthesia. When only the sural nerve is affected, combined nerve and muscle biopsy during the same procedure is also possible by sampling the sural nerve 3 cm more proximally than usual and a biopsy from the adjacent triceps surae muscle.

Biopsy specimens must be studied on **serial sections**, because arteritis usually occurs segmentally, and characteristic lesions may be present only on segments of a few tens of micrometers. Total nerve biopsy must be performed instead of fascicular biopsy because, almost invariably, only the epineurial arteries are affected, sometimes in association with inflammatory infiltration of perineurial vessels and with perineuritis. Epineurial and perineurial inflammatory infiltrates are common in the vicinity of characteristic arterial lesions, but they are seldom observed in the endoneurial space, except in the patients with NA occurring in the context of human immunodeficiency virus (HIV) infection.

Lesions of nerve fibers: ischemic neuropathy

Nerve ischemia, as observed in vasculitic neuropathy, induces acute axonal degeneration in most cases. In our series, Wallerian degeneration affected an average of 65±35% (standard deviation; SD) of the isolated fibers, with simultaneous degeneration of fibers in many cases (normal value<1%), a pattern which fits well with an ischemic lesion and may help to suspect vasculitis when characteristic arterial lesions have not been found. The average incidence of fibers showing segmental abnormalities of the myelin sheath was 1.9% (range 0–15%; normal <1%. Asymmetry of lesions between and within fascicles is also common in vasculitic neuropathy. Sometimes axon loss predominates in the centrofascicular area, which suggests an ischemic origin (Nukada and Dyck 1984).

Quantitative studies of epon embedded specimens and teased fiber preparations led to the following conclusions:

1. The intensity of axon loss and the incidence of degenerating fibers varied greatly from case to case, and between fascicles of individual nerves.
2. Axon loss predominated in myelinated fibers larger than 7 μm diameter.
3. Unmyelinated fibers were less affected.
4. Occasionally, even the Schwann cells seemed to undergo degeneration. This may preclude axonal regeneration and clinical recovery.
5. In most cases, the nerve lesions appeared to result from the summation of lesions of different age of nerve blood vessels (Fujimura et al. 1991).

Polysystemic and 'non-systemic necrotizing' arteritis

In our series of 200 patients, NA occurred in the context of multisystem disorders in 131 patients (65%), including 116 patients with connective tissue disorders.

Necrotizing arteritis and multisystem disorder

Patients in this group commonly manifested loss of weight, fever, asthenia, and myalgia in association with multisystem involvement like arthritis and cutaneous vasculitis.

Classic polyarteritis nodosa (PAN)

Classic PAN affected 36% of our patients. In these patients multisystem involvement was present with cutaneous vasculitis as the most common non-neurological manifestation. Specific skin involvement including livedo, cutaneous necrosis and nodules, were present in 22 patients (11%). In 17 patients (8.5%), non-specific edema, usually extreme in one limb, was present. In patients with cutaneous vasculitis and neuropathy, a nerve biopsy should be performed for diagnostic purposes only in those in whom the skin biopsy did not provide specific vasculitic lesions. Renal involvement was observed in 10% of patients. In another study of 95 patients seen in a department of internal medicine, asthma was present in 12 patients (12.6%) (Godeau and Guillevin 1982).

The Churg and Strauss variant of polyarteritis nodosa was diagnosed in 11 patients (5%) of our series. Whether the Churg–Strauss syndrome represents a separate entity is controversial. In 1951, Churg and Strauss reported a study of 14 cases of a form of disseminated necrotizing vasculitis occurring frequently among asthmatic patients, with fever, eosinophilia, and a fulminant multisystem disease with a pathology of NA, eosinophilic infiltration and extravascular granulomas. Fauci et al. (1978) classify this syndrome with PAN, whereas Chumbley et al. (1977) clearly differentiate their cases from PAN. Pulmonary infiltrates can be transient or nodular and chronic; the asthma may be of short or long duration; peripheral eosinophilia is observed routinely. Neurological involvement, usually mononeuritis multiplex, was found in 19 of 30 cases (Chumbley et al. 1977). In our experience, the vascular and nerve lesions observed in nerve biopsies from patients with this syndrome are similar to those observed in PAN, and peripheral eosinophilia and eosinophilic infiltration occur in classical PAN as well. The response of the so-called Churg–Strauss allergic granulomatosis to corticosteroid therapy is not different from that observed in classic PAN. Although pANCA (anti-neutrophil cytoplasmic autoantibodies) seem to be commonly found in this syndrome, the series studied are not large enough to make of this syndrome more than a variant of polyarteritis nodosa.

Necrotizing arteritis and neuropathy in patients with rheumatoid arthritis

NA is known to occur in patients with rheumatoid arthritis and represents a factor of poor prognosis

(Wattiaux et al. 1987). Forty-three patients of our series (21.5%) fitted into this group which represents the second largest group of patients with NA and multisystem connective tissue disorder. The occurrence of NA in the context of rheumatoid arthritis is classically associated with a poor outcome. Of the 32 patients with rheumatoid arthritis and neuropathy due to histologically proven necrotizing vasculitis in muscle and/or in nerve biopsy specimens (Puechal et al. 1995), 15 had a sensory and motor neuropathy, the others had a sensory neuropathy. Two-thirds of the patients had a multifocal pattern of neurological deficit, the other third manifested distal symmetrical sensory neuropathy. In this group of patients, Sjögren's syndrome was present in 22%, rheumatoid factor in 97%, nodules in 31% and articular erosions in all of them. NA, which was demonstrated in nerve and/or muscle biopsy specimens in all patients was more often found in the muscle (86%) than in the nerve biopsy specimen (64%). The survival rate was 57% at 5 years. Low CH50, C3 and C4 complement levels, which were found in 60% of the patients, were associated with a poorer outcome. Cryoglobulinemia was present in 13% of patients of this series. Search for hepatitis B antigens was negative in all of them.

Necrotizing arteritis associated with other connective tissue disorders

NA was associated with other connective tissue disorders including isolated Sjögren's syndrome in 4% of our patients, systemic lupus erythematosus in 1%, and systemic sclerosis in 1%. In 16 patients (8%) there was more than one connective tissue disorder associated with necrotizing arteritis and neuropathy, including the 12 patients with Sjögren's syndrome and rheumatoid arthritis.

The association of necrotizing vasculitis with primary Sjögren's syndrome has been reported by Molina et al. (1985), but the mechanism of neuropathy in this setting is not unique. Ataxic sensory neuropathy associated with autonomic dysfunction has been attributed to inflammatory lesions of dorsal root ganglia, presumably of immune origin (Griffin et al. 1990). Nevertheless, development of neuropathy in patients with Sjögren's syndrome, including sensory and sensorimotor symmetrical polyneuropathies can be due to vasculitis (Molina et al. 1985; Mellgren et al. 1989).

Necrotizing vasculitis and angiocentric lymphoproliferative disorders

This disorder encompasses the previously nosologic entities of lymphomatoid granulomatosis (Jaffe 1984); it represents an uncommon type of vasculitis which combines the angiodestructive and granulomatous features of Wegener's granulomatosis with the cellular atypicality of lymphoma (Liebow et al. 1972; Katzenstein et al. 1979; Winkelman 1980). At present, it may be concluded that lymphomatoid granulomatosis actually is a T cell lymphoma (Myers 1990).

Jaffe (1988) also provided a histological grading. Grade I is characterized by a predominant polymorphous lymphocytic infiltrate without cytologic atypia; grade II is characterized by a polymorphous infiltrate with clear cytologic atypia; grade III, also called angiocentric lymphoma, is clearly histologically malignant. The prognosis in this type of vasculitis is more severe than in most cases with NA; CNS involvement is frequently observed. This entity associates an angiocentric proliferation of T lymphocytes with lesions of blood vessels that induce nerve ischemia. Neuropathy associated with angiocentric proliferation of lymphocytes and necrosis of blood vessels, and infiltration of predominant $CD8^+$lymphocytes occurs in the course of HIV infection (Calabrese 1989).

Necrotizing arteritis and multisystemic non-connective tissue disorder

NA also occurs in the context of viral infection. In patients infected with HIV, inflammatory neuropathy can be associated with NA of the PAN type, but mononuclear cells predominate in the inflammatory infiltrate (Said et al. 1988; Calabrese et al. 1989). NA also occurs in association with hepatitis B infection. Infection with the virus of the hepatitis B was found in 19% of our patients, including two with chronic hepatitis. These figures confirm that infection with hepatitis B virus is more common in patients with NA than in controls and that it may play a role in the onset of NA (Sergent et al. 1976; Drüeke et al. 1980; Shusterman and London 1984; Editorial 1985). Recently, we observed patients with hepatitis C virus and necrotizing vasculitis.

Neuropathy as the only manifestation of vasculitis: the 'non-systemic' vasculitis

In a large proportion of patients first seen by neurologist for manifestations of peripheral neuropathy related to necrotizing arteritis, there is no other organ clinically involved than the peripheral nervous system (Harati and Niaken 1986; Dyck et al. 1987; Said et al. 1988; Hawke et al. 1991). The diagnosis of this 'non-systemic' vasculitis can be made only after nerve and/or muscle biopsy. This group of patients accounted for 35% of the 200 patients seen in our service with NA and neuropathy.

Is there such a syndrome as vasculitis restricted to the peripheral nervous system (PNS), as suggested by Dyck et al. (1987) who consider that these patients have a non-systemic, organ-specific vasculitis affecting only the PNS? In fact, silent involvement of other organs is common in such patients as shown by the frequent finding of NA in muscle biopsy specimens. In our series of patients with isolated vasculitic neuropathy, the muscle biopsy was as often diagnostic for vasculitis as the nerve biopsy, demonstrating that silent lesions of medium-sized muscle arteries was common in this context, and that vasculitis was not restricted to the nervous system. The same problem occurs in the so-called cutaneous vasculitis, in which 52% of the patients supposed to have a cutaneous variety of periarteritis nodosa actually had associated neuromuscular manifestations (Diaz-Perez and Winkelmann 1980). It is thus more appropriate to consider that the patients with apparently isolated vasculitic neuropathy are affected by a milder form of vasculitis, symptomatic in nerves only.

In this group of patients with isolated vasculitic neuropathy, the mean age of the patients was 61 years with 61% being female. General signs or symptoms, usually minor, including fever and loss of weight were present in half of them. Fifty-nine per cent of them complained of spontaneous pains of neurogenic or muscular origin. The erythrocyte sedimentation rate was normal in 33% of patients of this group. Patients with cryoglobulinemia were not included. From a neurological standpoint, approximately one-fourth of the patients presented with a distal symmetrical sensory or sensorimotor neuropathy, and the diagnosis of NA had seldom been considered before the results of the nerve and muscle biopsies.

Of the patients with isolated vasculitic neuropathy at the time of diagnosis whom we could follow for an average of 6 years, roughly one-third developed systemic manifestations; one-third died after an average of 3.3 years after the onset of the neuropathy, the majority of them (eight of 11) from systemic manifestations and three from infection. Twenty-four per cent had one or more relapses of neuropathy. The mean interval between the first and the second episodes of neuropathy was 3.5 years compared with 6 months to 1 year in patients who had had multisystem signs from the beginning; 31% did not relapse. These findings are in keeping with the better prognosis observed in the 'non-systemic' vasculitis than in the polysystemic forms (Dyck et al. 1987).

Vasculitic neuropathy in the elderly

We recently reviewed the clinicopathological data of 100 patients over 65 years of age who were referred for a disabling neuropathy. In 23% of them, necrotizing vasculitis was demonstrated in the nerve and/or muscle biopsies, whereas non-necrotizing vasculitis was found in 5%. In this group of patients, the neuropathy occurred in the context of a multisystem disorder in two-thirds of the patients, and as an isolated neuropathy in 10% (Chia et al. 1996). Vasculitis, both systemic and non-systemic, apppears therefore to be an important cause of neuropathy in the elderly, who usually respond well to treatment (Said et al. 1988).

Vasculitic neuropathy in diabetes mellitus

Vasculitis and ischemic nerve lesions were found in biopsies of the intermediate cutaneous nerve of the thigh in patients with severe forms of proximal diabetic neuropathy of the lower limbs (Said et al. 1993). The significance of this finding is not yet clear, but these patients had no signs of inflammation; vasculitis was restricted to the nerve specimens. We suggest that lesions of nerve fibers and of blood vessels due to diabetes mellitus may trigger an inflammatory reaction and reactive vasculitis in some patients. Alternatively, diabetes may make peripheral nerves more susceptible to an intercurrent inflammatory process. In both instances, lesions of epi- or perineurial blood vessels can result in ischemic nerve lesions responsible for severe forms of proximal diabetic neuropathy.

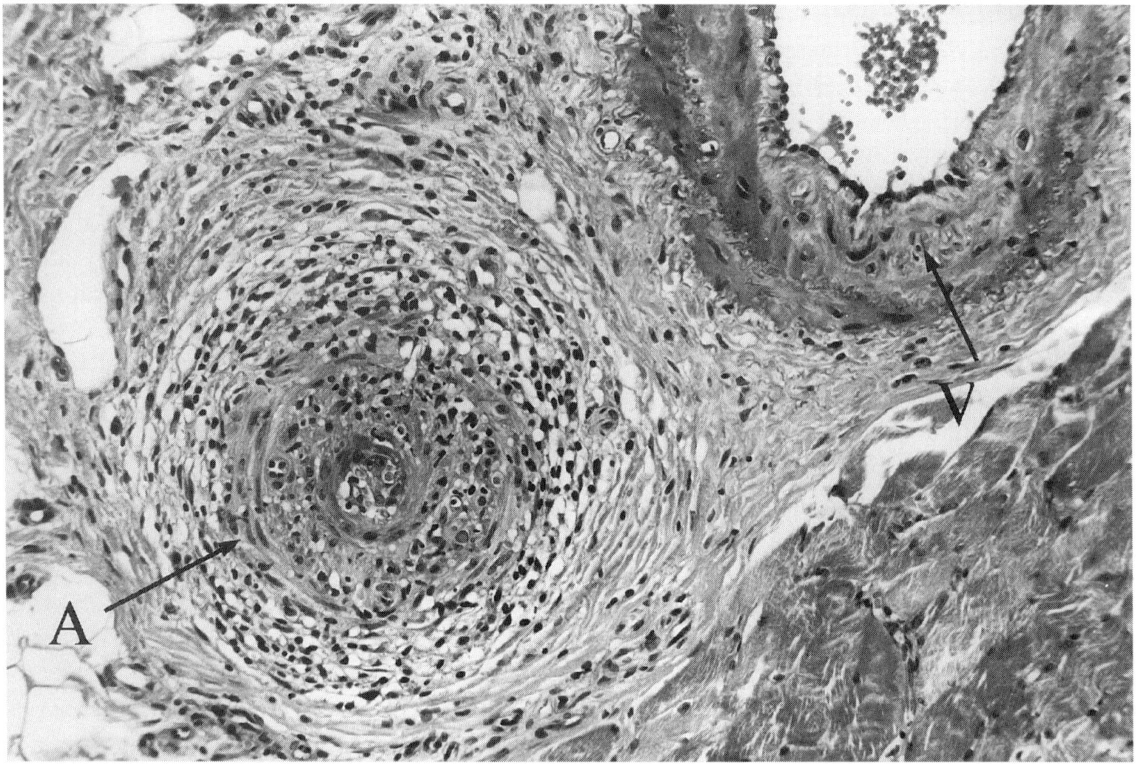

Figure 11.1 *Necrotizing vasculitis in a muscle biopsy specimen from a patient with multifocal neuropathy (150 x, H&E staining). Note the transparietal inflammatory infiltration and the presence of fibrinoid necrosis of the arterial wall (A) with sparing of the venule (V). Necrotizing arteritis is as often found in muscle biopsies as in nerve.*

Diagnosis of necrotizing vasculitis

The diagnosis of polyarteritis nodosa rests on histological criteria; these include transmural infiltration of small arteries with polymorphonuclear cells, often admixed with lymphocytes and eosinophils; leukocytoclasia; fibrinoid necrosis; destruction of the internal elastic lamina; occlusion of the lumen; and the usual sparing of adjacent venules (Figure 11.1). The arterial lesions progress to complete occlusion of the vessels followed by spontaneous recanalization. Transmural inflammatory infiltration with the presence of polymorphonuclear cells mixed with other cells, and the destruction of the arterial wall in necrotizing arteritis, must be differentiated from the inflammatory infiltrates which may be observed in chronic inflammatory demyelinating polyneuropathy. In this condition the infiltrates are formed exclusively by mononuclear cells without destruction of the vessel wall.

Pathophysiology of nerve lesions associated with vasculitis

In PAN the size of the blood vessels affected corresponds to that of most epineurial arteries; thus lesions and occlusion of a large number of such vessels induce nerve ischemia with subsequent axonal degeneration of the vast majority of nerve fibers. When nerve lesions are limited focal loss of axons occurs.

Necrotizing arteritis is the most common primary vasculitis responsible for vasculitic neuropathy. This process, which is related to local or systemic vascular inflammation, may involve large and small vessels, and produces vessel and tissue necrosis with typical leukocytic infiltration, leukocytoclasia, hemorrhage and fibrinoid change (Winkelmann 1980). Formation of soluble, circulating, immune complexes, which result from the binding of antibodies produced by stimulated plasma cells, to foreign or autoantigens, are suspected to play an important role in the lesions of blood vessels observed in PAN. But, in spite of the theoretical importance of circulating immune complexes in PAN, detection of circulating immune complexes is of no diagnostic or prognostic value (Nydegger 1985). The immune complexes are phagocytosed through the interaction of neutrophil Fc receptors with the Fc portion of the complexed antibody (Hogg 1988). A number of other factors including proteolytic enzymes, free radicals and inflammatory peptides released by neutrophilic polymorphonuclear cells (Moore, 1989; Smiley and Moore 1989) and complement attack complex (C5b-9) may also contribute to the vessel wall injury. The diagnostic value of immunoglobulins and fractions of complement, which are often found in the epineurial vessels of nerve biopsies from patients with vasculitic neuropathy (Panegyres et al. 1990; Hawke et al. 1991), is not established.

The role of anti-endothelial cells antibodies found in several connective tissue and systemic disorders, is still not clear (Panegyres et al. 1992). They are more often found in conditions that are seldom associated with PNS involvement such as scleroderma, Kawasaki's disease or systemic lupus erythematosus. Thus the role played by such antibodies and the usefulness of their detection in sera from patients with vasculitic neuropathy remains to be established (Brasile et al. 1989; Ferraro et al. 1990). ANCA can induce neutrophil degranulation and inactivate protease inhibitors (Frampton et al. 1990), and damage endothelial cells through activation of polymorphonuclear cells and the release of reactive oxygen species (Ewert et al. 1991). Such autoantibodies are commonly detected in patients with Wegener's granulomatosis, and their serum level seems to correlate with disease activity (Parlevliet et al. 1988; Goeken 1991), but the identification of this important marker of disease activity in Wegener's granulomatosis is not reliable in polyarteritis nodosa.

Cellular factors including macrophages and cytotoxic T lymphocytes are likely to play a role in vasculitic lesions (Kissel et al. 1989; Panegyres et al. 1990; Hawke et al. 1991). Cytotoxic lymphocytes specific for class 2 major histocompatibility complex also seem able to lyse endothelial cells in vitro, after action of interferon-gamma (Pober and Cotran 1990). Endothelial cells can serve as antigen presenting cells and can be induced to secrete a number of cytokines including IL-6, IL-1 and intercellular adhesion molecules, which can recruit and activate lymphocytes and increase cell damage (Panegyres et al. 1992).

Treatment

Since the use of corticosteroids in the treatment of polyarteritis nodosa, the 5-year survival improved from 13% in the control group to 48% in treated patients (Frohnert and Sheps 1967). It is widely admitted that one should start with prednisone at 1 mg kg^{-1} per day. Some authors start with 2 mg kg^{-1} per day. High doses of corticosteroids may not be well tolerated in the elderly. Simultaneous treatment with cyclophosphamide, 2 mg kg^{-1} per day, may help to reduce the dose of corticosteroids. In cases with severe general manifestations, pulses of intravenous prednisolone may help. It is difficult to tell how long this treatment should be maintained at full dose. This depends on the response to treatment, on the course and form of the disease, and on the tolerance to the treatment. We usually give a full dose of steroids for approximately 6–8 weeks and then taper prednisone in 6–10 months, or more. It is necessary to control the sedimentation rate periodically and to increase the doses of prednisone if the sedimentation rate increases, or if new manifestations of vasculitis appear. Many patients relapse either during reduction of steroid therapy or after treatment has been stopped. In our experience, up to half of the patients relapse during tapering of prednisone or after treatment has been stopped. Careful follow-up of patients is mandatory. In cases of Wegener's granulomatosis, some authors suggest using serial quantitation of ANCA levels for following and predicting disease activity (Cohen-Tervaert and Kallenberg, 1993).

In cases without clinical evidence of polysystemic involvement, in cases with normal sedimentation rate, and in elderly patients, the benefit of prolonged treatment with high doses of steroids is less certain. Indomethacin (100 mg per day) may be added to steroids when fever persists or when the sedimentation rate remains abnormal in spite of large doses of steroids.

A report on the usefulness of treatment with intravenous immunoglobulin (Jayne et al. 1991) needs to be confirmed in a comparative study with prednisone or other immunosuppressive drugs. In the evaluation of the efficacy of treatments of vasculitic neuropathies, it must be remembered that there is a wide range of modalities of evolution in NA, with spontaneous remissions of several years of the disease in some cases.

Sensorimotor deficit resulting from nerve ischemia takes months to recover because of the underlying axonal lesions. Motor recovery could benefit from physiotherapy. Persistence of residual pains is common.

References

Asbury, A.K. and Johnson P.C. (1978). Vasculitic neuropathy. In *Major Problems in Pathology*, vol. 9, *Pathology of Peripheral Nerve*, ed. J.L. Bennington, pp. 110–119. Philadelphia: W.B. Saunders.

Bonnin, H., Moretti, G.-F., and Riviere, J. (1948). La biopsie musculaire révélatrice des formes non cutanées de la périartérite noueuse. *J. Med. Bordeaux* **125**: 303–308.

Brasile, L., Kremer, J.M., and Clarke, J.L. (1989). Identification of an autoantibody to vascular endothelial cell-specific antigens in patients with systemic vasculitis. *Am. J. Med.* **87**: 74–80.

Calabrese, L.H., Estes, M., Yen-Lieberman, B. Proffitt, M.R., Tubbs, R., Fishleder, A.J., and Levin, K.H. (1989). Systemic vasculitis in association with human immunodeficiency virus infection. *Arthritis Rheum.* **32**: 569–576.

Chia, L., Fernandez, A., Lacroix, C., Adams, D., Planté, V., and Said, G. (1996). Contribution of nerve biopsy findings to the diagnosis of disabling neuropathy in the elderly: a retrospective review of 100 consecutive patients. *Brain.*

Chumbley, L.C., Harrison, Jr E.G., and Deremee, R.A. (1977). Allergic granulomatosis and angiitis (Churg–Strauss syndrome). *Proc. Mayo Clin.* **52**: 477–484.

Churg, J. and Strauss, L. (1951). Allergic granulomatosis, allergic angeitis, and periarteritis nodosa. *Am. J. Pathol.* **27**: 277–301.

Cohen-Tervaert, J.W. and Kallenberg, C. (1993). Neurologic manifestations of systemic vasculitides. *Rheum. Dis. Clin. N. Am.* **19**: 913–940.

Cornblath, D.R. and Sumner, A.J. (1991). Conduction block in neuropathies with necrotizing vasculitis. *Muscle Nerve* **14**: 185.

Davies, L. (1994). Vasculitic neuropathy. In *Inflammatory Neuropathies*, ed. J.G. Mcleod, *Ballière's Clinical Neurology* **3**: 193–210.

Diaz-Perez, J.L. and Winkelmann, R.K. (1980). Cutaneous periarteritis nodosa, a study of 33 cases. In *Vasculitis*, ed. K. Wolff and R.K. Winkelmann, pp. 273–284. London: Lloyd-Luke Ltd.

Drüeke, T., Barbanel C., Jungers, P., Digeon, M., Poisson, M., Brivet Trecan, G., Feldman, G. et al. (1980). Hepatitis B antigen associated periarteritis nodosa in patients undergoing long-term hemodialysis. *Am. J. Med.* **68**: 86–90.

Dyck, P.J., Benstead, T.J., Conn, D.L., Stevens, J.C., Windebank, A.J., and Low, P.A. (1987). Nonsystemic vasculitic neuropathy. *Brain* **110**: 843–854.

Editorial. (1985). Systemic vasculitis. *Lancet* **1**: 1252–1254.

Ewert, B.H., Jennette, J.C., and Falk, R.J. (1991). The pathogenetic role of antineutrophil cytoplasmic antibodies. *Am. J. Kidney Dis.* **18**: 188–95.

Fauci, A.S., Haynes, B.F., and Katz, P. (1978). The spectrum of vasculitis. *Ann. Intern. Med.* **89**: 660–676.

Ferraro, G., Meroni, P.L., Tincani, A., Sinico, A., Barcellini, W., Radice, A., et al. (1990). Anti-endothelial cell antibodies in patients with Wegener's granulomatosis and micropolyarteritis. *Clin. Exp. Immunol.* **79**: 47–53.

Frampton, G., Jayne, D.R.W., Perry, G.J., Lockwood, C.M., and Cameron, J.S. (1990). Autoantibodies to endothelial cells and neutrophil cytoplasmic antigens in systemic vasculitis. *Clin. Exp. Immunol.* **82**: 227–232.

Frohnert, P.P. and Sheps, S.G. (1967). Long-term follow up study of periarteritis nodosa. *Am. J. Med.* **43**: 8–13.

Fujimura, H., Lacroix, C., and Said, G. (1991). Vulnerability of nerve fibers to ischaemia. *Brain* **114**: 1929–1942.

Godeau, P. and Guillevin, L. (1982). Périartérite noueuse systémique. In *Maladies Dites Systémiques*, ed. M.-F. Kahn, and A.P. Peltier, pp. 414–445. Paris: Flammarion.

Goeken, J.A. (1991). Antineutrophil cytoplasmic antibody: a useful serological marker for vasculitis. *J. Clin. Immunol.* **11**: 161–74.

Griffin, J.W., Cornblath, D.R., and Alexander, E. (1990). Ataxic sensory neuropathy and dorsal root ganglionitis associated with Sjögren's syndrome. *Ann. Neurol.* **27**: 304–315.

Harati, Y. and Niakan, A. (1986). The clinical spectrum of inflammatory angiopathic neuropathy. *J. Neurol. Neurosurg. Psychiatry* **49**: 1313–1316.

Hawke, S.H.B., Davies, L., Pamphlett, R., Guo, Y.P., Pollard, J.D., and McLeod, J.G. (1991). Vasculitic neuropathy. A clinical and pathological study. *Brain* **114**: 2175–2190.

Hogg N. (1988). The structure and function of Fc receptors. *Immunol. Today* **9**: 185–187.

Jaffe, E.S. (1984). Pathologic and clinical spectrum of post-thymic T cell malignancies. *Cancer Invest.* **2**: 413–426.

Jaffe, E.S. (1988). Pulmonary lymphocytic angiitis: a nosologic quandary. *Mayo Clin. Proc.* **63**: 411–413.

Jayne, D.R.W., Davies, M.J., Fox, C.J.V., Black, C.M., and Lockwood, C.M. (1991). Treatment of systemic vasculitis with pooled intravenous immunoglobulin. *Lancet* **337**: 1137–9.

Jennette, J.C., Falk, R.J., Andrassy, K., Bacon, P.A., Churg, J., Gross, W.L., Hagen, E.C., Hoffman, G.S., Hunder, G.G., Kallenberg, C.G.M., McCluskey, R.T., Sinico, R.A., Rees, A.J., van ES, L.A., Waldherr, R., and Wiik, A. (1994). Nomenclature of systemic vasculitides. *Arthritis Rheum.* **37**: 187–192.

Katzenstein, A.A., Carrington, C.B., and Liebow, A.A. (1979). Lymphomatoid granulomatosis: a clinicopathologic study. *Cancer* **43**: 360–373.

Kissel, J.T., Riethman, J.L., Ormeza, J., Rammohan, K.W., and Mendell, J.R. (1989). Peripheral nerve vasculitis: immune characterization of the vascular lesions. *Ann. Neurol.* **93**: 129–145.

Kussmaul, A. and Maier, R. (1866). Ueber eine bisher nicht beschrebene eigenthumliche Arterienerkrankung (Periarteritis nodosa), die mit Morbus Brightii un rapid fortschreitender allgemeiner Muskellähmung einhergeht. *Dtsch. Arch. Klin. Med.* **1**: 484–517.

Lie, J.T. (1994). Nomenclature and classification of vasculitis: plus ça change, plus c'est la même chose. *Arthritis Rheum.* **2**: 181–186.

Liebow, A.A., Carrington, C.R.B., and Friedman, P.J. (1972). Lymphomatoid granulomatosis. *Hum. Path.* **3**: 457.

Lovshin, L.L. and Kernohan, J.W. (1948). Peripheral neuritis in periarteritis nodosa. *Arch. Intern. Med.* **82**: 321–338.

Maxeiner, S.R., McDonald, J.R., and Kirlklin, J.W. (1952). Muscle biopsy in the diagnosis of periarteritis nodosa: an evaluation. *Surg. Clin. N. Am.* **32**: 1225–1235.

Mellgren, S.J., Conn, D.L., Stevens, J.C., and Dyck, P.J. (1989). Peripheral neuropathy in primary Sjögren's syndrome. *Neurology* **39**: 390–394.

Molina, R., Provost, T.T., and Alexander, E.L. (1985). Peripheral inflammatory vascular disease in Sjögrens syndrome. *Arthritis Rheum.* **28**: 1341–1347.

Moore, P.M. (1989). Immune mechanisms in the primary and secondary vasculitides. *J. Neurol. Sci.* **93**: 129–145.

Moore, P.M. and Cupps, T.R. (1983). Neurological complications of vasculitis. *Ann. Neurol.* **14**: 155–167.

Myers, J.L. (1990). Lymphomatoid granulomatosis: past, present . . . future? *Mayo Clin. Proc.* **565**: 274.

Nukada, H. and Dyck, P.J. (1984). Microsphere embolization of nerve capillaries and fiber degeneration. *Am. J. Pathol.* **115**: 275–287.

Nydegger, U.E. (1985). A place for soluble immune complexes in clinical immunology. *Immunol. Today* **6**: 80–82.

Pages, M. and Pages, A.M. (1984). La biopsie nerveuse au cours de la périartérite noueuse. Son intêret diagnostique. *Semin. Hop. Paris* **60**: 3295–3299.

Panegyres, P.K., Blumbergs, P.C., Leong, A.S.-Y., and Bourne, A.J. (1990). Vasculitis of peripheral nerve and skeletal muscle: clinicopathological and immunopathic mechanisms. *J. Neurol. Sci.* **100**: 193–202.

Panegyres, P.K., Faull, R.J., Russ, G.R., Appleton, S.L., Wangel, A.G., and Blumbergs, P.C. (1992). Endothelial cell activation in vasculitis of peripheral nerve and skeletal muscles. *J. Neurol. Neursurg. Psychiatry* **55**: 4–7.

Parlevliet, K.J., Henzen-Logmans, S.C., Oe, P.L., Bronsveld, W., Balm, A.J., and Donker, A.J. (1988). Antibodies to components of neutrophil cytoplasm: a new diagnostic tool in patients with Wegener's granulomatosis and systemic vasculitis. *Q. J. Med.* **66**: 55–63.

Parry, G.J., Brown, M.J., and Asbury, A.K. (1981). Diagnostic value of nerve biopsy in mononeuritis multiplex. *Neurology* **31**: 129–130.

Pober, J.S. and Cotran, R.S. (1990). Cytokines and endothelial cell biology. *Physiol. Rev.* **70**: 427–451.

Puechal, X., Said, G., Hilliquin, P., Coste, J., Job-Deslandre, C., Lacroix, C., and Menkes, C.J. (1995). Peripheral neuropathy with necrotizing vasculitis in rheumatoid arthritis: a clinicopathological and prognostic study of 32 patients. *Arthritis Rheum.* **38**: 1618–1629.

Ropert, A. and Metral, S. (1990). Conduction block in neuropathies with necrotizing arteritis. *Muscle Nerve* **13**: 102–105.

Said, G. (1988). Vasculitic neuropathy in the elderly. In *Peripheral Nerve Changes in the Elderly. New Issues in Neurosciences* **1**: 199–204.

Said, G., Goulon-Goeau, C., Lacroix, C., and Moulonguet, A. (1993). Proximal diabetic neuropathy. Clinical aspects and morphological findings in biopsy specimens of the intermediate cutaneous nerve of the thigh. *Ann. Neurol.* **35**: 559–569.

Said, G., Lacroix, C., Fujimura, H., Blas, C., and Faux, N. (1988). The peripheral neuropathy of necrotizing arteritis: a clinicopathologic study. *Ann. Neurol.* **23**: 461–465.

Sergent, J.S., Lockshin, M.D., Christian, C.L., and Gocke, D.J. (1976). Vasculitis with hepatitis B antigenemia: long-term observations in nine patients. *Medicine* **55**: 1–18.

Shusterman, N. and London, W.T. (1984). Hepatitis B and immune-complex disease. *N. Engl. J. Med.* **313**: 43–45.

Smiley, J.D. and Moore, S.E. (1989). Immune complex vasculitis: role of complement and IgG-Fc receptor functions. *Am. J. Med. Sci.* **298**: 267–297.

Stern, G.M., Hoffbrand, A.V., and Urich, H. (1965). The peripheral nerves and skeletal muscles in Wegener's granulomatosis: clinicopathological study of four cases. *Brain* **88**: 151–164.

Wattiaux, M.J., Kahn, M.F., Thevenet, J.P., Sauvezie, B., and Imbert, J.C. (1987). L'atteinte vasculaire de la polyarthrite rhumatoide: etude retrospective de 37 polyarthrites rhumatoides avec atteinte vasculaire et revue de la littérature. *Ann. Med. Int.* **138**: 566–587.

Wees, S.J., Sunwood, L.N., and Oh, S.J. (1981). Sural nerve biopsy in systemic necrotizing vasculitis. *Am. J. Med.* **71**: 525–532.

Winkelmann, R.K. (1980). Classification of vasculitis. In *Vasculitis*, ed. K. Wolff and R.K. Winkelmann, pp. 1–24. London: Lloyd-Luke.

12 Neuropathies associated with anti-MAG antibodies and IgM monoclonal gammopathies

E. Nobile-Orazio

Introduction

IgM monoclonal gammopathies are a group of disorders characterized by the abnormal proliferation of a single clone of lymphoplasma cells, all producing an homogeneous immunoglobulin (M protein) of IgM isotype (Kyle 1987). They classically include Waldenström's macroglobulinemia (WM), which is a malignant lymphoproliferative disease, and benign IgM monoclonal gammopathy, which is also termed monoclonal gammopathy of undetermined significance (MGUS). The latter term is now preferred for the possible evolution of benign versus malignant forms after several years (Kyle 1984). Occasionally, IgM monoclonal gammopathy may result from other lymphoproliferative disorders, including chronic lymphocytic B cell leukemia or lymphoma (Azar et al. 1957; Chazot et al. 1976; Quian et al. 1984). In a recent hematological series of 65 patients with IgM monoclonal gammopathy followed at Milan University (Baldini et al. 1994), 15% of the patients had WM, 50% had MGUS while the remaining 35% did not fulfil the criteria for either WM or MGUS, reflecting the difficulty sometimes encountered in distinguishing between these forms. We classified this intermediate form as indolent or smouldering WM, following a similar definition (smoldering myeloma) introduced by some authorities (Kyle and Greipp 1980) in multiple myeloma.

IgM monoclonal gammopathies represent approximately 10–15% of all monoclonal gammopathies (Ritzmann et al. 1975; Kyle 1978). As monoclonal gammopathies occur in 1% of the population over age 50 years and 3% of those over 70 years (Kyle 1987), the overall prevalence of IgM monoclonal gammopathy in these cohorts may be from 100 to 450 per 100 000.

The association of peripheral neuropathy with IgM monoclonal gammopathies was highlighted in 1960 by Logothetis et al. who reviewed the neurological manifestations of 182 previously reported patients with Waldenström's macroglobulinemia and found that approximately 8% of them had symptoms of neuropathy. More recent prospective studies reported the presence of neuropathy in up to 50% of patients with Waldenström's macroglobulinemia (Arfmann et al. 1984; Nobile-Orazio et al. 1987) and 31% of those with IgM MGUS (Nobile-Orazio et al. 1992) half of whom were asymptomatic (subclinical neuropathy). The latter study also showed a significantly higher prevalence of neuropathy in patients with IgM MGUS than in those with IgG or IgA MGUS. This finding has been recently confirmed (Vrethem et al. 1993) and may explain the over representation of IgM MGUS in large series of patients with neuropathy associated with MGUS (Gosselin et al. 1991; Yeung et al. 1991; Suarez & Kelly 1993; Notermans et al. 1994). Combining the above mentioned figures, the prevalence of neuropathy associated with IgM monoclonal gammopathies in the population above 50 years of age may be of at least 30 per 100 000, half of whom may be asymptomatic.

Clinical syndromes

The neuropathies associated with IgM monoclonal gammopathy are clinically heterogeneous, probably reflecting the presence of different possible pathogenetic mechanisms for the neuropathy. Cranial nerve palsies, mononeuropathies or mononeuritis multiplex were reported in patients with WM and lymphoma (Logothetis et al. 1960; Fraser et al. 1976; Moulis and Mamus 1989) and were related to lymphoplasmacytic infiltration of nerves (Aarseth et al. 1961; Chazot et al. 1976; Ince et al. 1987), amyloid deposition (Bajada et al. 1980), cryoglobulinemic vasculitis (Chad et al. 1982; Thomas et al. 1992) or microangiopathy of endoneurial vessels (Lamarca et al. 1987). In most of these patients, however, as well as in the vast majority of those with IgM MGUS, the neuropathy is chronic, progressive, symmetric and predominantly distal. A number of different mechanisms have been originally implicated in the pathogenesis of this diffuse involvement including metabolic alterations (Endtz 1960), amyloid deposits (Nick et al. 1963; Le Bourhis et al. 1964), endoneurial accumulation of the M protein (Iwashita et al. 1974; Vital et al. 1985), diffuse microangiopathy (Powell et al. 1984) and, more recently, antineural antibody activity of the M protein (Latov 1987). The latter mechanism was first demonstrated by Latov et al. (1980) in a patient with sensorimotor neuropathy and an IgM monoclonal gammopathy reacting with a peripheral nerve myelin antigen that was later characterized to be the myelin-associated glycoprotein (MAG) (Braun et al. 1982). Since then reactivity of monoclonal IgM with MAG has been frequently reported in these patients (Steck et al. 1983; Stefansson et al. 1983; Melmed et al. 1983; Hafler et al. 1986; Nobile-Orazio et al. 1987; Pestronk et al. 1991), while several other neural antigens (Table 12.1) including different cytoskeletal proteins (Dellagi et al. 1982; Connolly et al. 1993; Nobile-Orazio et al. 1994), chondroitin sulfate C (Sherman et al. 1983), the gangliosides GM1 (Ilyas et al. 1988b; Nardelli et al. 1988), GM2 (Ilyas et al. 1988a), GD1a (Bollensen et al. 1989) and GD1b (Ben Younes-Chennoufi et al. 1992), sulfatide (Pestronk et al. 1991) and other glycolipids (Ilyas et al. 1985; Freddo et al. 1986a; Miyatani et al. 1987) were found to react, though less frequently, with IgM from other patients. IgM reactivity with one or more of these antigens was recently found in 65% of 75 patients with neuropathy and IgM monoclonal gammopathy but only 7% of 45 with IgM monoclonal gammopathy without neuropathy, and was more frequent in neuropathy patients with IgM MGUS (84%) than with WM (38%) (Nobile-Orazio et al. 1994). In this as in other series (Murray et al. 1986; Nobile-Orazio et al. 1987, 1989; Kelly et al. 1988). MAG was the more frequent target for IgM M proteins in patients with neuropathy (56%) followed by sulfatide (5%) and neurofilaments (5%) while IgM reactivities with the other neural antigens were only sporadically found. Cryoglobulinemia was the more frequent possible mechanism for the neuropathy (23%) in patients without antineural IgM reactivity. As some of these IgM reactivities have been associated with homogeneous neuropathy features, which suggests that the heterogeneity of the neuropathy in patients with IgM monoclonal gammopathy may partly reflect an immunological heterogeneity, the different clinical syndromes will be reviewed in relation to the antigen specificity of monoclonal IgM.

Neuropathy associated with anti-MAG IgM reactivity

MAG is a minor constituent of both CNS and PNS myelin membranes of approximate molecular weight (MW) of 100 kDa. It is mostly concentrated in the periaxonal region and other uncompacted regions of PNS myelin including Schmidt–Lanterman incisures, lateral loops and outer mesaxon, where it probably plays an important role in maintaining glial–axonal interactions (reviewed in Trapp 1990).

Table 12.1 *Anti-neural IgM reactivities in neuropathies associated with IgM monoclonal gammopathies*

Antigens	Frequency[a] (%) %	Clinical impairment[b]	Nerve pathology	Authors (see also text)
MAG/SGPG/P0	50–60%	S>M, SM	Dem.	Latov et al. (1980, 1988); Steck et al. (1983); Melmed et al. (1983); Nobile-Orazio et al. (1987)
Chondroitin sulfate C	1	SM	Axonal	Sherman et al. (1983)
Sulfatide	5	S, S>M, SM	Axonal, Dem.	Pestronk et al. (1991)
Cytoskeletal proteins: vimentin tubulin, 200k NF	5	variable	variable	Dellagi et al. (1982) Connolly et al. (1993) Nobile-Orazio et al. (1994)
Gangliosides				
GM1/GD1b	1	M, M>S, LMND	?	Freddo et al. (1986)
GM2	?	?	?	Ilyas et al. (1988)
GD1a	2	M	Dem.	Bollensen et al. (1989)
GD1b	1	SM	Axonal	Ben Younes-Chennoufi et al. (1992)
Disialosyl gangliosides	?	S>M	Dem.	Ilyas et al. (1986)
Phos. Ac.+ Gangliosides	?	SM	?	Freddo et al. (1986)
SGLPG	?	SM	?	Miyatani et al. (1987)

Notes:
[a] According to Nobile-Orazio et al. (1994) except GD1a (Carpo et al. 1996).
[b] Dem.: demyelinating; SM: sensory; M: motor; LMND: lower motor neuron disease; SM: sensorimotor neuropathy; S>M, M<S: predominantly sensory or motor.

In over 50% of patients with neuropathy associated with IgM monoclonal gammopathy and almost 70% of those with IgM MGUS the M protein binds to MAG (Figure 12.1) (Hafler et al. 1986; Murray et al. 1986; Nobile-Orazio et al. 1987, 1989, 1992, 1994; Kelley et al. 1988; Latov et al. 1988b; Gosselin et al. 1991; Yeung et al. 1991; Suarez and Kelly 1993). IgM reactivity with MAG is less frequent in patients with WM (38%) and is only sporadically found in patients with IgM-secreting lymphoma or leukemia (Latov 1987). Conversely, over 80% of patients with anti-MAG IgM have a IgM MGUS and most of the remaining patients have an indolent WM, which suggests that the finding of anti-MAG IgM in a patient with monoclonal gammopathy may be prognostically favourable for the presence of malignancy. IgM reactivity with MAG has also been reported in some patients with neuropathy without IgM monoclonal gammopathy (Nobile-Orazio et al. 1984b, 1989; Julien et al. 1989) but in these patients IgM reactivity was monoclonal, revealing the presence of an otherwise undetectable monoclonal gammopathy. In only few patients, reactivity with MAG was not associated with neuropathy (Nobile-Orazio et al. 1994), while in others it was associated with a subclinical neuropathy (Nobile-Orazio et al. 1989) that frequently, though not invariably, later became clinically manifest (personal observation). In only two cases the appearance of anti-MAG IgM was found to follow the development of neu ropathy (Gregory et al. 1993; Valldeoriola et al. 1993).

In patients with IgM monoclonal gammopathy IgM reactivity with MAG is specific or predominant for the light chain of the M protein, i.e. kappa in almost

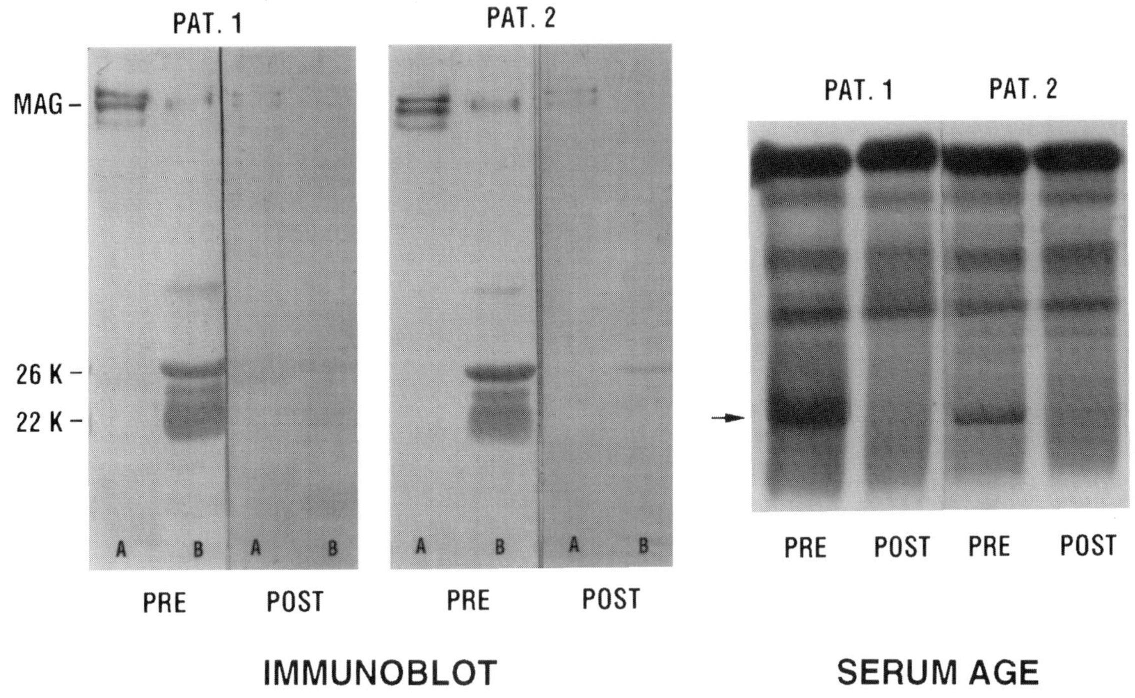

Figure 12.1 *Binding of patients' IgM antibodies to MAG and to the cross-reactive peripheral nervous system (PNS) myelin glycoproteins by immunoblot and patients' serum M proteins by agarose gel electrophoresis (AGE). For immunoblot, central nervous system (CNS) (A) and PNS (B) myelin proteins were separated by SDS polyacrylamide gel electrophoresis (PAGE), transferred onto nitrocellulose sheets, and immunostained with patients' sera using peroxidase conjugated goat immunoglobulins to human IgM. IgM from two patients with neuropathy and IgM monoclonal gammopathy bound to MAG in CNS and, faintly, in PNS myelin and to some PNS myelin glycoproteins with molecular weights of 22–26 KDa (K), recently found to include the myelin proteins Po and PMP-22 (PRE). In both patients serum absorbtion with PNS myelin (POST) almost completely removed IgM reactivity with MAG and with the cross-reactive glycoproteins. The same procedure also removed the circulating M proteins (arrows) as shown by serum AGE before and after absorbtion with PNS myelin.*

90% of positive patients, and is always directed against the same or closely related epitope(s) in the carbohydrate moiety in MAG (Frail et al. 1984; Shy et al. 1984; Lieberman et al. 1985; Ilyas et al. 1990). This epitope is also present in other glycoconjugates in nerve bound by anti-MAG M proteins, including the myelin glycoproteins Po and PMP-22 (Figure 12.1) (Nobile-Orazio et al. 1984a; Bollensen et al. 1988; Snipes et al. 1993) and the glycosphingolipids sulfoglucuronyl paragloboside (SGPG) and sulfoglucuronyl lactosaminyl paragloboside (SGLPG) (Figure 12.2) (Chou et al. 1986; Ariga et al. 1987) and is closely related if not identical to the HNK 1/L2 epitope expressed by human natural killer cell and by several neural cell adhesion molecules (McGarry et al. 1983; Kruse et al. 1984; Bollensen and Schachner 1987; Burger et al. 1990).

Clinical findings

The neuropathy in patients with anti-MAG M protein is quite homogeneous. Almost 80–90% of the patients are men. Even if the earliest reported patient with anti-MAG IgM developed his first symptoms at the age of 34 years (Latov et al. 1980), in most patients symptoms appear in the sixth or seventh decade and only occasionally after the age of 80 years (Nobile-Orazio et al. 1994; Smith 1994). In almost 90% of patients the neuropathy presents with sensory symptoms in the legs including paresthesias, hypodysestesia,

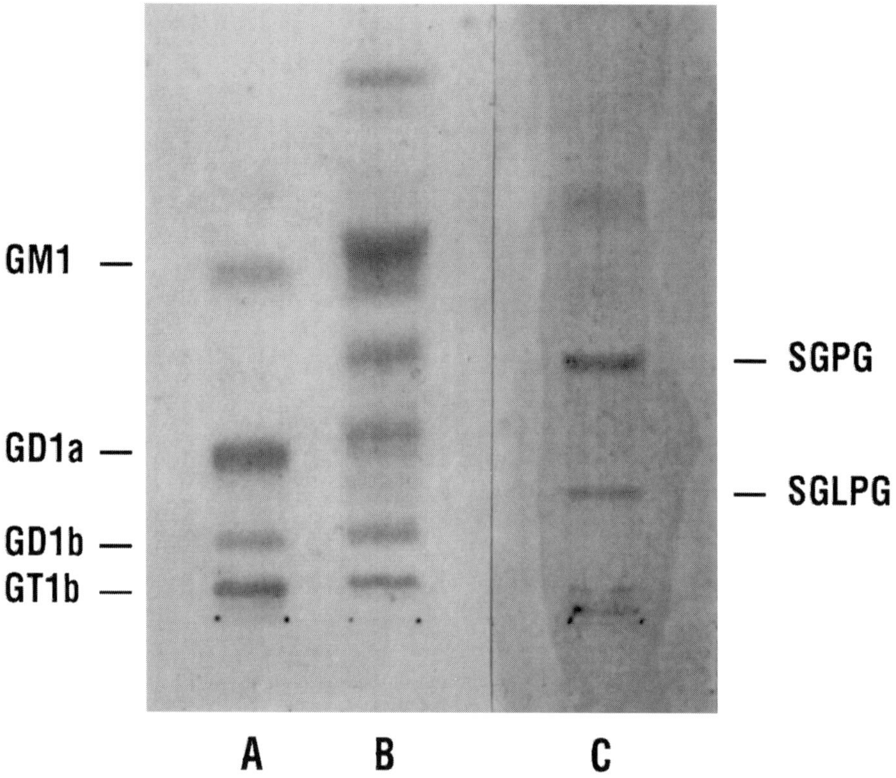

Figure 12.2 *Binding of human anti-MAG IgM antibodies to nerve glycolipids by immunostaining after high performance thin layer chromatography (overlay HPTLC). Pooled bovine brain gangliosides (GM1, GD1a, GD1b and GT1b, Fidia, Italy) (A) and human peripheral nerve glycolipids (B and C) were separated by HPTLC and stained with resorcinol (A and B) or incubated with serum from a patient with high titers of anti-MAG IgM antibodies and counterstained with a peroxidase conjugated goat immunoglobulins to human IgM (C). Patient's IgM bound to two nerve glycolipids migrating between GM1 and GD1a and between GD1a and GD1b corresponding, respectively, to glucuronylsulfate paragloboside (SGPG) and glucuronylsulfate lactosaminyl paragloboside (SGLPG).*

cramps or other pains and unsteadiness of gait, while weakness is frequently absent at onset (Table 12.2). A postural tremor in the upper limbs may be present at onset in 10% of patients, half of whom report it as the only initial symptom (Nobile–Orazio et al. 1994). After the onset, in the vast majority of patients the neuropathy run a slowly progressive course with a symmetric, distal impairment affecting the legs before and more severely than the arms. The neuropathy tends to stabilize after a few years (Smith 1994) but may later progress.

On clinical examination (Table 12.2), almost two-thirds of the patients have a predominant or selective sensory impairment and one-third of them have sensorimotor impairment whereas a predominant motor impairment has been only occasionally reported (Antoine et al. 1993; Nobile-Orazio et al. 1994). Some degree of ataxia with wide based and unsteady stance and gait is present in almost 80% of patients and correlates with a pronounced loss of position and vibration senses. Impairment of touch sensation in a sock-and-glove distribution is frequent but is rarely pronounced while pain sensation is generally preserved. Limb weakness and hypotrophy are found in two-thirds of patients but are prominent in a minority of them. Although a postural tremor in the upper limbs has been considered an hallmark of the neuropathy in these patients, its frequency in large series ranges from 36 to

Table 12.2 *Frequency of neuropathy symptoms and signs in 42 patients with IgM M protein reacting with MAG*

Symptoms and signs	Number of patients[a]
Symptoms at onset	
Paresthesias	24 (57)
Weakness	7 (17)
Gait unbalance	7 (17)
Upper limb tremor	4 (10)
Hypo/dysesthesias	4 (10)
Limb pain	2 (5)
Cramps	1 (2)
Symptoms at neurological examination	
Paresthesias	35 (74)
Weakness	30 (71)
Hypo/dysesthesias	27 (64)
Cramps	9 (21)
Neurological signs at examination	
Hypo/areflexia	41 (98)
Deep sensory loss: total	40 (95)
moderate or severe only	34 (81)
Ataxia	32 (76)
Superficial sensory loss: total	31 (74)
moderate or severe only	16 (38)
Weakness: total	27 (64)
moderate or severe only	16 (38)
Hypotrophy: total	21 (50)
moderate or severe only	9 (21)
Upper limb tremor	15 (36)

Note:
[a] Values in parentheses are percentages.
Source: From Nobile-Orazio et al. (1994).

89% (Yeung et al. 1991, Nobile-Orazio et al. 1994; Smith 1994). Deep tendon reflexes are almost invariably lost while cranial nerves and the autonomic system are not impaired.

Although these patients may develop some disability after several years, only few become severely disabled. In a recent prospective study on 18 patients followed for up to 14 years (mean 7.4 years) for instance, only two were unable to walk within 10 years from onset of symptoms (Smith 1994). This relatively low frequence of disability was confirmed in another prospective study with only one patient out of seven in a wheel chair within 5 years (Notermans et al. 1994).

Even if these patients do not have clinical impairment of the CNS a subclinical impairment may be revealed by electrophysiological studies including visual evoked potentials (VEPs) and magnetic stimulation and by magnetic resonance imaging (MRI) studies (Meier et al. 1984; Barbieri et al. 1987; Leger et al. 1992), and usually correlates with the presence of the anti-MAG M protein in the cerebrospinal fluid (CSF) (Barbieri et al. 1987).

Laboratory findings

CSF studies in these patients may reveal increased protein concentration with normal cell count, the presence of the monoclonal IgM and of anti-MAG antibodies (Barbieri et al. 1987; Cruz et al. 1991). Routine laboratory investigations are usually unrevealing in patients with IgM MGUS except for increased IgM levels (<30 g L^{-1}), the M protein by serum electrophoresis (Figure 11.1), and, occasionally, of an increased ethrocyte sedimentation rate. Higher levels of serum IgM (>30 g L^{-1}), anemia, lymphocytosis, thrombocytopenia, Bence–Jones proteinuria and diffuse bone marrow lymphoplasmacytic infiltrates are usually observed in patients with WM (Kyle 1987; Baldini et al. 1994).

In earlier studies serum IgM reactivity with myelin, corresponding in most instances to reactivity with MAG, was detected by a complement fixation assay (Latov et al. 1980) or by indirect immunohystochemistry on nerve sections (Dellagi et al. 1983; Smith et al. 1983; Harbs et al. 1985). IgM reactivity with MAG was first demonstrated by immunoblot (Western blot) after SDS-polyacrylamide gel electrophoresis (PAGE) of CNS myelin (Figure 11.1) (Braun et al. 1982; Steck et al. 1983; Stefansson et al. 1983; Nobile-Orazio et al. 1987) and later by ELISA (Nobile-Orazio et al. 1983; Pestronk et al. 1994) or radioimmunoassay (RIA) (Nobile-Orazio et al. 1985) using the purified MAG. IgM reactivity with the glycolipids SGPG and SGLPG was detected by immunostaining after HPTLC of nerve glycolipids (Figure 12.2) (Freddo et al. 1985a) and is currently measured by ELISA (McGinnis et al. 1988) using the purified SGPG. IgM reactivity with the low MW nerve glycoproteins cross-reacting with MAG, including Po and PMP-22, can be detected by immunoblot after SDS-PAGE of PNS myelin or nerve (Figure 12.1) (Nobile-Orazio et al. 1984a). In our experience the immunoblot system is the most sensitive and reliable method for measuring anti-MAG IgM antibodies and best correlates with the typical clinical syndrome (Nobile-Orazio et al. 1987, 1989; van den Berg et al. 1996). With this as well as with all the above mentioned systems it is mandatory to measure serum antibody titers by serial dilution and to establish normal reference values as low levels of anti-MAG or anti-SGPG IgM may be found both by ELISA and immunoblot in a consistent proportion or controls with and without circulating M protein, including some normal subjects (McGinnis et al. 1988; Nobile-Orazio et al. 1989, 1994), while high titers (over 1:6400 by immunoblot in our laboratory) are almost invariably associated with neuropathy (Nobile-Orazio et al. 1994; Pestronk et al. 1994; L.H. van den Berg et al. 1996).

Electrophysiological findings

In approximately 80% of patients with anti-MAG IgM, electrophysiological studies are consistent with a predominantly demyelinating neuropathy with slow motor and sensory conduction velocities, conduction block and prolonged F wave and distal latencies (Melmed et al. 1983; Nobile-Orazio et al. 1987; Kelly 1990). In two recent studies the mean motor conduction velocities in these patients were of 17.8 and 22.9 m s^{-1}, respectively (Nobile-Orazio et al. 1994; Smith 1994). A disproportionate prolongation of distal latencies for the degree of proximal conduction slowing has been recently shown in these patients suggesting a distal accentuation of conduction slowing (Kaku et al. 1994). This finding might help in distinguishing this neuropathy from other chronic acquired and inherited demyelinating polyneuropathies. Sensory nerve are usually more affected than motor nerves and are more severely affected in the lower than upper limbs reflecting the distribution of clinical impairment. Needle electromyography shows signs of chronic partial denervation with sparse fibrillation with a more severe involvement of intrinsic foot muscles (Nobile-Orazio et al. 1987).

Pathological findings

Morphological studies on sural nerve biopsies in these patients show loss of myelinated fibers on semithin sections without inflammatory infiltrates, amyloid deposits or vasculitis. Teased fiber studies almost invariably show segmental demyelination and remyelination sometimes associated with axonal degeneration (Meier et al. 1983; Melmed et al. 1983; Nemni et al. 1983; Steck et al. 1983; Stefansson et al. 1983; Nobile-Orazio et al. 1987, 1989, 1994; Vitel et al. 1989), whereas a predominant axonal degeneration is rarely found (Mendell et al. 1985). A peculiar finding on ultrastructural examination is the presence of a variable number of fibers with widely spaced myelin lamellae due to an increased distance between the major dense lines (Figure 12.3) (Meier et al. 1983; Melmed et al. 1983; Steck et al. 1983; Stefansson et al. 1983; Smith et al. 1983). This abnormality is often restricted to the outermost myelin lamellae and was found in over 90% of patients with anti-MAG IgM (Vital et al. 1989) but only rarely in other neuropathies. It is still debated whether this widening is due to the deposition of IgM between the major dense lines (Melmed et al. 1983; Tatum 1993) or to intramyelinic edema, possibly caused by the cytolytic effect of complement (Monaco et al. 1990). Direct immunohistochemical studies on sural nerve biopsies almost invariably reveal the presence of deposits of IgM (Figure 12.4) (Stefansson et al. 1983; Takatsu et al. 1985; Nobile-Orazio et al. 1987, 1994; Vital et al. 1989; Smith 1994) and, when examined, of complement, around the myelin sheaths (Hays et al. 1988; Monaco et al. 1990). A close correlation between the number of fibers with myelin splittings and that of fibers bound by the terminal cytolytic complex of complement has been demonstrated (Monaco et al. 1990).

Therapy

Treatment of patients with anti-MAG IgM is primarily directed at lowering anti-MAG IgM levels. This was attempted using several immunosuppressive regimens, either alone or in combination (Table 12.3) including prednisone, plasma exchange, cytotoxic agents (Latov et al. 1980; Melmed et al. 1983; Stefansson et al. 1983; Meier et al. 1984; Sherman et al. 1984; Ernerudh et al. 1986, 1992; Smith et al. 1987; Haas and Tatum 1988; Kelly et al. 1988; Nobile-Orazio et al. 1988) and, more recently, high-dose intravenous immunoglobulin (IVIG) (Cook et al. 1990; Hoang-Xuan et al. 1993) and fludarabine (Sherman et al. 1994). Even if these therapies did not always result in improvement of the neuropathy, possibly reflecting different responses

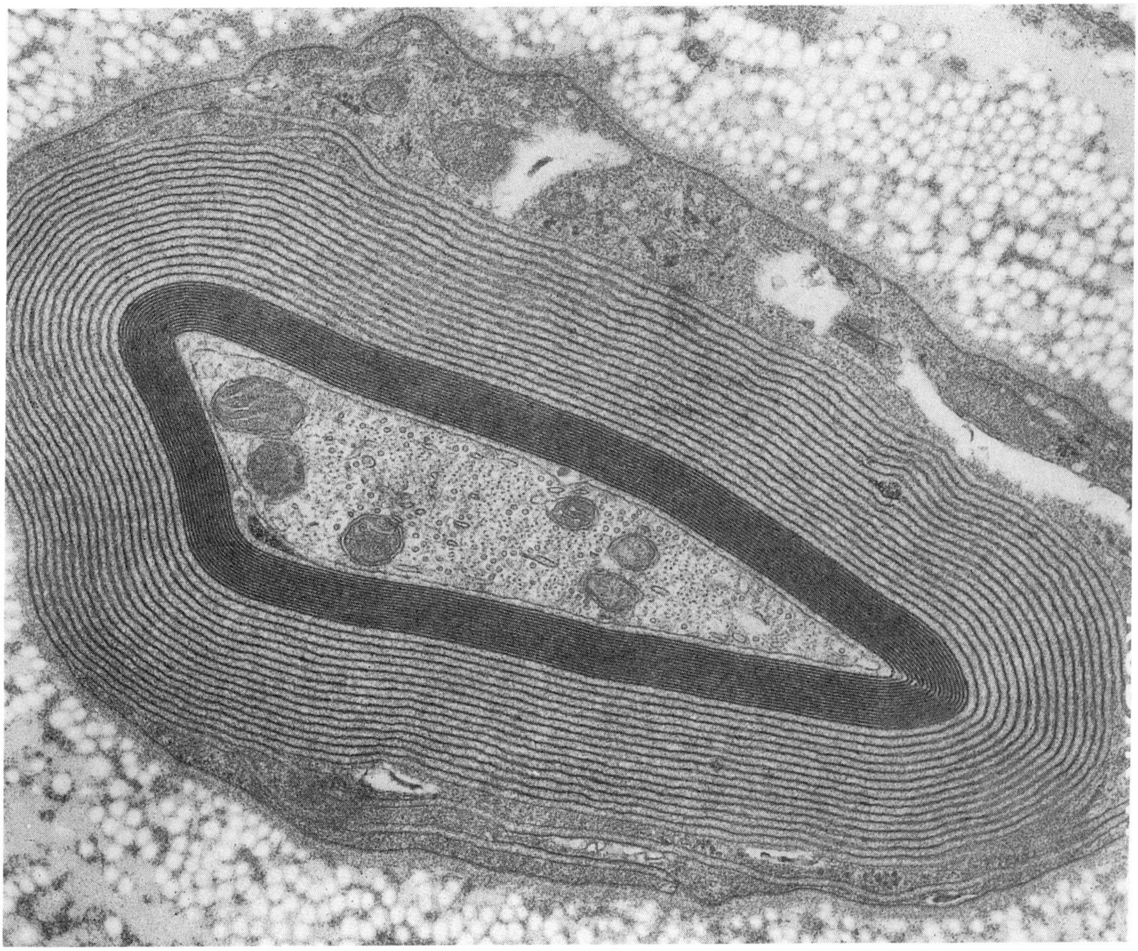

Figure 12.3 *Electron micrograph showing a myelinated nerve fiber in the sural nerve of a patient with neuropathy associated with IgM monoclonal gammopathy. There is a typical widening of peripheral myelin lamellae while the periodicity of the inner lamellae is normal. The patient had high titers of IgM antibodies reacting with sulfatide but not with MAG. Courtesy of Dr Maurizio Moggio, Milan University, Italy.*

to treatment of M protein-secreting clones, a 50% reduction of serum IgM or antibody levels was almost (Ernerudh et al. 1992; Melmed et al. 1983; Stefansson et al. 1983) invariably associated with clinical improvement (Latov et al. 1980; Kelly et al. 1988; Nobile-Orazio et al. 1988; Sherman et al. 1994). Plasma exchange is effective in rapidly lowering serum IgM M protein levels but its effects are transient as IgM rapidly rises to pretreatment levels after exchanges are suspended or delayed and needs to be associated with other immunosuppressants (Sherman et al. 1984; Haas and Tatum 1988). In our hands the alkylating agent chlorambucil, alone or in combination with prednisone, was effective in lowering anti-MAG M protein levels and in improving the neuropathy in 40% of patients while cyclophosphamide was not effective in patients who failed to respond to chlorambucil, and was less well tolerated (Nobile-Orazio et al. 1988). We currently treat our patients with oral chlorambucil (10 mg per day, reduced within 1–2 months to a maintenance regimen sufficient to keep the lymphocyte count between 500 and 1000/mm^3), alone or in combination with plasma exchange, for 6 months, after which we suspend chlorambucil if it is unable to lower IgM levels or to prevent their rise after plasma exchange and keep the patients in plasma exchange alone every 2–3 weeks.

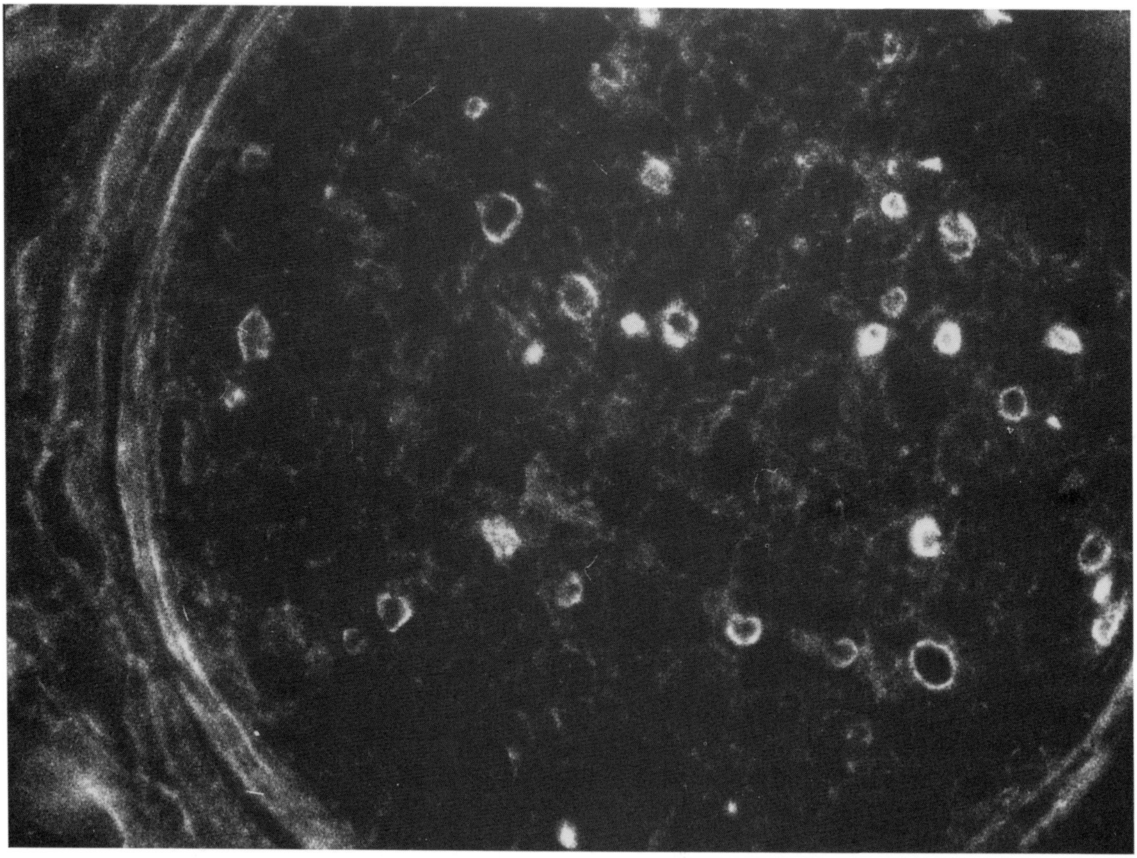

Figure 12.4 *Myelin deposits of IgM in the sural nerve of a patient with neuropathy and IgM monoclonal gammopathy reacting with MAG, by immunofluorescence microscopy. A 6 μm section of patient's nerve was incubated with fluorescein conjugated anti-human IgM rabbit immunoglobulins. Deposits of patient's IgM are found around the myelin sheath of several nerve fibers. Original magnification 400 ×. Courtesy of Dr Maurizio Moggio, Milan University, Italy.*

Better results were obtained with more intense immunosuppressive regimens (Kelly et al. 1988) but were frequently associated with severe side-effects. As these therapies may be harmful, especially in older patients, we prefer not to use them in patients with little or no restriction in their daily life or when the neuropathy is not progressive, unless treatment is required by hematological conditions. A symptomatic therapy for paresthesias and pain, if present, and reassurance concerning the slow progression of the disease (see above) may be sufficient in some patients. Fludarabine, a new immunosuppressive agent, was recently found to be extremely effective in these patients and associated with less adverse reaction than alkylating agents (Sherman et al. 1994).

Pathogenesis and animal models

There is considerable evidence that the neuropathy in these patients is an autoimmune disease caused by binding of anti-MAG IgM antibodies to one or more glycoconjugates in nerve bearing the HNK1/L2 epitope, including the glycoproteins MAG, P0, PMP-22 and the glycolipids SGPG and SGLPG: (1) High titers of anti-MAG antibodies have been almost invariably associated with a clinically homogeneous demyelinating neuropathy. These antibodies have also occasionally been found in asymptomatic patients, but most of them had a subclinical neuropathy (Nobile-Orazio et al. 1987, 1989) that frequently later became clinically manifest. Even if the lack of correlation between anti-MAG antibody titers and the severity of neuropathy among different individ-

Table 12.3 *Effect of immunosuppressive therapies in patients with neuropathy and anti-MAG IgM M proteins*

Authors	No. of patients	Therapy[a]	Improved
Latov et al. (1980)	1	PE+P+Ch	1
Stefansson et al. (1883)	1	PE+IS(?)	
Melmed et al. (1983)	3	P (1+Ch; 1+PE+Ch; 1PE+Az)	
Meier et al. (1984)	1	PE+P+Ch	1
Ernerudh et al. (1986)	3	PE	1
Smith et al. (1987)	4	3 PE(2+Ch)	2
		1 Ad+Cy, Ch	1
Kelly et al. (1988)	4	PE+P+Ch or Cy	4
Haas et al. (1988)	1	PE	1
Nobile-Orazio et al. (1988)	5	3 Ch (1+P)	2
		1 Ch, Cy	
		1 Ch, Cy+P	
Cook et al. (1990)	1	IVIg	1
Ernerudh et al. (1992)	5[b]	4 P (1+PE+Ch; 1+Ch)	3[b]
		1 Ch, M	
Hoang-Xuan et al. (1993)	2	IVIG	2
Sherman et al. (1994)	8	Fludarabine	7
Total	38		25 (66%)

Notes:
[a] P: prednisone; PE: plasma exchange; Ch: chlorambucil; Cy: cyclophosphamide; Az: azathioprine; M: melphalan; Ad: adriamycin; IS: immunosuppressive drugs not specified: IVIG: high dose intravenous immunoglobulins.
[b] Including one patient from Ernerudh et al. (1986).

uals may argue against a possible pathogenetic role of these antibodies (Gosselin et al. 1992), this discrepancy is not unusual in autoimmune diseases and may reflect different fine antibody specificities (Lieberman et al. 1985; Ilyas et al. 1990) or affinities (Ogino et al. 1994) for the antigen in vitro than in vivo. (2) Myelin deposits of IgM and, when examined, of complement have been found almost invariably in sural nerve biopsies in these patients. (3) With only few exceptions, therapeutic reduction of anti-MAG IgM levels, though difficult to achieve, was associated with improvement of the neuropathy. (4) Experimental demyelination of the nerve has been induced in animals by intraneural (Hays et al. 1987; Willison et al. 1988; Monaco et al. 1995) or systemic (Tatum 1993) injection of serum containing anti-MAG IgM antibodies.

Experimental studies of demyelination in animals were quite helpful in clarifying the possible mechanisms of the neuropathy in these patients. In earlier studies, injections of anti-MAG IgM antibodies in feline nerves caused demyelination only when added with fresh complement (Hays et al. 1987; Willison et al. 1988) suggesting that antibodies caused demyelination by complement fixation. Recently, however, demyelination of nerve with prominent widening of myelin lamellae superimposable to that observed in patients, was obtained in chickens by systemic injection of purified anti-MAG IgM without complement (Tatum 1993). This finding led to the hypothesis that antibodies may act by inhibiting myelin turnover or by altering the normal periodicity of myelin by separating or impeding the fusion of apposed leaflets of intraperiod lines, possibly explaining the slow progression of the neuropathy in these patients. It was not however investigated in this study whether human IgM was able to activate chicken complement. More recently, Monaco et al. (1995) induced demyelination with widely spaced myelin lamellae in rabbit nerve by intraneural injection of either anti-MAG IgM or the terminal complement complex (TCC).

They also demonstrated that in nerves treated with anti-MAG IgM, the abnormalities were concurrent with the activation of the rabbit's own complement to the formation of TCC. This finding together with the lack of effect of anti-MAG IgM in C6-deficient rabbit and the already mentioned correlation in nerve biopsies between the number of fibers with widened myelin lamellae and that of fibers showing TCC deposits seems to confirm the possible effector role of complement in the demyelination induced by anti-MAG IgM.

If the pathogenetic mechanisms of the neuropathy in patients with anti-MAG IgM have been, at least in part, elucidated, little is known about the cause of the development of IgM monoclonal gammopathy and its frequent reactivity with the same or closely related epitopes in the carbohydrate moiety of MAG. Low levels of anti-MAG IgM antibodies are found in approximately 20% of controls with and without circulating M protein, including some normal subjects (McGinnis et al. 1988; Nobile-Orazio et al. 1989) and B cells capable of secreting anti-MAG antibodies are present at birth (Lee et al. 1990), indicating that these antibodies are a common constituent of the human antibody repertoire (Dighiero et al. 1986). It is therefore possible that similar to the mechanism postulated for other M proteins with autoantibody activity (Avrameas et al. 1981; Dighiero et al. 1986) anti-MAG M proteins derive from monoclonal expansion of normally occurring anti-MAG IgM secreting clones. The reason for this expansion is not known but may be caused by transformations or mutations of anti-MAG secreting B cell clones disrupting normal regulatory interactions or by an activation of regulatory T cells, possibly induced by self or foreign antigens bearing the same or closely related carbohydrate epitopes (Latov 1987). Anti-MAG M protein secretion in vitro is subjected to T cell regulation (Latov et al. 1985; Spatz and Latov 1986) and anti-idiotypic antibodies to the M protein have been demonstrated in some patients (Nobile-Orazio et al. 1985; Page et al. 1985) suggesting that anti-MAG M-protein secretion, though abnormally increased, is somehow regulated as also indicated by the fact that in most patients anti-MAG M protein levels are stable for years and rapidly return to their original level when treatment directed at their reduction is suspended. Whether these antibodies may also have some as yet unknown regulatory role on the immune system (Tanaka et al. 1985) is not known but may prompt some caution on the risks of therapies directed at reducing M proteins levels in these patients.

Neuropathy with anti-chondroitin sulfate C IgM reactivity

Chondroitin sulfate C is a sulfated glycosaminoglycan widely represented in nerve endoneurium, axonal and neuronal membranes as well as in skin, cartilage and connective tissue (Margolis and Margolis 1989).

Sherman et al. (1983) first reported on two patients with a slowly progressive sensorimotor neuropathy, epidermolysis and an IgM monoclonal gammopathy reacting with chondroitin sulfate C. Since then, seven additional patients with neuropathy and IgM monoclonal gammopathy reacting with chondroitin sulfate C have been reported (Yee et al. 1989; Quattrini et al. 1991; Mamoli et al. 1992; Nemni et al. 1993; Nobile-Orazio et al. 1994). These patients had a chronic sensorimotor (Sherman et al. 1983; Yee et al. 1989) or predominantly sensory distal neuropathy (Quattrini et al. 1991; Mamoli et al. 1992; Nemni et al. 1993) often presenting with paresthesias and numbness in the legs. Some patients had a prominent deep sensory loss with gait ataxia. The neuropathy was often symmetrical with a glove-stocking distribution but was occasionally asymmetric (Yee et al. 1989).

Morphological studies on nerve biopsy in these patients showed axonal degeneration with deposits of IgM in the endoneurium (Takatsu et al. 1985; Yee et al. 1989; Nemni et al. 1993) and, in one patient, at Schmidt–Lanterman incisures (Quattrini et al. 1991). One patient improved with therapeutic reduction of IgM levels (Sherman et al. 1983) suggesting a possible pathogenetic role for this reactivity in the neuropathy. In some of these patients the M protein also bound by immunoblot to several bands, probably corresponding to mucopolysaccarides, in the endoneurium and other tissues (Freddo et al. 1985b; Yee et al. 1989; Quattrini et al. 1991), but only nerve was clinically affected in most of them.

Neuropathy with anti-sulfatide IgM reactivity

Sulfatide (galactosylceramide-3-*O*-sulfate) is the major acidic glycosphingolipid in central and periph-

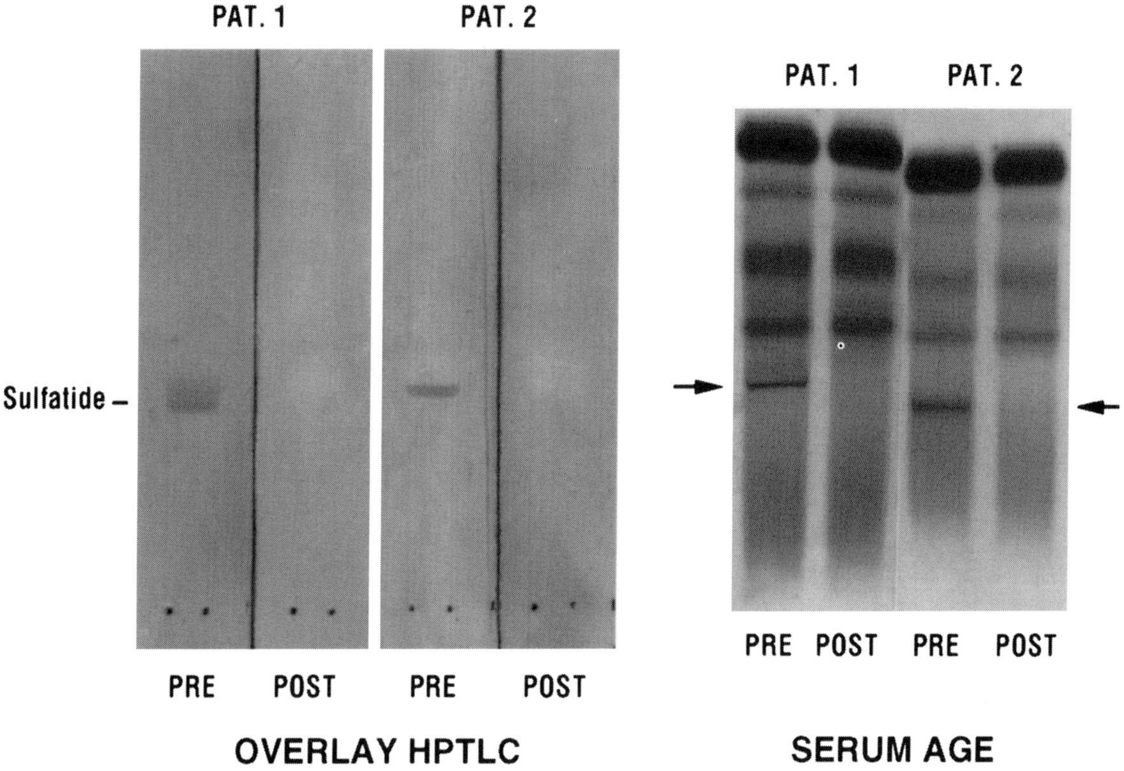

Figure 12.5 *Binding of patients' IgM antibodies to sulfatide by immunostaining after high performance thin layer chromatography (overlay HPTLC) and patients' serum M proteins by agarose gel electrophoresis (AGE). After migration by HPTLC, the purified sulfatide (Sigma, USA), was immunostained with patients' sera using peroxidase conjugated goat immunoglobulins to human IgM. IgM from two patients with neuropathy and IgM monoclonal gammopathy bound to sulfatide (PRE) while no reactivity with sulfatide was observed after serum absorbtion with sulfatide (POST). The same procedure also removed patients' M proteins (arrow) as shown by serum AGE before and after absorbtion with sulfatide.*

eral nerve myelin where its concentration is about 100 times higher than that of any ganglioside (Svennerholm & Fredman 1990).

Anti-sulfatide antibodies (see Chapter 14) were initially reported in patients with inflammatory demyelinating neuropathies (Fredman et al. 1991) while more recently high anti-sulfatide titers, mostly IgM, were associated with a chronic sensory axonal neuropathy (Pestronk et al. 1991). Since then more than 40 patients with neuropathy and high antisulfatide antibody titers, mostly IgM, have been reported, half of whom had an IgM monoclonal gammopathy (Ilyas et al. 1992; Quattrini et al. 1992; Nemni et al. 1993; van den Berg et al. 1993; Nobile-Orazio et al. 1994). In our series, IgM reactivity with sulfatide was present in 5% of patients with neuropathy and IgM monoclonal gammopathy and was always due to the M protein (Figure 12.5) (Nobile-Orazio et al. 1994). Most patients with antisulfatide IgM had a chronic progressive, predominantly sensory or sensorimotor neuropathy, often presenting with painful paresthesias and later affecting all sensory modalities (Ilyas et al. 1992; Quattrini et al. 1992; Nemni et al. 1993; van den Berg et al. 1993: Nobile-Orazio et al. 1994). Some patients also had prominent limb weakness and gait ataxia. The neuropathy was initially reported to be predominantly axonal (Pestronk et al. 1991; Quattrini et al. 1992; Nemni et al. 1993), but there are also reports of a demyelinating impairment

(Ilyas et al. 1992; van den Berg et al. 1993; Nobile-Orazio et al. 1994), and of selective small fiber involvement with normal electrophysiological or nerve biopsy studies (Pestronk et al. 1991; Quattrini et al. 1992).

Ultrastructural studies on sural nerve biopsy in all our patients showed abnormally spaced myelin lamellae identical to those observed in patients with anti-MAG IgM (Figure 11.3), while myelin deposits of the M protein and complement were found by direct immunofluorescence (Nobile-Orazio et al. 1994). The high concentration of sulfatide in myelin as well as the close correlation between the number of fibers with abnormally spaced myelin lamellae and that of fibers with deposits of the terminal cytolytic complex of complement in one patient (No. 6 in Monaco et al. 1990), support the hypothesis that, at least in some patients, myelin can be the target for these antibodies. Myelin deposits of IgM were not found in other patients, but their IgM bound to dorsal root ganglia (Quattrini et al. 1992; Nemni et al. 1993) possibly revealing a different site of attack for these antibodies. These differences may either reflect different fine specificities of anti-sulfatide antibodies or the presence in a consistent proportion of patients of other IgM reactivities, including MAG (Pestronk et al. 1991; Ilyas et al. 1992; van den Berg et al. 1993; Nobile-Orazio et al. 1994), GM1 (Quattrini et al. 1992) and chondroitin sulfate C (Nemni et al. 1993). No data are available on the clinical response to treatment in these patients, but two of our patients improved concomitantly with therapeutic reduction of serum IgM levels (unpublished observations) supporting the hypothesis that these antibodies may have pathogenetic relevance.

Neuropathy with IgM reactivity with cytoskeletal proteins

Several proteins constitute the main cytoskeletal organelles of neural cells including alpha and beta-tubulin for microtubules, neurofilaments (NF), glial fibrillary acidic protein and vimentin for intermediate filaments, and actin and myosin for microfilaments (Goldman and Yen 1986).

IgM reactivities with cytoskeletal proteins, including vimentin (Dellagi et al. 1982), beta-tubulin (Connolly et al. 1993) and the 200 kDa NF (Nobile-Orazio et al. 1994), have been occasionally reported in patients with neuropathy associated with IgM monoclonal gammopathy. In our series for instance IgM reactivity with the 200 kDa NF (Figure 12.6) was found in 5% of patients with neuropathy and IgM monoclonal gammopathy while one additional patient with a subclinical impairment had high anti-beta-tubulin IgM (Manfredini et al. 1994). Both patients with anti-200 kDa NF IgM had a sensorimotor demyelinating neuropathy, while the patient with IgM reacting with betatubulin had a relapsing-remitting chronic inflammatory demyelinating neuropathy (CIDP). This reactivity was also frequently observed by ELISA in CIDP patients without IgM monoclonal gammopathy (Connolly et al. 1993), but this finding was not confirmed using an immunoblot technique (Manfredini et al. 1994). Patients with anti-NF IgM had a clinically and electrophysiologically heterogeneous neuropathy presenting with paresthesias, cramps or weakness, and frequently had other concomitant possible mechanisms for the neuropathy, including anti-MAG IgM or cryoglobulinemia, casting some doubts on the pathogenetic relevance of this reactivity.

Neuropathy with anti-ganglioside IgM reactivity

Gangliosides are sialic acid-containing glycosphingolipids that are particularly abundant in neural membranes in CNS and PNS where they represent about 10% of the total lipid content (Wiegandt 1985).

Even if IgM reactivity with GM1 or other gangliosides was originally described in patients with IgM monoclonal gammopathy, these antibodies were subsequently found in several patients without monoclonal gammopathy. As the clinical correlates and pathogenetic aspects of these reactivities will be extensively reviewed elsewhere in this book, I will just briefly mention them in relation to IgM monoclonal gammopathies.

GM1

Freddo et al. (1986b) first reported on a patient with lower motor neuron disease associated with an IgM monoclonal gammopathy reacting with the gangliosides GM1 and GD1b. Since then several patients with predominantly motor syndromes and IgM monoclonal gammopathy reacting with GM1 have been

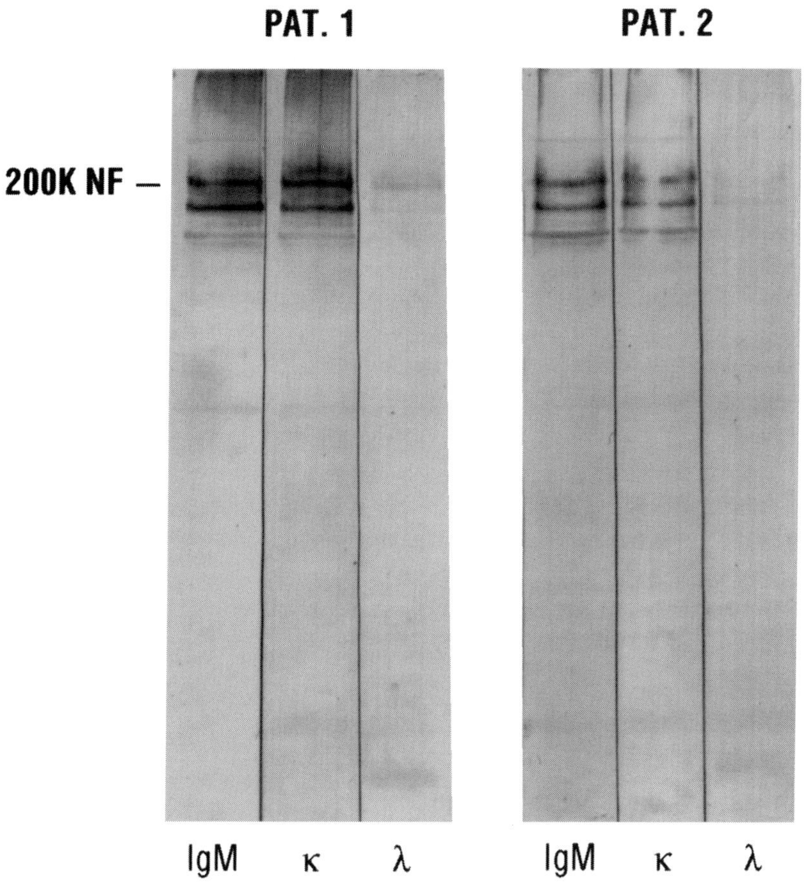

Figure 12.6 *Binding of patient IgM antibodies to the 200 KDa neurofilaments (200K NF) by immunoblot. Nerve proteins were separated by SDS polyacrylamide gel electrophoresis (PAGE), transferred onto nitrocellulose sheets, and immunostained with patients' sera using peroxidase conjugated goat immunoglobulins to human IgM, kappa (κ) or lambda (λ) light chains. IgM from two patients with neuropathy and IgM monoclonal gammopathy bound to the 200 K NF. In both patients IgM reactivity with the 200 K NF was specific for the light chain of the M proteins (kappa in both).*

reported including patients with motor neuron disease (Latov et al. 1988a; Nobile-Orazio et al. 1990; Sadiq et al. 1990; Kinsella et al. 1994), predominantly motor neuropathy with or without multifocal conduction block (Ilyas et al. 1988b; Nardelli et al. 1988; Kusunoki et al. 1989; Sadiq et al. 1990; Willison et al. 1994) but also, though less frequently, with sensorimotor neuropathy (Sadiq et al. 1990). In most of these patients the M protein also bound to GD1b and to asialo-GM1, sharing with GM1 the Gal(β1-3)GalNAc epitope (Latov et al. 1988a; Ilyas et al. 1988b; Nardelli et al. 1988; Nobile-Orazio et al. 1990; Sadiq et al. 1990). Therapeutic reduction of anti-GM1 antibody levels in some of these patients was associated with clinical improvement (Latov et al. 1988a; Kinsella et al. 1994) suggesting a possible pathogenetic role for these antibodies.

Gangliosides containing disialosyl groups

Six patients with neuropathy and an IgM monoclonal gammopathy reacting with gangliosides containing disialosyl groups, including GD1b, GT1b, GQ1b, and either GD3 or GD2 or both, have been reported (Ilyas et al. 1985; Arai et al. 1992; Daune et al. 1992; Obi et al. 1992; Yuki et al. 1992; Willison et al. 1993). In two of these patients the M protein also had cold agglutinin activity and bound to the Pr2 antigen on red cell membranes but none had anemia. These patients had an homogeneous clinical pattern with a large fiber sensory neuropathy characterized by paresthesias, numbness, prominent ataxia and areflexia and mild or no weakness. The neuropathy was chronic progressive in all but one patient (Yuki et al. 1992) who had an acute-relapsing course after an upper respiratory tract infection, with 10 relapses in 15 years. In all patients electrophysiological findings were consistent with a demyelinating process with reduced conduction velocities and prolonged distal and F wave latencies in motor nerves and absent or reduced sensory nerve action potentials. Morphological studies showed loss of large myelinated fibers in sural nerve biopsy with segmental demyelination and minimal or no axonal degeneration on teased fiber preparations. In none of these patients, though extensively investigated, were myelin deposits of M protein found in sural nerve. Treatment directed at reducing M protein levels, including plasma exchange, steroids and immunosuppressive agents in combination or alone was effective in two patients (Arai et al. 1992; Obi et al. 1992) but had minimal or no effect in the others (Ilyas et al. 1985; Yuki et al. 1992; Willison et al. 1993).

Other gangliosides

Monoclonal IgM reactivities with other gangliosides have been occasionally reported in patients with IgM monoclonal gammopathy. A selective IgM reactivity with GD1b but not with GM1 or other gangliosides was found in two patients, one with sensorimotor (Ben Younes-Chennoufi et al. 1992) and one with predominantly motor neuropathy (Nobile-Orazio et al. 1994). IgM reactivity with GD1a was found in three patients with predominantly motor neuropathy (Bollensen et al. 1989; Carpo et al. 1996) while two patients with a no better defined neuropathy had a monoclonal IgM reactivity with GM2 (Ilyas et al. 1988a) and one with a steroid responsive sensorimotor neuropathy associated with lymphoma had a monoclonal IgM reactivity with sialosyllactosaminil-paragloboside (SLPG) (Baba et al. 1985; Miyatani et al. 1987). IgM binding to a conformational epitope formed by a mixture of phosphatidic acid and gangliosides but not to the individual antigens was found in a patient with a slowly progressive sensorimotor neuropathy and chronic lymphocytic leukemia (Freddo et al. 1986a). The possible pathogenetic relevance of these unfrequent IgM reactivities remains unclear as in none of these patients was IgM deposits found in sural nerves. Both our patients with anti-GD1a antibodies (Carpo et al. 1996) improved with either/or prednisolone IVIG and cyclophosphamide and improvement correlated with a reduction of antibody levels (unpublished observations), while no reduction of IgM levels was observed in the only other patient responding to immunosuppressive therapy (Baba et al. 1985). In one patient a diffuse lymphocytic infiltration of perineurium and epineurium was found at autopsy (Bollensen et al. 1989) possibly indicating a different pathogenetic mechanism for the neuropathy.

Neuropathy with IgM not reacting with neural antigens

In approximately one-third of patients with neuropathy associated with IgM monoclonal gammopathy no reactivity of the M protein with nerve antigens can be detected (Nobile-Orazio et al. 1994). Over two-thirds of these patients have Waldenström's macroglobulinemia or lymphoma. Several non-immune mechanisms have been implicated in the pathogenesis of the neuropathy in this group of patients possibly explaining the heterogeneous clinical findings. Cryoglobulinemia is frequently found in these patients (Nobile-Orazio et al. 1994) and may cause mononeuropathy, mononeuritis multiplex or a symmetric neuropathy due to intravasal precipitation of cryoglobulins or vasculitis of vasa nervorum (Vallet et al. 1980; Chad et al. 1982; Lippa et al. 1986).

Neuropathy may be also caused by direct lymphoplasmacytic infiltration of nerves (Aarseth et al. 1961; Chazot et al. 1976; Ince et al. 1987), microangiopathy of vasa nervorum (Powell et al. 1984; Lamarca et al. 1987), endoneurial accumulation of the M protein (Iwashita et al. 1974; Vital et al. 1985) or amyloidosis (Nick et al. 1963; Le Bourhis et al. 1964; Baiada et al. 1980). In some patients these mechanisms were associated with cranial nerve palsies or mononeuritis multiplex while in other they caused a symmetric neuropathy (Le Bourhis et al. 1964; Iwashita et al. 1974; Powell et al. 1984; Vital et al. 1985; Ince et al. 1987). More than one possible mechanism for the neuropathy was occasionally found in some patients (Julien et al. 1984b; Meier et al. 1984; Thomas et al. 1992), while in others concomitant causes for the neuropathy were also present (Julien et al. 1984a; Nobile-Orazio et al. 1994) suggesting that, at least in some patients, the association of neuropathy with IgM monoclonal gammopathy may be coincidental. It is also possible that in some patients the M proteins react with still unidentified nerve antigens. Whatever the mechanism for the neuropathy in this heterogeneous group, treatment directed at reducing IgM M protein levels in some of these patients was associated with clinical improvement (Dalakas and Engel 1981; Dalakas et al. 1983; Sherman et al. 1984; Smith et al. 1987; Kelly et al. 1988).

Conclusions

There is now considerable evidence that the frequent occurrence of neuropathy in patients with IgM monoclonal gammopathies may be related to the frequent reactivity of IgM M proteins with antigens in peripheral nerve. IgM reactivities with some of these antigens, including MAG, sulfatide, chondroitin sulfate, GM1 and disialosyl ganglioside, were frequently though not invariably associated with homogeneous clinical findings supporting the hypothesis that a number of different clinical syndromes can be identified in this heterogeneous group of patients.

Even if the pathogenetic mechanisms of the neuropathy have been partially clarified, at least in the case of neuropathy associated with anti-MAG IgM, little is known on the cause for the monoclonal expansion of IgM with antineural activity. It is possible, however, that the understanding of the mechanisms underlying these monoclonal autoimmune responses might also help in understanding the etiopathogenesis of other autoimmune diseases.

There is not yet a general consensus on the possible clinical usefulness of the measurement of these antibodies (Gosselin et al. 1992; Latov 1992; Pestronk 1992). As the findings may be useful not only in understanding the possible pathogenetic mechanism of the neuropathy but also in monitoring the efficacy of therapy, it would be advisable to establish standardized protocols for the measurement of these antibodies in order to compare the results between different laboratories.

Treatment of these patients is frequently not effective and often relies on the use of cytotoxic agents not always well tolerated. Until more effective and, possibly, better tolerated therapies become available caution should be used in the treatment of these patients. A multicentric, double-blind controlled study on a large number of patients directed at comparing different therapeutic regimens is probably needed in order to identify the most effective and less toxic treatment.

Acknowledgements

I thank Drs Marinella Carpo, Nicoletta Meucci, Emanuela Manfredini and Miss Silvia Allaria for their valuable help and suggestions in preparing the manuscript. This work was made possible by the financial support of Associazione Italiana Sclerosi Multipla, Telethon (grants 486 and 674), IRCCS Ospedale Maggiore Policlinico and Associazione Amici Centro Dino Ferrari.

References

Aarseth, S., Ofstad, E., and Turvik, A. (1961). Macroglobulinemia Waldenström. A case with hemolytic syndrome and involvement of the nervous system. *Acta Med. Scand.* **169**: 691–699.

Antoine, J.C., Steck, A., and Michel, D. (1993). Neuropathie peripherique a predominance motrice associee a une IgM monoclonal anti-MAG. *Rev. Neurology* **149**: 496–499.

Arai, M., Yoshino, H., Kusano, Y., Yazaki, Y., Ohnishi, Y., and Miyatake, T. (1992). Ataxic polyneuropathy and anti-Pr_2 IgMk M proteinemia. *J. Neurol.* **239**: 147–151.

Ariga, T., Kohiriyama, T., Freddo, L., Latov, N., Saito, M., Kon, K., Ando, S., Suzuki, M., Hemling, M.E., Rinehart Jr, K.L., Kusunoki, S., and Yu, R.K. (1987). Characterization of sulfated glucuronic acid containing glycolipids reacting with IgM M-proteins in patients with neuropathy. *J. Biol. Chem.* **262**: 848–853.

Arfmann, M., Harbs, H., Deicher, H., Frick, E., Wurster, U., Stark, E., and Patzold, U. (1984). Polyneuropathye bei Makroglobulinamie Waldenström. *Aktuel. Neurol.* **11**: 7–12.

Avrameas, S., Guilbert, B., and Dighiero, B. (1981). Natural antibodies against tubulin, actin, myoglobulin, thyroglobulin, fetuin and transferrin are present in normal human sera and monoclonal immunoglobulins from multiple myeloma and Waldenström macroglobulinemia may express similar antibody specificities. *Ann. Immunol.* **132C**: 103–113.

Azar, H.A., Hill, W.T., and Osserman, E.F. (1957). Malignant lymphoma and lymphocytic leukemia associated with myeloma type serum proteins. *Am. J. Med.* **23**: 239–249.

Baba, H., Miyatani, N., Sato, S., Yuasa, T., and Miyatake, T. (1985). Antibody to glycolipid in a patient with IgM paraproteinemia and polyneuropathy. *Acta Neurol. Scand.* **72**: 218–221.

Baldini, L., Nobile-Orazio, E., Guffanti, A., Barbieri, S., Carpo, M., Cro, L., Cesana, B., Damilano, I., and Maiolo, A.T. (1994). Peripheral neuropathy in IgM monoclonal gammopathy and Waldenström macroglobulinemia: a frequent complication in males with low MAG-reactive serum monoclonal component. *Am. J. Hematol.* **45**: 25–31.

Bajada, S., Mastaglia, F.L., and Fisher, A. (1980). Amyloid neuropathy and tremor in Waldenström's macroglobulinemia. *Arch. Neurol.* **37**: 240–242.

Barbieri, S., Nobile-Orazio, E., Baldini, L., Fayoumi, Z., Manfredini, E., and Scarlato, G. (1987). Visual evoked potentials in patients with neuropathy and macroglobulinemia. *Ann. Neurol.* **22**: 663–666.

Ben Younes-Chennoufi, A., Leger, J.-M., Hauw, J.-J., Preud'homme, J.-J., Bouche, P., Aucouturier, P., Ratinahirana, H., Llubetzki, C., Lyon-Cain, O., and Baumann, N. (1992). Ganglioside GD1b is the target antigen for a biclonal IgM in a case of sensory-motor axonal polyneuropathy: involvement of N-acetylneuraminic acid in the epitope. *Ann Neurol.* **32**: 18–23.

Bollensen, E., Steck, A.J., and Schachner, M. (1988). Reactivity with the peripheral myelin glycoprotein Po in serum from patients with monoclonal IgM gammopathy and polyneuropathy. *Neurology* **38**: 1266–1270.

Bollensen, E. and Schachner, M. (1987). The peripheral myelin glycoprotein Po expresses the L2/HNK1 and L3 carbohydrate structure shared by neural adhesion molecules. *Neurosci. Lett.* **82**: 78–82.

Bollensen, E., Schipper, H.I., and Steck, A.J. (1989). Motor neuropathy with activity of monoclonal IgM antibody to GD1a ganglioside. *J. Neurol.* **236**: 353–355.

Braun, P.E., Frail, D.E., and Latov, N. (1982). Myelin associated glycoprotein is the antigen for a monoclonal IgM in polyneuropathy. *J. Neurochem.* **39**: 1261–1265.

Burger, D., Simon, M., Perruisseau, G., and Steck, A.J. (1990). The epitope(s) recognized by HNK-1 antibody and IgM paraprotein in neuropathies present on several *N*-linked oligosaccharide structures on human Po and myelin-associated glycoprotein. *J. Neurochem.* **54**: 1569–1575.

Carpo, M., Nobile-Orazio, E., Meucci, N., Gamba, M., Barbieri, S., Allario, S., and Scarlato, G. (1996). Anti-GDa antibodies in peripheral motor syndromes. *Ann. Neurol.* **39**: 539–543.

Chad, D., Pariser, K., Bradley, W.G., Adelman, L.S., and Pinn, V.W. (1982). The pathogenesis of cryoglobulinemic neuropathy. *Neurology* **32**: 725–729.

Chazot, G., Berger, B., Carrier, H., Barbaret, C., Bady, B., Dumas, R., Creyssel, R., and Schott, B. (1976). Manifestation neurologiques de gammopathies monoclonales. *Rev. Neurol.* **132**: 195–212.

Chou, D.K.H., Ilyas, A.A., Evans, J.E., Costello, C., Quarles, R.R.H., and Jungalwala, F.B. (1986). Structure of sulfated glucuronyl glycolipids in the nervous system reacting with HNK-1 antibody and some IgM paraproteins in neuropathy. *J. Biol. Chem.* **261**: 11 717–11 725.

Connolly, A.M., Pestronk, A., Trotter, J.L., Feldman, E.L., Cornblath, D.R., and Olney, R.K. (1993). High titer selective serum anti-beta-tubulin antibodies in chronic inflammatory demyelinating polyneuropathy. *Neurology* **43**: 557–562.

Cook, D., Dalakas, M., Galdi, A., Biondi, D., and Porter, H. (1990). High-dose intravenous immunoglobulin in the treatment of demyelinating neuropathy associated with monoclonal gammopathy. *Neurology* **40**: 212–214.

Cruz, M., Jiang, Y.-P., Ernerudh, J., Solders, G., Olsson, T., Osterman, P.-O., and Link, H. (1991). Antibodies to myelin-associated glycoprotein are found in cerebrospinal fluid in polyneuropathy associated with monoclonal serum IgM. *Arch. Neurol.* **48**: 66–70.

Dalakas, M.C. and Engel, W.K. (1981). Polyneuropathy with monoclonal gammopathy: studies of 11 patients. *Ann. Neurol.* **10**: 45–52.

Dalakas, M.C., Flaum, M.A., Rick, M., Engel, W.K., and Gralnick, H.R. (1983). Treatment of polyneuropathy in Waldenström's macroglobulinemia: role of paraproteinemia and immunologic studies. *Neurology* **33**: 1406–1410.

Daune, G.C., Farrer, R.G., Dalakas, M.C., and Quarles, R.H. (1992). Sensory neuropathy associated with monoclonal immunoglobulin M to GD1b ganglioside. *Ann. Neurol.* **31**: 683–685.

Dellagi, K., Brouet, J.C., Perreau, J., and Paulin, D. (1982). Human monoclonal IgM with autoantibody activity against intermediate filaments. *Proc. Natl. Acad. Sci. USA* **79**: 446–450.

Dellagi, K., Dupouey, P., Brouet, J.C., Billecocq, A., Gomez, D., Clauvel, J.P., and Seligmann, M. (1983). Waldenström's macroglobulinemia and peripheral neuropathy: a clinical and immunologic study of 25 patients. *Blood* **62**: 280–285.

Dighiero, G., Lymberi, P., Guilbert, B., Ternyck, T., and Avrameas, S. (1986). Natural autoantibodies constitute a substantial part of normal circulating immunoglobulins. *Ann. N.Y. Acad. Sci.* **475**: 135–145.

Endtz, L.J. (1960). Sur l'origine d'une polyneuropathie dans un cas de macroglobulinemia de Waldenström. *Presse Med.* **68**: 2181–2182.

Ernerudh, J., Brodtkorb, E., Olsson, T., Vedeler, C.A., Nyland, H., and Berlin, G. (1986). Peripheral neuropathy and monoclonal IgM with antibody activity against peripheral nerve myelin; effect of plasma exchange. *J. Neuroimmunol.* **11**: 171–178.

Ernerudh, J.H., Vrethem, M., Andersen, O., Lindberg, C., and Berlin, G. (1992). Immunochemical and clinical effects of immunosuppressive treatment in monoclonal IgM neuropathy. *J. Neurol. Neurosurg. Psychiatry* **55**: 930–934.

Frail, D.E., Edwards, A.M., and Braun, P.E. (1984). Molecular characteristics of the epitope in myelin associated glycoprotein that is recognized by a monoclonal IgM in human neuropathy patients. *Mol. Immunol.* **21**: 721–725.

Fraser, D.M., Parker, A.C., Amer, S., and Campbell, I.W. (1976). Mononeuritis multiplex in a patient with macroglobulinemia. *J. Neurol. Neurosurg. Psychiatry* 39: 711–715.

Freddo, L., Ariga, T., Saito, M., Macala, L.C., Yu, R.K., and Latov, N. (1985a). The neuropathy of plasma cell dyscrasia: binding of IgM M-proteins to peripheral nerve glycolipids. *Neurology* 35: 1420–1424.

Freddo, L., Hays, A.P., Sherman, W.H., and Latov, N. (1985b). Axonal neuropathy with IgM M protein reactive with nerve endoneurium. *Neurology* 35: 1321–1325.

Freddo, L., Hays, A.P., Nickerson, K.G., Spatz, L., McGinnis, S., Lieberson, R., Vedeler, C.A., Shy, M.E. Autilio-Gambetti, L., Graus, F.C., Petito, F., Chess, L., and Latov, N. (1986a). Monoclonal anti-DNA IgMk in neuropathy binds to myelin and to a conformational epitope formed by phosphatidic acid and gangliosides. *J. Immunol.* 137: 3821–3825.

Freddo, L., Yu, R.K., Latov, N., Donofrio, P.D., Hays, A.P., Greenberg, H.S., Albers, J.W., Allessi, A.G., Leavitt, A., Davar, G., and Keren, D. (1986b). Gangliosides GM1 and GD1b are antigens for IgM M-protein in a patient with motor neuron disease. *Neurology* 36: 454–458.

Fredman, P., Vedeler, C.A., Nyland, H., Aarli, J.A., and Svennerholm, L. (1991). Antibodies in sera from patients with inflammatory demyelinating polyradiculoneuropathy react with ganglioside LM1 and sulphatide of peripheral nerve myelin. *J. Neurol.* 238: 75–79.

Goldman, J.E. and Yen, S.-H. (1986). Cytoskeletal protein abnormalities in neurodegenerative diseases. *Ann. Neurol.* 19: 209–223.

Gosselin, S., Kyle, R.A., and Dyck, P.J. (1991). Neuropathy associated with monoclonal gammopathies of undetermined significance. *Ann. Neurol.* 30: 54–61.

Gosselin, S., Kyle, R.A., and Dyck, P.J. (1992). Monoclonal gammopathy and neuropathy. *Ann. Neurol.* 31: 690–691 (reply).

Gregory, R., Thomas, P.K., King, R.H.M., Hallam, P.L.J., Malcolm, S., Hughes, R.A.C. and Harding, A.E. (1993). Coexistance of hereditary motor and sensory neuropathy type Ia and IgM paraproteinemic neuropathy. *Ann. Neurol.* 33: 649–652.

Haas, D.C. and Tatum, A.H. (1988). Plasmapheresis alleviates neuropathy accompanying IgM anti-myelin-associated glycoprotein paraproteinemia. *Ann. Neurol.* 23: 394–396.

Hafler, D.A., Johnson, D., Kelly, J.J., Panitch, H., Kyle, R., and Weiner, H.L. (1986). Monoclonal gammopathy and neuropathy: myelin-associated glycoprotein reactivity and clinical characteristics. *Neurology* 36: 75–78.

Hays, A.P., Latov, N., Takatsu, M., and Sherman, W.H. (1987). Experimental demyelination of nerve induced by serum of patients with neuropathy and anti-MAG IgM M-proteins. *Neurology* 37: 242–256.

Hays, A.P., Lee, S.S.L., and Latov, N. (1988). Immune reactive C3d on the surface of myelin sheaths in neuropathy. *J. Neuroimmunol.* 18: 231–244.

Harbs, H., Arfmann, M., Frick, E., Hormann, Ch., Wurster, U., Patzold, U., Stark, E., and Deicher, H. (1985). Reactivity of sera and isolated monoclonal IgM from patients with Waldenström's macroglobulinemia with peripheral nerve myelin. *J. Neurol.* 232: 43–48.

Hoang-Xuan, K., Leger, J.M., Ben Younes-Chennoufi, A., Saidi, H., Bouche, P., Baumann, N., and Brunet, P. (1993). Traitment des neuropathies dysimmunitaire par immunoglobulin polyvalentes intraveineuses. *Rev. Neurol.* 149: 385–392.

Ilyas, A.A., Chou, D.K.H., Jungalwala, F.B., Costello, C., and Quarles, R.H. (1990). Variability in the structural requirement for binding of human monoclonal anti-myelin-associated glycoprotein immunoglobulin M antibodies and HNK-1 to sphingolipid antigens. *J. Neurochem.* 55: 594–601.

Ilyas, A.A., Cook, S.D., Dalakas, M.C., and Mithen, F.A. (1992). Anti-MAG IgM paraproteins from some patients with polyneuropathy associated with IgM paraproteinemia also react with sulfatide. *J. Neuroimmunol.* 37: 85–92.

Ilyas, A.A., Li, S.C., Chou, D.K.H., Li, Y.-T., Jungalwala, F.B., Dalakas, M.C., and Quarles, R.H. (1988a). Gangliosides GM2, IV⁴GalNAcGM1b and IV⁴GalNAcGD1a as antigens for monoclonal immunoglobulin M in neuropathy associated with gammopathy. *J. Biol. Chem.* 263: 4369–4373.

Ilyas, A.A., Quarles, R.H., Dalakas, M.C., Fishman, P.H., and Brady, R.O. (1985). Monoclonal IgM in a patient with paraproteinemic polyneuropathy binds to a carbohydrate containing disialosyl groups. *Ann. Neurol.* 18: 655–659.

Ilyas, A.A., Willison, H.J., Dalakas, M.C., Whitaker, J.N., and Quarles, R.H. (1988b). Identification and characterization of gangliosides reacting with IgM paraproteins in three patients with neuropathy associated with biclonal gammopathy. *J. Neurochem.* 51: 851–858.

Ince, P.G., Shaw, P.J., Fawcett, P.R.W., and Bates, D. (1987). Demyelinating neuropathy due to primary IgM kappa B cell lymphoma of peripheral nerve. *Neurology* 37: 1231–1235.

Iwashita, H., Argyrakis, A., Lowitzch, K., and Spaar, F.W. (1974). Polyneuropathy in Waldenström's macroglobulinemia. *J. Neurol. Sci.* 21: 341–354.

Julien, J., Vital, C., Vallat, J.M., Lagueny, A., Ferrer, X., Deminier, C., Leboutet, M.J., and Effroy, C. (1984a). IgM demyelinative neuropathy with amyloidosis and biclonal gammopathy. *Ann. Neurol.* 15: 395–399.

Julien, J., Vital, C., Vallat, J.M., Lagueny, A., Ferrer, X., and Leboutet, M.J. (1984b). Chronic demyelinating neuropathy with IgM-producing lymphocytes in peripheral nerve and delayed appearance of benign monoclonal gammopathy. *Neurology* 34: 1387–1389.

Julien, J., Vital, C., Vital, A., Lagueny, A., and Ferrer, X. (1989). Chronic progressive ataxic neuropathy with anti-MAG activity and delayed appearance of IgM monoclonal gammopathy. In *Peripheral Nerve Development and Regeneration: Recent Clinical Applications*, ed. E. Scarpini, M.G. Giori, D. Pleasure and G. Scarlato, pp. 289–294. Padova: Liviana Press.

Kaku, D.A., England, J.D., and Sumner, A.J. (1994). Distal accentuation of conduction slowing in polyneuropathy associated with antibodies to myelin-associated glycoprotein and sulphated glucuronyl paragloboside. *Brain* 117: 941–947.

Kelly, J.J. (1990). The electrodiagnostic findings in polyneuropathies associated with IgM monoclonal gammopathies. *Muscle Nerve* 13: 1113–1117.

Kelly, J.J., Adelman, L.S., Berkman, E., and Bhan, I. (1988). Polyneuropathies associated with IgM monoclonal gammopathies. *Arch. Neurol.* 45: 1355–1359.

Kinsella, L.J., Lange, D.J., Trojaburg, W., Sadiq, S.A., Younger, D.S., and Latov, N. (1994). Clinical and electrophysiologic correlates of elevated anti-GM1 antibody titers. *Neurology* **44**: 1278–1282.

Kruse, J., Mailhammer, R., Wernecke, H., Faissner, A., Sommer, I., Goridis, C., and Schachner, M. (1984). Neural cell adhesion molecules and myelin-associated glycoprotein share a common carbohydrate moiety recognized by monoclonal antibodies L2 and HNK-1. *Nature* **311**: 153–155.

Kusunoki, S., Shimizu, T., Matsumura, K., Maemura, K., and Mannen, T. (1989). Motor dominant neuropathy and IgM paraproteinemia: the IgM M-protein binds to specific gangliosides. *J. Neuroimmunol.* **21**: 177–181.

Kyle, R.A. (1978). Monoclonal gammopathy of undetermined significance: natural history in 241 cases. *Am. J. Med.* **64**: 814–826.

Kyle, R.A. (1984) 'Benign monoclonal gammopathy': A misnomer? *JAMA* **251**: 1849–1854.

Kyle, R.A. (1987). Plasma cell dyscrasia: definition and diagnostic evaluation. In *Polyneuropathies Associated with Plasma Cell Dyscrasia*, ed. J.J. Kelly, R.A. Kyle and N. Latov, pp. 1–28. Boston: Martinus Nijhoff Publishing.

Kyle, R.A. and Greipp, P.R. (1980). Smoldering multiple myeloma. *N. Eng. J. Med.* **302**: 1347–1349.

Lamarca, J., Casquero, P., and Pou, A. (1987). Mononeuritis multiplex in Waldenström's macroglobulinemia. *Ann. Neurol.* **22**: 268–272.

Latov, N. (1987). Waldenström's Macroglobulinemia and non-malignant IgM monoclonal gammopathies. In *Polyneuropathies Associated with Plasma Cell Dyscrasia*, ed. J.J. Kelly, R.A. Kyle and N. Latov, pp. 51–72. Boston: Martinus Nijhoff Publishing.

Latov, N. (1992). Monoclonal gammopathy and neuropathy. *Ann. Neurol.* **31**: 690 (letter).

Latov, N., Godfrey, M., Thomas, Y., Nobile-Orazio, E., Spatz, L., Abrams, J., Perman, J., Freddo, L., and Chess, L. (1985). Neuropathy and anti-myelin-associated glycoprotein IgM M-proteins: T cell regulation of M-protein secretion in vitro. *Ann. Neurol.* **18**: 182–188.

Latov, N., Hays, A.P., Donofrio, P.D., Kabat, E., Liao, J., Ito, H., McGinnis, S., Manoussous, K., Freddo, L., Shy, M.E., Sherman, W.H., Chang, H.W., Yu, R.K., and Rowland, L.P. (1988a). Monoclonal IgM with a unique specificity to gangliosides GM1 and GD1b and to lacto-*N*-tetraose associated with human motor neuron disease. *Neurology* **33**: 763–768.

Latov, N., Hays, A.P., and Sherman, W.H. (1988b). Peripheral neuropathy and anti-MAG antibodies. *Crit. Rev. Neurobiol.* **3**: 301–332.

Latov, N., Sherman, W.H., Nemni, R., Galassi, G., Shyong, J.S., Penn, A.S., Chess, L., Olarte, M.R., Rowland, L.P., and Ossermann, E.F. (1980). Plasma cell dyscrasia and peripheral neuropathy with a monoclonal antibody to peripheral nerve myelin. *N. Eng. J. Med.* **303**: 618–621.

Le Bourhis, J., Feve, J.-R., Besanon, C., and Leroux, M.-J. (1964). Neuropathie peripherique avec infiltration amyloid de nerfs au cours d'une macroglobulinemie de Waldenström's. *Rev. Neurol.* **111**: 474–478.

Lee, K.W., Inghirami, G., Sadiq, S.A., Thomas, F.A., Spatz, L., Knowles, D.M., and Latov, N. (1990). B-cells that secrete anti-MAG or anti-GM1 antibodies are present at birth and anti-MAG secreting B-cells are CD5$^+$. *Neurology* **40** (suppl. 1): 367 (abstract).

Leger, J.M., Ben Younes-Chenoufi, A., Zuber, M., Bouche, P., Jauberteau, M.O., Dormont, D., Danon, F., Baumann, N., and Brunet, P. (1992). Frequency of central lesions in polyneuropathy associated with IgM monoclonal gammopathy: an MRI, neurophysiological and immunochemical study. *J. Neurol. Neurosurg. Psychiatry* **55**: 112–115.

Lieberman, F., Marton, L.S., and Stefansson, K. (1985). Pattern of reactivity of IgM from the sera of eight patients with IgM monoclonal gammopathy and neuropathy with components of neural tissues: evidence for interaction with more than one epitope. *Acta Neuropathol. (Berl.)* **68**: 196–200.

Lippa, C.F., Chad, D.A., Smith, T.W., Kaplan, M.H., and Hammer, K. (1986). Neuropathy associated with cryoglobulinemia, **9**: 626–631.

Logothetis, J., Silverstein, P., and Coe, J. (1960). Neurological aspects of Waldenström's macroglobulinemia. *Arch. Neurol.* **3**: 574–573.

Mamoli, A., Nemni, R., Camerlingo, M., Quattrini, A., Casto, L., Lorenzetti, I., and Canal, N. (1992). A clinical electrophysiological, morphological and immunological study of chronic sensory neuropathy with ataxia and paresthesia. *Acta Neurol. Scand.* **85**: 110–115.

Manfredini, E., Nobile-Orazio, E., Allaria, S., and Scarlato, G. (1994). Anti-beta tubulin IgM antibodies in demyelinating neuropathy. *Clin. Neuropathol.* **13**: 1455 (abstract).

Margolis, R.K. and Margolis, R.U. (1989). Structure and localization of glycoproteins and proteoglycans. In *Neurobiology of Glycoconjugates*, ed. R.U. Margolis and R.K. Margolis, pp. 85–26. New York: Plenum Press.

McGarry, R.C., Helfand, S.L., Quarles, R.H., and Roder, J.C. (1983). Recognition of myelin-associated glycoprotein by the monoclonal antibody HNK-1. *Nature* **306**: 376–378.

McGinnis, S., Kohriyama, T., Yu, R.K., Pesce, M.A., and Latov, N. (1988). Antibodies to sulfated glucuronic acid containing glycosphingolipids in neuropathy associated with anti-MAG antibodies and in normal subjects. *J. Neuroimmunol.* **17**: 119–126.

Meier, C., Roberts, K., Steck, A., Hess, C., Miloni, E., and Tschopp, L. (1984). Polyneuropathy in Waldenström's macroglobulinemia: reduction of endoneurial IgM deposits after treatment with chlorambucil and plasmapheresis. *Acta Neuropathol. (Berl.)* **64**: 297–307.

Meier, C., Vandevelde, M., Steck, A., and Zurbriggen, A. (1983). Demyelinating polyneuropathy associated with monoclonal IgM paraproteinemia. Histological, ultrastructural and immunocytochemical studies. *J. Neurol. Sci.* **63**: 353–367.

Melmed, C., Frail, D., Duncan, I., Braun, P., Danoff, D., Finlayson, M., and Stewart, J. (1983). Peripheral neuropathy with IgM monoclonal immunoglobulin directed against myelin-associated glycoprotein. *Neurology* **33**: 1397–1405.

Mendell, J.R., Sahenk, Z., Whitaker, J.N., Trapp, B.D., Yates, A.J., Griggs, R.C., and Quarles, R.H. (1985). Polyneuropathy and IgM monoclonal gammopathy: studies on the pathogenetic role of anti-myelin-associated glycoprotein antibody. *Ann. Neurol.* **17**: 243–254.

Miyatani, N., Baba, H., Sato, S., Kanamura, K., Yuasa, T., and Miyatake, T. (1987). Antibody to sialosyllactosaminylparagloboside in a patient IgM with paraproteinemia and polyradiculoneuropathy. *J. Neuroimmunol.* **14**: 189–196.

Monaco, S., Bonetti, B., Ferrari, S., Moretto, G., Nardelli, E., Tedesco, F., Mollnes, T.E., Nobile-Orazio, E., Manfredini, E., Bonazzi, L., and Rizzuto, N. (1990). Complement-mediated demyelination in patients with IgM monoclonal gammopathy and polyneuropathy. *N. Engl. J. Med.* **322**: 649–652.

Monaco, S., Ferrari, S., Bonetti, B., Moretto, G., Kirshfink, M., Nardelli, E., Nobile-Orazio, E., Zanusso, G., Rizzuto, N., and Tedesco, F. (1995). Experimental induction of myelin changes by anti-MAG antibodies and terminal complement complex. *J. Neuropathol. Exp. Neurol* (in press).

Moulis, H. and Mamus, S.W. (1989). Isolated trochlear nerve palsy in a patient with Waldenström's macroglobulinemia: complete recovery with combination therapy. *Neurology* **39**: 1399.

Murray, N., Page, N., and Steck, A.J. (1986). The human anti-myelin-associated glycoprotein IgM system. *Ann. Neurol.* **19**: 473–478.

Nardelli, E., Steck, A.J., Barkas, T., Schluep, M., and Jerusalem, F. (1988). Motor neuron syndrome and monoclonal IgM with antibody activity against gangliosides GM1 and GD1b. *Ann. Neurol.* **23**: 524–528.

Nemni, R., Fazio, R., Quattrini, A., Lorenzetti, I., Mamoli, D., and Canal, N. (1993). Antibodies to sulfatide and to chondroitin sulfate C in patients with chronic sensory neuropathy. *J. Neuroimmunol.* **43**: 79–86.

Nemni, R., Galassi, G., Latov, N., Sherman, W.H., Olarte, M.R., and Hays, A.P. (1983). Polyneuropathy in nonmalignant IgM plasma cell dyscrasia: a morphological study. *Ann. Neurol.* **14**: 43–54.

Nick, J., Contamin, F., Brion, S., Guillard, A., and Guiraudon, M. (1963). Macroglobulinemie de Waldenström avec neuropathie amyloid. *Rev. Neurol.* **109**: 21–30.

Nobile-Orazio, E., Baldini, L., Barbieri, S., Marmiroli, P., Spagnol, G., Francomano, E., and Scarlato, G. (1988). Treatment of patients with neuropathy and anti-MAG IgM M-proteins. *Ann. Neurol.* **24**: 93–97.

Nobile-Orazio, E., Barbieri, S., Baldini, L., Marmiroli, P., Carpo, M., Premoselli, S., Manfredini, E., and Scarlato, G. (1992). Peripheral neuropathy in monoclonal gammopathy of undetermined significance: prevalence and immunopathogenetic studies. *Acta Neurol. Scand.* **85**: 383–390.

Nobile-Orazio, E., Francomano, E., Daverio, R., Barbieri, S., Marmiroli, P., Manfredini, E., Carpo, M., Moggio, M., Legname, G., Baldini, L., and Scarlato, G. (1989). Anti-myelin-associated glycoprotein IgM antibody titers in neuropathy associated with macroglobulinemia. *Ann. Neurol.* **26**: 543–550.

Nobile-Orazio, E., Hays, A.P., Latov, N., Perman, G., Golier, J., Shy, M.E., and Freddo, L. (1984a). Specificity of mouse and human monoclonal antibodies to myelin associated glycoprotein. *Neurology* **34**: 1336–1342.

Nobile-Orazio, E., Latov, N., Hays, A.P., Takatsu, M., Abrams, G.M., Sherman, W.H., Miller, J.R., Messito, M.J., Saito, T., Tamoush, A., Lovelace, R.E., and Rowland, L.P. (1984b). Neuropathy and anti-MAG antibodies without detectable serum M-protein. *Neurology* **34**: 218–221.

Nobile-Orazio, E., Legname, G., Daverio, R., Carpo, M., Giuliani, A., Sonnino, S., and Scarlato, G. (1990). Motor neuron disease in a patient with a monoclonal IgMk directed against GM1, GD1b and high-molecular-weight neural-specific glycoproteins. *Ann. Neurol.* **28**: 190–194.

Nobile-Orazio, E., Manfredini, E., Carpo, M., Meucci, N., Monaco, S., Ferrari, S., Bonetti, B., Cavaletti, G., Gemignani, F., Durelli, L., Barbieri, S., Allaria, S., Sgarzi, M., and Scarlato, G. (1994). Frequency and clinical correlates of anti-neural IgM antibodies in neuropathy associated with IgM monoclonal gammopathy. *Ann. Neurol.* **36**: 416–424.

Nobile-Orazio, E., Marmiroli, P., Baldini, L., Spagnol, G., Barbieri, S., Moggio, M., Polli, N., Polli, E., and Scarlato, G. (1987). Peripheral neuropathy in macroglobulinemia: incidence and antigen specificity of M-proteins. *Neurology* **37**: 1506–1514.

Nobile-Orazio, E., McIntosh, C., and Latov, N. (1985). Anti-MAG antibody and antibody complexes: detection by radioimmunoassay. *Neurology* **35**: 988–992.

Nobile-Orazio, E., Vietorisz, T., Messito, M.J., Sherman, W.H., and Latov, N. (1983). Anti-MAG IgM antibodies in patients with neuropathy and IgM M-proteins: detection by ELISA. *Neurology* **33**: 939–942.

Notermans, N.C., Wokke, J.H.J., Lokhorst, H., Franssen, H., van der Graaf, Y., and Jennekens, F.G.I. (1994). Polyneuropathy associated with monoclonal gammopathy of undetermined significance (MGUS). A prospective study of the prognostic value of clinical and laboratory abnormalities. *Brain* **117**: 1385–1393.

Obi, T., Kusunoki, S., Takatsu, M., Mizoguchi, K., and Nishimura, Y. (1992). IgM M-protein in a patient with sensory dominant neuropathy binds preferentially to polysialogangliosides. *Acta Neurol. Scand.* **86**: 215–218.

Ogino, M., Tatum, A.H., and Latov, N. (1994). Affinity of human anti-MAG antibodies in neuropathy. *J. Neuroimmunol.* **52**: 41–46.

Page, N., Murray, N., Perruisseau, G., and Steck, A.J. (1985). A monoclonal anti-idiotypic antibody against a human monoclonal IgM with specificity for myelin-associated glycoprotein. *J. Immunol.* **134**: 3094–3099.

Pestronk, A. (1992). Monoclonal gammopathy and neuropathy. *Ann. Neurol.* **31**: 689 (letter).

Pestronk, A., Li, F., Bieser, K., Choksi, R., Whitton, A., Kornberg, A.J., Goldstein, J.M., and Yee, W.-C. (1994). Anti-MAG antibodies: major effects of antigen purity and antibody cross-reactivity on ELISA results and clinical correlation. *Neurology* **44**: 1131–1137.

Pestronk, A., Li, F., Griffin, J., Feldman, E.L., Cornblath, D., Trotter, J., Zhu, S., Yee, W.C., Phillips, D., Peeples, D.M., and Winslow, B. (1991). Polyneuropathy syndromes associated with serum antibodies to sulfatide and myelin-associated glycoprotein. *Neurology* **41**: 357–362.

Powell, H.C., Rodriguez, M., and Hughes, R.A.C. (1984). Microangiopathy of vasa nervorum in dysglobulinemic neuropathy. *Ann. Neurol.* **15**: 386–394.

Quattrini, A., Corbo, M., Dhaliwal, S.K., Sadiq, S.A., Lugaresi, A., Oliveira, A., Uncini, A., Abouzahr, K., Miller, J.R., Lewis, L., Estes, D., Cardo, L., Hays, A.P., and Latov, N. (1992). Anti-sulfatide antibodies in neurological disease: binding to rat dorsal root ganglia neurons. *J. Neurol. Sci.* **112**: 152–159.

Quattrini, A., Nemni, R., Fazio, F., Iannaccone, S., Lorenzetti, I., Grassi, F., and Canal, N. (1991). Axonal neuropathy in a patient with monoclonal IgM kappa reactive with Schmidt–Lantermann incisures. *J. Neuroimmunol.* **33**: 73–79.

Quian, G.-X., Fu, S.M., Solank, D.L., and Rai, K.R. (1984). Circulating monoclonal IgM proteins in B-cell chronic lymphocytic leukemia. Their identification, characterization and relationship membrane IgM. *J. Immunol.* **133**: 980–988.

Ritzmann, S.E., Loukas, D., Sakai, H., Daniels, J.C., and Levin, W.C. (1975). Idiopathic (asymptomatic) monoclonal gammopathies. *Arch. Intern. Med.* **135**: 95–106.

Sadiq, S.A., Thomas, F.P., Kilidireas, K., Protopsaltis, S., Hays, A.P., Lee, K.W., Romas, S.N., Kumar, N., van den Berg, L., Santoro, M., Lange, D.J., Younger, D.S., Lovelace, R.E., Troyaborg, W., Sherman, W.H., Miller, J.R., Minuk, J., Fehr, M.A., Roelofs, R.I., Hollander, D., Nichols, F.T. III, Mitsumoto, H., Kelly, J.J. Jr, Swift, T.R., Munsat, T.L., and Latov, N. (1990). The spectrum of neurologic disease associated with anti-GM1 antibodies. *Neurology* **40**: 1067–1072.

Sherman, W.H., Latov, N., Hays, A.P., Takatsu, M., Nemni, R., Galassi, G., and Ossermann, E.F. (1983). Monoclonal IgM-k antibody precipitating with chondroitin sulphate C from patients with axonal polyneuropathy and epidermolysis. *Neurology* **33**: 192–201.

Sherman, W.H., Latov, N., Lange, D., Hays, R., and Younger, D. (1994). Fludarabine for IgM antibody-mediated neuropathies. *Ann. Neurol.* **36**: 326–327 (abstract).

Sherman, W.H., Olarte, M.R., McKiernan, G., Sweeney, K., Latov, N., and Hays, A.P. (1984). Plasma exchange treatment of peripheral neuropathy associated with plasma cell dyscrasia. *J. Neurol. Neurosurg. Psychiatry* **47**: 813–819.

Shy, M.E., Vietorisz, T., Nobile-Orazio, E., and Latov, N. (1984). Specificity of human IgM M-proteins that bind to myelin-associated glycoprotein: peptide mapping, deglycosylation and competitive binding studies. *J. Immunol.* **133**: 2509–2512.

Smith, I.S. (1994). The natural history of chronic demyelinating neuropathy associated with benign IgM paraproteinemia. *Brain* **117**: 949–957.

Smith, I.S., Kahn, S.N., Lacey, B.W., King, R.H.M., Eames, R.A., Whybrew, D.J., and Thomas, P.K. (1983). Chronic demyelinating neuropathy associated with benign IgM paraproteinemia. *Brain* **106**: 169–195.

Smith, T., Sherman, W., Olarte, M.R., and Lovelace, R.E. (1987). Peripheral neuropathy associated with plasma cell dyscrasia: a clinical and electrophysiological follow-up study. *Acta Neurol. Scand.* **75**: 244–248.

Snipes, G.J., Suter, U., and Shooter, E.M. (1993). Human peripheral myelin protein-22 carries the L2/HNK1 carbohydrate adhesion epitope. *J. Neurochem.* **61**: 1961–1964.

Spatz, L. and Latov, N. (1986). Secretion of anti-myelin associated glycoprotein antibodies by B-cells from patients with neuropathy and nonmalignant monoclonal gammopathy. *Cll. Immunol.* **1**: 434–440.

Steck, A.J., Murray, N., Meier, C., and Perruisseau, G. (1983). Demyelinating neuropathy and monoclonal IgM antibody to myelin-associated glycoprotein. *Neurology* **33**: 19–23.

Stefansson, K., Marton, L., Antel, J.P., Wollmann, R.L., Roos, R.P., Chejfec, G., and Arnason, B.G.W. (1983). Neuropathy accompanying IgM lambda monoclonal gammopathy. *Acta Neuropathol. (Berl).* **59**: 255–261.

Suarez, G.A. and Kelly, J.J. (1993). Polyneuropathy associated with monoclonal gammopathy of undetermined significance: further evidence that IgM-MGUS neuropathies are different from IgG-MGUS. *Neurology* **43**: 1304–1308.

Svennerholm, L. and Fredman, P. (1990). Antibody detection in Guillain–Barré syndrome. *Ann. Neurol.* **27** (suppl.): 36–40.

Tanaka, M., Nishizawa, M., Inuzuka, T., Baba, H., Sato, S., and Miyatake, T. (1985). Human natural killer cell activity is reduced by treatment of anti-myelin-associated glycoprotein (MAG) monoclonal mouse IgM antibody and complement. *J. Neuroimmunol.* **10**: 115–127.

Takatsu, M., Hays, A.P., Latov, N., Abrams, G.M., Sherman, W.H., Nemni, R., Nobile-Orazio, E., Saito, T., and Freddo, L. (1985). Immunofluorescence study of patients with neuropathy and IgM M-proteins. *Ann. Neurol.* **18**: 173–181.

Tatum, A.H. (1993). Experimental paraprotein neuropathy: demyelination by passive transfer of human anti-myelin-associated glycoprotein. *Ann. Neurol.* **33**: 502–506.

Thomas, F.A., Lovelace, R.E., Ding, X.-S., Sadiq, S.A., Petty, G.W., Sherman, W.H., Latov, N., and Hays, A.P. (1992). Vasculitic neuropathy in a patient with cryoglobulinemia and anti-MAG IgM monoclonal gammopathy. *Muscle Nerve* **15**: 891–898.

Trapp, B.D. (1990). Myelin-associated glycoprotein. Location and potential functions. *Ann. N.Y. Acad. Sci.* **605**: 29–43.

Valldeoriola, F., Graus, F., Steck, A.J., Munoz, E., de la Fuente, M., Gallart, T., Ribalta, T., Bombi, J.A., and Tolosa, E. (1993). Delayed appearance of anti-myelin associated glycoprotein in a patient with chronic demyelinating polyneuropathy. *Ann. Neurol.* **34**: 394–396.

Vallat, J.M., Desproges-Gotteron, R., Leboutet, M.J., Loubet, A., Gaulde, N., and Treves, R. (1980). Cryoglobulinemic neuropathy: a pathological study. *Ann. Neurol.* **8**: 179–185.

Van den Berg, L.H., Lankamp, C.L.A.M., de Jager, A.E.J., Notermans, N.C., Sodaar, P., Marrink, J., de Jong, H.J., and Wokke, J.H.J. (1993). Anti-sulphatide antibodies in peripheral neuropathy. *J. Neurol. Neurosurg. Psychiatry* **56**: 1164–1168.

Van den Berg, L., Hays, A.P., Nobile-Orazio, E., Kinsella, L.J., Manfredni, E., Corbo, M., Rosoklija, G., Younger, D.S., Lovelace, R.E., Trojaburg, W., Lange, D.E., Goldstein, S., Delfiner, J.S., Sadiq, S., Sherman, W.H., and Latov, N. (1996). Anti-MAG and anti-SGPG antibodies in neuropathy. Muscle Nerve **19**: 637–643.

Vital, C., Deminiere, C., Bourgouin, B., Lagueny, A., David, B., and Loiseau, P. (1985). Waldenström's macroglobulinemia and peripheral neuropathy: deposition of M-component and kappa light chain in the endoneurium. *Neurology* **35**: 603–606.

Vital, A., Vital, C., Julien, J., Baquey, A., and Steck, A.J. (1989). Polyneuropathy associated with IgM monoclonal gammopathy. Immunological and pathological study in 31 patients. *Acta Neuropathol.* **79**: 160–167.

Vrethem, M., Cruz, M., Wen-Xin, H., Malm, C., Holmgren, H., and Ernerudh, J. (1993). Clinical, neurophysiological and immunological evidence of polyneuropathy in patients with monoclonal gammopathies. *J. Neurol. Sci.* **114**: 193–199.

Wiegandt, H. (1985). Gangliosides. In *Glycolipids*, ed. H. Wicgandt, pp. 199–260. Amsterdam: Elsevier.

Willison, H.J., Paterson, G., Kennedy, P.G.E., and Veitch, J. (1994). Cloning of human anti-GM1 antibodies from motor neuropathy patients. *Ann. Neurol.* **35**: 471–478.

Willison, H.J., Paterson, G., Veitch, J., Inglis, G., and Barnett, S.C. (1993). Peripheral neuropathy associated with monoclonal IgM anti-Pr2 cold agglutinins. *J. Neurol. Neurosurg. Psychiatry* **56**: 1178–1183.

Willison, H.J., Trapp, B.D., Bacher, J.D., Dalakas, M.C., Griffin, J.W., and Quarles, R.H. (1988). Demyelination induced by intraneural injection of human anti-myelin-associated glycoprotein antibodies. *Muscle Nerve* **11**: 1169–1176.

Yee, W.C., Hahn, A.F., Hearn, S.A. and Rupar, A.R. (1989). Neuropathy in IgM lambda paraproteinemia. Immunoreactivity to neural proteins and chondroitin sulfate. *Acta Neuropathol.* **78**: 57–64.

Yeung, K.B., Thomas, P.K., King, R.H.M., Waddy, H., Will, R.G., Hughes, R.A.C., Gregson, N.A., and Leibowitz, S. (1991). The clinical spectrum of peripheral neuropathies associated with benign monoclonal IgM, IgG and IgA paraproteinemia. *J. Neurol.* **238**: 388–391.

Yuki, N., Miyatani, N., Sato, S., Hirabayashi, M., Yamazaki, M., Yoshimura, N., Hayashi, Y., and Miyatake, T. (1992). Acute relapsing sensory neuropathy associated with IgM antibody against B-series gangliosides containing a GalNAcbeta1-4(Gal3-2alfaNeuAc8-alfaNeuAc)beta1 configuration. *Neurology* **42**: 686–689.

13 Motor neuropathies associated with anti-GM1 ganglioside antibodies

T. Kuntzer and A.J. Steck

Introduction

For almost 10 years attention has been drawn to a relationship between motor syndromes and serum autoantibodies binding to one or more gangliosides. During this period, an increasing number of patients have been described with a clinical syndrome of motor weakness and electrophysical evidence of focal motor nerve conduction abnormalities as well as axonal loss. Some of these patients have been shown to have anti-GM1 antibodies in high titers, yet these antibodies have also been found in patients with amyotrophic lateral sclerosis and other motor neuron syndromes, Guillain-Barré syndrome (GBS), and sometimes in autoimmune diseases. Whether these antibodies are pathogenic or are associated factors is a matter of a considerable debate (for reviews see Kornberg and Pestronk 1994; Lange and Trojaborg, 1994; Parry, 1994). The different views lie in part in the difficulty in identifying specific electrodiagnostic and immune features in patients with similar clinical conditions. Recent experimental evidence suggests, however, that anti-GM1 antibodies can cause a motor syndrome with abnormal nerve conduction tests and supports the view of the proponents of the autoimmune theory, who showed earlier a beneficial response in some of those patients to immunosuppressive therapy. This chapter summarizes the roles of gangliosides, discusses the clinical, electrophysiological, histological and immunological findings and reports the therapeutic responses seen in patients with motor syndromes and anti-GM1 ganglioside antibodies, excluding GBS or its variants (see Chapter 7).

Definitions

Gangliosides: background

Gangliosides are complex acidic glycolipids composed of a lipid moiety (ceramide) attached to one or more sugars that by definition must contain at least one sialic acid residue. They are important components of nerve membranes in the peripheral (PNS) and central nervous system (CNS), concentrated at the nodes of Ranvier and at synaptic terminals. Four gangliosides are especially abundant in the brain: GM1, GD1a, GD1b, GT1b. They each contain the same 4-sugar chain, but vary in the number of sialic acid molecules (for reviews see Pestronk 1991; Merrill et al. 1993; Tettamanti and

Riboni 1993; Willison 1994). In the peripheral nerve, a fifth ganglioside, LM1, containing a different carbohydrate structure occurs in relative abundance. Numerous minor gangliosides in brain, nerve and myelin have been described. GM1 is one of the most abundant gangliosides in neuronal membranes.

Gangliosides are synthesised in the Golgi apparatus, transported down the axons at fast rates of axoplasmic flow to become inserted in the axolemma and at synaptic terminals. Gangliosides reside in the outer layer of plasma membrane. The hydrophilic sugars are located on the outer surface of the membrane. They are linked to the cell by the hydrophobic lipid moiety, which is inserted into the membrane. It has been postulated that gangliosides play a role in membrane and cell functions by interacting with receptors, ion channels, adhesion molecules or signal transducing systems. There is evidence which suggests that administration of exogenous GM1 gangliosides enhances neurite outgrowth and recovery from injury. GM1 and other gangliosides can function as cellular receptors. The binding of cholera toxin to GM1 gangliosides is well documented. Gangliosides on nerve terminals may also serve as receptors for tetanus and botulinum toxins.

Motor syndromes

The evaluation of a patient with weakness implies clinical and laboratory investigations to determine whether the weakness is caused by upper (cortical) motor neuron (UMN) dysfunction, manifested by slowed rapid movements, hyperreflexia, Babinski's sign and spasticity, or by lower (spinal and brainstem) motor neuron (LMN) dysfunction, manifested by atrophy, fasciculations or cramps, and loss or diminution of reflexes. Having clinically concluded that the damage is in the motor unit, defined as a motor neuron, its axon and all the muscle fibers which it innervates, one must decide whether the LMN, motor axon, neuromuscular junction or muscle fibers is affected. This decision is usually uncomplicated as the clinical, electrophysiologic and biochemical data offer abundant evidence that the LMN, their axons or myelin sheaths have been damaged. Electromyography and nerve conduction studies are important aids to the differential diagnosis and can exclude a myopathy, a predominant motor demyelinating neuropathy or a neuromuscular transmission block (reviewed in Kimura 1989). Separating motor neuron diseases (MND), which include UMN diseases and LMN syndromes, from motor neuropathy (motor axonopathies and myelinopathies) may not be always possible (see Laboratory investigations, below).

There is some ambiguity in the common terminology for MND, e.g. the use of MND and amyotrophic lateral sclerosis (ALS) as synonyms because they are defined by semiology. ALS is defined clinically as the combination of LMN and definite UMN signs. Although ALS is usually easy to recognise, it still remains a diagnosis of exclusion (World Federation of Neurology Research Group on Neuromuscular Diseases 1994). Of the remaining MND (for reviews see Kuncl et al. 1992; Harding, 1993), spinal muscular atrophy (SMA) are among the most common childhood neuromuscular diseases, in which there are only LMN signs. These are inherited diseases as an autosomal recessive trait. Although the pathogenesis of these syndromes is unknown, progress in understanding the genetics of SMA is occurring, e.g. identification of linkage to chromosome 5q in Werdnig–Hoffman and Kugelberg–Welander diseases. The various SMA syndromes are broadly divided into those with generalised or diffuse weakness and those with regional involvement of a restricted distribution (X-linked bulbospinal SMA or Kennedy's syndrome, in which mutation of the androgen receptor gene was demonstrated, some patients with a Charcot Marie Tooth disease-like phenotype, SMA and hexosaminidase abnormalities, juvenile bulbar palsy or Fazio-Londe disease, facio-scapulo-humeral or scapulo-peroneal SMA). Not studied in linkage analysis are a small number of adult-onset cases.

Immunological aspects

The abundance of gangliosides in the nervous system and the extracellular location of their sugars, makes it attractive to speculate that they could be targets in autoimmune neurological disorders. The terminal disaccharide on GM1, Gal(beta 1–3)GalNac, including galactose (Gal) and galactosamine (GalNac), was known to be antigenic when it occurred on systemic glycoproteins (for a review see Pestronk 1991). Several investigators have tested sera of presumed autoimmune disorders for antibody binding to panels of gangliosides, looking for possible targets of the immune process. The first report of ganglioside GM1 antibodies occurring in association with a motor syndrome came from the laboratory of Dr N. Latov (Freddo et al. 1986). That patient had LMN signs and abnormally elevated titers of monoclonal IgM antibody that recognised gangliosides GM1 and GD1 as antigens. This suggested that a specific antibody might be capable of producing MND; however, the mechanism of action remained uncertain. The inclusion of a serum from a patient with motor neuropathy with abnormal conduction studies, as a control in a study of antiglycolipid reactivity in GBS, led to the discovery by Pestronk et al. that high titers of polyclonal anti-gangliosides GM1 activity were common in motor neuropathies, but not in most other neuropathies (Ilyas et al. 1988; Pestronk et al. 1988). They showed that patients previously thought to have MND may improve with immunosuppressive therapy. High titers of IgM and IgG anti-gangliosides GM1 antibodies have then been found in 18–84% of patients with motor neuropathy and multifocal persistent conduction block (for reviews see Pestronk et al. 1990; Adams et al. 1991; Lamb and Patten, 1991; Pestronk, 1991; Lange et al. 1992; Sanders et al. 1993; Kinsella et al. 1994; Bouche et al. 1995), yet high titers of these antibodies have also been found in 5–85% of patients with amyotrophic lateral sclerosis and LMN syndromes (Freddo et al. 1986; Latov et al. 1988; Pestronk et al. 1988; Pestronk 1991; Sanders et al. 1993), GBS, the acute motor axonal neuropathy (AMAN), also known as the Chinese paralysis syndrome, the acute axonal form of GBS associated with *Campylobacter jejuni* infection, and patients with autoimmune diseases, including myasthenia gravis and polymyositis (Pestronk 1991) or paraneoplastic pure sensory neuropathy (Kinsella et al. 1994). The IgM anti-GM1 antibodies are usually seen in high titers in motor neuropathy and multifocal persistent conduction block (Pestronk, 1991; Kornberg et al. 1994), whereas selective serum IgG anti-GM1 antibody reactivity is rarely associated with this neuropathy. The chronic LMN syndromes with selective IgG antibodies do not have conduction block. The sum of these studies indicate that mild or moderate increased titers of anti-GM1 antibodies are clinically non-specific and not associated with particular clinical syndromes or diseases.

Clinical description of the diseases

Most of the published studies have shown that there is a relationship between high titers of anti-GM1 antibodies and at least two acquired motor syndromes, a motor neuropathy with multifocal conduction blocks (MN with CB), and a distal LMN syndrome.

Motor neuropathy with conduction block

This neuropathy was simultaneously described by different groups; Parry and Clarke (1988) reported five cases, Chad et al. (1986) and Roth et al. (1986) a single patient each. Their cases were young (less than 45 years old) males. It has subsequently been reported by many other investigators (Pestronk et al. 1990; Case records MGH, 1992; Kaji et al. 1992, 1993; Lange et al. 1992; Parry 1992, 1993a; Bouche et al. 1995). Its incidence is not known, but probably low; three cases out of 6000 patients having been seen in 5 consecutive years in our Electromyography (EMG) laboratory, and ten cases were reported out of 169 MND patients (Lange et al. 1992). The onset is usually insidious and asymmetrical, but not always (van den Bergh et al. 1989), more frequent in the upper limbs, with weakness associated with fasciculations and myokymia. The disorder is suspected on clinical grounds by finding motor weakness initially localized to one or more nerve trunks territory, with slight muscular wasting contrasting to the severity and duration of the weakness, and abnormal spontaneous activity of the affected muscles (Chad et al. 1986; Roth et al. 1986; Roth and Magistris, 1987b). The presence of these signs should lead to the electrophysiological search of persistent conduction block (CB) on the nerves innervating the weak muscles (see Laboratory investigations). In these muscles, frequent asynchronous fasciculations can be recorded (Roth and Magistris 1987b). During maximal effort, the number of motor unit potentials is reduced according to the severity of the CB. Signs of moderate chronic denervation can be seen in clinically unaffected muscles (Roth et al. 1986). CB are multifocal; proximal nerve segments are frequently affected as often as distal segments (Chad et al. 1986; Roth et al. 1986; Parry and Clarke, 1988; van den Bergh et al. 1989; Lange et al. 1992; Kaji et al. 1993). Upper limbs are always clinically affected and cramps are frequent.

Cranial involvement is rare (Kaji et al. 1992; Magistris and Roth 1992a; Roberts et al. 1995). The deep reflexes are absent or diminished in the affected muscle groups. Although transient paresthesia may be reported, objective sensory deficit are usually absent. The course is slowly progressive over months or years (Parry and Clarke, 1988; Krarup et al. 1990; Magistris and Roth, 1992a; Parry, 1992, 1993b), yet variable, from spontaneous remission without treatment (Chad et al. 1986) and one case out of 24 (Bouche et al. 1995) to development of tetraplegia within years, and with respiratory failure and death (Magistris and Roth 1992a). A stepwise evolution may be encountered, but relapsing course had never been reported.

Lower motor neuron syndromes

Non-familial LMN syndromes have asymmetrical patterns of weakness that may begin in distal muscles (for a review see Pestronk 1991). These syndromes are, in our experience, more frequent than MN with CB. In one study, 27% of 152 MND patients presented this syndrome (Lange et al. 1992). Distal LMN syndromes (Latov et al. 1988; Pestronk et al. 1990, 1994; Shy et al. 1990; Lange et al. 1992; Adams et al. 1993; Tsai et al. 1993) begin with asymmetrical weakness in a hand or foot. Differences from MN with CB include more frequent onset in the legs and more extensive muscle wasting. Reflexes may be present and there are no UMN signs. Cramps are frequent, fasciculations being rarely reported. The course is slowly progressive over months or years. Electrophysiological studies show prominent evidence of axonal loss without CB (see Laboratory investigations).

Laboratory investigations in motor neuropathy with conduction block and lower motor neuron syndromes

The usual biological parameters are within normal ranges. Serum immunoelectrophoresis rarely shows a monoclonal peak (Kinsella et al. 1994), but a polyclonal profile may be seen, either IgM or IgG. Serum IgM concentration may be elevated or normal. Cerebrospinal fluid (CSF) analysis is generally unremarkable.

Electrophysiological studies

Electromyographic recordings are useful to know if the abnormal denervation-reinnervation process, observed in MND and motor axon diseases, is localized or is outside the distribution of a single peripheral nerve or nerve root. It is therefore also useful to test paraspinal muscles. In MN conduction studies may reveal (for reviews see Kaji and Kimura, 1991; Kuntzer and Magistris, 1995) reduced conduction velocities, localized failure of transmission of the nerve impulses (*CB*; see below) or long latency motor axon reflex, a sign of axonal regeneration following Wallerian degeneration, that is never seen in MND and can help localizing the damage to the motor axons (Roth 1979; Roth et al. 1986; Magistris and Roth 1992b). In some circumstances, nerve biopsy can help in the diagnosis of a MN (see Histological examination, below).

In MN with CB, persistent (more than 4–5 months) or permanent CB have to be demonstrated concomitantly with the underlying motor weakness. The underlying possible mechanisms include paranodal and segmental demyelination, and physical or chemical dysfunction of the ionic channels (Brown 1984; Kaji and Kimura 1991; Kuntzer and Magistris 1995). Different electrodiagnostic (Ex) criteria of CB have been published, but are still discussed (Kaji and Kimura 1991; Kuntzer and Magistris 1995). Restrictive criteria of partial CB have been proposed when the amplitude or area of the motor evoked response had been reduced by 50%, or more on proximal compared with distal stimulation (Rhee et al. 1990). The required reduction in the amplitude and the area of the negative peak between the proximal and distal sites depends on the distance between these two sites and the presence or absence of desynchronization (Rhee et al. 1990; Kaji and Kimura 1991; Kuntzer and Magistris 1995). In all cases, CB should only be considered: (1) if there are concordant clinical signs, i.e. motor weakness, (2) after supramaximal proximal stimuli, (3) if the results are obtained after the acute period, as a study of less than 10 days can locate the lesion but cannot yield information on its nature, (4) if there is no evidence of innervation abnormalities (Sonck et al. 1991; Gutman 1993), an effect of volume conduction (Dumitru and Delisa 1991), severe axonal loss, all of which are associated with possible interpotential phase cancellation of individual action potentials (for reviews see Rhee et al. 1990; Kaji and Kimura 1991; Kuntzer and Magistris 1995). It may be useful to compare results with the other side and to carry out very distal and segmental proximal stimulations to differentiate CB from axonal (Wallerian) degeneration. In general, it is advisable to use surface monopolar electrodes to stimulate proximal nerves (Roth and Magistris 1987a), as the intensity of the stimuli is more bearable for the patient, and the stimuli can be applied more accurately at these sites. Small stimulators, such as those used for small children or babies, may be useful for very short distance (e.g. 1 cm apart) segmental stimulation. Distal motor latencies are usually normal, as are conduction velocities measured over nerve segments without CB. Sensory nerve action potentials and conduction are usually preserved.

In LMN syndromes, segmental nerve conduction studies are usually normal except where prominent axon loss exists in motor nerves, resulting in reduced compound muscle action potential area, and slight reduction in motor conduction velocities. On electromyography, fibrillation potentials and positive sharp waves are recorded. Fasciculation potentials can be seen, but are never grouped as in MN with CB. Recruitment of motor unit potentials is invariably reduced in weak muscles. Most motor units are large, consistent with the underlying pathophysiological process of denervation and reinnervation. When sampled, similar abnormalities can be found in uninvolved or less affected muscles in the upper or lower limbs, substantiating a more diffuse process than is suspected clinically.

Anti-gangliosides titers

The enzyme linked immunosorbent assay (ELISA) system is the most commonly used for quantification of anti-GM1 antibody titers. Microwells in the titer plates are coated with the glycolipid antigen, the patient serum added to the antigen coated microwells, and the serum antibodies that bind are a measured in a colorimetric reaction. Results are usually reported as titers and when interpreting an assay result, consideration must be given to the normal range established for that laboratory. Titers are usually expressed as the highest serum dilution at which binding is detected, or in comparison to standard curves.

Low levels of circulating anti-GM1 antibodies are present in many normal individuals, so elevated titers are defined in comparison to normal subjects and to patients with other neurological and immunological diseases (Adams et al. 1991; Willison 1994; Zielasek et al. 1994; Latov and Steck 1995). Available antibody assays only approximate the in vivo conditions and do not measure such variables as the state of blood–nerve barrier, the concentration of antibodies in the endoneurial compartment, the ability of these antibodies to activate complement or recruit effector cells. Estimates of the frequency of increased anti-GM1 antibody titers in patients with MN with CB range from 18 to 82% and 1.3 to 55% in distal LMN syndromes (see Immunological aspects, above). Although they are usually polyclonal, the antibodies appear to be remarkably selective, reacting with only a limited epitope on the carbohydrate moeity of GM1. Some antibodies are highly specific for GM1 or recognize internal determinants shared by GM1 or GM2, but in most patients the anti-GM1 antibodies recognise the Gal(beta 1–3)GalNac determinant which is shared by GM1 and the ganglioside GD1b.

Histological examinations

Motor neuropathy with conduction block

Auer et al. (1989) and Kaji et al. (1993) biopsed nerves at identified sites of CB (ulnar nerve high in the axilla and medial pectoral nerve, respectively) and found well demarcated areas where axons have thin myelin sheaths in relation to axonal caliber and onion bulb formations (Auer et al. 1989) or scattered demyelinated axons surrounded by small onion bulbs (Kaji et al. 1993). Sural nerve biopsy may be normal (Roth et al. 1986; van den Bergh et al. 1989; Lange et al. 1992), but despite normal sensory nerve conduction parameters, changes have been seen (Latov et al. 1988; Parry and Clarke 1988; Pestronk et al. 1988; Krarup et al. 1990), with mild loss of myelinated axons or slightly increased incidence in segmental demyelination. Usually, there is no inflammation and blood vessels are normal. Immune deposits are not found in the nerve biopsy specimens. In a recent study with 12 radial cutaneous nerve biopsies, five cases showed no abnormalities, four signs of several clusters of regenerating fibres, one signs of active fascicular axonal lesions and two signs of demyelination and remyelination on teased fiber preparations (Bouche et al. 1995). Biopsy of the motor branch of the obturator nerve supplying the gracilis muscle has been partially described, but the method has not been validated (Corbo et al. 1995).

Lower motor neuron syndromes

The conclusions regarding the pathological abnormalities in these syndromes must be regarded with caution in view of the small number of necropsies reported in SMA and motor neuropathies (Hays, 1991). We have studied a patient with distal onset LMN syndrome and high titers of anti-GM1 antibodies in whom death occurred 6 years after first symptoms (Adams et al. 1993). A predominantly motor radiculoneuropathy was found with multisegmental IgG and IgM deposits on the nerve fibers. There was also an ascending retrograde degeneration of the spinal motor neurons with a corresponding severe endstage neurogenic muscular atrophy. In favor of a primary axonal lesion was the presence of evenly distributed phosphorylated neurofilaments within the perikarya of spinal motor neurons with central chromatolysis (ubiquitine negative), suggesting impaired axonal transport, and deposits of immunoglobulins on the nerve fibers. We did not find demyelinative features, onion bulbs or inflammatory cells in peripheral nerves.

Experimental data with summary of relevant patient-oriented research

It is not known whether the anti-GM1 antibodies cause or contribute to the disease or are only an associated abnormality (Latov and Steck 1995). Anti-GM1 antibodies might directly cause a disease by binding to GM1, or cross-reactive antigens in nerve and activating proinflammatory pathways or creating a functional block of GM1-modulated processes (Thomas et al. 1989, 1991; Santoro et al. 1990, 1992; Corbo et al. 1993; Willison et al. 1994; Roberts et al. 1995; Waxman, 1995).

Early studies have demonstrated deleterious effects of antisera against a variety of gangliosides in isolated and cultured neuronal cells (Roth et al. 1985; Schwerer et al. 1986), but several recent observations are important to the view of a direct pathological relevance of anti-GM1 antibodies:

1. In rabbits immunized with Gal(beta 1–3)GalNac or GM1, antibodies to these antigens can bind to the nodes of Ranvier and cause a neuropathy characterized by impaired nerve conduction (decline in the ratio of the amplitudes of the motor responses evoked by proximal versus distal stimulation) and mild axonal changes (Thomas et al. 1991). The distribution of immunoglobulin deposits in the rabbit model was similar to that reported in a case of amyotrophic lateral sclerosis (ALS) with CB and anti-GM1 antibodies (Santoro et al. 1990). When injected with fresh human complement into rat sciatic nerve, the serum of the ALS patient induces CB with temporal dispersion and deposits of immunoglobulin are detected at the nodes of Ranvier (Santoro et al. 1992). While Gal(beta 1–3)GalNac antibodies have also been shown to bind to the surface of motor neurons, no immunoglobulin deposits are detected in the spinal cord of immunized rabbits.
2. In an in vitro preparation of a rat sciatic nerve, human and rabbit sera with high titers of anti-ganglioside antibodies applied to a restricted segment of the nerve induce blocking of the nerve conduction in myelinated nerve fibres only (Arasaki et al. 1993).
3. It has been postulated that anti-GM1 antibodies and impaired blood–nerve barrier may interfere with remyelination (Kaji et al. 1994).
4. GM1 and Gal(beta 1–3)GalNac bearing glycoproteins that crossreact with anti-GM1 antibodies are present at the nodes of Ranvier in human peripheral nerve (Gregson et al. 1991; Corbo et al. 1993). The human anti-GM1 antibodies also bind to and damage or kill mammalian spinal motor neurons in culture (Heiman-Patterson et al. 1993) and block conduction at the motor endplate (Willison et al. 1994).
5. Human monoclonal anti-GM1 antibodies can be cloned from peripheral blood of motor neuropathy patients (Willison et al. 1994). The combination of affinity chromatography, ELISA and isoelectric focusing has shown that the sera from three patients contains a mixture of anti-

Gal(beta 1–3)GalNac moiety antibodies derived from different B cell clones. In two sera, an anti-GM1 antibody clone was quantitatively dominant such it could be resolved into a distinct paraprotein, which was not visible in the whole sera.

6. Using intracellular microelectrodes in the mouse phrenic nerve-hemidiaphragm preparation, it has been demonstrated that sera from eight patients with MN with CB and high anti-GM1 antibodies in six cases caused complete CB with absence of a detectable endplate potential in three cases (Roberts et al. 1995). The effects were antibody-mediated and did not appear to involve complement. It is worth noting that the serum of a patient that did not have detectable anti-GM1 antibodies also interfered with motor nerve function. In this study, one explanation could be a direct or indirect effect on Na^+ channel function in the distal nerve.

7. It was shown that antibodies against GM1 antibodies can have two distinct effects on an isolated rat myelinated nerve fibers, depending on whether complement is present (Takigawa et al. 1995). One is due to the action of anti-GM1 itself that increases the K^+ current and may induce demyelination in the paranodal region and the other, in the presence of complement, decreases the Na^+ current, increases membrane leakiness, and may be due to the formation of antibody–complement complexes. If Na^+ channels can be the targets of immune attack, the diversity and distribution of Na^+ channels in different types of axons may provide a basis for selective axonal pathology as it is now clear that sensory and motor axons express ion channels with different properties (Waxman 1995).

Differential diagnosis

Erythrocyte sedimentation rate (ESR) hematologic and biochemical screening, chest radiograph and electrocardiogram (ECG), antinuclear antibodies, thyroid function tests, serum creatine kinase levels, protein electrophoresis and Venereal Disease Research Laboratory (VDRL) should be undertaken in all patients with a motor syndrome. These tests are performed mainly to exclude thyroid and parathyroid disorders and autoimmune disorders that may be associated with motor neuropathy and spinal cord syndromes. Electromyography and nerve conduction studies should be carried out by an experienced neurophysiologist to exclude neuromuscular junction disorders, myopathy and to localize the damage to the LMN or motor axons or their myelin sheaths (see Laboratory investigations, above). As spinal magnetic resonance imaging (MRI) and lumbar puncture with analysis of CSF help to exclude common disorders such as spondylotic polyradiculopathy or myelopathy or neoplasm, many neurologists would now regard them as mandatory in patients with motor syndromes. A search for antibodies to GM1 should be carried out in a reference laboratory. Occasionally the following investigations may be relevant: a search for antibodies to *B. burgdorferi*, HIV, leukocyte or fibroblast hexosaminidase A and B activity.

Motor neuropathy with conduction block

The acute or chronic inflammatory demyelinating neuropathies, primary or secondary (human immunodeficiency virus (HIV), Lyme-related, autoimmune disorders, including some forms with monoclonal gammopathies, toxic or pharmaceuticals-related, some lymphomas) are the most frequent forms of motor neuropathies with CB (for reviews see Chance and Reilly 1994; Mendell et al. 1994; Kuntzer and Magistris 1995). It is worth noting that CB is not a feature of a generalized neuropathy, particularly if it is only present at common sites of compression. The relationship between chronic inflammatory demyelinating poly-radiculo-neuropathies (CIDP) and anti-GM1 antibodies is controversial, several authors arguing that MN with CB can be considered as a predominantly motor variant of CIDP. There are indeed clinical, electrophysiological, morphologic and immunologic similarities between MN with CB and CIDP (Parry 1994; Hughes 1995). In general, CIDP with predominant motor involvement tend to have more widespread abnormalities of demyelination and sensory conduction than MN with CB, but purely motor CIDP have been reported (Hughes, 1990). In CIDP, CSF protein is generally elevated (usually normal in MN with CB), high anti-GM1 antibodies titers have been demonstrated (Lamb and Patten 1991), not all CIDP patients respond to prednisone, and a patient with chronic relapsing axonal neuropathy has been observed (Chroni et al. 1995). The chronic progressive forms of CIDP are rare (Hughes 1990) and no relapsing MN with CB has been reported. Other neuropathies with CB are either acquired, such as certain vasculitic neuropathies with transient CB (Magistris et al. 1994), or genetically determined. In the latter group, persistent (more than 4–5 months) or permanent motor CB, fluctuating in severity, may be seen in the usual sites of entrapment (e.g. peroneal at the fibular head, ulnar at the wrist or elbow, median at the carpal tunnel), but other proximal sites are possible. In this neuropathy, known as the hereditary neuropathy with liability to pressure palsies (HNPP), motor and sensory nerve conduction may be prolonged in clinically affected patients as well as in asymptomatic gene carrier. The HNPP locus has been assigned to chromosome 17p11.2–12 and is associated with a PMP22 gene deletion. DNA tests are available for the diagnosis (Chance and Reilly 1994).

Lower motor neuron syndromes

In late onset SMA, the illness may begin in adult life (Brooke 1986; Kuncl et al. 1992; Harding 1993). Sporadic cases are common. The onset is gradual and the muscles around the hip are among the first to be involved. Shoulder and arm weakness becomes troublesome in the late stages of the illness. As already mentioned, no linkage analysis was carried out in these forms of adult-onset SMA. These patients have symmetrical proximal or generalized weakness and progress slowly. The usual varieties of SMA seldom spare the proximal muscles and the patient who presents with distal weakness and wasting should first be suspected of having a MN. Over 100 patients have been described with focal MND (for reviews see Brooke 1986; Donofrio 1994). The disease begins insidiously with wasting and fasciculations involving one or several groups of muscles of the shoulder girdle, forearm, hand or thigh. The disease is usually unilateral and may be rapidly progressive initially, whereas further progression appears to be slow or absent. When there is such localized involvement, it is important to rule out other possible diagnoses such as root compression, spinal cord tumors or various forms of 'neuralgic amyotrophy'.

Therapy, both in current use and experimental

Some patients with MN with CB can be treated effectively, yet not unanimously recognized (Lange et al. 1992). Patients usually do not benefit from prednisone and plasma exchange (Krarup et al. 1990). Certain respond to monthly intravenous cyclophosphamide (1 gm/body surface area, preceded on each occasion by plasma exchange) (Pestronk et al. 1994). Recent studies (Chaudhry et al. 1993; Nobile-Orazio et al. 1993; Azulay et al. 1994; Elliott and Pestronk 1994; van den Berg et al. 1995) have shown that human immunoglogulin (HIG) therapy in MN with CB usually has a temporary beneficial effect. Dose–response curves and the optimal frequency of HIG infusions are unknown. In one patient (van den Berg et al. 1995), who improved after an initial infusion of 0.4 g kg^{-1} for 5 consecutive days, HIG maintenance of 0.4 g kg^{-1} every week for 11 months, lead to further improvement. It appears therefore that a sufficient dosage and frequency of HIG infusions as maintenance therapy is necessary. In a large series, the response to HIG therapy seems to be correlated with the absence of amyotrophy. Based on these observations, it is appropriate to initiate treatment with HIG and continue if patients respond. If no benefit is obtained, the use of IV cyclophosphamide is appropriate, depending on the degree of disability and the patient's understanding of the seriousness of potential side-effects.

There are relatively few descriptions of the effects of treatment of patients with MN with CB but without detectable anti-GM1 antibodies. One patient almost completely recovered with prednisone and plasma exchanges (van den Bergh et al. 1989). HIG infusions were followed by improvement in strength in some patients (Chaudhry et al. 1993) and two patients improved after treatment with high doses of cyclophosphamide (Tan et al. 1994).

The decision concerning whether to treat patients with LMN syndromes and anti-GM1 antibodies without CB is often difficult. The presence of high serum anti-GM1 antibodies titers and some pathological findings in the biopsed nerve (see Histological examinations, above) or electrodiagnostic evidence of demyelination (Ad hoc subcommittee of the American Academy of Neurology AIDS Task Force 1991) are useful indications that a motor syndrome may be potentially treatable. Measureable improvement after treatment with HIG, although unusual in this group (Azulay et al. 1994) may provide support for additional immunotherapy, with agents such as cyclophosphamide, or further periodic HIG infusions. Studies that evaluated the effects of cyclophosphamide or chlorambucil treatment for patients with LMN syndromes over short periods of time, up to 6 months, failed to find evidence of benefit (Kuntzer et al. 1992; Tsai et al. 1993; Tan et al. 1994), yet an early improvement was reported in a single case (Shy et al. 1990). Initial benefit may begin as late as 6–9 months after treatment was stopped (Pestronk et al. 1994).

There is no convincing evidence that immunomodulating therapy of any kind alters the progression of disability in patients with motor syndromes that include upper motor signs (Drachman et al. 1994; Leigh and Ray-Chauhuri 1994).

References

Ad hoc subcommittee of the American Academy of Neurology AIDS Task Force. (1991). Research criteria for the diagnosis of chronic inflammatory demyelinating polyneuropathy (CIDP). *Neurology* **41**: 617–618.

Adams, D., Kuntzer, T., Burger, D., Magistris, M.R., Chofflon, M., Regli, F., and Steck, A.J. (1991). Predictive value of anti-GM1 ganglioside antibodies in neuromuscular diseases: a study of 181 sera. *J. Neuroimmunol.* **32**: 223–230.

Adams, D., Kuntzer, T., Steck, A.J., Lobrinus, A., Janzer, R.C., and Regli, F. (1993). Motor conduction block and high titres of anti-GM1 ganglioside antibodies: pathological evidence of a motor neuropathy in a patient with lower motor neuron syndrome. *J. Neurol. Neurosurg. Psychiatry* **56**: 982–987.

Arasaki, K., Kusunoki, S., Kudo, N., and Kanazawa, I. (1993). Acute conduction block in vitro following exposure to antiganglioside sera. *Muscle Nerve* **16**: 587–593.

Auer, R.N., Bell, R.B., and Lee, M.A. (1989). Neuropathy with onion bulb formations and pure motor manifestations. *Can. J. Neurol. Sci.* **16**: 194–197.

Azulay, J.P., Blin, O., Pouget, J., Boucraut, J., Billé-Tuc, F., Charles, G., and Serratrice, G. (1994). Intravenous immunoglobulin treatment in patients with motor neuron syndromes associated with anti-GM1 antibodies: a double-blind, placebo-controlled study. *Neurology* **44**: 429–432.

Bouche, P., Moulonguet, A., Ben Younes-Chennoufi, A., Adams, D., Baumann, N., Meininger, V., Léger, J.M., and Said, G. (1995). Multifocal motor neuropathy with conduction block, a study of 24 patients. *J. Neurol. Neurosurg. Psychiatry* **59**: 38–45.

Brooke, M.H. (1986). *A Clinician's View of Neuromuscular Diseases*, 2nd edn. Baltimore: Williams & Wilkins.

Brown, W.F. (1984). *The Physiological and Technical Basis of Electromyography.* Boston: Butterworths.

Case records 43–1992 (1992). *N. Engl. J. Med.* **327**: 1298–1305.

Chad, D.A., Hammer, K., and Sargent, J. (1986). Slow resolution of multifocal weakness and fasciculations: a reversible motor neuron syndrome. *Neurology* **36**: 1260–1263.

Chance, P.F. and Reilly, M. (1994). Inherited neuropathies. *Curr. Opin. Neurol.* **7**: 372–380.

Chaudhry, V., Corse, A.M., Cornblath, D.R., Kuncl, R.W., Drachman, D.B., and Freimer, M.L. (1993). Multifocal motor neuropathy: response to human immune globulin. *Ann. Neurol.* **33**: 237–242.

Chroni, E., Hall, S.M., and Hughes, R.A.C. (1995). Chronic relapsing axonal neuropathy: a first case report. *Ann. Neurol.* **37**: 112–115.

Corbo, M., Iannaccone, S., Latov, N., Abouzhar, K., Quathini, A., Lazzerini, A., Nemmi, R., Canal, N., and Hays, A.P. (1995). Pathological studies of motor nerve biopsies in motor neuropathy and motor neuron disease. *J. Neurol.* **242(S2)**: S53.

Corbo, M., Quattrini, A., Latov, N., and Hays, A.P. (1993). Localization of GM1 and Gal(B1–3)GalNac antigenic determinants in peripheral nerve. *Neurology* **43**: 809–814.

Donofrio, P.D. (1994). AAEM Case report 28: monomelic amyotrophy. *Muscle Nerve* **17**: 1129–1134.

Drachman, D.B., Chaudhry, V., Cornblath, D.R., Kuncl, R.W., Pestronk, A., Clawson, L., Mellits, E.D., Quaskey, S., Quinn, T., Calkins, A., and Order, S. (1994). Trial of immunosuppression in amyotrophic lateral sclerosis using total lymphoid irradiation. *Ann. Neurol.* **35**: 142–150.

Dumitru, D. and Delisa, J.A. (1991). AAEM minimonograph 10: volume conduction. *Muscle Nerve* **14**: 605–624.

Elliott, J.L. and Pestronk, A. (1994). Progression of multifocal motor neuropathy during apparently successful treatment with human immunoglobulin. *Neurology* **44**: 967–968.

Freddo, L., Yu, R.K., Latov, N., Donofrio, P.D., Hays, A.P., Greenberg, H.S., Albers, J.W., Allessi, A.G., and Keren, D. (1986). Gangliosides GM1 and GD1b are antigens for IgM M-proteins in a patient with motor neuron disease. *Neurology* **36**: 454–458.

Gregson, N.A., Jones, D., Thomas, P.K., and Willison, H.J. (1991). Acute motor neuropathy with antibodies to GM1 ganglioside. *J. Neurol.* **238**: 447–451.

Gutman, L. (1993). AAEM minimonograph 2: important anomalous innervations of the extremities. *Muscle Nerve* **16**: 339–347.

Harding, A.E. (1993). Inherited neuronal atrophy and degeneration predominantly of lower motor neurons. In *Peripheral Neuropathy*, 3rd edn, ed. P.J. Dyck, J.W. Griffin, P. Low and J.F. Poduslo, pp. 1051–1064. Philadelphia: W.B. Saunders.

Hays, A.P. (1991). Separation of motor neuron diseases from pure motor neuropathies. In *Amyotrophic Lateral Sclerosis and Other Motor Neuron Diseases*, ed. L.P. Rowland, *Adv. Neurol.* **56**: 385–398. New York: Raven Press.

Heiman-Patterson, T., Krupa, T., Thompson, P., Nobile-Orazio, E., Tahmoush, A.J., and Shy, M.E. (1993). Anti-GM1/GD1b M-proteins damage human spinal cord neurons co-cultured with muscle. *J. Neurol. Sci.* **120**: 38–45.

Hughes, R.A.C. (1990). *Guillain-Barré Syndrome.* London: Springer-Verlag.

Hughes, R.A.C. (1995). The concept and classification of Guillain-Barré syndrome and related disorders. *Rev. Neurol.* **151**: 291–294.

Ilyas, A.A., Willison, H.J., Quarles, R.H., Jungalwala, F.B., Cornblath, D.R., Trapp, B.D., Griffin, J.W., and McKhann, G.M. (1988). Serum antibodies to ganglioside in Guillain-Barré syndrome. *Ann. Neurol.* **23**: 440–447.

Kaji, R. and Kimura, J. (1991). Nerve conduction block. *Curr. Opin. Neurol.* **4**: 744–748.

Kaji, R., Hirota, N., Oka, N., Kohara, N., Watanabe, T., Nishio, T., and Kimura, J. (1994). Anti-GM1 antibodies and impaired blood-nerve barrier may interfere with remyelination in multifocal motor neuropathy. *Muscle Nerve* **17**: 108–110.

Kaji, R., Oka, N., Tsuji, T., Mezaki, T., Nichio, T., Akiguchi, I., and Kimura, J. (1993). Pathological findings at the sites of conduction block in multifocal motor neuropathy. *Ann. Neurol.* **35**: 152–158.

Kaji, R., Shibasaki, H., and Kimura, J. (1992). Multifocal demyelinating motor neuropathy: cranial nerve involvement and immunoglobulin therapy. *Neurology*, **42**: 506–509.

Kimura, J. (1989). *Electrodiagnosis in Disease of Nerve and Muscle: Principles and Practice*, 2nd edn. Philadelphia: F.A. Davis.

Kinsella, L.J., Lange, D.J., Trojaborg, W., Sadiq, S.A., Younger, D.S., and Latov, N. (1994). Clinical and electrophysiologic correlates of elevated anti-GM1 antibody titers. *Neurology* **44**: 1278–1282.

Kornberg, A.J. and Pestronk, A. (1994). The clinical and diagnostic role of anti-GM1 antibody testing. *Muscle Nerve* **17**: 100–104.

Kornberg, A.J., Pestronk, A., Bieser, K., Ho, T.W., McKhann, G.M., Wu, H.S., and Jiang, Z. (1994). The clinical correlates of high-titer IgG anti-GM1 antibodies. *Ann. Neurol.* **35**: 234–237.

Krarup, C., Stewart, J.D., Sumner, A.J., Pestronk, A., and Lipton, S.A. (1990). A syndrome of asymmetric limb weakness with motor conduction block. *Neurology* **40**: 118–127.

Kuncl, R.W., Crawford, T.O., Rothstein, J.D., and Drachman, D.B. (1992). Motor neuron diseases. In *Diseases of the Nervous System: Clinical Neurobiology*, ed. A.K. Asbury, G.M. McKhann and W.I. McDonald, pp. 1179–1208. Philadelphia: W.B. Saunders.

Kuntzer, T. and Magistris, M.R. (1995). Blocs de conduction et neuropathies périphériques. *Rev. Neurol.* **151**: 368–382.

Kuntzer, T., Steck, A.J., Adams, D., and Regli, F. (1992). Chlorambucil fails to improve patients with motor neuropathies and antibodies to gangliosides. *J. Neurol. Neurosurg. Psychiatry* **55**: 857–858.

Lamb, N.L. and Patten, B.M. (1991). Clinical correlations of anti-GM1 antibodies in amyotrophic lateral sclerosis and neuropathies. *Muscle Nerve* **14**: 1021–1027.

Lange, D.J. and Trojaborg, W. (1994). Do GM1 antibodies induce demyelination? *Muscle Nerve* **17**: 105–107.

Lange, D.J., Trojaborg, W., Latov, N., Hays, A.P., Younger, D.S., Uncini, A., Blake, D.M., Hirano, M., Burns, S.M., Lovelace, R.E., and Rowland, L.P. (1992). Multifocal motor neuropathy with conduction block: is it a distinct clinical entity? *Neurology* **42**: 497–505.

Latov, N., Hays, A.P., Donofrio, P.D., Liao, J., Ito, H., McGinnis, S., Manoussos, K., Freddo, L., Shy, M.E., Sherman, W.H., Chang, H.W., Greenberg, H.S., Albers, J.W., Alessi, A.G., Keren, D., Yu, R.K., Rowland, L.P., and Kabat, E.A. (1988). Monoclonal IgM with unique specificity to gangliosides GM1 and GD1b and to lacto-*N*-tetraose associated with human motor neuron disease. *Neurology* **38**: 763–768.

Latov, N. and Steck, A.J. (1995). Neuropathies associated with anti-glycoconjugate antibodies and IgM monoclonal gammopathies. In *Peripheral Nerve Disorders*, 2nd edn, ed. A.K. Asbury and P.K. Thomas, Boston: Butterworth-Heinemann.

Leigh, P.N. and Ray-Chauhuri, K. (1994). Motor neuron disease. *J. Neurol. Neurosurg. Psychiatry* **57**: 886–896.

Magistris, M.R., Kohler, A., and Estade, M. (1994). Conduction block in vasculitic neuropathy. *Eur. Neurol.* **34**: 283–285.

Magistris, M.R. and Roth, G. (1992a). Motor neuropathy with multifocal persistent conduction blocks. *Muscle Nerve* **15**: 1056–1057.

Magistris, M.R. and Roth, G. (1992b). Motor axon reflex and indirect double discharge: ephaptic transmission? *Electroencephal. Clin. Neurophysiol.* **85**: 124–130.

Mendell, J.R., Barohn, R.J., Peter Bosch, E., and Kissel, J.T. (1994). Peripheral neuropathy. *Continuum* **1**: 13.

Merrill, A.H., Hannun, Y.A., and Bell, R.M. (1993). Introduction: sphingolipids and their metabolites in cell regulation. *Adv. Lipid Res.* **25**: 1–21.

Nobile-Orazio, E., Meucci, N., Barbieri, S., Carpo, M., and Scarlato, G. (1993). High-dose intravenous immunoglobulin therapy in multifocal motor neuropathy. *Neurology* **43** (Pt 1): 537–544.

Parry, G.J.G. (1992). Motor neuropathy with multifocal persistent conduction blocks. *Muscle Nerve* **15**: 1057–1058.

Parry, G.J.G. (1993a). Motor neuropathy with multifocal conduction block. *Sem. Neurol.* **13**: 269–275.

Parry, G.J.G. (1993b). Motor neuropathy with multifocal conduction block. In *Peripheral Neuropahty*, 3rd edn, ed. P.J. Dyck, P.K. Thomas, J.W. Griffin, P.A. Low and J.F. Poduslo, 3rd edn, pp. 1518–1524. Philadelphia: W.B. Saunders.

Parry, G.J.G. (1994). Antiganglioside antibodies do not necessarily play a role in multifocal motor neuropathy. *Muscle Nerve* **17**: 97–99.

Parry, G.J.G. and Clarke, S. (1988). Multifocal acquired demyelinating neuropathy masquerading as motor neuron disease. *Muscle Nerve* **30**: 103–107.

Pestronk, A. (1991). Invited review: motor neuropathies, motor neuron disorders, and antiglycolipid antibodies. *Muscle Nerve* **14**: 927–936.

Pestronk, A., Cornblath, D.R., Ilyas, A.A., Baba, H., Quarles, R.H., Griffin, J.W., Alderson, K., and Adams, R.N. (1988). A treatable multifocal motor neuropathy with antibodies to GM1 ganglioside. *Ann. Neurol.* **24**: 73–78.

Pestronk, A., Chaudhry, V., Feldman, E.L., Griffin, J.W., Cornblath, D.R., Denys, E.H., Glasberg, M., Kuncl, R.W., Olney, R.K., and Yee, W.C. (1990). Lower motor neuron syndromes defined by pattern of weakness, nerve conduction abnormalities and high titers of antiglycolipid antibodies. *Ann. Neurol.* **27**: 316–326.

Pestronk, A., Lopate, G., Kornberg, A.J., Elliott, J.L., Blume, G., Yee, W.C., and Goodnough, L.T. (1994). Distal lower motor neuron syndrome with high-titer serum IgM anti-GM1 antibodies: improvement following immunotherapy with monthly plasma exchange and intravenous cyclophosphamide. *Neurology* **44**: 2027–2031.

Rhee, E.K., England, J.D., and Sumner, A.J. (1990). A computer simulation of conduction block: effects produced by actual block versus interphase cancellation. *Ann. Neurol.* **28**: 146–156.

Roberts, M., Willison, H.J., Vincent, A., and Newsom-Davis, J. (1995). Multifocal motor neuropathy human sera block distal motor nerve conduction in mice. *Ann. Neurol.* **38**: 111–118.

Roth, G. (1979). Intranervous regeneration: the study of motor axon reflexes. *J. Neurol. Sci.* **41**: 139–148.

Roth, G. and Magistris, M.R. (1987a). Detection of conduction block by monopolar percutaneous stimulation of the brachial plexus. *Electromyogr. Clin. Neurophysiol.* **27**: 45–53.

Roth, G. and Magistris, M.R. (1987b). Neuropathies with prolonged conduction block, single and grouped fasciculations, localized limb myokymia. *Electroencephal. Clin. Neurophysiol.* **67**: 428–438.

Roth, G.A., Roeyttae, M., Yu, R.K., and Raine, C.S. (1985). Antisera to different glycolipids induce myelin alterations in mouse spinal cord tissue cultures. *Brain Res.* **339**: 9–18.

Roth, G., Rohr, J., Magistris, M.R., and Ochsner, F. (1986). Motor neuropathy with proximal mutifocal persistent conduction block, fasciculations, and myokymia. *Eur. Neurol.* **25**: 416–423.

Sanders, K.A., Rowland, L.P., Murphy, P.L., Younger, D.S., Latov, N., Sherman, W.H., Pesce, M., and Lange, D.J. (1993). Motor neuron diseases and amyotrophic lateral sclerosis: GM1 antibodies and paraproteinemia. *Neurology* **43**: 418–420.

Santoro, M., Thomas, F.P., Fink, M.E., Lange, D.L., Uncini, A., Wadia, N.H., Latov, N., Hays, A.P. (1990). IgM deposits at nodes of Ranvier in a patient with amyotrophic lateral sclerosis, anti-GM1 antibodies and multifocal motor conduction block. *Ann. Neurol.* **28**: 373–377.

Santoro, M., Uncini, A., Corbo, M., Staugaitis, S.M., Thomas, F.P., Hays, A.P., and Latov, N. (1992). Experimental conduction block induced by serum from a patient with anti-GM1 antibodies. *Ann. Neurol.* **31**: 385–390.

Schwerer, B., Lassman, H., Kitz, K., and Bernheimer, H. (1986). Ganglioside GM1, a molecular target for immunological and toxic attacks: similarity of neuropathological lesions induced by ganglioside-antiserum and cholera toxin. *Acta Neuropathol.* **72**: 55–61.

Shy, M.E., Heiman-Patterson, T., Parry, G.J.G., Tahmoush, A., Evans, V.A., and Schick, P.K. (1990). Lower motor neuron disease in a patient with auto-antibodies against Gal(B1–3)GalNac in gangliosides GM1 and GD1b: improvement following immunotherapy. *Neurology* **40**: 842–844.

Sonck, W.A., Franck, M.M., and Engels, H.L. (1991). Innervation anomalies in upper and lower extremities: potential clinical implications. How to identify with electrophysiologic techniques. *Electromyogr. Clin. Neurophysiol.* **31**: 67–80.

Takigawa, T., Yasuda, H., Kikkawa, R., Shigeta, Y., Saida, T., and Kitasato, H. (1995). Antibodies against GM1 ganglioside affect K^+ and Na^+ currents in isolated rat myelinated nerve fibers. *Ann. Neurol.* **37**: 436–442.

Tan, E., Lynn, D.J., Amato, A.A., Kissel, J.T., Rammohan, K.W., Sahenk, Z., Warmolts, J.R., Jackson, C.E., Barohn, R.J., and Mendell, J.R. (1994). Immunosuppressive treatment of motor neuron syndromes. Attempts to distinguish a treatable disorder. *Arch. Neurol.* **51**: 194–200.

Tettamanti, G. and Riboni, L. (1993). Gangliosides and modulation of the function of neuronal cells. *Adv. Lipid Res.* **25**: 235–265.

Thomas, F.P., Lee, A.M., Romas, S.N., and Latov, N. (1989). Monoclonal IgMs with anti-Gal(B1–3)GalNac activity in lower motor neuron disease: identification of glycoprotein antigens in neural tissue and cross-reactivity with serum immunoglobulins. *J. Neuroimmunol.* **23**: 167–174.

Thomas, F.P., Trojaborg, W., Nagy, C., Sadiq, S.A., Latov, N., and Hays, A.P. (1991). Experimental autoimmune neuropathy with anti-GM1 antibodies and immunoglobulin deposits at the nodes of Ranvier. *Acta Neuropathol.* **82**: 378–383.

Tsai, C.P., Lin, K.P., Liao, K.K., Wang, S.J., Wang, V., Kao, K.P., and Wu, Z.A. (1993). Immunosuppressive treatment in lower motor neuron syndrome with autoantibodies against GM1 ganglioside. *Eur. Neurol.* **33**: 446–449.

Van den Berg, L.H., Franssen, H.J., and Wokke, J.H.J. (1995). Improvement of multifocal motor neuropathy during long term weekly treatment with human immunoglobulin. *Neurology* **45**: 987–988.

Van den Bergh, P., Logigian, E.L., and Kelly, J.J. (1989). Motor neuropathy with multifocal conduction blocks. *Muscle Nerve* **11**: 26–31.

Waxman, S.G. (1995). Sodium channel blockade by antibodies: a new mechanism of neurological disease? *Ann. Neurol.* **37**: 421–423.

Willison, H.J. (1994). Antiglycolipid antibodies in peripheral neuropathy: fact or fiction? *J. Neurol. Neurosurg. Psychiatry* **57**: 1303–1307.

Willison, H.J., Paterson, G., Kennedy, P.G., and Veitch, J. (1994). Cloning of human anti-GM1 antibodies from motor neuropathy patients. *Ann. Neurol.* **35**: 471–478.

World Federation of Neurology Research Group on Neuromuscular Diseases. (1994). El Escorial World Federation of Neurology Criteria for the Diagnosis of Amyotrophic Lateral Sclerosis. *J. Neurol. Sci.* **124** (suppl.): 96–107.

Zielasek, J., Ritter, G., Magi, S., Hartung, H.P., Toyka, K.V., and Steck, A.J. (1994). A comparative trial of anti-glycoconjugate antibody assays: IgM antibodies to GM1. *J. Neurol.* **241**: 475–480.

14 Neuropathies associated with anti-sulfatide and other glycoconjugate antibodies

L.H. van den Berg

Introduction

Besides the extensively studied antibodies to the myelin-associated glycoprotein (MAG) or the GM1 ganglioside (Chapters 12 and 13), antibodies to other glycoconjugates have been reported. A possible role of antibodies against the ganglioside GQ1b in the Miller Fisher variant of the Guillain-Barré syndrome (GBS) is discussed in Chapter 7. In this chapter antibodies to sulfatide, the GD1b ganglioside and chondroitin sulfate C will be discussed.

Anti-sulfatide antibodies

Sulfatide is a common glycolipid found in central and peripheral nerve tissue, and is highly enriched in myelin (Norton and Cammer 1984; Svennerholm and Fredman 1990). Sulfatide (sulfa-galactosylceramide, galactosylceramide-3-*O*-sulfate) is galactocerebroside sulfated in the carbon-3 position and is a potential autoantigen in predominantly sensory neuropathies.

Polyneuropathy associated with anti-sulfatide antibodies

Elevated titers of serum anti-sulfatide antibodies were initially reported in patients with multiple sclerosis, idiopathic thrombocytopenic purpura, and chronic active hepatitis (Ryberg 1978; van Vliet et al. 1987; Toda et al. 1990). In 1991 Pestronk et al. described the presence of anti-sulfatide antibodies in the serum of patients with polyneuropathy, followed by several other studies. Elevated anti-sulfatide antibodies are usually detected in patients with predominantly sensory neuropathy frequently associated with an IgM monoclonal gammopathy (Pestronk et al. 1991; Nemni et al. 1992; Quattrini et al. 1992; van den Berg et al. 1993). Neuropathy associated with elevated anti-sulfatide antibodies does not however appear to constitute one clinical syndrome, while anti-sulfatide antibodies may crossreact with several other glycoconjugates. The different clinical presentations associated with elevated anti-sulfatide antibodies are summarized in Table 14.1. The role of the anti-sulfatide antibodies in the pathogenesis of the associated neuropathies is unknown, and has not yet been examined in experimental systems. No reports are available on treatment

Table 14.1 *Antibodies to sulfatide*

	Type neuropathy	antibody characteristics
Pestronk et al (1991)	– axonal, predominantly sensory	– polyclonal and monoclonal IgM, polyclonal IgG
	– demyelinating sensorimotor	– polyclonal and monoclonal IgM, polyclonal IgG (associated with anti-MAG antibodies)
Ilyas et al (1991)	– GBS	– polyclonal IgG, IgM
Fredman et al (1991)	– GBS and CIDP	– polyclonal IgG
Quattrini et al (1992)	– axonal sensory	– polyclonal IgM
	– axonal sensorimotor	– monoclonal IgM
	– demyelinating sensorimotor	– monoclonal IgM (associated with anti-GM1 antibodies)
Ilyas et al (1992)	– demyelinating sensorimotor	– monoclonal IgM (associated with anti-MAG antibodies)
Van den Berg et al (1993)	– axonal sensory	– monoclonal IgM
	– demyelinating sensorimotor	– monoclonal IgM (associated with anti-MAG antibodies)
	– GBS	– polyclonal IgM, IgG, IgA
Nemni et al (1992)	– axonal sensory	– polyclonal and monoclonal IgM, polyclonal IgG (associated with anti-chondroitin sulfate antibodies)
Fredman et al (1993)	– demyelinating sensorimotor	– monoclonal IgM
Nobile-Orazio et al (1994)	– demyelinating sensorimotor	– monoclonal IgM

of patients with polyneuropathy associated with elevated anti-sulfatide antibodies.

Axonal, predominantly sensory, neuropathy

In the first report on antibodies to sulfatide in neuropathy, elevated titers were found in seven patients with chronic axonal predominantly sensory neuropathy (Pestronk et al. 1991). In all these patients, sensory loss was distal and involved both large and small fiber modalities. Four of these patients had anti-sulfatide antibodies of the IgG isotype, whereas three patients had antibodies of the IgM isotype, two of which were monoclonal. Several studies have confirmed the presence of elevated titers of anti-sulfatide antibodies in the serum of patients with a predominantly sensory axonal neuropathy.

In a large study in our laboratory anti-sulfatide antibodies in patients with polyneuropathy were compared with antibody titers in normal and disease controls: elevated titers were detected in two patients with a mild predominantly axonal sensory neuropathy associated with an IgM monoclonal gammopathy (van den Berg et al. 1993). The patients had identical presenting complaints of painful nocturnal paresthesiae, but neurological deficit was minimal and the clinical course was very slowly progressive. In contrast to other studies antibody titers were not elevated in a group of 63 patients with a chronic idiopathic axonal polyneuropathy (CIAP) without monoclonal gammopathy (Notermans et al. 1993, 1994). Another study also reported two patients with a mild sensory axonal neuropathy with painful paresthesias (Quattrini et al. 1992). In both patients electrophysiological studies were normal, as well as light and electron microscopy of the sural nerve biopsy. In this study elevated antibody titers were also found in a patient with a progressive sensorimotor neuropathy associated with IgM monoclonal gammopathy. Electromyography (EMG) and nerve conduction revealed a moderately severe, predominantly axonal peripheral neuropathy.

Anti-sulfatide antibodies were crossreactive with chondroitin sulfate C (ChS C) in four patients. Absorption studies with each of the two compounds strongly reduced the reactivity against both sulfatide and ChS C showing the crossreactive nature of the antibodies (Nemni et al. 1992). Morphological studies of sural nerve biopsies in these four patients showed that axonal degeneration was the main feature of nerve injury (Nemni et al. 1992). Deposits of IgM were demonstrated by direct immunocytochemistry in two patients: in one patient IgM was localized at the Schmidt–Lanterman incisures, and in another patient in the endoneurium and at the outer surface of the myelin sheaths.

Demyelinating sensorimotor neuropathy

Anti-sulfatide antibodies in demyelinating sensorimotor neuropathy are usually present in association with an IgM monoclonal gammopathy. In a study by Nobile-Orazio et al. on the frequency and clinical correlates of anti-neural IgM antibodies in 75 patients with neuropathy associated with IgM monoclonal gammopathy, four patients (5%) had high anti-sulfatide IgM antibodies. These patients had a sensorimotor neuropathy with morphological evidence of predominant demyelination and myelin deposits of IgM (Nobile-Orazio et al. 1994).

In other studies highly elevated anti-sulfatide antibodies were associated with demyelinating sensorimotor neuropathy with anti-MAG antibodies (Pestronk et al. 1991; Ilyas et al. 1992; van den Berg et al. 1993). In some of these patients the anti-MAG and anti-sulfatide were both of the IgM kappa isotype and absorption of patient serum with sulfatide resulted in a substantial reduction of antibody binding to sulfatide as well as to MAG, which suggests that the IgM kappa monoclonal antibody reacted with both antigens (Ilyas et al. 1992; van den Berg et al. 1993). Other patients with neuropathy associated with anti-MAG IgM monoclonal gammopathy also had polyclonal IgM or IgG anti-sulfatide antibodies (Pestronk et al. 1991; Ilyas et al. 1992). The clinical and pathological features of patients with polyneuropathy with anti-MAG as well as anti-sulfatide antibodies were similar to patients with anti-MAG polyneuropathy without anti-sulfatide antibodies.

One patient had a sensorimotor neuropathy with multifocal motor conduction block associated with elevated anti-sulfatide and anti-GM1 ganglioside antibodies (Quattrini et al. 1992). Morphological studies in this patient showed demyelination in the motor nerve. The anti-sulfatide and anti-GM1 antibody activities were both IgM lambda, but the anti-sulfatide activity was selectively immunoabsorbed by sulfatide and not by GM1, indicating that there were two different antibodies present. In this patient there was electrophysiological and morphological evidence for demyelination in motor but not sensory nerves. The patient could have had a mild sensory neuropathy in addition to the demyelinating motor neuropathy with multifocal conduction block which is frequently associated with anti-GM1 antibodies.

Inflammatory demyelinating polyneuropathy

By using thin-layer chromatography (TLC) anti-sulfatide antibodies were detected in 65% of GBS cases and 87% of patients with chronic inflammatory demyelinating polyneuropathy (CIDP) (Fredman et al. 1991). In this study disease controls were not included and 15% of healthy controls also had anti-sulfatide antibodies. In contrast, Ilyas et al. did not find elevated anti-sulfatide antibodies in GBS by TLC and enzyme linked immunosorbent assay (ELISA), when titers were compared with normal and disease controls. In our study only one of 21 GBS patients had elevated anti-sulfatide antibody titers (van den Berg et al. 1993). Of the 21 GBS patients, the patient with elevated anti-sulfatide antibodies had the most extensive sensory loss. The anti-sulfatide antibodies were of the IgM, IgG and IgA isotypes, and titers were highest in the acute phase of the disease and returned to the normal range within 3 weeks, which suggests that the antibodies were related to the disease. Elevated anti-sulfatide antibodies may be an infrequent finding in inflammatory neuropathies patients and may be peculiar to patients with extensive sensory loss.

The role of anti-sulfatide antibodies in the pathogenesis of neuropathy

In order to study possible binding sites in peripheral nerve tissue of the anti-sulfatide antibodies in serum of patients with neuropathy, indirect immunofluorescence studies were performed (Nemni et al. 1992; Quattrini et al. 1992; Nardelli et al. 1994). The human anti-sulfatide antibodies bound to the surface of unfixed rat dorsal root ganglia (DRG) neurons and to human neuroblastoma cells. The antibodies bound to central white matter and peripheral nerve myelin only following fixation, and they did not bind to the surface of peripheral myelin following injection into rat sciatic nerve, which suggests that sulfatide may be shielded on the surface of the myelin sheath in normal peripheral nerve. Sulfatide appears to become exposed following fixation, and might also become exposed following nerve injury (Nemni et al. 1992; Quattrini et al. 1992). In patients with anti-sulfatide antibodies crossreactive with ChS C, the antibodies immunostained unfixed axons and the outer surface of the myelin sheaths. In one of these patients antibodies reacted with Schmidt–Lanterman incisures.

It is likely that the anti-sulfatide antibodies differ in their fine specificities and crossreactivities and the orientation of the sulfatide molecule on the surface of the target cells. Several sulfated molecules are present in peripheral nerve tissue and crossreactivity with antibodies binding to sulfatide may occur. The binding site and the fine specificity of anti-sulfatide antibodies may determine the particular clinical syndrome. Thus in patients who have predominantly axonal sensory neuropathy, binding may occur to sensory axons whereas in patients with demyelinating neuropathy (anti-MAG associated or GBS) antibodies may be directed against the sulfatide in myelin. Sensory loss as the common feature of all six patients with raised anti-sulfatide antibodies may be explained by antibody binding to dorsal root ganglia. Additional motor deficit or demyelination may result from binding of these antibodies to crossreactive sulfated epitopes, the presence of associated anti-MAG activity or to other underlying immune abnormalities. The number of patients so far reported is too small to make definite clinical or pathological correlations.

It is not known whether the anti-sulfatide antibodies have a role in the sensory impairment, or whether they are only an associated abnormality. The blood–nerve barrier is relatively permeable at the DRG (Ollson 1984), and the DRG neurons are potentials targets for the autoantibodies. The antibodies could disrupt the interaction of sulfatide with extracellular adhesion molecules (Holt et al. 1990), interfere with the function of associated endorphin receptors (Wu et al. 1986), or damage the cells through complement fixation (Quattrini et al. 1992). It is unlikely that the antibodies arise as a result of tissue breakdown, as raised anti-sulfatide antibodies were not found in the disease controls, who also had nerve damage. In addition, in the patient with GBS, the antibodies were present in high titres early in the acute phase of the disease prior to significant tissue breakdown. In a substantial number of patients the anti-sulfatide antibodies occurred as monoclonal gammopathy suggesting a primary B-cell response. In GBS the presence of IgG and IgA antibodies suggest T cell involvement. The significance of anti-sulfatide antibodies in neurological disease, however, remains to be demonstrated in experimental systems.

Anti-GD1b antibodies

Several studies reported patients with a sensory ataxic neuropathy (sensory ganglionopathy) associated with an IgM monoclonal gammopathy in which the IgM reacted with the GD1b ganglioside and other gangliosides containing disialosyl groups, such as GD3, GD2, and GT1b, but not GM1, GM3 or GD1a (Ilyas et al. 1985; Arai et al. 1992; Daune et al.1992; Obi et al. 1992; Yuki et al. 1992; Willison et al. 1993). Although antibodies against GD1b are also seen in patients with motor neuron syndromes and mixed sensorimotor neuropathies (Latov 1995), in these cases the IgM also recognizes GM1 or other gangliosides without disialosyl moieties. In patients with sensory ataxic neuropathy, the anti-GD1b antibodies exhibited anti-Pr2 and cold agglutinin activity (Arai et al. 1992; Willison et al. 1993). All patients with sensory ataxic neuropathy associated with anti-GD1b antibodies had large-fiber sensory loss with areflexia, and most had gait ataxia and elevated CSF protein levels. Sural nerve biopsies demonstrate loss of large myelinated fibers with segmental demyelination, but IgM deposits were not detected in biopsied nerves using direct immunofluorescence. One of the patients developed an acute neuropathy as in GBS, but following initial improvement, the disease progressed in a stepwise fashion (Yuki et al. 1992). Response to therapy was generally poor, although some improvement was reported with plasmapheresis and prednisone (Arai et al. 1992; Obi et al. 1992).

There is substantial evidence for an antibody

response to GD1b localized in dorsal root ganglia leading to a sensory ataxic neuropathy: immunization of rabbits with GD1b caused a sensory ataxic neuropathy with areflexia, ataxia, and normal strength, as clinically seen in the human disease. The DRG neurons of the immunized rabbits expressed GD1b as shown by a mouse monoclonal anti-GD1b antibody (Dalakas and Quarles 1996; Kusunoki et al. 1996). It was also shown that anti-GD1b antibodies from a patient with acute relapsing sensory neuropathy caused cell death of rat DRG neurons in culture (Ohsawa et al. 1993).

Anti-chondroitin sulfate C antibodies

Several patients with monoclonal or polyclonal IgM anti-ChS C antibodies and predominantly sensory or sensorimotor axonal neuropathy have been described (Nemni et al. 1992; Sherman et al. 1983; Kabat et al. 1984; Freddo et al. 1985, 1986; Yee et al. 1989; Quattrini et al. 1991). In three patients with monoclonal IgM anti-ChS C antibodies and axonal neuropathy, sural nerve biopsies showed endoneurial deposits of the monoclonal IgM (Freddo et al. 1985). Another patient had binding of IgM to the Schmidt–Lanterman incisures (Nemni et al. 1992). Some of the chondroitin C antibodies crossreacted with sulfatide (Nemni et al. 1992). The role of the anti-ChS C antibodies in the pathogenesis of the associated neuropathies is unknown, and has not yet been examined in experimental systems.

Neuropathy and other glycoconjugate antibodies

Neuropathy associated with IgM antibodies to other glycoconjugates has been reported. One patient had a monoclonal IgM that bound to sialosyllactosaminyl paragloboside (Baba et al. 1985; Miyatani et al. 1987). Two patients had IgM M proteins specific for GM2, GM1b-GalNAc, and GD1a-GalNAc (Ilyas et al. 1988). Three patients had a motor neuropathy with antibodies to the GD1a ganglioside (Bollensen et al. 1989; Carpo et al. 1996). Another monoclonal IgM from a patient with chronic lymphocytic leukemia and neuropathy bound to myelin and crossreacted with denatured DNA and with a conformational epitope of phosphatic acid and gangliosides (Freddo et al. 1986; Spatz et al. 1990). Several patients with neuropathy and IgM antibodies to intermediate filaments have also been described (Dellagi et al. 1982).

References

Arai, M., Yoshino, H., Kusano, Y., Yazaki, Y., Ohnishi, Y., and Miyatake, T. (1992). Ataxic polyneuropathy and anti-Pr2 IgMkappa M proteinemia. *J. Neurol.* **239**: 147–151.

Baba, H., Miyatani, N., and Sato, S. (1985). Antibody to glycolipid in a patient with IgM paraproteinemia and polyradiculoneuropathy. *Acta Neurol. Scand.* **72**: 218–221.

Bollensen, E., Schipper, H.I., and Steck, A.J. (1989). Motor neuropathy with activity of monoclonal IgM antibody to GD1a ganglioside. *J. Neurol.* **236**: 353–355.

Carpo, M., Nobile-Orazio, E., Meucci, N., Gamba, M., Barbieri, S., Allaria, S., and Scarlato, G. (1996). Anti-GD1a ganglioside antibodies in peripheral motor syndromes. *Ann. Neurol.* **39**: 539–543.

Dalakas, M.C., and Quarles, R.H. (1996). Autoimmune ataxic neuropathies (sensory ganglionopathies): are glycolipids the responsible autoantigens? *Ann. Neurol.* **39**: 419–422.

Daune, G.C., Farrer, R.G., Dalakas, M.C., and Quarles, R.H. (1992). Sensory neuropathy associated with monoclonal immunoglobulin M to GD1b ganglioside. *Ann. Neurol.* **31**: 683–685.

Dellagi, K., Brouet, J., Perreau, J., and Paulin, D. (1982). Human monoclonal IgM with autoantibody activity against intermediate filaments. *Proc. Natl Acad. Sci.* **79**: 446–450.

Fredman, P., Lycke, J., Andersen, O., Vrethem, M., Ernerudth, J., and Svennerholm, L. (1993). Peripheral neuropathy associated with monoclonal IgM antibody to glycolipids with a terminal glucuronyl-3–sulfate epitope. *J. Neurol.* **240**: 381–387.

Fredman, P., Vedeler, C.A., Nyland, H., Aarli, J.A., and Svennerholm, L. (1991). Antibodies in sera from patients with inflammatory demyelinating polyradiculoneuropathy react with ganglioside LM1 and sulphatide of peripheral nerve myelin. *J. Neurol.* **238**: 75–79.

Freddo, L., Hays, A.P., Nickerson, K.G., and Latov, N. (1986). Monoclonal anti-DNA IgMkappa in neuropathy binds to myelin and to a conformational epitope formed by phosphatidic acid and gangliosides. *J. Immunol.* **137**: 3821–3825.

Freddo, L., Hays, A., Sherman, W.H., and Latov, N. (1985). Axonal neuropathy in a patient with IgM M-protein reactive with nerve endoneurium. *Neurology* **35**: 1321–1325.

Freddo, L., Sherman, W.H., and Latov, N. (1986). Glycosaminoglycan antigens in peripheral nerve; studies with antibodies from a patient with neuropathy and monoclonal gammopathy. *J. Neuroimmunol.* **12**: 57–64.

Holt, G.D., Pangburn, M.K., and Ginsburg, V. (1990). Properdin binds to sulfatide and has a sequence homology with other proteins that bind sulfated glycoconjugates. *J. Biol. Chem.* **265**: 2852–2855.

Ilyas, A.A., Cook, S.D., Dalakas, M.C., and Mitchen, F.A. (1992). Anti-MAG IgM paraproteins from some patients with polyneuropathy associated with IgM paraproteinemia also react with sulfatide. *J. Neuroimmunol.* **37**: 85–92.

Ilyas, A.A., Li, S.C., and Chou, D.K.H. (1988). Gangliosides GM2, IVGal-NAcGm1b, and IVGalNAcGd1a as antigens for monoclonal immunoglobulin M in neuropathy associated with gammopathy. *J. Biol. Chem.* **263**: 4369–4373.

Ilyas, A.A., Mithen , F.A., Dalakas, M.C., Wargo, M., Bielory, L., and Cook, S.D. (1991). Antibodies to sulfated glycolipids in Guillain-Barré syndrome. *J. Neurol. Sci.* **105**: 108–117.

Ilyas, A.A., Quarles, R.H., Dalakas, M.C., Fishman, P.H., and Brady, R.O. (1985). Monoclonal IgM in a patient with paraproteinemic polyneuropathy binds to gangliosides containing disialosyl groups. *Ann. Neurol.* **18**: 655–659.

Kabat, K.A., Liao, J., Sherman, W.H., and Osserman, E.F. (1984). Immunological characterization of the specificities of two human monoclonal IgMs reacting with chondroitin sulfates. *Carbohydrate Res.* **130**: 289–298.

Kusunoki, S., Shimizu, J., Chiba, A., Yoshikazu, U., Hitoshi, S., and Kanazawa, I. (1996). Experimental sensory neuropathy induced by sensitization with ganglioside GD1b. *Ann. Neurol.* **39**: 424–431.

Latov, N. (1995). Pathogenesis and therapy of neuropathies associated with monoclonal gammopathies. *Ann. Neurol.* **37** (Suppl. 1): S32–S42.

Miyatani, N., Baba, H., Sato, S., Nakamura, K., Yuasa, T., and Miyatake, T. (1987). Antibody to sialosyllactos-aminylparagloboside in a patient with IgM paraproteinemia and polyradiculoneuropathy. *J. Neuroimmunol.* **14**: 189–196.

Nardelli, E., Anzini, P., Moretto, G., Rizzuto, N., and Steck, A.J. (1994). Pattern of nervous tissue immunostaining by human anti-glycolipid antibodies. *J. Neurol. Sci.* **122**: 220–227.

Nemni, R., Fazio, R., Quattrini, A., Lorenzetti, I., Mamoli, A., and Canal, N. (1992). Antibodies to sulfatide and to chrondroitin sulfate C in patients with chronic sensory neuropathy. *J. Neuroimmunol.* **43**: 79–86.

Nobile-Orazio, E., Manfredini, E., Carpo, M., Meucci, N., Monaco, S., Ferrari, S., Bonetti, B., Cavaletti, G., Gemignani, F., Durelli, L., Barbieri, S., Allaria, S., Sgarzi, M., and Scarlato, G. (1994). Frequency and clinical correlates of anti-neural IgM antibodies in neuropathy associated with IgM monoclonal gammopathy. *Ann. Neurol.* **36**: 416–424.

Norton, W.T. and Cammer, W. (1984). Isolation and characterization of myelin. In *Myelin.* ed. P. Morell. New York: Plenum Press.

Notermans, N.C., Wokke, J.H.J., Franssen, H., van der Graaf, Y., Vermeulen, M., van den Berg, L.H., Bär, P.R., and Jennekens, F.G.I. (1993). Chronic idiopathic polyneuropathy presenting in middle and old age: a clinical and electrophysiological study of 75 patients. *J. Neurol. Neurosurg. Psychiatry* **56**: 1066–1071.

Notermans, N.C., Wokke, J.H.J., van der Graaf, Y., Franssen, H., van Dijk, G.W., and Jennekens, F.G.I. (1994). Chronic idiopathic axonal polyneuropathy: a 5 year follow-up. *J. Neurol. Neurosurg. Psychiatry* **57**: 1525–1527.

Obi, T., Kusunoki, S., Takatsu, M., Mizoguchi, K., and Nishimura, Y. (1992). IgM M-protein in a patient with sensory-dominant neuropathy binds preferentially to polysialogangliosides. *Acta Neurol. Scand.* **86**: 215–218.

Ohsawa, T., Miyatake, T., and Yuki, N. (1993). Anti-B-series ganglioside-recognizing autoantibodies in an acute sensory neuropathy patient cause cell death of rat dorsal root ganglion neurons. *Neurosci. Lett.* **157**: 167–170.

Ollson, Y. (1984). Vascular permeability in the peripheral nervous system. In *Peripheral Neuropathy,* ed. P.J. Dyck, P.K. Thomas, E.H. Lambert and R. Bunge, pp. 579–599. Philadelphia: W.B. Saunders.

Pestronk, A., Li, F., Griffin, J.W., Feldman, E.L., Cornblath, D.R., Trotter, J., Zhu, S., Yee, W.C., Philips, D., Peeples, D.M., and Winslow, B. (1991). Polyneuropathy syndromes associated with serum antibodies associated with serum antibodies to sulfatide and MAG. *Neurology* **41**: 357–362.

Quattrini, A., Corbo, M., Dhaliwal, S.K., Sadiq, S.A., Lugaresi, A., Oliviera, A., Uncini, A., Abouzahr, K., Miller, J.R., Lewis, L., Estes, D., Cardo, L., Hays, A., and Latov, N. (1992). Anti-sulfatide antibodies in neurological disease: binding to rat dorsal root ganglia neurons. *J. Neurol. Sci.* **112**: 152–159.

Quattrini, A., Nemni, R., Fazio, R., Iannaccone, S., Lorenzetti, I., Grassi, F., and Canal, N. (1991). Axonal neuropathy in a patient with monoclonal IgM kappa reactive with Schmidt–Lanterman incisures. *J. Neuroimmunol.* **33**: 73–79.

Ryberg, B. (1978). Multiple specificities of anti-brain antibodies in multiple sclerosis and chronic myelopathy. *J. Neurol. Sci.* **38**: 357–382.

Sherman, W.H., Latov, N., and Hays, A. (1983). Monoclonal IgM kappa antibody precipitating with chondroitin sulfate C from patients with axonal polyneuropathy and epidermolysis. *Neurology* **33**: 192–201.

Spatz, L., Wong, K.K., Williams, M., and Latov, N. (1990). Cloning and sequence analysis of the variable heavy and light chain regions of an anti-myelin/DNA antibody from a patient with peripheral neuropathy and chronic lymphocytic leukemia. *J.Immunol.* **144**: 2821–2828.

Svennerholm, L., and Fredman, P. (1990). Antibody detection in Guillain-Barré syndrome. *Ann. Neurol.* **27**(suppl.): S36–S40.

Toda, G., Ikeda, Y., Kashiwagi, M., Iwamori, M., and Oka, H. (1990). Hepatocyte plasma membrane glycosphingolipid reactive with sera from patients with autoimmune chronic active hepatitis: its identification as sulphatide. *Hepatology* **12**: 664–670.

Van den Berg, L.H., Lankamp, C.L.A.M., de Jager, A.E.J., Notermans, N.C., Sodaar, P., Marrink, J., de Jong, H.J., Bär, P.R., and Wokke, J.H.J. (1993). Anti-sulphatide antibodies in peripheral neuropathy. *J. Neurol. Neurosurg. Psychiatry* **56**: 1164–1168.

Van Vliet, H.H.D.M., Kappers, M.C., and van der Hel, J.W.B. (1987). Antibodies against glycosphingolipids in sera of patients with idiopathic purpura. *Br. J. Haematol.* **67**: 103–108.

Willison, H.J., Paterson, G., Veitch, J., Inglis, G., and Barnett, S.C. (1993). Peripheral neuropathy associated with monoclonal IgM anti-Pr2 cold agglutinins. *J. Neurol. Neurosurg. Psychiatry* **56**: 1178–1183.

Wu, C.S.C., Lee, N.M., Loh, H.H., and Yang, J.T. (1986). Competitive binding of dynorphin-(1–13) and B-endorphin to cerebroside sulfate in solution. *J. Biol. Chem.* **261**: 3687–3691.

Yee, W.C., Hahn, A.F., Hearn, S.A., and Rupar, A.R. (1989). Neuropathy in IgM paraproteinemia: immunoreactivity to neural proteins and chondroitin sulfate. *Acta Neuropath. (Berl.)* **78**: 57–64.

Yuki, N., Miyatani, N., Sato, S., Hirabayashi, Y., Yamazaki, M., Yoshimura, N., Hayashi, Y., and Miyatake, T. (1992). Acute relapsing sensory neuropathy associated with IgM antibody against B-series gangliosides containing a GalNAcB1–4(Gal3–2aNeuAc8–2aNeuAc)B1 configuration. *Neurology* **42**: 686–689.

15 Paraneoplastic peripheral neuropathy

P.S. Smitt and J.B. Posner

Introduction

Paraneoplastic peripheral neuropathies are disorders of the peripheral nerve or its primary neuron that are caused by cancer but are not ascribable to invasion or compression of peripheral nerves by the cancer or to clearly identifiable secondary effects of the cancer or its treatment such as malnutrition or nerve damage from radiation or chemotherapy (Posner 1995) (Table 15.1).

Paraneoplastic disorders of peripheral nerves can be extremely variable. (1) The nerves may be affected focally as in paraneoplastic brachial plexopathy (Lachance et al. 1991), or mononeuritis multiplex (Johnson et al. 1979), or may be part of a more widespread disorder as, for example, encephalomyelitis (Dalmau et al. 1992), necrotizing myelopathy (Ojeda 1984), or Lambert–Eaton syndrome combined with cerebellar degeneration (Clouston et al. 1992). (2) The disorder may have discrete and identifiable clinical, laboratory and pathological fingerprints such as subacute sensory neuronopathy associated with the anti-Hu antibody and with inflammatory destruction of dorsal root ganglia (Dalmau et al. 1992), or be more vague and less easily identifiable as seen in the neuromyopathy of cancer (Croft and Wilkinson 1965). (3) The peripheral nerve disorder may occur before identification of cancer and its presence be highly suggestive that an underlying cancer is the cause as, for example, the Lambert–Eaton myasthenic syndrome (LEMS) (O'Neill et al. 1988) or subacutely developing sensory neuronopathy (Dalmau et al. 1992). Conversely, the disorder may occur only slightly more often in cancer patients than in patients without cancer and, thus, rarely warrant a search for an underlying cancer; examples are Guillain-Barré syndrome (GBS) (Lisak et al. 1977) associated with Hodgkin's disease, or motor neuron disease associated with lymphoma (Schold et al. 1979). A peripheral nerve disorder that occurs no more commonly in patients with cancer than in the general population may, in an individual instance, be so clearly associated with cancer as to make the diagnosis of a paraneoplastic syndrome mandatory. One example is amyotrophic lateral sclerosis associated with solid tumors (Rosenfeld and Posner 1991).

The physician confronted by a patient with a possible paraneoplastic peripheral neuropathy has a twofold task. The first is to determine in the patient

Table 15.1 *Some causes of peripheral neuropathy in cancer patients*

Mechanism	Examples
Neoplastic invasion or compression	Leptomeningeal metastases Peripheral nerve or nerve plexus Neurolymphomatosis
Chemotherapeutic agents	Vinca alkaloids (vincristine) Platinum compounds (*cis*-platin) Taxol
Radiation therapy	Myelopathy Plexopathy
Nutritional neuropathies	Cancer cachexia Specific vitamin deficiencies (vitamins B1, B12) Pressure neuropathies
Metabolic disorders	Uremia (pelvic tumors) Hypothyroidism (post-radiation therapy) Multiorgan failure (critical illness polyneuropathy)
Not related to cancer	Diabetes mellitus

not known to have cancer whether the peripheral neuropathy is paraneoplastic and, if so, the site of the causal tumor. The second is, in a patient known to have cancer, to determine whether the peripheral neuropathy is paraneoplastic in origin or results from metastasis, non-metastatic complications of the cancer, or a complication of treatment (Table 15.1).

This chapter considers the diagnosis and management of paraneoplastic peripheral neuropathies. Not considered here are the paraproteinemic peripheral neuropathies discussed in detail in Chapter 12 and neuromyotonia and the Lambert–Eaton syndrome considered in Chapter 17.

General considerations

History

Auche in 1890 was probably the first to describe the association of peripheral neuropathy with cancer. Although Oppenheim's (1888) report of a patient with a cavitary lesion in the lung and peripheral neuropathy preceded Auche's report, Oppenheim attributed his patient's peripheral neuropathy to tuberculosis. Nevertheless, Oppenheim clearly recognized that non-metastatic nervous system abnormalities could be encountered in patients with cancer in his reports published in 1888 (Oppenheim 1888). Despite these early descriptions, textbooks written as late as the 1930s give scant reference to non-metastatic peripheral neuropathy.

In 1933, Weber and Hill described the clinical and pathological findings in a patient with a peripheral neuropathy associated with esophageal cancer, illustrating demyelination in the posterior columns. Denny-Brown's (1948) report of two patients with sensory neuropathy associated with small-cell lung cancer finally established the relationship between peripheral neuropathies of the sensory type and lung cancer, and began the modern era of the study of paraneoplastic syndromes. Attempts to classify paraneoplastic peripheral neuropathies on the basis of clinical findings, pathological abnormalities or presumed pathophysiological mechanisms soon followed (Henson and Urich 1982) (Table 15.2). The term paraneoplastic was first applied to a peripheral neuropathy by Guichard (1949) to distinguish polyneuropathies associated with metastases from those occurring in the absence of metastases.

Classification

Several different types of peripheral neuropathy are associated with cancer (Table 14.2). Clinically, paraneoplastic neuropathies can be divided into four major groups:

1. Motor neuropathy including disorders of the neuromuscular junction and anterior horn cells.
2. Sensory neuropathy including disorders of the dorsal root ganglion or posterior horns.
3. Sensorimotor neuropathy. The sensorimotor neuropathies can be divided into two clinical groups: (a) acute neuropathies mimicking GBS or relapsing and remitting neuropathies and, (b) subacute or chronic sensorimotor neuropathies.
4. Autonomic neuropathy including abnormalities of the intermediolateral cell column of the spinal cord or of autonomic ganglia.

Table 15.2 *Classification of paraneoplastic peripheral neuropathy*

MOTOR NEUROPATHY
Motor-neuron disease (ALS)
isolated
associated with encephalomyelitis
Subacute motor neuronopathy
Lambert–Eaton syndrome
Myasthenia gravis
Neuromyotonia
Stiff-man syndrome
SENSORY NEUROPATHY
Subacute sensory neuronopathy
isolated
associated with encephalomyelitis
Chronic distal sensory neuropathy
SENSORIMOTOR NEUROPATHY
Acute
Guillain-Barré syndrome
Subacute/chronic
disabling
mild
AUTONOMIC NEUROPATHY
isolated
associated with encephalomyelitis
FOCAL NEUROPATHY
acute brachial plexopathy
NEUROMYOPATHY

Furthermore, paraneoplastic neuropathies may be either focal, involving single or multiple discrete nerves, or generalized (polyneuropathy). Pathologically, the disorder may involve primarily the cell body, the axon, the myelin sheath, or a combination (see below).

Prevalence

The frequency of paraneoplastic peripheral neuropathies can be viewed from two perspectives. The first is the prevalence of peripheral neuropathy in patients known to have cancer. Several clinical, pathological and electrophysiological studies have addressed this aspect (Table 15.3). Unfortunately, in most of the studies, it is difficult to identify what percentage of patients were suffering from metabolic or nutritional disorders associated with cancer rather than true paraneoplastic peripheral neuropathy because evidence concerning nutritional status as presented is often inadequate or conflicting. Taken together, however, the data indicate that although many patients (perhaps 30–40%) with cancer give evidence of peripheral nerve dysfunction when laboratory investigations are used, only a few (approximately 1%) are clinically affected by peripheral nerve symptoms not ascribable to cachexia or malnutrition.

Other studies address the likelihood that a patient with a clinically apparent peripheral neuropathy has cancer as the underlying cause (Table 15.4). In these patients, because the cancers are often small, nutritional and metabolic disorders probably do not play a role; however, the data are often biased by referral patterns in which only undiagnosed or very severe peripheral neuropathies are likely to be referred to specialty centers and therefore enhance the apparent incidence of paraneoplastic peripheral neuropathies. Nevertheless, a gross estimate suggests that 10–15% of patients with peripheral neuropathy not caused by diabetes will eventually prove to have a paraneoplastic neuropathy.

Pathology

The pathological changes in the peripheral nerve vary. In general, demyelinating lesions are uncommon except when associated with antibodies against myelin-associated glycoprotein (Chapter 12). Most of the peripheral neuropathies are axonal of the dying-back type with secondary demyelination in some. Neuronal neuropathies are also common. Neuropathies, either involving anterior horn cells or dorsal root ganglion cells, are a common finding in the pure motor and pure sensory neuropathies often associated with more widespread central nervous system (CNS) disease as occurs in the encephalomyelitis associated with cancer (Henson and Urich 1982). In a few instances of paraneoplastic peripheral neuropathy, the nerve is damaged indirectly as, for example, when paraneoplastic vasculitis causes nerve ischemia (Chapter 11). These disorders are usually focal or multifocal, resembling mononeuritis multiplex, but may be generalized.

Table 15.3 *Incidence of neuropathies in patients with cancer*

Cancer diagnosis	Patients in study (*n*)	Diagnostic criteria for neuropathy	*n*	%	Reference
Clinical studies					
Lung	299	Peripheral neuritis	5	1.7	Lennox and Prichard (1950)
Lung	501	Peripheral neuritis	11	2.2	Lea (1952)
Lung	250	Any peripheral nervous system disorder	40	16	Croft and Wilkinson (1963)
		Polyneuritis	4	1.6	
Breast	250	Any peripheral nervous system disorder		4.4	
		Polyneuritis	2	0.8	
All cancer	1465	Neuromyopathy	62	4.2	Croft and Wilkinson (1963)
		Mixed peripheral neuropathy	18	1.2	
		Motor neuropathy	3	0.2	
		Sensory neuropathy	0		
		Myopathy and myasthenia	15	1	
All cancer	1500	Proximal symmetrical weakness and wasting	52	3.5	Shy and Silverstein (1965)
Lung	3843	Clinical neuropathy (excluding sensory neuronopathy)	27	0.7	Henson and Urich (1982)
All cancer	171	Quantitative vibration threshold	21	12	Lipton et al. (1987)
Non-lung	29	Quantitative vibration threshold	9	31	Lipton et al. (1991)
	14	Quantitative temperature threshold	6	43	
SCLC	150	Neuromuscular signs	66	44	Erlington et al. (1991)
Lymphoma	229	Clinical neuropathy	4	1.7	Hutchinson et al. (1958)
All	774	Clinical peripheral neuropathy	11	1.4	Currie et al. (1970)
Reticuloses myeloma	125		4	3.2	Currie et al. (1970)
Hodgkin's	210		3	1.4	
NHL	228		1		
CLL	41		1		
CML	36		1		
PCV	68		1		
Acute leukemia	66		—		
Electrophysiological studies					
Cancer	82	Nerve conduction and needle EMG criteria for PNP	14	17	Moody (1965)
Lung	55	Clinical neuropathy	3	5.5	Trojaborg et al. (1969)
		Denervation and normal MNCV	20	36	
Lymphoma	62	Clinical neuropathy	5	8	Walsh (1971)
		Electrophysiological polyneuropathy	22	35	
Lung	28	Proximal muscle weakness	16	57	Campbell and Paty (1974)
		Sluggish reflexes	10	36	
	26	EMG: small amplitude short duration MUP	16	53	
		Denervation on EMG	11	42	
		Spontaneous activity	9	30	
All cancer	195	Wasting or objective sensory loss	56	30	Paul et al. (1978)
		Generalized wasting	27	14	
		Proximal wasting	14	7	
		Slowed NCV	50	26	
		Denervation EMG	63	32	
		Mainly axonal change EMG and NCV			

Table 15.3 (*cont.*)

Cancer diagnosis	Patients in study (n)	Diagnostic criteria for neuropathy	n	%	Reference
All cancer		Sensory polyneuropathy	21	11	
		Motor polyneuropathy	16	8	
		Sensorimotor polyneuropathy	14	7	
SCLC	71	Cachexia and symmetrical			Hawley et al. (1980)
		Peripheral neuropathy			
		early stage	as in control		
		15% weight loss		100	
Lung	80	Clinically only minor neurological abnormalities			Lenman et al. (1981)
		EMG signs of denervation		35	
		Slowed nerve conduction velocity		13	
Lung	60	Clinically mild peripheral neuropathy	8	13	Graus et al. (1983)
		Electrophysiological axonal neuropathy	11	18	
Lymphoma	30	Severe sensorimotor dymyelinating PNP	2	6	Graus et al. (1983)
		Electrophysiological mild axonal neuropathy	3	10	
Breast	61	Electrical stimulation			Bruera et al. (1988)
		Relaxation velocity			
Breast cancer	43	Clinical neuropathy	0	0	Hormigo et al. (1993)
		Electrophysiological	5	12	
	18	Sensorimotor neuropathy			
Benign breast		Clinical neuropathy	0	0	
Biopsy		Electrophysiological	3	17	
		Sensorimotor neuropathy			
Pathological studies					
All cancer	46	Clinical peripheral motor neuropathy	2	4.5	Hildebrand and Coers (1967)
		Pathologic terminal axonal motor innervation	20	44	
	27	Patients with weight loss	17	63	
	19	Patients without weight loss	3	16	
Lung	33	Clinical polyneuropathy	16	48	Teravainen and Larsen (1977)
		Diabetes/cytoxic therapy excluded	11	33	
	19	Nerve conduction velocity lowered	10	52	
	13	Intercostal muscle biopsy			
		Altered presynaptic ACh release			
All cancer	210	Deltoid muscle autopsy samples contain more scattered and small group atrophy			Schmitt (1978)
		Related to cachexia			
Lung	100	Proximal myopathy	15	15	Gomm et al. (1990)
SCLC	35	Cachectic myopathy (10% weight loss)	18	18	
Non-SCLC	65	Muscle biopsy:	74	74	
		Type II atrophy	12	12	
		Type I and II atrophy	1	1	
		Type I atrophy	12	12	
		Necrosis			

Notes:

ACh: acetylcholine; EMG: electromyograph; MNCV: motor nerve conduction velocities; MUP: motor unit potentials; NCV: nerve conduction velocities; PNP: peripheral neuropathy.

Pathophysiology

The pathophysiology of most paraneoplastic peripheral neuropathies is unknown. Early investigators, such as Oppenheim (1888), believed that nonmetastatic complications of cancer arose from toxic substances secreted by the tumor or from other metabolic disorders caused by the tumor. Although it is now recognized that tumors can make or induce normal cells to synthesize cytokines (Tracey and Cerami 1992), a true peripheral nervous system toxin secreted by the tumor has never been identified. Furthermore, in most paraneoplastic peripheral neuropathies, removal of the tumor does not alter the neurological disorder.

Denny-Brown proposed that the sensory neuronopathy he described arose from competition between the tumor and the dorsal root ganglion cell for a vital nutrient such as pantothenic acid (Denny-Brown 1948). Tumors associated with paraneoplastic peripheral neuropathy are usually too small to compete successfully for an important substrate and, as indicated above, removal of the tumor does not cause resolution of the neurological deficit.

Although neither of the above hypotheses accounts for most of the florid paraneoplastic peripheral neuropathies outlined in Table 15.2, it may be that many of the subclinical neuropathies encountered by careful clinical, electrophysiological or pathological examination result from: (1) cachexia, weight loss and malnutrition, (2) substances produced by the cancer, or (3) competition between the cancer and the body for vital nutrients.

Henson and colleagues, identifying inflammatory infiltrates in the CNS of patients with encephalomyelitis associated with cancer (many of whom had sensory neuropathy as well) suggested that a viral infection had caused the disorder (Henson et al. 1965). This hypothesis was supported when the paraneoplastic syndrome, progressive multifocal leukoencephalopathy (PML), was found to result from an opportunistic infection with a papova virus. Most untreated cancer patients who suffer from opportunistic infections have cancers of the immune system such as Hodgkin's disease, leukemia and lymphoma, the setting in which PML occurs. On the contrary, most patients with paraneoplastic peripheral neuropathy suffer from solid tumors such as lung cancer that are not associated with immune suppression. Exceptions are the increased incidence of GBS in patients with Hodgkin's disease (Lisak et al. 1977) and subacute motor neuronopathy (Schold et al. 1979), usually associated with Hodgkin's disease and non-Hodgkin's lymphoma.

In 1961, Russell suggested that the inflammatory infiltrates in the nervous systems of patients with paraneoplastic syndromes may be a result of "a carcinoma even of small size that elaborates some products which could, in certain subjects, provoke the formation of antibodies" (Russell 1961). Her remarks initiated the current hypothesis for the pathogenesis of most, if not all, paraneoplastic neuropathies. The current paradigm suggests that immunologically privileged self-antigens found in the nervous system are aberrantly expressed in the growing cancer. The patient must have a genetically determined propensity to generate self-reactive T lymphocyte clones and the tumor must contain on its surface the major histocompatibility complex of 'susceptibility alleles' which allow binding and presentation of the autoantigen to T cells. Finally, the patient must have inherited or acquired abnormalities in immunoregulation that lead to activation of self-reactive T cells and deficient suppression of self-reactive T and B cells (Sinha et al. 1990). The result of this complicated process is that an immune reaction against an autoantigen(s), present in both the nervous system and the tumor, causes both suppression of growth of the tumor and damage to the nervous system. Because the tumor is kept in check and the nervous system symptoms are so prominent, the patient usually presents to a neurologist without evidence of an underlying cancer (Dalmau et al. 1990). The cancer may be very small and sometimes is identified only at autopsy.

An immune pathogenesis has clearly been demonstrated in the LEMS (Chapter 17). Evidence that LEMS is actually an autoimmune disease includes the clinical response to immunosuppression and, most compelling, the passive transfer of the disorder to experimental animals that are injected with IgG from patients with LEMS (Lang et al. 1981; Fukunaga et al. 1983). Patients with small-cell cancer produce IgG antibodies against calcium channels that are expressed both by the cancer and the neuromuscular junction. The antibodies so produced bind specifically to calcium

Table 15.4 *Cancer in patients with peripheral neuropathy*

Author	n	Study type	Neuropathy	Cancer n (%)	Remarks
Cancer in patients presenting with peripheral neuropathy					
Lennox and Prichard (1950)	28	Hospital chart review	Peripheral neuritis	5 (18)	All had carcinoma of bronchus
Matthews (1952)	46	Hospital chart review	Polyneuritis	2 (4)	Carcinoma of bronchus and breast
Rose (1960)	80	Hospital chart review	Peripheral neuropathy	3 (4)	
Prineas (1970)	278	Hospital chart review	Polyneuropathy	15 (5.4)	Follow-up of idiopathic cases revealed carcinomas in 4/15 cases: 2×repeat X-chest; 1×retroperitoneal sarcoma; 1×autopsy only
Huang (1981)	59	Neurology unit chart review	Clinical and electrophysiological peripheral neuropathy	7 (12)	Elderly patients (>60 years old) leukemia (2), myeloma, lymphoma, sclerotic multiple myeloma, gastric, and renal carcinoma. Two of the patients presented with the polyneuropathy
George and Twomey (1986)	74	Electrophysiology Unit chart review	Electrophysiological Polyneuropathy	10 (13)	Elderly population (65 years old) carcinomas of bronchus (5), stomach (2), colon (1), and multiple myeloma (2)
Cancer in patients with cryptogenic polyneuropathy					
Fagius (1983)	91	Chart review; follow-up of cryptogenic cases	Chronic cryptogenic polyneuropathy	1 (1)	Gastric carcinoma with anemia
McLeod et al. (1984)	47	Chart review; follow-up of case, >1 year	Biopsy proven polyneuropathy	5 (11)	Carcinoma of lung (2), pancreas (1), colon (1), and seminoma of the testis (1)
Grahamm et al. (1991)	41	Chart review with outpatient follow-up	Cryptogenic poly-neuropathy after inpatient evaluation	1 (2)	Non-Hodgkin's lymphoma with IgM-I paraproteinemia
Cancer in patients with specific neuropathies					
Chalk et al. (1992) Windebank et al. (1990)		Chart review	Subacute sensory neuronopathy	SCLC	±20 High selection bias of studied population makes determination of relative incidence less meaningful (statement authors)
Shy et al. (1986) Younger et al. (1990)	326	Chart review	Motor neuron disease	Lymphoma	5 (1.5) Marked association between lymphoma in MND with increased CSF protein or

						serum paraproteinemia
Rowland et al. (1992)	37	Prospective study	Motor neuron disease	lymphoma	2 (5.4)	
Notermans et al. (1993) Notermans et al. (1994)	75	Prospective description and prognostic cohort study	Chronic idiopathic polyneuropathy of middle and older age	—	0 (0)	Mildly progressive axonal polyneuropathy, often reaching plateau

Note:
CSF: cerebrospinal fluid; MND: motor neuron disease; SCLC: small cell lung cancer.

channels of the presynaptic neuromuscular junction (Hewett and Atchison 1992), causing an electron microscopically visible disarray (Fukuoka et al. 1987). The failure of calcium entry leads to diminished acetylcholine release. A gene coding for a protein similar in structure to the beta subunit of the calcium channel has been cloned and characterized. The protein reacts with antibodies in the sera of about 30% of LEMS patients (Rosenfeld et al. 1993).

Although an autoimmune process is probably the cause of most paraneoplastic peripheral neuropathies, opportunistic infections may also play a role. The two mechanisms could potentially coexist; 'molecular mimicry' between viral and CNS proteins could cause an immune response to an opportunistic virus to damage the nervous system (Sculier et al. 1987).

The evidence for an autoimmune pathogenesis is less clear in other paraneoplastic peripheral neuropathies. The evidence is strongest in paraneoplastic sensory neuronopathy accompanied by the Hu antibody (Dalmau et al. 1992). In this disorder, a highly conserved, otherwise strictly neuronal gene (HuD), is expressed in all small-cell lung cancers, many neuroblastomas, and in a few other cancers. In some patients whose tumors contain the HuD gene and express the Hu antigen, an immune response to the antigen is characterized by a serum anti-Hu autoantibody. If the titer of the anti-Hu antibody is low, the patient appears to remain asymptomatic but his tumor grows more slowly and metastasizes less regularly than that of patients with the same histological tumor who do not raise an anti-Hu antibody response (Dalmau et al. 1990). In patients with high titers of the anti-Hu antibody, a neurological syndrome characterized by the subacute development of a sensory neuronopathy, sometimes associated with encephalomyelitis, develops. An inflammatory response appears to destroy dorsal root ganglion cells, leading to the clinical syndrome which is usually but not always irreversible (Dalmau et al. 1992).

Diagnosis

In most instances, there is no clinical, electrodiagnostic or pathological difference between peripheral neuropathies that are paraneoplastic and those that arise in the absence of cancer. The best examples are GBS occurring in patients with Hodgkin's disease, which runs a similar clinical course to the more common non-paraneoplastic GBS (Lisak et al. 1977), and LEMS, two-thirds of which occurs in the setting of cancer (usually small-cell lung cancer) in which patients do not differ clinically from the one-third in whom no cancer exists (O'Neill et al. 1988). Thus, the neurologist confronted with a patient with a polyneuropathy who is not known to have cancer will only be able to decide whether the disorder is paraneoplastic or non-paraneoplastic if he searches for and finds a cancer. Even if the physician suspects an underlying cancer, an initial search may be negative because the tumor may be too small to be detected.

The physician confronted with a patient suffering a peripheral neuropathy of unknown cause should consider the possibility of an underlying cancer in all patients but especially in those patients in whom the disorder has developed rapidly over weeks and months rather than years, and in those in whom the neuropathy has caused significant disability. More slowly developing mild weakness or sensory loss is less likely to be paraneoplastic in origin. When the peripheral neuropathy is associated with additional signs of CNS disease, an underlying cancer should also be considered. In addition, specific clinical syndromes, such as a pure sensory neuropathy or the Lambert–Eaton myasthenic syndrome are more likely to be paraneoplastic than a sensorimotor peripheral neuropathy.

The history may give clues to an underlying cancer. Weight loss (if not deliberate), malaise and fatigue suggest that the disorder involves more than just the peripheral nerves. A history of heavy smoking suggests the possibility of lung cancer. Heavy alcohol intake is associated with squamous cancers of the mouth, pharynx, larynx and esophagus. A strong family history of ovarian or breast cancer also suggests the need for further workup.

The general physical examination may also be helpful. Signs of recent weight loss might suggest an underlying cancer. Enlarged lymph nodes should be searched for. Breasts and testes should be examined carefully and the abdomen palpated. Rectal examination may yield evidence of an underlying cancer of the prostate or colon.

Although a careful history and physical examination are mandatory in the workup of a patient with a peripheral neuropathy, a question is how extensive the laboratory examination should be. Sometimes, the nature of the peripheral neuropathy mandates certain laboratory tests. For example, the Lambert–Eaton myasthenic syndrome and subacute sensory neuropathy both require a careful examination of the lungs by CT scan for an underlying small-cell lung cancer. For most patients with sensorimotor neuropathy of unknown cause, no clues as to the nature of the cancer are available. In general, most patients should have a chest radiograph and routine blood studies. Additional blood studies that may give a clue to the underlying nature of the disorder include measurements of immunoglobulins looking for paraproteinemia (Chapter 11), erythrocyte sedimentation rate suggesting a disorder more widespread than an idiopathic peripheral neuropathy, measurement of biochemical tumor markers including, in specific patients, carcino-embryonic antigen, prostate specific antigen, CA-125 and antineuronal antibodies (anti-Hu). Mammography should be considered in patients with a slowly developing sensory motor neuropathy associated with itching and muscle cramps (Peterson et al. 1994).

Specific disorders

Motor neuropathies

Weakness without sensory symptoms can be caused by paraneoplastic disorders that involve the lower motor neuron anywhere along its course from the anterior horn cell to the postsynaptic neuromuscular junction. In some disorders the site of pathology is unknown. It is doubtful that paraneoplastic damage to axons or myelin sheaths is ever exclusively motor. Although some axonal or demyelinating paraneoplastic neuropathies are clinically predominantly motor with minimal sensory symptoms, they are considered below under the topic 'Sensorimotor neuropathies'.

Subacute motor neuronopathies/motor neuron disease

Epidemiological studies of motor neuron disease (MND) (amyotrophic lateral sclerosis) do not show an increased incidence of that disorder in patients with cancer (Henson and Urich 1982); clinical evidence, however, suggests that in rare instances, motor neurons may be affected in a paraneoplastic process either as an isolated finding or as part of a more widespread paraneoplastic encephalomyelitis. The evidence that paraneoplastic anterior horn cell disease exists is based on three findings. (1) Occasional patients with a clinical syndrome indistinguishable from MND recover after treatment of an underlying cancer (Rosenfeld and Posner 1991). (2) Serum protein assays and bone marrow examination of patients with MND suggest a higher than expected incidence of lymphoma (Younger et al. 1991; Rowland et al. 1992). (3) Evidence that paraneoplastic encephalomyelitis can begin as an illness clinically indistinguishable from MND (Dalmau et al. 1992).

A disorder called by Schold et al. (1979), subacute motor neuropathy, associated with Hodgkin's disease and non-Hodgkin's lymphoma, is a variant of motor neuron disease. Characteristically, a patient already known to have a lymphoma develops a subacute and progressive, painless and often patchy lower motor neuron weakness which usually affects legs more than arms. Atrophy is present but fasciculations are not prominent; the bulbar musculature is usually spared. Although patients sometimes complain of paresthesias, sensory loss is mild despite often profound weakness. Motor and sensory nerve conduction velocities are normal or only mildly decreased; electromyography gives evidence of denervation. The cerebrospinal fluid (CSF) is acellular with a mildly elevated protein concentration. The magnetic resonance scan of the cord is normal. The course is usually benign and independent of the activity of the underlying neoplasm. Unlike MND, the neurological defect usually does not incapacitate the patient; instead, it often stabilizes or improves spontaneously after months or years. Treatment does not hasten recovery.

The main pathological findings are degeneration of neurons in the anterior horns of the spinal cord. Sometimes patchy and mild demyelination of the spinal cord is seen in the white matter, particularly that surrounding the gray matter columns. The lateral columns of the spinal cord, unlike in typical MND, are spared.

Indirect evidence suggests that the disorder may be caused by an opportunistic viral infection of anterior horn neurons. (1) The disorder is associated with a lymphoma, which results in immunosuppression and favors opportunistic viral infections. Of patients reported with the disorder, one died of progressive multifocal leukoencephalopathy and another of an opportunistic nocardia infection. (2) The pathological abnormalities resemble those of burnt-out poliomyelitis. Viral-like particles were identified in the anterior horns of one patient although a specific virus had not been isolated (Walton et al. 1968). (3) A similar neurological disorder affecting spinal anterior horn cells in a strain of mice is caused by the murine leukemia virus (Rosenfeld and Posner 1991).

There is controversy over whether this disorder is a separate illness or is a manifestation of MND associated with cancer. In a review of 422 patients with MND, Younger et al. (1991) found eight who also had lymphoma. Some of these patients had upper motor neuron as well as lower motor neuron signs, casting doubt on the specificity of subacute motor neuronopathy. In a more recent report of 37 consecutive patients with MND who underwent bone marrow biopsy, two were found to have evidence of lymphoma (Rowland et al. 1992). The relevant clinical implications are two: (1) patients with MND should probably be screened by immunofixation analysis for paraprotein and bone marrow biopsy should be considered; (2) if a lymphoma is discovered, the course of the patient's neurological disease, although probably independent of treatment of lymphoma, may be more benign and possibly remitting.

Sensory neuropathies

Subacute sensory neuronopathy

Subacute sensory neuronopathy is so named because the major pathology affects neurons of the dorsal root ganglion, with secondary degeneration of sensory fibers of peripheral nerves. Motor nerves are unaffected. Although the disorder is rare, the likelihood that a patient who has a subacutely developing sensory neuronopathy has cancer is about 20% and, thus, all patients with the disorder deserve a careful workup for the cancer (Horwich et al. 1977; Chalk et al. 1992). Paraneoplastic sensory neuronopathy (PSN) can occur as an isolated disorder or as a manifestation of paraneoplastic encephalomyelitis.

Two-thirds of patients with PSN have lung cancer, particularly small-cell lung cancer (Chalk et al. 1992; Dalmau et al. 1992). PSN is predominantly a female illness despite the continuing slight preponderance of males with the underlying small-cell cancer. The neuronopathy precedes the diagnosis of cancer by an average of about a year. Sometimes the cancer is discovered only at autopsy. If the disorder appears after the diagnosis of cancer, it usually does so within 6 months. There are a few instances of the cancer disappearing as the paraneoplastic syndrome develops (Darnell and DeAngelis 1993).

The symptoms usually begin with paresthesias and often painful dysesthesias. Clumsiness and unsteady gait then develop and usually become the most predominant signs. Usually the sensory symptoms start distally and asymmetrically in the limbs but a proximal distribution in the extremities, trunk and sometimes the face occurs. In a few patients, the symptoms remain stable for months with mild neurological deficits (Graus et al. 1994) but in the majority, symptoms progress rapidly leaving the patient substantially disabled in a few weeks to a few months. The symptoms then stabilize. Henson reports a single patient whose symptoms developed overnight (Henson and Urich 1982).

All sensory modalities are affected but the most striking abnormality is severe sensory ataxia with pseudoathetosis of the hands. Deep tendon reflexes are depressed or absent. Motor power is normal or only mildly impaired.

Electrophysiological studies demonstrate small or absent sensory action potentials. Motor nerve conduction studies and F waves may remain entirely normal and electromyography does not give evidence of denervation. The CSF usually has an increased protein concentration with elevated IgG and oligoclonal bands. Early in the course of the disease there is mild pleocytosis.

Those patients with subacute sensory neuronopathy complicating small-cell lung cancer and a few with other cancers demonstrate the anti-Hu antibody in their serum. This antibody that reacts with the nuclei of neurons and of small cell lung cancers identifies a nuclear antigen that is an RNA binding protein (Dalmau et al. 1990; Szabo et al. 1991).

PATHOLOGY. The dorsal root ganglia are the main site of pathological damage. Most of the ganglia are affected although involvement may be patchy. If the patient dies early during the course of the disease, lymphocytes and macrophages are found in the dorsal root ganglion. The majority of cells in the infiltrates are T lymphocytes, predominantly cytotoxic T lymphocytes. In later stages sensory neurons are lost and replaced by a proliferation of satellite cells (nodules of Nageotte). Secondary changes are noted in posterior nerve roots, peripheral sensory nerves, and posterior columns of the spinal cord (Denny-Brown 1948; Horwich et al. 1977; Graus et al. 1990; Dalmau et al. 1992).

TREATMENT. The disorder runs a course independent of that of the cancer, usually developing rapidly and then stabilizing. Occasional patients have been reported to respond either to treatment of the tumor or to immunosuppressive therapy (Sagar and Read 1982; Graus et al. 1992); however, plasmapheresis and intravenous gammaglobulin, as well as corticosteroids, are ineffective in most patients (Graus et al. 1992).

Distal sensory neuropathy

Distal progressive peripheral neuropathies often begin with sensory symptoms and remain sensory for a considerable period of time. The reasons are twofold. The first is that sensory fibers are longer than motor fibers and dying-back neuropathies are likely to cause sensory damage before they do motor damage. The second is that involvement of peripheral nerves becomes symptomatic earlier (paresthesias and numbness), than mild motor weakness, particularly in the small muscles of the feet that may not be apparent until it becomes substantial. For that reason, a number of patients suffering from terminal dying-back axonal neuropathies have been classified as having sensory neuropathy although the neuropathies are usually mixed. These neuropathies are discussed below under the heading Chronic sensorimotor neuropathy.

Sensorimotor neuropathies

Sensory motor neuropathies can be divided into two main categories. (1) Acute neuropathies mimicking GBS, or relapsing and remitting neuropathies analogous to the chronic inflammatory demyelinating polyneuropathies. (2) Subacute or chronic sensorimotor neuropathies usually axonal but sometimes demyelinating. The disorders may be mild and non-disabling, usually appearing in patients with far advanced cancer where they are usually considered to be nutritional in origin, or they may appear early in the course of the disease and cause either mild or, more commonly, severe disability.

Sensorimotor peripheral neuropathies, in general, are much more common as a paraneoplastic syndrome than either motor or pure sensory neuropathies; however, they are also much more common as a non-paraneoplastic syndrome. Thus, in a patient presenting to the neurologist with any of these neuropathies, although cancer should be considered, it is only in the subacutely developing severe sensorimotor neuropathies that a paraneoplastic syndrome should be a major diagnostic consideration.

Acute sensorimotor neuropathy

GUILLAIN-BARRÉ SYNDROME. An acutely developing, predominantly motor peripheral neuropathy indistinguishable clinically or pathologically from GBS can occur in patients with cancer. Most investigators consider its occurrence in patients with solid tumors as coincidental, the coincidental association of two common diseases. The link between Hodgkin's disease and the GBS, however, is more firmly established (Cameron et al. 1958; Klingon 1965; Currie et al. 1970; Lisak et al. 1977; Henson and Urich 1982; Shy et al. 1986; Halls et al. 1988). The majority of patients have known Hodgkin's disease at the time GBS develops. Severe paralysis is present in most patients, requiring artificial ventilation in some. Electrophysiological and pathological findings are indistinguishable from idiopathic GBS and most patients, including some not reported, have responded to plasma exchange but not to corticosteroids. This disorder has also been reported with leukemias, non-Hodgkin's lymphoma and multiple myeloma (Barron et al. 1962).

When occurring with leukemia and lymphoma, infiltration of peripheral nerves or roots (in the leptomeninges) by tumor must be ruled out. In some patients, diagnosis can only be made by biopsy (Sumi et al. 1983).

RELAPSING AND REMITTING PERIPHERAL NEUROPATHY. These disorders are clinically and pathologically similar to idiopathic relapsing and remitting peripheral neuropathy. They are probably demyelinating (Croft et al. 1967) but may sometimes be axonal (Schlaepfer 1974). Only 15% of patients with this neuropathy have lung cancer. Other sites of primary growth include breast, stomach, cervix, uterus, bladder, testes, and thymus (Croft et al. 1967). The disorder is also associated with osteosclerotic myeloma (Chapter 11), Hodgkin's disease (Croft et al. 1967; Lisak et al. 1977), and lymphoma (Croft et al. 1967; Sumi et al. 1983). The neuropathy precedes clinical evidence of the cancer in half the patients by 2–8 years. In the other half, it occurs after the cancer is diagnosed and may occur as long as 6 years after diagnosis (Croft et al. 1967). Characteristically, the patients develop an acute or subacute neuropathy that waxes and wanes, sometimes resulting in complete recovery. These are monophasic in some, while in others, two or more episodes of neuropathy occur. Some believe that steroids may cause the remission. In others, improvement follows removal of the tumor (Croft and Wilkinson 1969; Littler 1970; Enevoldson et al. 1990; Evans and Kaufman 1994). As with the idiopathic form, in some patients the symptoms are predominantly motor.

CSF protein content is frequently elevated but CSF cell counts are normal. Electrophysiological studies demonstrate reduced nerve conduction velocities and denervation (Croft et al. 1967; Sumi et al. 1983). Whether this disorder is simply a coincidence of idiopathic inflammatory polyneuropathy occurring in a patient with cancer is not clear.

Subacute and chronic sensorimotor polyneuropathy

SUBACUTE SENSORIMOTOR POLYNEUROPATHY. Unlike more chronically developing sensorimotor polyneuropathies, the development of a subacute and severe sensorimotor polyneuropathy, for which a cause cannot immediately be determined, warrants a careful workup for cancer. The majority of patients have lung cancer although patients with other neoplasms including colon, pancreas, myeloma and sarcoma have been described (Croft and Wilkinson 1969). In two-thirds of the patients with paraneoplastic subacute sensorimotor polyneuropathy, the symptoms develop before or simultaneously with other manifestations of the neoplasm (Croft and Wilkinson 1969). The onset and progression may be acute (developing over days) or run a more protracted course (weeks or months). Usually the legs are more affected than the arms. In some cases, the symptoms are almost exclusively motor (Lennox and Prichard 1950). Cranial nerves and autonomic involvement are rare although trigeminal sensory loss may develop. This disorder may be part of a more widespread encephalomyelitis but also may occur as a purely peripheral process.

CSF protein is often elevated. Pleocytosis is usually absent. Eletrophysiological tests demonstrate slowing of nerve conduction velocities in some patients but not to the degree suggesting demyelination (Croft et al. 1967).

Autopsy specimens generally show both loss of axons and myelins in peripheral nerves and sometimes nerve roots. Lymphocytic infiltration in peripheral nerve may be observed as well.

The course of the disorder is often progressive, with relentless deterioration, independent of the course of the tumor. Some patients stabilize and many go on to become incapacitated. Rarely spontaneous remission occurs (Croft et al. 1967).

SENSORIMOTOR NEUROPATHY. This disorder occurs in two settings. (1) A mild, predominantly sensory polyneuropathy develops, often during terminal phases of the disease. It may appear several years after the diagnosis of cancer is made. It is characterized mainly by a distal polyneuropathy with sensory symptoms in a glove and stocking distribution, diminished reflexes and some mild weakness. The lower extremities are more affected and sometimes exclusively affected. In half of the patients in one series, there was some proximal muscle weakness raising the question of myopathy ('neuromyopathy') (Henson et al. 1954; Hildebrand and Coers 1967). Electrophysiological evidence, however, demonstrates a mixed sensorimotor axonal polyneuropathy. The disorder is not disabling and, as the patients are known to have cancer and usually are in the terminal stages of the disease, rarely require medical intervention for either diagnosis or therapy. The pathogenesis is probably malnutrition and cachexia. (2) A distal sensorimotor polyneuropathy is frequently found in patients in the earlier stages of cancer when tested electrophysiologically or with quantitative sensory testing. Most of these patients are asymptomatic but some have chronic and slowly progressive symptoms that are predominantly sensory. Peterson et al. (1994) identified nine patients with breast cancer and a slowly progressive sensorimotor, but predominantly sensory polyneuropathy, sometimes with features suggestive of myopathy (proximal weakness) or CNS dysfunction (hyperreflexia and extensor plantar responses). The disorder progressed very slowly over many years, was not disabling and was frequently heralded by itching and/or muscle cramps. In one patient, itching initially over the left breast and later diffusely, preceded the identification of the cancer by a year and a half. Most patients remained fully functional as neither the neuropathy nor the breast cancer were disabling.

Autonomic neuropathies

Paraneoplastic autonomic neuropathy is rare but may occur either alone or as part of a more widespread encephalomyelitis. Usually associated with small-cell lung cancer, it also occurs with other cancers and may present prior to or after the cancer diagnosis. The patients usually present with a subacute onset of postural hypotension (van Lieshout et al. 1986), intestinal immobility (Chinn and Schuffler 1988; Lennon et al. 1991), pupillary abnormalities (Maitland et al. 1985) and a neurogenic bladder. The syndrome is generally progressive but may stabilize or improve with treatment of the underlying tumor. The disorder usually occurs as a manifestation of a more widespread encephalomyelitis associated with the anti-Hu antibody. If the anti-Hu antibody is present, the underlying cancer is small-cell lung cancer (Dalmau et al. 1992).

Focal or multifocal neuropathies

Most sensory and sensorimotor neuropathies are symmetrical although they can be asymmetrical, at least at onset, and some can remain asymmetrical throughout the course of the disease. A few patients develop clearly focal or multifocal neuropathies (mononeuritis multiplex) which differ from the usual paraneoplastic sensorimotor neuropathy. Johnson et al. (1979) described three cases of a paraneoplastic mononeuritis multiplex caused by vasculitis of vasa nervorum. There was no vasculitis in other organs. Oh et al. (1991) reported a patient with endometrial carcinoma who developed a paraneoplastic vasculitic neuropathy that responded to cyclophosphamide. Vincent et al. (1986) in a series of 50 patients with nerve and/or muscle microvasculitis seen on biopsy, found seven associated with malignancy. In two patients the cancer was found after the discovery of the vasculitis. All the patients exhibited sensory motor neuropathy which was often painful and asymmetrical. Harati and Niakan (1986), studying 33 patients with inflammatory angiopathic neuropathy, discovered malignant neoplasms in three. CSF protein levels are often elevated. Steroids and cyclophosphamide are effective in some whereas spontaneous improvement occurs in others.

The second characteristic focal neuropathy is a paraneoplastic brachial plexopathy. This disorder occurs more commonly in patients with Hodgkin's disease than in patients with solid tumors. It is clinically, electrophysiologically and pathologically indistinguishable from idiopathic acute brachial neuritis. As with that disorder, it runs a benign course although exploration of the brachial plexus in one patient revealed a slight decrease in the density of myelinated fibers, mononuclear cells distributed between nerve bundles and conspicuous subperineural edema. Most of the infiltrating cells were T cell in origin. Evidence of demyelination and remyelination was present suggesting an inflammatory demyelinating plexopathy. The disorder must be differentiated from radiation injury, traumatic injury surgery and anesthesia and ischemic brachial neuritis (Lachance et al. 1991).

Acknowledgments

Supported in part by NIH Grant NS2606. Dr Smitt is the recipient of a Clinical and Research Fellowship from the Dutch Cancer Society.

References

Auche, M. (1890). Des nevrites peripheriques chez les cancereux. *Medicine* 10: 785–807.

Barron, K.D., Rowland, L.P., and Zimmerman, H.M. (1962). Neuropathy with malignant tumor metastases. *Neur. Met. Dis.* 56: 10–31.

Cameron, D.G., Howell, D.A., and Hutchison, J.L. (1958). Acute peripheral neuropathy in Hodgkin's disease. Report of a fatal case with histologic features of allergic neuritis. *Neurology* 8: 575–577.

Campbell, M.J. and Paty, D.W. (1974). Carcinomatous neuromyopathy: 1. Electrophysiological studies. An electrophysiological and immunological study of patients with carcinoma of the lung. *J. Neurol. Neurosurg. Psychiatry* 37: 131–141.

Chalk, C.H., Windebank, A.J., Kimmel, D.W., and McManis, P.G. (1992). The distinctive clinical features of paraneoplastic sensory neuronopathy. *Can. J. Neurol. Sci.* 19: 346–351.

Chinn, J.S. and Schuffler, M.D. (1988). Paraneoplastic visceral neuropathy as a cause of severe gastrointestinal motor dysfunction. *Gastroenterology* 95: 1279–1286.

Clouston, P.D., Saper, C.B., Arbizu, T., Johnston, I., Lang, B., Newsom-Davis, J., and Posner, J.B. (1992). Paraneoplastic cerebellar degeneration. III. Cerebellar degeneration, cancer and the Lambert–Eaton myasthenic syndrome. *Neurology* 42: 1944–1950.

Croft, P.B., Urich, H., and Wilkinson, M. (1967). Peripheral neuropathy of sensorimotor type associated with malignant disease. *Brain* 90: 31–66.

Croft, P.B. and Wilkinson, M. (1963). Carcinomatous neuromyopathy. Its incidence in patients with carcinoma of the lung and breast. *Lancet* i: 184–188.

Croft, P.B. and Wilkinson, M. (1965). The incidence of carcinomatous neuromyopathy in patients with various types of carcinomas. *Brain* 88: 427–434.

Croft, P.B. and Wilkinson, M. (1969). The course and prognosis in some types of carcinomatous neuromyopathy. *Brain* 92: 1–8.

Currie, S., Henson, R.A., Morgan, H.G., and Poole, A.J. (1970). The incidence of the non-metastatic neurological syndromes of obscure origin in the reticuloses. *Brain* 93: 629–640.

Dalmau, J., Furneaux, H.M., Gralla, R.J., Kris, M., and Posner, J.B. (1990). Detection of the anti-Hu antibody in the serum of patients with small cell lung cancer: a quantitative western blot analysis. *Ann. Neurol.* 27: 544–552.

Dalmau, J., Graus, F., Rosenblum, M.K., and Posner, J.B. (1992). Anti-Hu-associated paraneoplastic encephalomyelitis/sensory neuronopathy. A clinical study of 71 patients. *Medicine* 71: 59–72.

Darnell, R.B. and DeAngelis, L.M. (1993). Regression of small-cell lung carcinoma in patients with paraneoplastic neuronal antibodies. *Lancet* 341: 21–22.

Denny-Brown, D. (1948). Primary sensory neuropathy with muscular changes associated with carcinoma. *J. Neurol. Neurosurg. Psychiatry* 11: 73–87.

Enevoldson, T.P., Ball, J.A., and McGregor, J.M. (1990). Resolution of a severe sensorimotor neuropathy following resection of an associated asymptomatic gastric lymphoma. *J. Neurol. Neurosurg. Psychiatry* 53: 267–268.

Erlington, G.M., Murray, N.M., Spiro, S.G., and Newsom-Davis, J. (1991). Neurological paraneoplastic syndromes in patients with small cell lung cancer. A prospective survey of 150 patients. *J. Neurol. Neurosurg. Psychiatry* 54: 764–767.

Evans, C.C. and Kaufman, H.D. (1994). Unusual presentation of seminoma of the testis. *Br. J. Surg.* 58: 703–704.

Fagius, J. (1983). Chronic cryptogenic polyneuropathy. The search for a cause. *Acta Neurol. Scand.* 67: 173–180.

Fukunaga, H., Engel, A.G., Lang, B., Newsom-Davis, J., and Vincent, A. (1983). Passive transfer of Lambert–Eaton myasthenic syndrome with IgG from man to mouse depletes the presynaptic membrane active zones. *Proc. Natl. Acad. Sci. USA* 80: 7636–7640.

Fukuoka, T., Engel, A.G., Lang, B., Newson-Davis, J., Prior, C., and Wray, D. (1987). Lambert–Eaton myasthenic syndrome. I. Early morphological effects of IgG on the presynaptic membrane active zones. *Ann. Neurol.* 22: 193–199.

George, J. and Twomey, J.A. (1986). Causes of polyneuropathy in the elderly. *Age Ageing* 15: 247–249.

Gomm, S.A., Thatcher, N., Barber, P.V., and Cummings, W.J.K. (1990). A clinicopathological study of the paraneoplastic neuromuscular syndromes associated with lung cancer. *QJM – Monthly Journal of the Association of Physicians*, 278: 577–595.

Grahamm, F., Winterholler, M., and Neundorfer, B. (1991). Cryptogenic polyneuropathies: an out-patient follow-up study. *Acta Neurol. Scand.* 84: 221–225.

Graus, F., Bonaventura, I., Uchuya, M., Valls-Sole, J., Rene, R., Leger, J.M., Tolosa, E. and Delattre, J. (1994). Indolent anti-Hu-associated paraneoplastic sensory neuropathy. *Neurology* 44: 2258–2261.

Graus, F., Cordon-Cardo, C., and Posner, J.B. (1985). Neuronal antinuclear antibody in sensory neuronopathy from lung cancer. *Neurology* 35: 538–543.

Graus, F., Ferrer, I., and Lamarca, J. (1983). Mixed carcinomatous neuropathy in patients with lung cancer and lymphoma. *Acta Neurol. Scand.* 68: 40–48.

Graus, F., Ribalta, T., Campo, E., Monforte, R., Urbano, A., and Rozman, C. (1990). Immunohistochemical analysis of the immune reaction in the nervous system in paraneoplastic encephalomyelitis. *Neurology* 40: 219–222.

Graus, F., Vega, F., Delattre, J.-Y., Bonaventura, I., Rene, R., Arbaiza, D., and Tolosa, E. (1992). Plasmapheresis and antineoplastic treatment in CNS paraneoplastic syndromes with antineuronal autoantibodies. *Neurology* 42: 536–450.

Guichard, A. and Vignon, G. (1949). La polyradiculonevrite cancereuse metastatique. Paralysies multiples des nerfs craniens et rachidiens par generalisation microscopique d'un epithelioma du col uterin. *J. Med.* 00: 197–207.

Halls, J., Bredkjaer, C., and Friis, M.L. (1988). Guillain-Barré syndrome: diagnostic criteria, epidemiology, clinical course and prognosis. *Acta Neurol. Scand.* 78: 118–122.

Harati, Y., and Niakan, E. (1986). The clinical spectrum of inflammatory-angiopathic neuropathy. *J. Neurol. Neurosurg. Psychiatry* 49: 1313–1316.

Henson, R.A., Hoffman, H.L., and Urich, H. (1965). Encephalomyelitis with carcinoma. *Brain* 88: 449–464.

Henson, R.A., Russell, D.S., and Wilkinson, M. (1954). Carcinomatous neuropathy and myopathy: a clinical and pathological study. *Brain* **77**: 82–121.

Henson, R.A. and Urich, H. (1982). *Cancer and the Nervous System: The Neurological Manifestations of Systemic Malignant Disease.* London: Blackwell Scientific.

Hewett, S.J. and Atchison, W.D. (1992). Specificity of Lambert–Eaton myasthenic syndrome immunoglobulin for nerve terminal calcium channels. *Brain Res.* **599**: 324–332.

Hildebrand, J. and Coers, C. (1967). The neuromuscular function in patients with malignant tumours. Electromyographic and histological study. *Brain* **90**: 67–82.

Hormigo, A., and Lieberman, F. (1994). Nuclear localization of anti-Hu antibody is not associated with in vitro cytotoxicity. *J. Neuroimmunol* **55**: 205–212.

Hormigo, A., Luis, M.L., and Alves, M. (1993). Electrophysiological evaluation of the paraneoplastic syndrome in early stages. *Muscle Nerve* **16**: 1419–1420.

Horwich, M.S., Cho, L., Porro, R.S., and Posner, J.B. (1977). Subacute sensory neuropathy: a remote effect of carcinoma. *Ann. Neurol.* **2**: 7–19.

Huang, C.Y. (1981). Peripheral neuropathy in the elderly: a clinical and electrophysiologic study. *J. Am. Geriatr. Soc.* **29**: 49–54.

Hutchinson, E.C., Leonard, B.J., Maudsley, C., and Yates, P.O. (1958). Neurological complications of the reticuloses. *Brain* **81**: 75–92.

Johnson, P.C., Rolak, L.A., Hamilton, R.H., and Laguna, J.F. (1979). Paraneoplastic vasculitis of nerve: a remote effect of cancer. *Ann. Neurol.* **5**: 437–444.

Keating, J.W. and Cormwell, L.D. (1978). Remote effects of neuroblastoma. *J. Roentgenol.* **131**: 299–303.

Klingon, G.H. (1965). The Guillain-Barré syndrome associated with cancer. *Cancer* **18**: 157–163.

Lachance, D.H., O'Neill, B.P., Harper, C.M., Jr, Bauks, P.M., and Cascino, T.L. (1991). Paraneoplastic brachial plexopathy in a patient with Hodgkin's disease. *Mayo Clin. Proc.* **66**: 97–101.

Lang, B., Newsom-Davis, J., and Wray, D. (1981). Autoimmune aetiology for myasthenic (Eaton–Lambert) syndrome. *Lancet* **1**: 224–226.

Lea, A.J. (1952). A survey of 501 cases of bronchogenic carcinoma. *Thorax* **7**: 305–309.

Lenman, J.A., Fleming, A.M., Robertson, M.A.H., Abbott, R.J., Clee, M.D., Ferguson, I.F., and Wright, D.S. (1981). Peripheral nerve function in patients with bronchial carcinoma. Comparison with matched controls and effects of treatment. *J. Neurol. Neurosurg. Psychiatry* **44**: 54–61.

Lennon, V.A., Sas, D.F., Busk, M.F., Scheithauer, B., Matagelada, J.-R., Camilleri, M., and Miller, L.J. (1991). Enteric neuronal autoantibodies in pseudoobstruction with small-cell lung carcinoma. *Gastroenterology* **100**: 137–142.

Lennox, B. and Prichard, S. (1950). The association of bronchial carcinoma and peripheral neuritis. *Q. J. Med.* **74**: 97–109.

Lipton, R.B., Galer, B.S., Dutcher, J.P., Portenoy, R.K., Berger, A., Arezzo, J.C., Mizruchi, M., Wiernik, P.H., and Schaumburg, H.H. (1987). Quantitative sensory testing demonstrates that subclinical sensory neuropathy is prevalent in patients with cancer. *Arch. Neurol.* **44**: 944–946.

Lipton, R.B., Galer, B.S., Dutcher, J.P., Portenoy, R.K., Pahmer, V., Meller, F., Arezzo, J.C., and Wiernik, P.H. (1991). Large and small fibre type sensory dysfunction in patients with cancer. *J. Neurol. Neurosurg. Psychiatry* **54**: 706–709.

Lisak, R.P., Mitchell, M., Zweiman, B., Orrechio, E. and Asbury, A.K. (1977). Guillain-Barré syndrome and Hodgkin's disease: three cases with immunological studies. *Ann. Neurol.* **1**: 72–78.

Littler, W.A. (1970). Peripheral sensorimotor neuropathy in association with a seminoma of an undescended testicle. *Postgrad. Med. J.* **46**: 166–167.

Maitland, C.G., Scherokman, B.J., Schiffman, J., Harlan, J.W., and Galdi, A.P. (1985). Paraneoplastic tonic pupils. *J. Clin. Neuro-Ophthalmol.* **5**: 99–104.

Matthews, W.B. (1952). Cryptogenic polyneuritis. *Proc. R. Soc. Med.* **45**: 667–669.

McLeod, J.G., Tuck, R.R., Pollard, J.D., Cameron, J., and Walsh, J.C. (1984). Chronic polyneuropathy of undetermined cause. *J. Neurol. Neurosurg. Psychiatry* **47**: 530–535.

Moody, J.F. (1965). Electrophysiological investigations into the neurological complications of carcinoma. *Brain* **88**: 1023–1036.

Notermans, N.C., Wokke, J.H., Franssen, H., van der Graf, Y., Vermeulen, M., Van den Berg, L.H., Bar, P.R., and Jennekens, F.G.I. (1993). Chronic idiopathic polyneuropathy presenting in middle or old age: a clinical and electrophysiological study of 75 patients. *J. Neurol. Neurosurg. Psychiatry* **56**: 1066–1071.

Notermans, N.C., Wokke, J.H., Franssen, H., Vermeulen, M., Busch, H.F., and Jennekens, F.G. (1994). Course of chronic idiopathic polyneuropathy during middle age and older: 2-year follow-up study. *Ned. Tijdschr. Geneeskd.* **138**: 1281–1285.

O'Neill, J.H., Murray, N.M., and Newsom-Davis, J. (1988). The Lambert–Eaton myasthenic syndrome. A review of 50 cases. *Brain* **111**: 577–596.

Oh, S.J., Slaughter, R., and Harrell, L. (1991). Paraneoplastic vasculitic neuropathy: a treatable neuropathy. *Muscle Nerve* **14**: 152–156.

Ojeda, V.J. (1984). Necrotizing myelopathy associated with malignancy. A clinicopathologic study of two cases and literature review. *Cancer* **53**: 1115–1123.

Oppenheim, H. (1888). Uber Hirnsymptome bei Carcinomatose ohne nachweisbare. Veranderungen im Gehirn. *Charite-Ann (Berl.)* **13**: 335–344.

Paul, T., Katiyar, B.C., Misra, S., & Pant, C.G. (1978). Carcinomatous neuromuscular syndromes. A clinical and quantitative electrophysiological study. *Brain* **101**: 53–63.

Peterson, K., Forsyth, P.A., and Posner, J.B. (1994). Paraneoplastic sensorimotor neuropathy associated with breast cancer. *J. Neuro-Oncol.* **21**: 159–170.

Posner, J.B. (1995). *Neurological Complications of Cancer.* Philadelphia: F.A. Davis.

Prineas, J. (1970). Polyneuropathies of undetermined cause. *Acta Neurol. Scand. Suppl.* **44**: 1–72.

Rose, F.C. (1960). Discussion on neuropathies in rheumatic disease and steroid therapy. *Proc. Royal Soc. Med.* **53**: 51–53.

Rosenfeld, M.R. and Posner, J.B. (1991). Paraneoplastic motor neuron disease. In *Advances in Neurology*, vol. 56, *Amyotrophic Lateral Sclerosis and Other Motor Neuron Diseases*, ed. L.P. Rowland, pp. 445–459. New York: Raven Press.

Rosenfeld, M.R., Wong, E., Dalmau, J., Manley, G., Posner, J.B., Sher, E., and Furneaux, H.M. (1993). Cloning and characterization of a Lambert–Eaton myasthenic syndrome antigen. *Ann. Neurol.* **33**: 113–120.

Rowland, L.P., Sherman, W.H., Latov, N.,Lange, D.J., McDonald, T.D., Younger, D.S., Murphy, P.L., Hays, A.P., and Knowles, D. (1992). Amyotrophic lateral sclerosis and lymphoma: bone marrow examination and other diagnostic tests. *Neurology* **42**: 1101–1102.

Russell, D.S. (1961). Encephalomyelitis and carcinomatous neuropathy. In *The Encephalitides*, ed. L. van Bogaert, J. Radermecker, J. Hozay and A. Lowenthal, pp. 131–135. Amsterdam: Elsevier.

Sagar, H.J. and Read, D.J. (1982). Subacute sensory neuropathy with remission: an association with lymphoma. *J. Neurol. Neurosurg. Psychiatry* **45**: 83–85.

Schlaepfer, W.W. (1974). Axonal degeneration in the sural nerves of cancer patients. *Cancer* **34**: 371–381.

Schmitt, H.P. (1978). Quantitative analysis of voluntary muscles from routine autopsy material with special reference to the problem of remote carcinomatous changes ('neuromyopathy'). *Acta Neuropathol*, **43**: 143–152.

Schold, S.C., Cho, E.S., Somasundaram, M., and Posner, J.B. (1979). Subacute motor neuronopathy: a remote effect of lymphoma. *Ann. Neurol.* **5**: 271–287.

Sculier, J.-P., Feld, R., Evans, W.K., DeBoer, G., Shepherd, F.A., Payne, D.G., Pringle, J.F., Yeoh, J., Quirt, I. C., Curtis, J.E., Myers, R., and Herman, J.G. (1987). Neurologic disorders in patients with small-cell lung cancer. *Cancer* **60**: 2275–2283.

Shy, M.E., Rowland, L.P., Smith, T., Trojaborg, W., Latov, N., Sherman, W., Pesce, M.A., Lovelace, R.E., and Osserman, E.F. (1986). Motor neuron disease and plasma cell dyscrasia. *Neurology* **36**: 1429–1436.

Shy, B.M. and Silverstein, I. (1965). A study of the effects upon the motor unit by remote malignancy. *Brain* **88**: 515–528.

Sinha, A.A., Lopez, M.T., and McDevitt, H.O. (1990). Autoimmune diseases: the failure of self tolerance. *Science* **248**: 1380–1388.

Sumi, S.M., Farrell, D.F. and Knauss, T.A. (1983). Lymphoma and leukemia manifested by steroid-responsive polyneuropathy. *Arch. Neurol.* **40**: 577–582.

Szabo, A., Dalmau, J., Manley, G., Rosenfeld, M., Wong, E., Henson, J., Posner, J., and Furneaux, H. (1991). HuD, a paraneoplastic encephalomyelitis antigen, contains RNA-binding domains and is homologous to Elav and Sex-lethal. *Cell* **67**: 325–333.

Teravainen, H. and Larsen, A. (1977). Some features of the neuromuscular complications of pulmonary carcinoma. *Ann. Neurol.* **2**: 495–502.

Tracey, K.J. and Cerami, A. (1992). Tumor necrosis factor in the malnutrition (cachexia) of infection and cancer. *Am. J. Trop. Med. Hyg.* **47**: 2–7.

Trojaborg, W., Frantzen, E., and Andersen, I. (1969). Peripheral neuropathy and myopathy associated with carcinoma of the lung. *Brain* **92**: 71–82.

Van Lieshout, J.J., Wieling, W., Van Montfrans, G.A., Settels, J.J., Speelman, J.D., Endert, E., and Karemaker, J.M. (1986). Acute dysautonomia associated with Hodgkin's disease. *J. Neurol. Neurosurg. Psychiatry* **49**: 830–832.

Van Lieshout, J.J., Wieling, W., van Montfrans, G.A., Settels, J.J., Speelman, J.B., Endert, E., and Karenmaker, J.M. (1986). Acute dysautonomia associated with Hodgkin's disease. *J. Neurol. Neurosurg. Psychiatry* **49**: 830–832.

Vincent, D., Dubas, F., Hauw, J.J., Godeau, P., Lhermitte, F., Buge, A., and Castaigne, P. (1986). Nerve and muscle microvasculitis in peripheral neuropathy: a remote effect of cancer? *J. Neurol. Neurosurg. Psychiatry* **49**: 1007–1010.

Walsh, J.C. (1971). Neuropathy associated with lymphoma. *J. Neurol. Neurosurg. Psychiatry* **34**: 42–50.

Walton, J.N., Tomlinson, B.E., and Pearce, G.W. (1968). Subacute 'poliomyelitis' and Hodgkin's disease. *J. Neurol. Sci.* **6**: 435–445.

Weber, F.P., and Hill, T.R. (1993). Complete degeneration of the posterior columns of the spinal cord with chronic polyneuritis in a case of widespread carcinomatous disease elsewhere. *J. Neurol. Psychopathol.* **14**: 57–60.

Windebank, A.J., Blexrud, M.D., Dyck, P.J., Daube, J.R., and Karnes, M.S. (1990). The syndrome of acute sensory neuropathy: Clinical features and electrophysiologic and pathologic changes. *Neurology.* **40**: 584–591.

Younger, D.S., Rowland, L.P., Latov, N., Hays, A.P., Lange, D.J., Sherman, W., Inghirami, G., Pesce, M.A., Knowles, D.M., Powers, J., Miller, J.R., Fetell, M.R., and Lovelace, R.E. (1991). Lymphoma, motor neuron diseases, and amyotrophic lateral sclerosis. *Ann. Neurol.* **29**: 78–86.

Younger, D.S., Rowland, L.P., Latov, N., Sherman, W., Pesce, M., Lange, D.J., Trojaborg, W., Miller, J.R., Lovelace, R.E., Hays, A.P., and Kim, T.S. (1990). Motor neuron disease and amyotrophic lateral sclerosis: relation of high CSF protein content to paraproteinemia and clinical syndromes. *Neurology* **40**: 595–599.

16 Polyneuropathies associated with myeloma, POEMS, and non-malignant IgG and IgA monoclonal gammopathies

J.J. Kelly, Jr

Myeloma neuropathy

Introduction

There have been reports of neurological involvement with multiple myeloma (MM) for many years. The most common neurological complications reported have been encephalopathies due to metabolic factors and spinal cord and nerve root compression syndromes due to spinal bony involvement. Peripheral neuropathies are rare. Davison and Balser (1937) first reported peripheral neuropathy in a review of the neurological complications in a large series of patients with MM. Other studies followed (Scheinker 1938; Crow 1956; Victor et al. 1958). Despite their rarity, MM patients can on occasion present with dramatic neuropathies and some of these syndromes serve as models for the remote complications of malignancy; therefore, these neuropathies are important. They are best approached by division into those associated with typical lytic MM and those associated with osteosclerotic myeloma (OSM).

Typical lytic multiple myeloma

In large series of patients with MM, peripheral neuropathy only occurred in 3–5% of patients (Silverstein and Doniger 1963); however, when the prevalence of polyneuropathy was studied prospectively, the prevalence increased to 40–60% (Hesselvik 1969; Walsh 1971), especially when electrophysiological testing and histopathological studies were added. Although perhaps important in understanding the biology of peripheral neuropathy, these subclinical cases are not important to the clinician.

Careful studies of polyneuropathy in MM (Kelly et al. 1981a) have indicated marked heterogeneity (Table 16.1), and thus different mechanisms are likely, much like the neuropathy associated with carcinoma (Croft et al. 1967; Croft and Wilkinson 1969). The most common syndrome is a relatively mild sensorimotor neuropathy, often preterminal. These patients complain of pain and paresthesias and have mild distal sensory loss, areflexia and often insignificant weakness. Electrophysiological studies and nerve histopathology usually indicate an axonopathy. The mechanism of this neuropathy, although unknown, likely relates to metabolic factors associated with advanced malignancy and weight loss.

Another rare neuropathy syndrome in MM patients is pure sensory neuropathy, which is similar in all aspects to the sensory neuronopathy syndrome associated

Table 16.1 *Major features of lytic myeloma neuropathy*

Type	Pain	Autonomic	Mainly sensory, motor or mixed	Slow nerve conduction velocity	Carpal tunnel syndrome	Cerebrospinal fluid protein	Nerve biopsy	Course
Sensorimotor	+	No	Mixed	+	No	No	AD, SD	Slow
Sensory	+	No	Sensory	No	No	+	AD	Stable
Motor	No	Yes	Motor	Yes	No	+++	SD	Progressive
Amyloid	Yes	Yes	Sensory>motor	No	Yes	+	AD	Progressive

Note:
AD: axonal degeneration; SD: segmental demyelination.
Source: Reprinted from Kelly Jr, J.J. et al. (1984). The spectrum of peripheral neuropathy in myeloma. *Neurology* **31**: 31, with permission.

with carcinoma (Horwich et al. 1977). This disorder is likely due to pathology at the level of the dorsal root ganglion, possibly immunological in nature. In addition, these patients can develop a severe motor neuropathy or polyradiculoneuropathy, similar to Guillain-Barré syndrome (GBS) or chronic inflammatory demyelinating polyradiculoneuropathy (CIDP). The course of the motor neuropathy and the pure sensory neuropathy are independent of the status of the malignancy and likely represent triggering of the autoimmune process due to perturbation of the immune system by the malignancy.

MM patients can also develop amyloid neuropathy due to the deposition of light chain fragments of the circulating M protein. The clinical presentation is similar to that of primary systemic amyloidosis (Kelly et al. 1979), except that these patients may have associated myeloma complications, including encepatholopathy or spinal involvement, which may complicate the clinical picture.

In all cases, there is no effective treatment, with the exception of the motor neuropathies which may respond to treatments effective in idiopathic GBS and CIDP. See Kelly et al. (1987) for a more detailed discussion of this topic.

Osteosclerotic multiple myeloma

Scheinker (1938) reported a 39-year-old man with a progressive sensorimotor neuropathy beginning in the legs. The patient had a solitary plasmacytoma of the sternum and two large areas of thickened, deeply pigmented skin on the anterior chest wall. The cerebrospinal fluid (CSF) protein level was elevated, but the nervous system was not directly involved by the plasmacytoma. Subsequent cases were then described by Crow (1956) and Victor et al. (1958). In an excellent report, Morley and Schwieger (1967) reviewed 23 cases with OSM and peripheral neuropathy from the literature and added four more of their own. They also noted that radiotherapy was beneficial for some patients. Takatsuki and Sanada (1983) described the diverse features of the syndrome and emphasized its frequency in Japanese males. Although most of the early cases were reported from Japan, and it was felt that the syndrome was mainly limited to the Japanese, many cases have been recognized in the western world in the last decade. Bardwick et al. (1980) suggested the acronym POEMS (*p*olyneuropathy, *o*rganomegaly, *e*ndocrinopathy, *m*-protein, *s*kin changes). The major shortcoming of the eye-catching title is that many patients with OSM and peripheral neuropathy will not have all of the features of the POEMS syndrome (Miralles et al. 1992; Kelly et al. 1983). It is better to consider this diagnostic possibility in any patient with a typical peripheral neuropathy and one or more of the systemic features known to occur with this disease. This syndrome is characterized by osteosclerotic bone lesions, sensorimotor peripheral neuropathy with predominantly motor disability, high CSF protein levels, low motor nerve conduction velocities, monoclonal gammopathy usually of lambda light-chain type and a variable mix of organomegaly, skin, and endocrine abnormalities (see below).

CLINICAL FEATURES. Based on studies by a number of groups (Bardwick et al. 1980; Driedger and

Table 16.2 *Non-neurological abnormalities in patients with osteosclerotic myeloma*

Abnormality	1 M	2 M	3 M	4 F	5 M	6 F	7 M	8 M	9 F	10 F	11 M	12 F	13 M	14 M	15 M	16 F
Gynecomastia	+												+			
Hepatomegaly		+	+	+		+	+						+			
Splenomegaly				+		+										
Hyperpigmentation		+						+	+				+			+
Edema		+	+					+								
Lymphadenopathy		+	+													
Papilledema			+	+			+									
Digital clubbing			+								+		+			
White nails													+			
Hypertrichosis			+					+					+			+
Atrophic testes								+					+		+	
Impotence		+						+					+		+	
Polycythemia	+					+		+			+				+	
Leukocytosis	+										+				+	
Thrombocytosis			+		+		+	+	+	+	+	+	+	+	+	+
Low plasma testosterone		+		+				+					+		+	
High serum estrogen		+						+					+			
Low serum thyroxine		+													+	
Hyperglycemia		+														

Note:
F: female; M: male.
Source: Reprinted from Kelly Jr, J.J., Kyle, R.A., Miles, J.M. and Dyke, P.J. (1983). Osteosclerosis myeloma and peripheral neuropathy. *Neurology* **33**:202–210, with permission et al. (1984).

Pruzanski 1980; Kelly et al. 1983; Takatsuki and Sanada 1983; Miralles et al. 1992), the following clinical picture has emerged. Osteosclerotic myeloma occurs in about 2% of patients with multiple myeloma. About one-half of these patients are less than 51 years of age at diagnosis. Symptoms of peripheral neuropathy generally precede the diagnosis of OSM by a median of 1.5 years. The diagnosis of myeloma is usually made during the evaluation of a cryptogenic peripheral neuropathy in most instances. Sensory symptoms, seldom painful, are usually noticed first by the patients. They consist of tingling, pins and needles, and coldness and always begin in the feet. Motor involvement follows the sensory symptoms and both are distal, symmetric, and progressive with a gradual proximal spread. Severe weakness occurs in more than one-half of the patients and results in an inability to climb stairs, rise from a chair, or grip objects firmly with the hands. Patients may become bedfast or wheelchair-bound. The course is slowly progressive. In our experience, patients do not have sudden improvement or worsening unrelated to therapy, as occurs in chronic inflammatory neuropathies. Autonomic symptoms are not a feature. Impotence may occur but is probably from an endocrinological cause. Anorexia and weight loss occur rarely. Bone pain is rarely a feature of the condition.

Physical examination reveals symmetrical motor and sensory deficits in the extremities which are worse distally. Cranial nerves are not involved except for occasional papilledema. Weakness is more marked than sensory loss, with more than one-half of patients having severe muscle weakness with areflexia. Sensory loss usually affects touch-pressure, vibratory and joint position sense, but affects temperature discrimination and nociception to a lesser degree.

Non-neurological features of organomegaly or an endocrinopathy are common (Tables 16.2 and 16.3). Hepatomegaly occurs in almost one-half of patients,

Table 16.3 *Clinical and biochemical features of 38 patients with plasma cell dyscrasia and polyneuropathy*

	No. of features of POEMS syndrome				
	1–2	3	4	all 5	Total
Characteristic	*n*=10	*n*=12	*n*=11	*n*=5	*n*=38
Clinical features					
Any skin changes	0	7	10	5	22 (58%)
Hyperpigmentation	0	5	7	5	17 (45%)
Lymphadenopathy	0	4	7	5	16 (42%)
Papilledema	3	2	7	2	14 (37%)
Edema	1	3	5	2	11 (29%)
Hepatomegaly	0	1	4	4	9 (24%)
Splenomegaly	0	2	3	3	8 (21%)
Ascites	0	0	2	2	4 (11%)
Pleural effusion	0	1	1	1	3 (8%)
Biochemical findings					
Bone lesions	10	12	10	4	36 (95%)
Sclerotic	10	10	7	4	31 (82%)
M protein					
IgA–1	4	5	6	2	17 (45%)
IgG–1	3	6	1	2	12 (32%)
1 light chain	0	0	2	1	3 (8%)
IgG–k	0	1	0	0	1 (3%)
Indeterminate	0	0	1	0	1 (3%)
None	3	0	1	0	4 (11%)
Hypothroidism	0	1	5	1	7 (18%)

Source: Reprinted from Miralles et al. (1992), with permission.

while splenomegaly and lymphadenopathy are less common. Hyperpigmentation is frequent. Hypertrichosis, characterized by the development of prominent, stiff, coarse hair on the extremities, may be striking. Idiopathic flushing reminiscent of carcinoid syndrome has been reported (Myers et al. 1991). Gynecomastia and atrophic testes can occur, as well as clubbing of the fingers and toes and white nails.

LABORATORY FEATURES

General. Routine laboratory abnormalities are often not prominent (Table 16.4). Anemia is not a feature of OSM. In fact, polycythemia is often present (Delauche et al. 1981; Kelly et al. 1983). Thrombocytosis occurs in more than one-half of patients (Kelly et al. 1983), and leukocytosis is also seen. In contrast to MM, renal insufficiency and hypercalcemia are rarely found in OSM. Examination of the bone marrow aspirate and biopsy is either normal or shows a modest increase (less than 5%) in normal-appearing plasma cells, so that the diagnosis of myeloma can rarely be made solely on the basis of the bone marrow examination.

A monoclonal protein is found in the serum in three-fourths of patients. The size of the M-spike is usually modest (median 11 g L^{-1}) and is rarely more than 30 g L^{-1} (Kelly et al. 1983). Frequently, the M protein is obscured by a normal gamma or beta component and is not detected unless immunoelectrophoresis or immunofixation is carried out. In our experience, all patients have had a lambda light chain with either an A or G heavy chain. We are not aware of any documented case with an M heavy chain; however, well-documented rare instances of monoclonal kappa proteins have been reported (Reitan et al. 1980). The presence of monoclonal light chain in the urine (Bence-Jones proteinuria) and, when present, is of modest amount.

Table 16.4 *Presenting laboratory abnormalities in patients with osteosclerotic myeloma*

Abnormality	Result
Anemia (Hb< 120 g^{-1})	0/16
Increased ESR (>30 mm/h)	2/15*b*
Increased serum creatinine (>1.20 mg^{-1})	2/16
Hypercalcemia (>101 mg^{-1})	1/16
Serum M component	12/16
Urine M component	2/15*b*
M component type	8 G, 3 A 1G+A 4 none
Myeloma in marrow[a]	1/16
Bone lesions	
Multiple sclerotic	5
Multiple mixed sclerotic+lytic	4
Solitary mixed sclerotic+lytic	7
Increased hemoglobin	
(>170 g^{-1} males)	
(>150 g^{-1} females)	
Leukocytosis (>10.9×10^{3}L)	3/16
Thrombocytosis (>370×10^{3}L)	12/15[b]

Notes:
[a] More than 10% plasma in bone marrow.
[b] Not done in one.
Source: From Kelly Jr, J.J., Kyle, R.A., Miles, J.M., and Dyck, P.J. (1983). Osteosclerosis myeloma and peripheral neuropathy. *Neurology* **33**:202–210.

Endocrinological findings include low plasma testosterone levels in males, likely accounting for the impotence, which is frequent. Occasionally, high serum estrogen levels may be recognised. Also, mild hyperglycemia is occasionally seen. Hyperprolactinemia has also been reported (Bardwick et al. 1980).

Radiographic findings. Osteosclerotic lesions (Figure 16.1) are seen, by definition, in all cases. The lesions may be modest in size and be misinterpreted as benign bony sclerosis, or they may be prominent and produce a striking ivory sclerotic vertebral body. Frequently the lesions consist of both osteosclerotic and lytic features. There is a report of a 'benign' localized rib lytic lesion which became osteosclerotic over several years, leading to eventual biopsy with establishment of the diagnosis (Simmons et al. 1994). Multiple bone lesions are more common than single lesions. Typically, the bone lesions involve the spine, pelvis, ribs, and proximal extremities and usually spare the distal extremities and skull. Resnick et al. (1981) have emphasized a ring-like appearance of the osteosclerotic lesions. They also pointed out that irregular and spiculated bony contours may be evident about the apophyseal joints, laminae, and transverse processes of vertebrae. Approximately one-half of patients with a plasma cell dyscrasia and osteosclerotic lesions have peripheral neuropathy (Driedger and Pruzanski 1979).

These bone lesions may be difficult to diagnose as the radioactive bone scan may be negative in these patients and radiography is more reliable in their detection (Kelly et al. 1983), which is the opposite of most malignant bone lesions. In addition, the radiologist may not be able to distinguish benign from neoplastic lesions based solely on the radiographic appearance. Thus, we advocate biopsy of any suspicious lesion in the appropriate clinical setting, especially if there are osteosclerotic features. We have had several patients with benign interpretations of sclerotic bony lesions (hemagioma of spine and fibrous dysplasia of rib). We insisted on biopsy because of the clinical picture and the presence of a serum M protein with discovery of a solitary osteosclerotic plasmacytoma.

The diagnosis of osteosclerotic myeloma depends upon demonstration of the presence of increased numbers of abnormal plasma cells in a biopsy specimen from the osteosclerotic lesion. These cells stain with a single type of heavy chain and a single class of light chain by the immunoperoxidase technique, which indicates monoclonal plasma cell proliferation.

Electromyography (EMG)

Nerve conduction studies reveal moderate slowing of the conduction velocities (CV), with prolonged distal latencies and prolonged distal latencies and progressive dispersion of the compound muscle action potential (CMAP) with stimulation of motor

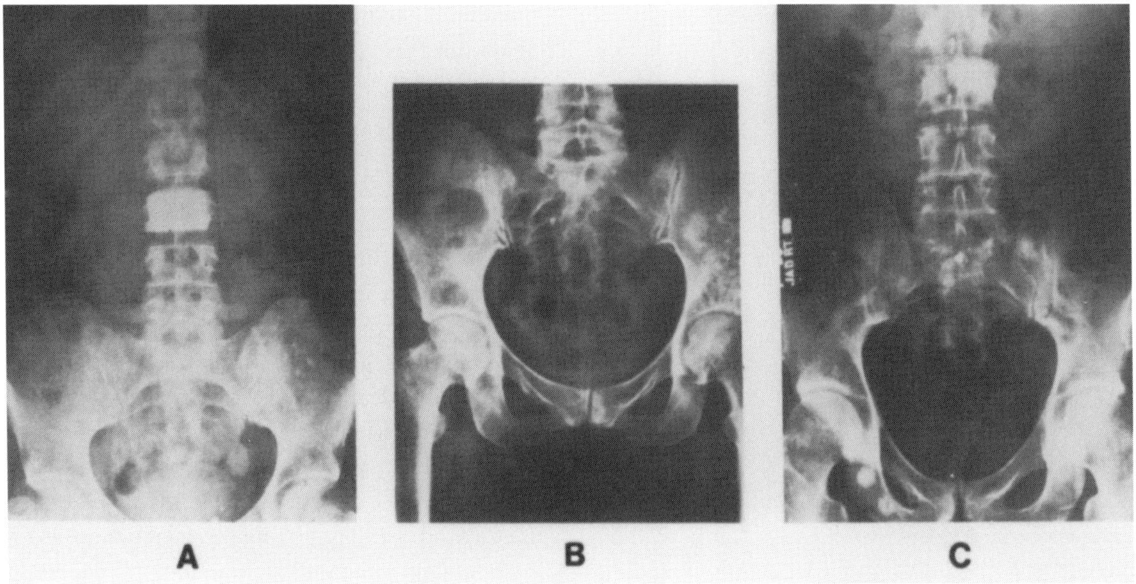

Figure 16.1 *(A) Ivory sclerotic L3 vertebra in a 47-year-old woman with widespread mixed lytic and sclerotic lesions. (B) Multiple sclerotic lesions involving vertebral bodies, sacrum, ischium and pelvis in a 42-year-old woman. (C) Solitary mixed lytic and sclerotic lesions of the left ilium in a 56-year-old woman.*

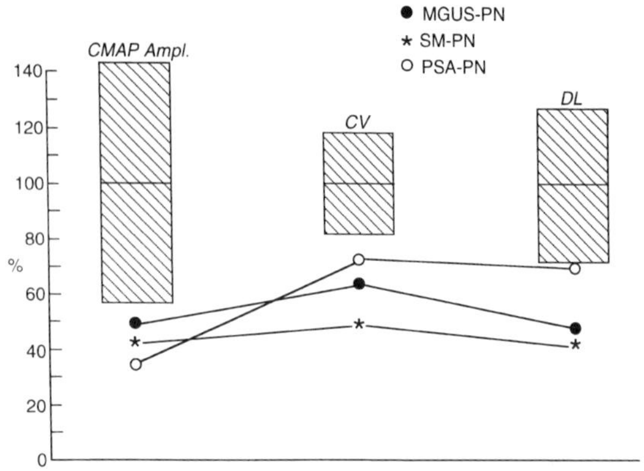

Figure 16.2 *Ulnar nerve conduction studies in patients with plasma cell dyscrasia and peripheral neuropathy. Note the relative preservation of amplitude in osteosclerotic myeloma but marked reduction in CV. CMAP Ampl.: compound muscle action potential amplitude; CV: conduction velocity; DL: distal latency; MGUS-PN: MGUS with polyneuropathy; SM-PN: osteosclerotic myeloma with polyneuropathy; PSA-PN: primary systemic amyloidosis with polyneuropathy.*

nerves more proximally. In general, lowering of motor nerve CV is proportionately greater than reduction in the CMAP amplitude (Figure 16.2). On needle EMG, distal fibrillation potentials and enlarged, polyphasic voluntary motor unit action potentials with decreased recruitment are found (Kelly 1983). These findings suggest a polyneuropathy with a prominent demyelinating component as well as features of axonal degeneration. Rare cases with axonal features without much evidence of demyelination have been reported but we have not seen such a case (Ropper and McKee 1993).

Cerebrospinal fluid. Protein levels are elevated in all instances. Approximately one-half of our cases had a CSF protein level more than 100 mg L^{-1} (Kelly et al. 1983). The cell count is almost always normal. Plasma cells are not found.

Nerve biopsy. Nerve biopsies are not particularly helpful in this disorder. They generally show a mixture of demyelinating and axonal changes with no or sparse mononuclear cell infiltration in the perineurium (Kelly et al. 1983). Biopsy is important if amyloid is a consideration but this diagnosis can generally be excluded by the clinical picture and electrodiagnostic studies.

OTHER FEATURES. Sessile or polypoid cutaneous lesions ranging from flesh to wine-red in color have been reported in OSM with peripheral neuropathy. Histological examination revealed multiple, haphazardly arranged small vessels lined by a single layer of endothelial cells confirming the diagnosis of multiple capillary hemangiomas (Puig et al. 1985). Ono et al. (1985) also reported hemangiomatous proliferation of small blood vessels in the skin, kidneys, brain and lymph nodes. Biopsy of the skin confirmed the presence of capillary hemangiomas. In addition, proliferation of glomerular capillaries resembling membranoproliferative glomerulonephritis was found. Imayama and Urabe (1984) reported that the cutaneous hemangiomas had histological features of a globulated cellular capillary hemangioma as well as pyogenic granuloma and a cherry angioma. Extensive cutaneous necrosis from diffuse leukocytoclastic vasculitis with calcium deposition has been described(Raper and Ibels 1985). Jeha et al. (1981) reported a patient with osteosclerotic myeloma and chronic lymphocytic leukemia, but no evidence of peripheral neuropathy.

Case study

The patient was a 72-year-old woman who was referred for progressive weakness and inability to walk. She had a 3-year history of leg and arm weakness and numbness with loss of the ability to walk, even with aids, in the last year. Her health was otherwise good. Examination disclosed an elderly woman who otherwise appeared fit. She was seated in a wheelchair and was unable to stand and walk. The cranial nerves, including fundi, were normal. She had diffuse muscle weakness graded around 4+ (MRC scale) in the proximal arms, 2-3 in the hands, 3 in the hips, and 0 in the distal legs. She was areflexic and had a stocking/glove loss of sensation, primarily for vibration and position sense. She had mild hepatomegaly and hyperpigmentation of skin that was unexplained. Laboratory data disclosed normal routine studies of blood and organ function. Serum protein electrophoresis disclosed a small gamma peak that on immunofixation electrophoresis was a monoclonal IgA lambda protein. There were no light chains detected in the urine. Bone marrow biopsy was normal. Metastatic skeletal survey disclosed only 'fibrous dysplasia' in the second rib. The radionuclide bone scan was normal. The hematologist classified the monoclonal gammopathy as a MGUS (undetermined significance). Electromyography (EMG) disclosed a demyelinating polyradiculoneuropathy. CSF examination revealed a high protein concentration (1350 mg L^{-1}) with a normal cell count. She was diagnosed as CIDP and treated with high-dose prednisone (60 mg per day orally). After 3 months, she returned and was worse. Further consultation was sought.

When seen by us, she had worsened and was cushingoid. We reviewed the radiographs with a radiologist experienced in the evaluation of myeloma who felt that he could not exclude OSM as the lesion had a sclerotic rim, although it looked benign. We requested a bone biopsy which revealed a plasmacytoma which stained for IgA lambda. Based on this, radiotherapy was administered to the lesion (4000 rad) with substantial improvement over the ensuring months. By 6 months, she had gained at least one MRC grade in her proximal muscles and by 9 months could walk with a cane. By 1 year, she was walking with bilateral ankle-foot orthosis (AFOs) without a cane and was fairly independent. At 2 years, by phone, she reported that except for persistent bilateral foot dorsiflexor weakness, requiring the continued use of AFOs, she otherwise considered herself normal. She was then lost to further follow-up.

Comment: It is easy to see in retrospect why this patient was felt to have CIDP; however, the systemic features were not noted and the radiologic interpretation of the bony lesion was taken at face value. The clinician has to have a high index of suspicion to detect these patients and any of the elements of the POEMS syndrome should be a 'red flag.'

PATHOLOGY AND PATHOGENESIS. Waldenström et al. (1978) raised pertinent questions concerning whether these patients really had MM and whether the osteosclerosis or the myeloma played a role in the peripheral neuropathy. The number of cases reported and the common features indicate that this is a recognizable entity. It might best be classified as a variant of MM.

Dayan and Stokes (1972) produced a demyelinating peripheral neuropathy in rats by implanting plasma cell tumors that produced an excess of light chains and caused a mixed peripheral neuropathy. Lavenstein et al. (1979) noted the deposition of IgG in the perineurium of a patient with polyneuropathy and OSM. However, the authors could not tell whether the immunoglobulin played a role in the neuropathy or whether it was simply deposited in the damaged nerve. A demyelinating polyneuropathy developed in mice injected with monoclonal IgG protein from patients with myelomatous polyneuropathy but not with immunoglobulin from normal donors (Besinger et al. 1981). The type of neuropathy in these patients with OSM and polyneuropathy into rat sciatic nerves failed to produce abnormal slowing of motor conduction velocity when compared with control rats (J.J. Kelly et al. unpublished observations). The possibility of an autoimmune process has been entertained by some investigators (Reitan et al. 1980). None of 17 patients with osteosclerotic myeloma and peripheral neuropathy demonstrated anti-myelin associated glycoprotein (MAG) activity which is frequently detected in patients with a monoclonal IgM protein and peripheral neuropathy (Hafler et al. 1986). Reactivity of serum from patients against other antigens has not been studied.

The endocrinological changes have been of interest to a number of investigators. Serum estrogen levels are commonly elevated in OSM. Matsumine (1985) reported an accelerated conversion of androgen to estrogen in two patients with osteosclerotic myeloma by intravenous loading with dehydroepiandrosterone sulfate. Hypercalcitoninemia was found in a patient with OSM and peripheral neuropathy (Rousseau et al. 1978). Others have found normal levels of calcitonin in patients with OSM and peripheral neuropathy (Pruzanski and Williams 1980). Limited endocrinological studies in some of our patients suggested disturbed hypothalamic–pituitary dysfunction rather than endorgan failure (Kelly et al. 1983). Indeed, Reulecke et al. (1988) found antibody activity directed at neuroendocrine tissue in the hypothalamic–pituitary axis in one patient. These studies need to be repeated and expanded.

Despite the 'demyelinating' appearance of the polyneuropathy by EMG testing (Kelly 1983), recent studies suggest that axonopathy with secondary segmental demyelination may be the primary histopathological finding. In a study of five patients with OSM and peripheral neuropathy, Ohi et al. (1985) noted a loss of myelinated fibers. The peaks of histograms of myelinated fiber diameters were displaced to smaller categories suggesting fiber atrophy. In addition, there was a lack of noticeably increased numbers of demyelinated axons, a clustered rather than random distribution of segmental demyelination, and axonal attenuation relative to myelin thickness, all suggesting a special axonal vulnerability with secondary segmental demyelination. Although superficially compelling, these techniques do not reliably separate axonal from demyelinating polyneuropathy and it is most likely that this polyneuropathy is indeed primarily demyelinating.

Small foci of mononuclear cells in a perivascular location in the epineurium are common. Amyloid deposition is absent. Borges et al. (1983) presented evidence from a patient with myeloma neuropathy of unstated type that retrograde transport of M protein light chains from serum to nerve cell body was associated with disruption of normal axonal transport and axonal dysfunction.

The cause of the peripheral neuropathy and systemic manifestations in OSM is unknown. Presumably the plasma cells secrete an immunoglobulin or another substance that is toxic to peripheral nerves and may also cause more widespread abnormalities in some patients. It is tempting to incriminate the role of lambda light chains in the pathogenesis because they occur in almost all patients. It is possible that the multiple manifestations of OSM are due to a common surface receptor on diverse tissue recognized by the circulating immunoglobulin or perhaps some other secretary product of the plasmacytoma. Bardwick et al. (1980), however, were unable to demonstrate anti-nerve antibodies in their patients; however, Reulecke et al. (1988) demonstrated the occurrence of antibody activity directed at neuroendocrine tissues in their patients. Clearly, more work needs to be done on the recognition of antibodies directed at peripheral nerves and neuroendocrine tissues.

MANAGEMENT AND THERAPY. Patients with OSM differ significantly from those with classic MM, which has a peak frequency in the seventh decade of life and commonly presents with bone pain, weakness, and fatigue. In addition, anemia, renal insufficiency, and hypercalcemia are often found. The bone marrow is usually heavily infiltrated with malignant plasma cells, and large M-components are apparent in the serum and/or urine. The average duration of survival is 2–3 years.

In contrast, OSM occurs at an earlier age and the patients rarely complain of bone pain. These patients usually present because of peripheral neuropathy, and the bony lesions are discovered only when sought. Anemia, hypercalcemia, and renal insufficiency are rare. The bone marrow is rarely infiltrated with plasma cells, and M-components (usually lambda) are small in the serum, may occasionally be absent, and are infrequently found in the urine. Patients can survive for many years and death may be due to polyneuropathy or other systemic features not typically seen in lytic MM.

Peripheral neuropathy is infrequent in MM but occurs in approximately 50% of patients with OSM. In addition, organomegaly and endocrinopathy are common in OSM. In contrast to amyloid neuropathy, progressive sensory (dysesthetic) and autonomic involvement are rare in OSM. IN the latter, CSF protein is usually very high and nerve conduction studies reveal moderate slowing of motor CV.

It must be emphasized that patients with OSM usually present with sensorimotor peripheral neuropathy. Thus, unless the bony lesion is discovered, often fortuitously, the clinical picture very much resembles the slowly progressive variant of idiopathic CIDP. For this reason, we advocate mandatory bone radiographs in any patients with a progressive, primary motor neuropathy whether or not there is a recognized M protein. A metastatic bone survey must be carried out to detect osteosclerotic lesions as the radioactive bone scan may be negative (Kelly et al. 1983). Open biopsy of suspicious bone lesions is mandatory. The M protein in the serum and urine is frequently small and may often be missed unless immunoelectrophoresis or immunofixation is carried out. Patients with OSM and peripheral neuropathy have progression of their disease when untreated usually until the patients are unable to walk and death may occur.

If the patient has single or multiple osteosclerotic lesions in a limited area, they should be treated with radiation (4000–5000 rads). Resection of an isolated lesion can also bring about improvement (Simmons et al. 1994). More than one-half of patients will show substantial improvement of the neuropathy (Table 16.5). The improvement is gradual but slow and may not be evident for 3–6 months. Some patients have showed continued improvement for up to 2 years after radiation therapy. Unfortunately, most of these patients eventually relapse with recurrent bony lesions and worsening polyneuropathy.

If the patient has widespread osteosclerotic lesions, chemotherapy is necessary. We prefer melphalan (0.15 mg kg^{-1}) daily plus prednisone (20 mg three times daily) for 7 days every 6 weeks. We and others (Donofrio et al. 1984) have seen responses with this regimen, but they are usually not as impressive as radiation for solitary lesions. Prednisone alone is relatively ineffective (Kelly et al. 1983; Miralles et al. 1992). There is no evidence that the addition of azathioprine is beneficial. In addition, these patients generally do not respond to plasma exchange therapy (Silberstein et al. 1985; Miralles et al. 1992).

FUTURE DIRECTIONS. The etiology of these related syndromes likely lies in the secretion of some substance by the plasma cells which is toxic to peripheral nerves and other tissues. The discovery of a common cell surface receptor which is an epitope of the monoclonal antibody would help to establish this theory. It should be possible to use the monoclonal antibody secreted by the plasmacytes in these patients as a probe to study nerve and other involved tissues. Preliminary studies have shown deposition of antibodies from these patients in neuroendocrine tissues but it is not known if this is a primary or secondary event (Reulecke et al. 1988). Screening of serum from these patients against a panel of peripheral nerve and myelin antigens would also be useful. So far, we know that these patients do not have anti-MAG activity in their sera (Hafler et al. 1986) but other surface proteins have not been studied. The

Table 16.5 *Results of treatment*

	Multiple lesions	Solitary lesions
Number of patients	9	7
Median follow-up (months)		
Median	48	29
Range	4–79	3–98
Treatment modality	Melphalan and prednisone in 7	Radiotherapy in 6
	None in 2	Excision in 1
Result		
Improvement:		
Substantial		3
Moderate		1
Slight	3	2
Stabilization	2	1
No response	2	
Current status		
Dead	1	2
Alive	8	5

Source: From Kelly Jr, J.J., Kyle, R.A., Miles, J.M., and Dyck, P.J. (1993), Osteosclerotic myeloma and peripheral neuropathy, *Neurology* **33**:202–210.

possibility that there is an immune reaction against the plasmacytoma in these patients with the antibodies crossreacting with identical epitopes on other tissues, an anology with the Lambert–Eaton myasthenic syndrome, should also be studied. Production of other factors such as IL-2 (Mandler et al. 1992) and other cytokines should also be explored further.

Clearly, there are many avenues for further study of these patients; however, their scarcity makes such study difficult.

POEMS syndrome

The POEMS syndrome (Bardwick et al. 1980) is a peculiar multisystem disorder with many systemic features of unclear etiology. It occurs most commonly in the setting of OSM but may also occur in the presence of non-malignant lymphoid hyperplasia syndromes (angiofollicular lymph node hyperplasia, Castleman's disease) or even a less well-characterized non-malignant monoclonal gammopathies. Patients usually have an M protein which, like OSM, is IgA or G heavy chain and lambda light chain. The syndrome has occasionally been reported in the presence of polyclonal gammopathy. One patient had peripheral neuropathy and osteosclerotic bone lesions, as well as lymphadenopathy and involvement of the salivary glands with an angiofollicular lymphoid lesion (Castleman's disease) (Kobayashi et al. 1985). In the non-myeloma cases, the non-hematologic manifestations of the disorder (Tables 16.2 and 16.3) are identical to the OSM cases and the patient must be carefully evaluated for underlying myeloma. For reasons mentioned above, we and others (Kelly et al. 1983; Miralles et al. 1992; Ropper and McKee 1993) consider the acronym POEMS a poor name as it focuses attention on a small subgroup of these patients. Most patients with OSM have one or more manifestations of the POEMS syndrome (Tables 16.2 and 16.3) without having the full syndrome. I favor the eponym Crow–Fukase syndrome (Nakanishi et al. 1984) named after the two investigators who first described the syndrome.

The etiology of this peculiar syndrome is unclear. As in OSM, it is tempting to ascribe the systemic manifestations to the interaction of the monoclonal immunoglobulin with a common surface epitope on widespread neurological and non-neurological tissues.

Non-malignant IgG and IgA monoclonal gammopathies

The neuropathies associated with IgG- and IgA-monoclonal gammopathy of undetermined significance (MGUS) are much less uniform and less well understood than those associated with IgM-MGUS and the malignant gammopathies. A limited number of studies have examined these neuropathies and, in general, the following points can be made.

1. They are less frequent than the IgM-MGUS neuropathies (Gosselin et al. 1991; Suarez and Kelly 1993; Vrethem 1994).
2. They are less likely to be associated with anti-nerve antibody activity. In fact, only rare cases of non-IgM-MGUS neuropathies have been found to have antibody activity against defined neural antigens (Sewell et al. 1981; Sadiq et al. 1991; Nemni et al. 1990; Vrethem 1994).
3. As a corollary, they are much less likely to evidence positive immunofluorescent staining of the nerve either by direct or indirect immunofluoresence.
4. They are much more heterogeneous in their clinical presentations, with primarily motor, primarily sensory and mixed varieties. In addition, some are mostly demyelinating by electrophysiological and morphological criteria, others are mostly axonal and others mixed (Read et al. 1978; Dalakas and Engel 1981; Mahonen et al. 1982; Hoogstraten et al. 1983; Nemni et al. 1990; Suarez and Kelly 1993; Vrethem 1994).
5. Their response to therapy is highly variable with some responding to treatments normally effective in CIDP while others respond poorly to any therapy. In the only controlled study of treatment in this group, a subgroup of IgG and IgA-MGUS neuropathies responded to plasmapheresis better than the IgM group (Dyck et al. 1991).

Three large studies have compared IgM with non-IgM-MGUS neuropathies (Gosselin et al. 1991; Suarez and Kelly 1993; Vrethem 1994). There seems to be a clearcut difference between the two groups with the IgA and IgG-MGUS patients showing less sensory involvement, less evidence of demyelination, and a reduced prevalence versus the IgM group. It is unlikely that there is a single cause as in osteosclerotic and amyloid neuropathies because of the heterogeneity of this group. In addition, other causes need to be excluded by carrying out proper studies, which is less of an issue in the IgM neuropathies. As a general rule, the finding of a mainly demyelinating process on electrodiagnostic testing predicts response to treatment. Whether the monoclonal protein in IgA and IgG MGUS-neuropathies is of primary pathogenetic importance or simply represents the co-occurence of two rare disorders is a question which is unresolved in most of these cases.

References

Bardwick, P.A., Zvaifler, N.J., Gill, G.N., Newman, D., Greenway, G.D., and Resnick, D.L. (1980). Plasma cell dyscrasia with polyneuropathy, organomegaly, endocrinopathy, M protein, and skin changes: the POEMS syndrome. *Medicine* **59**: 311–322.

Besinger, U.A., Toyka, K.V., Anzil, A.P., Fateh-Moghadam, A., Neumeier, D., Rauscher, R., and Heininger, K. (1981). Myeloma neuropathy: passive transfer from man to mouse. *Science* **213**: 1027–1030.

Borges, L.F., Busis, N., and Zervas, N. (1983). Axonal transport of myeloma proteins (abstract). *Ann. Neurol.* **14**: 120.

Croft, P.B. and Wilkinson, M. (1969). The course and prognosis in some types of carcinomatous neuromyopathy. *Brain* **92**: 1–8.

Croft, P.B., Urich, H., and Wilkinson, M. (1967). Peripheral neuropathy of sensorimotor type associated with malignant disease. *Brain* **90**: 31–66.

Crow, R.S. (1956). Peripheral neuritis in myelomatosis. *Br. Med. J.* **2**: 802–804.

Dalakas, M.C. and Engel, W.K. (1981). Polyneuropathies with monoclonal gammopathy: studies of 11 patients. *Ann. Neurol.* **10**: 45–52.

Davison, C. and Balser, B.H. (1937). Myeloma and its neural complications. *Arch. Surg.* **35**: 913–936.

Dayan, A.D. and Stokes, M.I. (1972). Peripheral neuropathy and experimental myeloma in the mouse. *Nature (New Biol.)* **236**: 117–118.

Delauche, M.C., Clauvel, J.P., and Seligmann, M. (1981). Peripheral neuropathy and plasma cell neoplasias: a report of 10 cases. *Br. J. Haematol.* **48**: 383–392.

Donofrio, P.D., Albers, J.W., Greenberg, H.S., and Mitchell, B.S. (1984). Peripheral neuropathy in osteosclerotic myeloma: clinical and electrodiagnostic improvement with chemotherapy. *Muscle Nerve* **7**: 137–141.

Driedger, H. and Pruzanski, W. (1979). Plasma cell neoplasia with osteosclerotic lesions: a study of five cases and a review of the literature. *Arch. Intern. Med.* **139**: 892–896.

Driedger, H. and Pruzanski, W. (1980). Plasma cell neoplasia with peripheral polyneuropathy: a study of five cases and a review of the literature. *Medicine* **59**: 301–310.

Dyck, P.J., Low, P.A., Windebank, A.J., Jaradeh, S.S., Gosselin, S., Bourque, P., Smith, P.E., Kastz, K.M., Karnes, J.L., and Evans, B.A. (1991). Plasma exchange in polyneuropathy associated with monoclonal gammopathy of undetermined significance. *N. Engl. J. Med.* **325**: 1482–1486.

Gosselin, S., Kyle, R.A., and Dyck, P.J. (1991). Neuropathies associated with monoclonal gammopathy of undetermined significance. *Ann. Neurol.* **30**: 54–61.

Hafler, D.A., Johnson, D., Kelly, J.J., Panitch, H., Kyle, R., and Weiner, H.L. (1986). Monoclonal gammopathy and neuropathy: myelin associated glycoprotein reactivity and clinical characteristics. *Neurology*, **36**: 75–78.

Hesselvik, M. (1969). Neuropathological studies on myelomatosis. *Acta Neurol. Scand.* **45**: 95–108.

Hoogstraten, M.C., de Jager, A.E.J., van den Berg, H.M., and Suurmeyer, A.J. (1983). Polyneuropathy and benign monoclonal gammopathy. *Clin. Neurol. Neurosurg.* **85**: 101–111.

Horwich, M.S., Cho, L., Proor, R.S., and Posner, J.B. (1977). Subacute sensory neuropathy: a remote effect of carcinoma. *Ann. Neurol.* **2**: 7–19.

Imayama, S. and Urabe, H. (1984). Electron microscope study on the hemangiomas in POEMS syndrome. *J. Dermatol. (Tokyo)* **11**: 550–559.

Jeha, M.T., Hamblin, T.J., and Smith, J.L. (1981). Coincident chronic lymphocyte leukemia and osteosclerotic multiple myeloma. *Blood* **57**: 517–619.

Kelly Jr, J.J. (1983). The electrodiagnostic findings in peripheral neuropathy associated monoclonal gammopathy. *Muscle Nerve* **6**: 504–509.

Kelly Jr, J.J., Kyle, R.A., and Latov, N. (1987). *Polyneuropathies Associated with Plasma Cell Dyscrasias*, Chapter 6. Boston: Martinus-Nijhoff.

Kelly Jr, J.J., Kyle, R.A., Miles, J.M., O'Brien, P.C., and Dyck, P.J. (1981a). The spectrum of peripheral neuropathy in myeloma. *Neurology* **31**: 24–31.

Kelly Jr, J.J., Kyle, R.A., Miles, J.M., and Dyck, P.J. (1983). Osteosclerotic myeloma and peripheral neuropathy. *Neurology* **33**: 202–210.

Kelly Jr, J.J., Kyle, R.A., O'Brien, P.C., and Dyck, P.J. (1979). The natural history of peripheral neuropathy in primary systemic amyloidosis. *Ann. Neurol.* **6**: 1–7.

Kelly Jr, J.J., Kyle, R.A., O'Brien, P.C., and Dyck, P.J. (1981b). Prevalence of monoclonal protein in peripheral neuropathy. *Neurology* **31**: 1480–1483.

Kobayashi, H., Ii, K., Sano, T., Sakaki, A., Hizawa, K., and Ogushi, F. (1985). Plasma cell dyscrasia with polyneuropathy and endocrine disorders associated with dysfunction of salivary glands. *Am. J. Surg. Pathol.* **9**: 759–763.

Lavenstein, B., Dalakas, M., and Engel, W.K. (1979). Polyneuropathy in 'non-secretory' osteosclerotic multiple myeloma with immunoglobulin deposition in peripheral nerve tissue. *Neurology (Minneap.)* **29**: 611 (abstract).

Mahonen, M., Partanen, J., Collan, Y., Naukkarien, A., Sorri, T., Sivenius, J., and Riekkinon, P. (1982). Monoclonal gammopathy with neurological signs and symptoms: a clinical, neurophysiological and muscle biopsy study. *Acta Neurol. Scand.* **66**: 643–651.

Mandler, R.N., Kerrigan, D.P., Smart, J., Kuis, W., Villegert, P., and Lotz, M. (1992). Castleman's disease in POEMS syndrome with elevated interleukin 6. *Cancer* **69**: 2697–2703.

Matsumine, H. (1985). Accelerated conversion of androgen to estrogen in plasma-cell dyscrasia associated with polyneuropathy anasarca, and skin pigmentation. *N. Engl. J. Med.* **313**: 1025–1026 (letter to the editor).

Miralles, G.D., O'Fallon, J.R., and Talley, N.J. (1992). Plasma cell dyscrasia with polyneuropathy: the spectrum of the POEMS syndrome. *N. Engl. J. Med.* **327**: 1919–1923.

Morley, J.B. and Schwieger, A.C. (1967). The relation between chronic polyneuropathy and osteosclerotic myeloma. *J. Neurol. Neurosurg. Psychiatry* **30**: 432–442.

Myers, B.M., Miralles, G.D., Taylor, C.A., Castineau, D.A., Pisani, R.J., and Tally, N.J. (1991). POEMS syndrome with idiopathic flushing mimicking carcinoid. *Am. J. Med.* **90**: 646–648.

Nakanishi, T., Sobue, I., Toyokura, Y., Nishitani, H., Kuroiwa, Y., Satoyoshi, E., Tsubaki, T., Igata, A., and Ozaki, Y. (1984). The Crow–Fukase syndrome: a study of 102 cases in Japan. *Neurology* **34**: 712–720.

Nemni, R., Feltri, M.I., Fazio, R., Quatini, A., Lorenzetti, I., Corbo, M., and Canal, N. (1990). Axonal neuropathy with monoclonal IgG kappa that binds to a neurofibrillary protein. *Ann. Neurol.* **28**: 361–364.

Ohi, T., Kyle, R.A., and Dyck, P.J. (1985). Axonal attenuation and secondary segmental demyelination in myeloma neuropathies. *Ann. Neurol.* **17**: 225–261.

Ono, K., Ito, M., Hotchi, M., Katsuyama, T., Komiya, I., and Yamada, T. (1985). Polyclonal plasma cell proliferation with systemic capillary hemangiomatosis, endocrine disturbance, and peripheral neuropathy. *Acta Pathol. Jpn* **35**: 251–267.

Pruzanski, W., and Williams, C. (1980). Role of calcitonin in osteosclerosis of myeloma? *Arch. Intern. Med.* **140**: 1554 (letter).

Puig, L., Moreno, A., Domingo, P., Llistosella, E., and de Moragas, J.M. (1985). Cutaneous angiomas in POEMS syndrome. *J. Am. Acad. Dermatol.* **12**: 961–964.

Raper, R.F. and Ibels, L.S. (1985). Osteosclerotic myeloma complicated by diffuse arteritis, vascular calcification, and extensive cutaneous necrosis. *Nephron* **39**: 389–392.

Read, D.J., van Hegan, R.I., and Mathews, W.B. (1978). Peripheral neuropathy and benign IgG paraproteinemia. *J. Neurol. Neurosurg. Psychiatry* **41**: 215–219.

Reitan, J.B., Pape, E., Fossa, S.D., Julsrud, O.-J., Slettnes, O.N., and Solheim, O.P. (1980). Osteosclerotic myeloma with polyneuropathy. *Acta Med. Scand.* **208**: 137–144.

Resnick, D., Greenway, G.D., Bardwick, P.A., Zvaifler, N.J., Gill, G.N., and Newman, D.R. (1981). Plasma cell dyscrasia with polyneuropathy, organomegaly, endocrinopathy, M protein, and skin changes: the POEMS syndrome: distinctive radiographic abnormalities. *Radiology* **140**: 17–22.

Reulecke, M., Dumas, M., and Meier, C. (1988). Specific antibody activity against neuroendocrine tissue in a case of POEMS syndrome with IgG gammopathy. *Neurology* **38**: 614–616.

Ropper, A.H., and McKee, A.C. (1993). Case Records of the Massachusetts General Hospital: Case 21–1993. *N. Engl. J. Med.* **328**: 1550–1558.

Rosseau, J.J., Franck, G., Grisar, T., Reznick, M., Heynen, G., and Salmon, J. (1978). Osteosclerotic myeloma with polyneuropathy and ectopic secretion of calcitonin. *Eur. J. Cancer* **14**: 133–140.

Sadiq, S.A., van den Berg, L.H., Thomas, F.P., Kilidreas, K., Hays, A.P., and Latov, N. (1991). Human monoclonal anti-neurofilament antibody crossreacts with a neuronal surface protein. *J. Neurosci. Res.* **29**: 319–325.

Scheinker, I. (1938). Myelom und Nervensystem: Uber eine bisher nicht beschriebene mit eigentumlichen Hautveranderungen einhergehende Polyneuritis bei einem plasmazellulaaren Myelom des Sternums. *Dtsch. Z. Nervenheilkd.* **147**: 247–273.

Sewell, H.F., Mathews, J.B., Gooch, E., Millac, P., Willox, A., Stain, M.A., and Walker, F. (1981). Autoantibody to nerve tissue in a patient with a peripheral neuropathy and an IgG paraprotein. *J. Clin. Pathol.* **34**: 1163–1166.

Silberstein, L.E., Duggan, D., and Berkman, E.M. (1985). Therapeutic trial of plasma exchange in osteosclerotic myeloma associated with the POEMS syndrome. *J. Clin. Apheresis* **2**: 253–247.

Silverstein, A. and Doniger, D.E. (1963). Neurologic complication of myelomatosis. *Arch. Neurol.* **9**: 534–544.

Simmons, Z., Bromberg, M.B., Feldman, E.L., and Blairis, M. (1993). Polyneuropathy associated with IgA monoclonal gammopathy of undetermined significance. *Muscle Nerve* **16**: 77–83.

Simmons, Z., Wald, J., Albers, J.W., and Feldman, E.L. (1994). The natural history of a 'benign' rib lesion in a patients with a demyelinating polyneuropathy and an unusual variant of POEMS syndrome. *Muscle Nerve* **17**: 1055–1059.

Suarez, G.A. and Kelly Jr, J.J. (1993). Polyneuropathy associated with monoclonal gammopathy of undetermined significance. Further evidence that IgM-MGUS neuropathies are different from IgG-MGUS. *Neurology* **43**: 1304–1308.

Takatsuki, K. and Sanada, Z. (1983). Plasma cell dyscrasia with polyneuropathy and endocrine disorder: Clinical and laboratory features of 109 reported cases. *Jpn J. Clin. Oncol.* **13**: 543–556.

Victor, M., Banker, B.Q., and Adams, R.D. (1958). The neuropathy of multiple myeloma. *J. Neurol. Neurosurg. Psychiatry* **21**: 73–88.

Vrethem, M. (1994). *Polyneuropathies associated with monoclonal gammopathies.* Linkoping University Dissertation No. 409, Linkoping.

Waldenström, J.G., Adner, A., Gydell, K., and Zettervall, O. (1978). Osteosclerotic 'plasmocytoma' with polyneuropathy, hypertrichosis, and diabetes. *Acta Med. Scand.* **203**: 297–303.

Walsh, J.C. (1971). The neuropathy of multiple myeloma. *Arch. Neurol.* **25**: 404–414.

17 Neuromyotonia and the Lambert–Eaton myasthenic syndrome

J. Newsom-Davis

Introduction

The motor nerve terminal is vulnerable to autoimmune attack for two reasons. First, it is rich in transmembrane molecules concerned either in generating the action potential or in synaptic transmission, whose extracellular domains are potentially accessible to the immune system. Second, unlike the remainder of the nerve, the terminal lacks the protection provided by the blood–nerve barrier from circulating autoantibodies that might crossreact with neural antigens. For the same reasons, the nerve–muscle preparation is an informative site at which to investigate the actions of sera or immunoglobulins from patients with myasthenic or peripheral nerve disorders of uncertain etiology but suspected of being mediated by autoantibodies.

The clinical and laboratory features pointing to an antibody-mediated autoimmune disease are exemplified by the postsynaptic disorder myasthenia gravis. Clinical features in favor of such an etiology include: (1) demonstration of improvement following plasmapheresis (although failure to respond does not exclude such an etiology), (2) response to immunosuppressive drugs, and (3) precipitation by, or association with, infections. Laboratory criteria (adapted from Koch's postulates for infectious diseases) are: (1) detection of serum antibody to the specified antigen at some stage in the illness, (2) 'passive transfer' of the pathophysiological features to experimental animals by repeated injections of the patients' plasma or immunoglobulin fraction, and (3) induction of the disease in animals by immunization with the purified antigen.

This chapter will be concerned with two disorders in which the antigenic targets are voltage-gated ion channels. In acquired neuromyotonia (NMT), the dominant target appears to be voltage-gated K^+ channels (VGKCs) that normally serve to control peripheral nerve excitability, while in the Lambert–Eaton myasthenic syndrome (LEMS) it is the voltage-gated Ca^{2+} channels (VGCCs) on which acetylcholine release depends (Figure 17.1). In the present context, it may be noted that the use of the nerve–muscle preparation has, in two further disorders, recently elucidated the role of antibodies to particular gangliosides that are known to be enriched at synapses. In the Miller Fisher syndrome, a variant of the Guillain-Barré syndrome (GBS), IgG antibodies to GQ1b ganglioside have been detected by

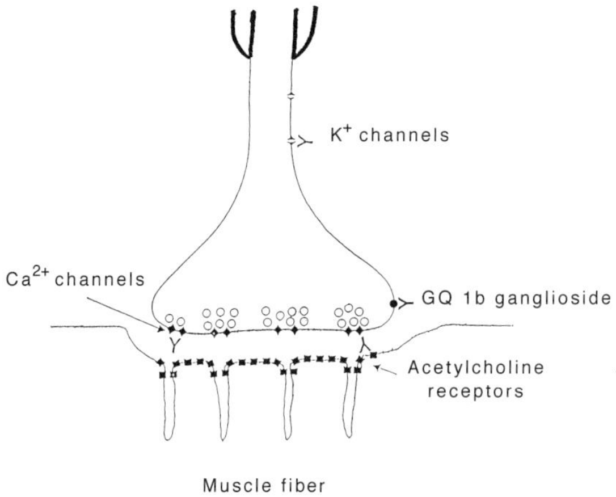

Figure 17.1 *Diagram of the neuromuscular junction showing targets for antibody-mediated autoimmunity.*

several groups (for a review see Willison 1994); application of anti-GQ1b positive sera to the nerve–muscle preparation in vitro produced complete block of acetylcholine release by 3 hours, convalescent anti-GQ1b negative sera being without effect (Roberts et al. 1994). In multifocal motor neuropathy, anti-GM1 positive plasma, or monoclonal anti-GM1 antibodies derived from such patients, were shown to block nerve conduction in distal motor nerves using the nerve–muscle preparation either on direct application or following passive transfer (Willison et al. 1994).

Acquired myotonia

Acquired neuromyotonia is one of several types of myokymia (muscle twitching). Although probably described clinically by Morvan (1890), who also noted accompanying insomnia and hallucinations in his cases, the peripheral aspects of the disorder were first clearly defined by the pioneering electromyographical studies of Denny-Brown and Foley (1948) in two patients, one of whom was a 37-year-old physician. Clinically, the patients exhibited an 'undulating myokymia' that was characterized electromyographically by the occurrence of individual motor units often firing as triplets or multiplets at high instantaneous frequencies. The peripheral nerve origin of these spontaneous motor unit discharges was established by Isaacs (1961) who showed that the motor unit discharges persisted during complete proximal nerve block but were abolished by curare, which suggests that they were arising in the terminal arborization of the motor nerves. The discharges also continued during sleep or general anesthesia, distinguishing them from the spasms occurring in stiff-man syndrome. He proposed the term 'continuous muscle fiber activity' to describe the disorder but Mertens and Zschocke (1965) preferred the term 'Neuromyotonie' which more accurately describes its nature. Subsequently the disorder has become known as neuromyotonia, the prefix 'acquired' being used to distinguish this form of neuromyotonia from that observed in patients with hereditary neuropathies (Newsom-Davis and Mills 1993).

Clinical features

Onset is typically insidious. Muscle twitching, muscle aching or excessive cramps are usually the first symptom, but in some it may be pseudomyotonia, resembling tetany. Symptoms are often provoked by voluntary muscle contraction. The muscle twitching is occasionally noticed first by an observer other than the patient. As the symptoms become more severe, so disability increases and may significantly interfere with normal activity. In particular, the first few seconds of an activity, such as walking, may be difficult because of pain and stiffness. Pseudomyotonia (slow relaxation) of hand grip is observed in some patients, or slowness of retraction of the tongue following protrusion. Myokymia and/or pseudomyotonia can be readily provoked by limb ischemia, e.g. by a blood pressure cuff. Chvostek's sign may be present. Some patients may be aware of muscle weakness and also of muscle hypertrophy that is often evident to the observer. Sweating may be excessive. A few patients experience occasional tingling or shock-like sensory symptoms. Some cases have been reported to experience insomnia, hallucinations or altered behavior (Newsom-Davis and Mills 1993).

There is an increased association with thymoma and with myasthenia gravis. A literature survey over the last 20 years revealed five cases of thymoma in about 40 cases of NMT (Newsom-Davis and Mills 1993). Penicillamine has been reported to induce NMT in one case (as it can in myasthenia gravis), and several cases

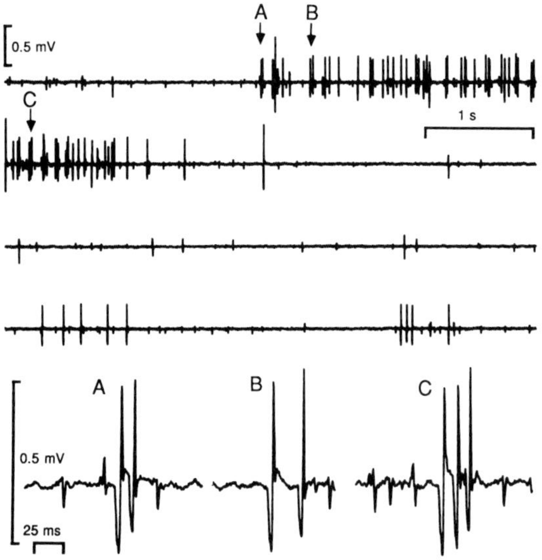

Figure 17.2 *Needle recording from the first dorsal interosseous muscle of a patient with acquired neuromyotonia. The upper four traces are continuous and show a neuromyotonic discharge lasting some 4 s. Within the discharge, single motor units fire as doublets (at A and B) or triplets (at C). Reprinted with permission from Newsom-Davis and Mills,* Brain, *1993.*

have been observed in association with lung cancer, proved to be small-cell lung cancer in one case. Thus NMT can, like LEMS, occur as a spontaneous disorder or as a paraneoplastic syndrome.

Case history of a patient with neuromyotonia

An 18-year-old girl developed generalized muscle twitching, cramps and spasms at the age of 11 years, shortly after an illness diagnosed as glandular fever. The twitching involved muscles of the eyelids, face, neck, limbs and trunk. Muscle spasms were made worse by muscle activity, and the twitching was observed to continue during sleep. She was often woken by cramp. She complained of excessive sweating. She was considerably disabled, and had been unable to attend school since the age of 12 years. She had very great difficulty in climbing stairs and had to use crutches when walking.

She had been investigated at several hospitals, and at one time her symptoms were attributed to a psychological cause.

On initial examination, there was evident widespread myokymia, readily increased by voluntary muscle contraction. She was underweight, and the development of secondary sexual characteristics was delayed. Muscle hypertrophy was not evident.

Electromyography (Dr K. R. Mills) revealed neuromyotonic discharges characterized by individual motor units firing as doublets or triplets at high instantaneous frequency (more than 90/s) and spontaneous discharges lasting from 100 ms to several tens of seconds at similar high frequencies. Serum creatine kinase was raised.

A course of ten daily plasmapheresis over 12 days was associated with a substantial decline in myokymia from day 8, confirmed by the patient who commented that twitching had greatly decreased and that she had become free of muscle cramps. Symptoms began to increase again in severity about 2 weeks after the last day of exchange.

Electromyographic features

Spontaneous repetitive firing of single motor units as doublets, triplets or in longer bursts with high intraburst frequencies (typically more than 40/s) is the hallmark of NMT. A typical pattern is illustrated in Figure 17.2. These spontaneous bursts occur at irregular intervals. The abnormal discharges are often triggered by voluntary contraction, and can also be provoked by nerve stimulation that may elicit a prolonged after-discharge. Fasciculation or fibrillation potentials are often present. Neuromyotonic discharges can sometimes be detected in the absence of visible myokymia. The discharges are readily provoked by limb ischemia. Curare abolishes the discharges, thereby excluding their muscular origin. The discharges may continue despite

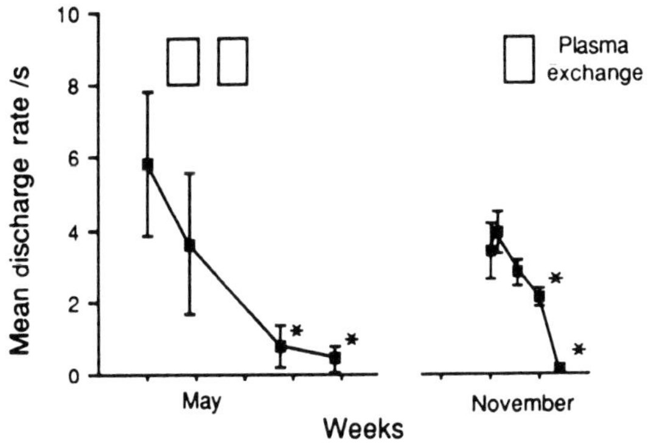

Figure 17.3 *Mean (±SD) discharge rate of motor units in medial gastrocnemius muscle in a patient with acquired neuromyotonia during two admissions for plasma exchange 6 months apart. Each block represents a 5-day course of plasma exchange. The rate of spontaneous discharges is significantly reduced by the procedure* *$p<0.01$. *Reprinted, with permission, from Sinha et al.,* The Lancet, *1991.*

peripheral nerve block with local anesthetic (e.g. ulnar nerve block at the elbow) indicating in such cases that they arise in the terminal portion of the motor nerve as originally described by Isaacs (1961). Proximal block may reduce the discharges in some patients, which suggests sites of origin both above and below the block. In other cases, proximal block may abolish all activity pointing to a more proximal site of initiation (Newsom-Davis and Mills 1993). In one such case, activity was completely abolished by epidural block (Hosokawa et al. 1987). Nerve conduction studies may be normal or show evidence of demyelinating or axonal neuropathy.

Etiology

Several clinical features of acquired NMT point to a possible autoimmune causation. These include the already mentioned associations with thymoma and with myasthenia gravis, the report of its provocation by penicillamine treatment, and the finding of oligoclonal bands in the cerebrospinal fluid (CSF) in some patients (for a review see Newsom-Davis and Mills 1993).

The reduction in myokymia and in neuromyotonic discharges following plasmapheresis provides direct evidence for a circulating factor (Sinha et al. 1991; Newsom-Davis and Mills 1993; Ishii et al. 1994). Figure 17.3 shows the significant decline in the quantified electromyographical discharges in a patient of ours with NMT, following two 5-day courses of plasmapheresis. Over the following months, the discharges returned, but a further course of plasma exchange at 6 months resulted in a similar decline in discharge frequency.

Spontaneous or repetitive firing of motor nerves could result either from a decrease in the number of functional VGKCs or from interference with sodium channel function. The former appears more likely, by analogy with the effects of antibodies to other ion channels (for example the reduction in the number of functional acetylcholine receptors in myasthenia gravis). A decrease in the number of functional VGKCs would be expected to cause prolongation of the action potential at the nerve terminal and thereby facilitate neuromuscular transmission by increasing the quantal content of the endplate potential (i.e. the number of acetylcholine quanta released by each nerve impulse). This was shown to be the case in experiments in which mice were injected intraperitoneally either with NMT plasma or its IgG fraction for up to 21 days, and the in vitro resistance to *d*-tubocurarine investigated (Sinha et al. 1991). Resistance was significantly increased compared with control mice, consistent with the hypothesis. In further similar passive transfer studies, the quantal content of the endplate potential was measured directly by intracellular microelectrode recording. Quantal content was significantly increased by some NMT preparations, again implying prolongation of the action potential at the nerve terminal and suggesting that some NMT sera contain antibodies that can reduce the number of functional VGKCs (Shillito et al. 1992).

Antibodies to voltage-gated potassium channels

Alpha-dendrotoxin, a component of the venom of the green mamba, is a ligand for VGKCs. Four of our NMT sera have precipitated human brain VGKCs, labelled with ^{125}I-alpha-dendrotoxin, although some NMT sera have been negative in this assay. One NMT sera also precipitated two types of ^{125}I-alpha-dendrotoxin-labeled Shaker-like human brain VGKC, extracted from *Xenopus* oocytes that had been injected with the relevant VGKC cRNA (Hart et al. 1994). These preliminary studies show that antibodies to human VGKCs can be detected in some NMT sera and, together with the electrophysiological data, suggest that such antibodies may be the primary pathological element in these patients.

Diagnosis

The diagnosis is based on the clinical features outlined above and the characteristic electromyographical changes. The detection of anti-VGKC antibodies would be a confirmatory finding. A positive family history and evidence of impaired nerve conduction velocity point to a hereditary neuropathy as the cause (Hahn et al. 1991). Benign myokymia is excluded by its focal and short-lived nature. In the cramp-fasciculation syndrome, the calf-muscles are predominantly affected; neuromyotonia is not evident on electromyography, but after-discharges can be elicited (Tahmoush et al. 1991). There are however similarities between this syndrome and NMT in that patients may respond to carbamazepine.

Therapy

The first treatment was introduced by Isaacs (1961) who used phenytoin in two cases of NMT with strikingly beneficial results. It was later shown that carbamazepine was also effective in this condition (Hughes and Matthews 1969), and these two drugs given at anticonvulsant doses have been the mainstay of treatment since then. Some patients, however, fail to respond adequately to this medication and should be considered for immunological treatment. Several cases have now been reported to respond to plasmapheresis (see above). Intravenous immunoglobulin therapy caused an increase of symptoms in one case (Ishii et al. 1994). Two of the authors' cases have improved substantially following treatment with prednisolone and either azathioprine or methotrexate for about 1 year. More data are needed before such treatment can be confidently recommended, but in patients with severe NMT that has failed to respond to carbamazepine and phenytoin, immunosuppressive drug treatment should be considered. When a thymoma is present, surgical removal will normally be necessary although it is not clear whether this results in neurological improvement.

Future developments

Judging by the cases that have recently come to our notice, we believe that NMT may be more common than its rare reporting suggests, particularly in patients with thymoma or myasthenia gravis, but also in association with lung cancer. At present, diagnosis is primarily based on clinical observation and electromyography, but developments in the assay for anti-VGKC antibodies may provide an additional and specific aid to diagnosis. It may also help to show whether there is more than one form of aquired NMT, that might reflect the VGKC subtype being targeted. Further studies will be needed to evaluate the role of immunosuppressive drug treatment in patients failing to respond adequately to carbamazepine and phenytoin.

Lambert-Eaton myasthenic syndrome

A myasthenic syndrome that associated with cancer was first recognized by Anderson et al. (1953). Remarkably, in view of subsequent discoveries, they suggested that the oat cell (small-cell) tumour in their case might have given rise to 'an unusual form of peripheral neuropathy, possibly similar to myasthenia gravis'. Its distinction electrophysiologically from myasthenia gravis was established by Lambert and his colleagues (Eaton and Lambert 1957). It was also soon recognized that the syndrome could occur in the apparent absence of small-cell cancer and in non-smokers. In our analysis of 50 consecutive cases of LEMS seen at a single hospital, a lung tumor was present in 24, and proven histologically to be small-cell lung carcinoma in 21 cases (O'Neill et al. 1988). Of the remainder, 14 had been followed for between 5 and more than 10 years. Thus the syndrome can occur in those with lung cancer (C-LEMS) and those in whom no cancer can be detected (NC-LEMS).

Clinical features

Onset age can be from the first decade to extreme old age. The onset is usually insidious, but is occasionally subacute, maximum severity developing within 2–3 months. The commonest presenting symptoms are fatiguable leg weakness and difficulty in walking, and at presentation these symptoms affect virtually all patients (O'Neill et al. 1988). Gait takes on a rolling quality. One patient describes his difficulties as being like 'walking through treacle'. Arm weakness is common, and occasionally there is severe involvement of respiratory muscles. Drooping eyelids are usually bilateral and affect about 20% of patients. Mild double vision can occur. Weakness is worse in hot weather or after a hot bath, and can be relieved by cold. Symptoms are occasionally first revealed by the use of a calcium antagonist such as diltiazem. Autonomic symptoms are common, affecting 80% of patients, but are not always spontaneously reported. Dry mouth is the commonest but constipation and impaired sexual function (failure of erection or ejaculation) are also frequent.

On examination, weakness (without wasting) is more evident proximally than distally. There is a characteristic augmentation of strength during the first few seconds of a maximum voluntary contraction that is easy to overlook. Continued testing usually provokes fatigue and increased weakness. The tendon reflexes may also exhibit post-tetanic potentiation, the responses being depressed or absent in resting muscle in 90% of patients, but enhancing following 15 seconds of maximum voluntary contraction. Pupillary responses are occasionally sluggish.

Case history

A 43-year-old woman presented with an 18 month history of fatigue on walking, difficulty in climbing stairs and general lethargy. When initially examined, weakness was not obvious but the tendon reflexes were noted to be very depressed. She was at first thought to have a myopathy. Further direct questioning revealed that she had a dry mouth for several months and was also aware of blurred vision. She had smoked 15 cigarettes a day for 30 years.

Examination revealed bilateral ptosis and positive Cogan's sign (upward twitch of the eyelid on attempted up-gaze). There was weakness of neck flexion and proximal weakness of upper and lower limbs, with well-marked augmentation of strength during the first few seconds of a voluntary effort. Tendon reflexes were depressed but showed post-tetanic potentiation. There was no sensory loss.

Electromyography (EMG) revealed a greatly reduced compound muscle action potential amplitude (1.2 mV; normal >8.4 mV) in a hand muscle, that increased tenfold following 15 seconds of maximum voluntary contraction. Single-fiber electromyography showed increased jitter with blocking. Initial investigations in a chest unit appeared to suggest a right lower lobe lesion, but further tests including computed tomography (CT) chest scan and bronchoscopy failed to identify a lung tumor.

She was treated initially with 3,4-diaminopyridine, which improved muscle strength but resulted in episodes suggesting temporal lobe seizures. This treatment was therefore withdrawn and she received a course of plasma exchange and alternate day prednisolone therapy. There was a return of strength and improvement in walking. She was seen regularly at the chest clinic for follow-up with repeated CT chest scan and radiographs.

About 5.5 years after the onset of muscle weakness, and 6 months after her last normal chest radiograph, she developed marked increase in weakness and a productive cough. Bronchoscopy revealed a tumor in the right intermediate bronchus which proved histologically to be a small-cell lung cancer. She underwent right pneumonectomy and excision of hilar nodes.

Following surgery, without change in prednisolone therapy, there was improvement in strength and in the compound muscle action potential amplitude. Examined about 5 years after her pneumonectomy, she showed only mild proximal weakness.

Pathology

An unexpected finding in two patients with NC-LEMS who underwent muscle biopsy was a selective, and in one case progressive, loss of type 1 muscle fibers (Squier et al. 1991), leading to an overwhelming type 2 predominance. Light microscopic studies of the end-plate in five patients (four had associated cancer) showed enlargement of the area of contact between nerve and muscle, that was interpreted as being

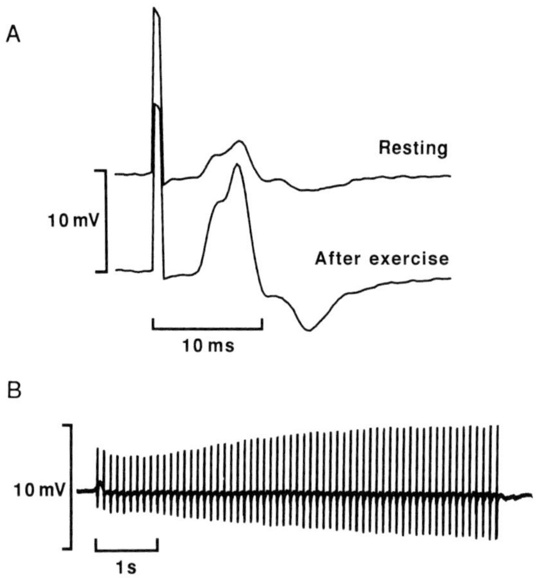

Figure 17.4 *Compound muscle action potential in abductor digiti minimi elicited by supramaximal nerve stimulation in a patient with the Lambert–Eaton myasthenic syndrome, showing (A) a large increase in amplitude following 15 s maximum voluntary contraction and (B) similar facilitation during nerve stimulation at 10 Hz. Courtesy of Dr K.R. Mills.*

compensatory (Hesselmans et al. 1992). Ultrastructural studies revealed no presynaptic abnormality, but post-synaptic membrane length and area were decreased, possibly because of newly formed nerve sprouts.

Cancer associations

About 60% of patients with LEMS have an underlying small-cell lung cancer (SCLC). Almost all of these will have a history of smoking. There is a weak association with lymphoma and thymoma. The interval between the onset of LEMS and radiological evidence of SCLC is typically less than 2 years but in occasional cases the neurological syndrome may precede evidence of tumor by 5 years. There appears to be no difference between the clinical features of C-LEMS and NC-LEMS.

From a prospective study of 150 cases with SCLC, and a literature review, Elrington et al. (1991) estimated the overall prevalence of LEMS at about 3% giving an approximate annual incidence of 250 new cases in the UK.

Immunological associations

Other autoimmune disease occur at increased frequency in LEMS, especially thyroid disease, pernicious anemia, vitiligo and celiac disease (Willcox et al. 1985). About 50% of the series of 50 LEMS patients studied by O'Neill et al. (1988) had a past or family history of autoimmunity and/or detectable serum antibodies. Lennon et al. (1982) studied sera from 64 patients, detecting organ-specific autoantibodies in 45%, compared with 17% in age-matched controls. MG occasionally associates with LEMS. A study of HLA and Ig heavy chain gene associations in a group of 30 patients showed a significant association with HLA-B8, especially in NC-LEMS, and with G1m(2) especially in C-LEMS (Willcox et al. 1985). These associations need to be confirmed in a larger series.

Electromyography

The hallmark of LEMS is a reduced amplitude of the compound muscle action potential (CMAP) measured in a resting muscle, that declines at low rates of stimulation but which shows an increase, typically exceeding 100% of the resting value, following 10–15 s of maximum voluntary contraction (Figure 17.4). High frequency (10–40 Hz) electrical nerve stimulation will produce a similar increase, but is less well tolerated by the patient.

An increase in jitter on single fiber EMG is present in LEMS as in myasthenia gravis. In 29 patients studied by this technique, jitter and/or blocking was found in all, while in some muscles every potential examined showed these characteristics (O'Neill et al. 1988). As would be expected of a presynaptic disorder, jitter and blocking improve at higher stimulation rates during axonal microstimulation but, as Trontelj and Stålberg (1990) point out, this can also occur in the primarily postsynaptic disorder myasthenia gravis.

Etiology

The nature of the electrophysiological abnormality was identified by Lambert and Elmqvist (1971), in studies of biopsied muscle from LEMS patients. They showed that the quantal content of the endplate potential, i.e. the number of quanta (packages) of acetylcholine released by each nerve impulse, was substantially reduced in resting muscle, often failing to trigger an action potential. Miniature endplate potential amplitudes, however, were normal. Quantal content increased during repetitive nerve stimulation, and following an increasing external Ca^{2+} concentration. These studies established the presynaptic nature of LEMS, and its similarities with the effects of lower external concentrations of Ca^{2+} or high Mg^{2+}. Direct measurement of acetylcholine content and release, and of acetylcholinesterase, were consistent with the view that the defect in LEMS lay in the acetylcholine release mechanism (Molenaar et al. 1982).

A clue to the autoimmune nature of LEMS was its association with other autoimmune diseases (see above), as in myasthenia gravis. Plasma exchange (which removes circulating antibodies) was followed by short-term clinical improvement that reached its peak at about 15 days, supporting the hypothesis (Lang et al. 1981). Immunosuppressive drug therapy was also found to be effective in patients with NC-LEMS (Newsom-Davis and Murray 1984). The IgG fraction of LEMS plasma injected intraperitoneally into mice, or the plasma itself, reproduced the physiological changes of LEMS, inducing a reduction in the quantal content of the endplate potential, implying that antibodies binding to nerve terminal determinants, possibly voltage-gated calcium channels, were likely to be responsible for the disorder in humans (Lang et al. 1981, 1983). This was confirmed in the passive transfer model by direct measurements of resting and evoked release of acetylcholine (Lang et al. 1984).

Paucity of the presynaptic active zones and disorganization of active zone particles (that are believed to represent voltage-gated calcium channels) were reported by Fukunaga et al. (1982) in freeze-fracture electron microscopic studies of LEMS nerve–muscle preparations, and it was suggested that the active zone particles might be the targets for the pathogenic autoantibodies in LEMS reported by Lang et al. (1981). In collaborative studies between the two groups, it was then shown that the characteristic morphological changes could, like the pathophysiological changes, be passively transferred to mice by injection of LEMS IgG (for a review see Engel et al. 1989). The effects of the IgG appeared to depend on crosslinking of adjacent active zone particles by the divalent antibody; monovalent (Fab) fragments were ineffective. The earliest changes observed were clustering of the particles, followed by a reduction in their numbers. These changes were in accord with the reduction in the quantal content of the endplate potentials observed in parallel studies on the diaphragm in these mice. Importantly also, LEMS IgG could be localized at motor nerve terminal active zones by immunoelectron microscopy. Further passive transfer studies using LEMS IgG, in which quantal content was studied over a range of calcium concentrations, indicated that the reduced quantal content was likely to be due to an approximately 40% reduction in the number of functional voltage-gated calcium channels (Lang et al. 1987).

Anti-voltage-gated calcium channel (VGCC) antibodies

VGCC antibodies may be classified pharmacologically and electrophysiologically into at least four subtypes (T,L,N and P/Q). A radioimmunoassay to detect anti-VGCC antibodies was first reported by Sher et al. (1989), who used the radio-iodinated toxin from a cone snail (*Conus geographus*; ^{125}I-ω-CgTx GVIA) that labels N-type VGCCs. Although a large proportion of LEMS cases were positive, so also were some controls. Leys et al. (1991) detected raised titers in about 44% of patients, but again also in a number of disease controls. Antibodies against L-type VGCCs were detected using ^{3}H-PN200-110 in a proportion of patients, but tended to be positive only in those with high-anti-N-type VGCC antibody activity (El Far et al. 1995). Electrophysiological studies on cell lines confirms anti-L type activity in some LEMS sera (Kim and Neher 1988; Peers et al. 1990).

The demonstration that acetylcholine release in the mammalian neuromuscular junction is blocked by the P-type channel blocker ω-Aga IVA (derived from the

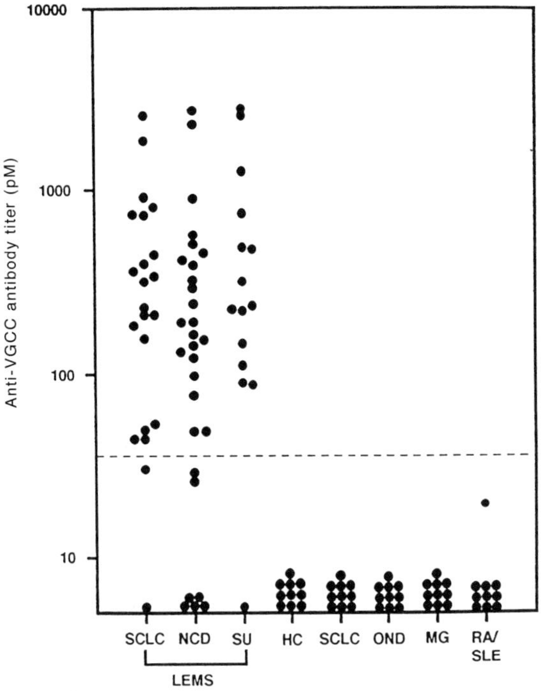

Figure 17.5 *Serum anti-voltage-gated calcium channel antibodies in the Lambert–Eaton myasthenic syndrome and controls measured by immunoprecipitation using ^{125}I-ω-conotoxin MVIIC. Non-specific binding of each serum, measured in the presence of excess cold toxin, has been subtracted. Antibody titers were considered positive if greater than 40 pM (mean+3 SD for the healthy controls; dashed line). SCLC: small-cell lung carcinoma; NCD: no cancer detected; SU: status uncertain; HC: healthy controls; OND: other neurological disease: MG: myasthenia gravis; RA/SLE: rheumatoid arthritis/systemic lupus erythematosus. Reprinted, with permission, from Motomura et al.,* Journal of Neurology, Neurosurgery and Psychiatry, *1995.*

American bird-eating spider), rather than an N-type or L-type channel blocker (Uchitel et al. 1992), stimulated the search for alternative ligands. We have used the toxin from *Conus magus* (CmTx MVIIC), which binds P/Q-type VGCCs. In a series of 66 patients with clinically and electromyographically definite LEMS, a raised antibody titer was detected in 85% (Figure 17.5). The lack of positivity in healthy individuals and in patients with other neurological diseases and the high incidence of positivity in the patients indicates that this new assay will be very useful in diagnosis. It also suggests that these antibodies may be the principal pathogenic agent in this disorder.

The site of the antigenic determinants on the VGCC, in particular which subunit of the VGCC is targeted, have not yet been established although antibodies directed to the beta-subunit have been identified (Rosenfeld et al. 1993; El Far et al. 1995); however the beta-subunit is believed to be cytoplasmic and may not therefore be the primary target.

Antibodies to synaptotagmin

Antibodies to the synaptic vesicle protein synaptotagmin have been detected in a few patients who also have high anti-N-type VGCC antibody activity (Leveque et al. 1992), but their significance is not yet clear. Takamori et al. (1994) were able to induce the physiological changes of LEMS (reduced quantal content and facilitation at high stimulation frequencies) in some but not all rats immunized with a synthetic peptide corresponding to synaptotagmin residues 20–53. Immunization with another peptide (residues 1–30) had no effect.

Role of the small-cell lung cancer

The likely neuroectodermal origin of SCLC, which expresses neuroendocrine markers such as neuron-specific enolase, clearly raises the possibility that it may express antigenic determinants which could elicit crossreactive immune responses with nervous system determinants. Significantly, perhaps, SCLC is the commonest cancer to associate with paraneoplastic syndromes. These syndromes include, in addition to LEMS, encephalomyelitis, cerebellar degeneration, subacute sensory neuropathy, and retinal degeneration. In the context of LEMS, it may be noted that SCLC shows electrical excitability and can generate Ca^{2+} spikes. Roberts et al. (1985) used a $^{45}Ca^{2+}$ flux assay in an SCLC line to investigate the actions of LEMS IgG. It was first shown

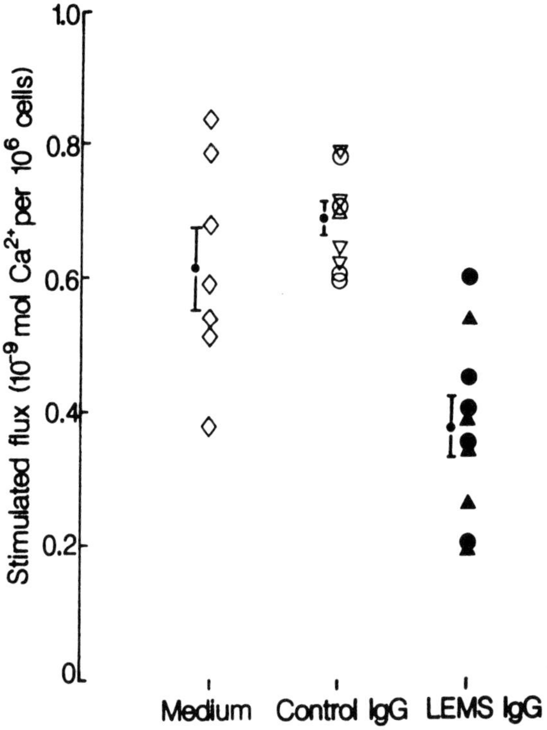

Figure 17.6 *Effects of Lambert–Eaton myasthenic syndrome (LEMS) IgG and control IgG on 96 mM K^+-stimulated $^{45}Ca^{2+}$ flux in small-cell lung cancer (SCLC) cells. In each experiment, five separate sets of cells were usually assayed: one set cultured in medium alone (◊), two sets in control IgG and two sets in LEMS IgG. Control IgG was obtained from healthy laboratory workers (○), other neurological disease control (▽), and a SCLC patient without LEMS (△). LEMS IgG was obtained from patients with associated SCLC (▲) or with no tumor evident (●). Reprinted, with permission, from Roberts et al.,* Nature, *1985.*

that an increasing external concentration of K^+ to depolarize the cells resulted in a corresponding increasing influx of Ca^{2+}; however, when the cells were incubated for several days in LEMS IgG at physiological concentrations, there was a substantial and highly significant decline in Ca^{2+} influx compared with control IgG from healthy individuals or from patients with other neurological diseases (Figure 17.6). NC-LEMS IgG was as effective in reducing Ca^{2+} influx as C-LEMS. These findings suggested that, in C-LEMS, tumor VGCCs were provoking the crossreactive anti-VGCC antibody response. They leave unanswered the question of what stimulates the response in NC-LEMS.

In further support of the hypothesis that tumor VGCCs provoke the antibody response is the finding that within individuals disease severity (as measured by CMAP amplitude) correlates positively with reduction of Ca^{2+} influx by their IgG (Lang et al. 1989). Moreover, an analysis of the effects of specific tumor therapy in a group of LEMS patients with SCLC, who had survived treatment by more than 2 months, showed that in all of them the CMAP amplitude increased into the normal range 6–12 months after starting treatment (Chalk et al. 1990). One patient, who had a right lower lobectomy and local radiotherapy, is surviving 9 years later without signs of LEMS or of tumor recurrence.

Morris et al. (1992) undertook an immunocytochemical characterization of SCLC in patients with LEMS, comparing the findings with those in patients with SCLC but no neurological disorder. In the LEMS cases there was a greater infiltration of the tumor by activated macrophages. In addition, expression of a 200 kDa neurofilament antigen and of MHC class I antigen by the tumor were reduced in LEMS-associated SCLCs compared with controls (non-LEMS SCLC). The latter finding might be explained by cytotoxic T cell killing of tumor cells expressing high levels of class I. The results lend support to the view that a more vigorous immune response is generated in SCLC patients with LEMS than in those without LEMS.

Diagnosis

LEMS can often be confidently diagnosed on the association of proximal muscle weakness, depressed tendon reflexes, post-tetanic potentiation and autonomic features. Electromyographical studies should confirm this, as indicated in a previous section. The improvement in the radioimmunoassay for anti-VGCC antibodies makes this a valuable means of confirming the diagnosis as it appears to be positive in over 85% of patients and false-positives appear to be very rare (Motomura et al. 1995).

Other disorders need to be excluded, however. Myasthenia gravis can be distinguished by differences in its electromyographical features, and by the presence of anti-acetycholine esterase antibodies in most patients. Patients with botulism may have a similar electromyographic finding but their serum will be negative for anti-VGCC antibodies. Congenital or hereditary presynaptic causes of myasthenia can usually be distinguished by a positive family history, early onset, and absence of specific antibodies.

Therapy

The introduction of 3,4-diaminopyridine (3,4-DAP) in the treatment of LEMS has proved valuable in both C-LEMS and NC-LEMS (McEvoy et al. 1989). The compound acts by partially blocking K^+ flux through voltage-gated K^+ channels in peripheral nerve, thereby prolonging the action potential at the nerve terminal, enhancing Ca^{2+} influx and thus increasing acetylcholine release. Adults are usually started on an oral dose of 10 mg four or five times daily, increasing to a maximum of 20 mg five times daily. Most patients experience perioral or distal parasthesiae about an hour after ingestion. Excessive doseage leads to central excitation and seizures. The drug is contraindicated in epilepsy. It is preferred to guanidine which has a high incidence of side-effects.

SCLC should be treated promptly and vigorously not only for its own sake, but because this may improve the associated neurological disorder (Chalk et al. 1990). Where tumor is suspected (i.e. in smokers with a history of less than 5 years) regular radiological follow-up is needed so that the appearance of the tumor is detected early. In SCLC patients who have failed to improve satisfactorily with tumor therapy and 3,4-diaminopyridine, alternate day prednisolone should be considered.

In cases where an underlying SCLC is not expected, treatment with alternate day prednisolone and azathioprine can be exceptionally effective, although the response is typically slow (Newsom-Davis and Murray 1984). Initially, the prednisolone dose should be 1 mg kg^{-1} bodyweight, and the azathioprine dose 2.5 mg kg^{-1} bodyweight.

Plasma exchange (plasmapheresis) is useful in patients who have severe symptoms but, because such treatment is passive, it should be used in conjunction with immunosuppressive drug therapy (Newsom-Davis and Murray 1984) or with treatment of the associated tumour. Bird (1992) reported improvement following treatment with intravenous immunoglobulin (400 mg kg^{-1} per day for 5 days) in a single LEMS patient without malignancy. The patient relapsed at 10 weeks but responded to repeat treatment at a lower dose. Our recently completed double-blind cross-over trial of intravenous immunoglobulin in ten patients with NC-LEMS showed a significant improvement in several strength measures during the active treatment (Bain et al. 1994). The dose used in the trial was 1 g kg^{-1} per day for 2 days. It is not yet clear what the optimal long-term dose would be, but intravenous immunoglobulin treatment should be considered for patients with moderately severe symptoms that fail to respond to other treatment.

Future developments

More needs to be known about the cause of the autonomic symptoms in LEMS, and in particular the subtype(s) of VGCC being targeted. Further studies will be required to establish the features of the SCLC, and the inherited susceptibility factors (immune response genes), that result in LEMS developing in some patients but not in others. The use of long-term intravenous immunoglobulin treatment, possibly in conjunction with other immunosuppresive drugs, needs to be evaluated.

References

Anderson, H.J., Churchill-Davidson, H.C., and A.T. Richardson. (1953). Bronchial neoplasm with myasthenia. *Lancet* **ii**: 1291–1293.

Bain, P., Elrington, G., Goodger, E., Misbah, S., Panegyres, P., MacPherson, K., Chapel, H., and J. Newsom-Davis. (1994). A randomised double blind controlled study of intravenous immunoglobulin in the Lambert–Eaton myasthenic syndrome. In *Proceedings of the Association of British Neurologists and Nederlandse Vereniging voor Neurologie*, Aviemore, 4–6 May 1994. *J. Neurol. Neurosurg. Psychiatry* **57**: 1287.

Bird, S.J. (1992). Clinical and electrophysiologic improvement in Lambert-Eaton syndrome with intravenous immunoglobulin therapy. *Neurology* **42**: 1422–1423.

Chalk, C.H., Murray, N.M., Newsom-Davis, J., O'Neill, J.H., and Spiro, S.G. (1990). Response of the Lambert–Eaton myasthenic syndrome to treatment of associated small-cell lung carcinoma. *Neurology* **40**: 1552–1556.

Denny-Brown, D. and Foley, J.M. (1948). Myokymia and the benign fasciculation of muscular cramps. *Trans. Assoc. Am. Physicians* **61**: 88–96.

Eaton, L.M. and Lambert, E.H. (1957). Electromyography and electric stimulation of nerves in diseases of motor unit. Observations on myasthenic syndrome associated with malignant tumors. *JAMA* **163**: 1117–1124.

El Far, O., Marqueze, B., Leveque, C., Martin-Moutot, N., Lang, B., Newsom-Davis, J., Yoshida, A., Takahashi, M., and Seagar, M.J. (1995). Antigens associated with N and L type calcium channels in Lambert–Eaton myasthenic syndrome. *J. Neurochem.* **64**: 1696–1702.

Elrington, G.M., Murray, N.M.F., Spiro, S.G., and Newsom-Davis, J. (1991). Neurological paraneoplastic syndromes in patients with small cell lung cancer: a prospective survey of 150 patients. *J. Neurol. Neurosurg. Psychiatry* **54**: 764–767.

Engel, A.G., Nagel, A., Fukuoka, T., Fukunaga, H., Osame, M., Lang, B., Newsom-Davis, J., Vincent, A., Wray, D.W., and Peers, C. (1989). Motor nerve terminal calcium channels in Lambert–Eaton myasthenic syndrome. Morphologic evidence for depletion and that the depletion is mediated by autoantibodies. *Ann. NY Acad. Sci.* **560**: 278–290.

Fukunaga, H., Engel, A.G., Osame, M., and Lambert, E.H. (1982). Paucity and disorganisation of presynaptic membrane active zones in the Lambert–Eaton myasthenic syndrome. *Muscle Nerve* **5**: 686–697.

Hahn, A.F., Parkes, A.W., Bolton, C.F., and Stewart, S.A. (1991). Neuromyotonia in hereditary motor neuropathy. *J. Neurol. Neurosurg. Psychiatry* **54**: 230–235.

Hart, I.K., Vincent, A., Leys, K., Laux, V., Pongs, O., Lorra, C., and Newsom-Davis, J. (1994). Serum autoantibodies bind to voltage-gated potassium channels in acquired neuromyotonia. *Ann. Neurol.* **36**: 325.

Hesselmans, L.F.G.M., Jennekens, F.G.I., Kartman, J., Wokke, J.H.J., De Visser, Klaver-Krol, M.E.G., De Baets, M., Spaans, F., and Veldman, H. (1992). Secondary changes of the motor endplate in Lambert-Eaton myasthenic syndrome: a quantitative study. *Acta Neuropathol.* **83**: 202–206.

Hosokawa, S., Shinoda, H., Sakai, T., Kato, M., and Kuroiwa, Y. (1987). Electrophysiological study on limb myokymia in three women. *J. Neurol. Neurosurg. Psychiatry* **50**: 877–881.

Hughes, R.C. and Matthwes, W.B. (1969). Pseudomyotonia and myokymia. *J. Neurol. Neurosurg. Psychiatry* **32**: 11–14.

Isaacs, H. (1961). A syndrome of continuous muscle-fibre activity. *J. Neurol. Neurosurg. Psychiatry* **24**: 319–325.

Ishii, A., Hayashi, A., Ohkoshi, N., Oguni, E., Maeda, M., Ueda, Y., Ishii, K., Arasaki, K., Mizusawa, H., and Shoji, S. (1994). Clinical evaluation of plasma exchange and high dose intravenous immunoglobulin in a patient with Isaacs' syndrome. *J. Neurol. Neurosurg. Psychiatry* **57**: 840–842.

Kim, Y.I. and Neher, E. (1988). IgG from patients with Lambert–Eaton syndrome blocks voltage dependent calcium channels. *Science* **239**: 405–408.

Lambert, E.H. and Elmqvist, D. (1971). Quantal components of end-plate potentials in the myasthenic syndrome. *Ann. NY Acad. Sci.* **183**: 183–199.

Lang, B., Molenaar, P.C., Newsom-Davis, J., and Vincent, A. (1984). Passive transfer of Lambert–Eaton myasthenic syndrome in mice: decreased rates of resting and evoked release of acetylcholine from skeletal muscle. *J. Neurochem.* **42**: 658–662.

Lang, B., Newsom-Davis, J., Peers, C., Prior, C., and Wray, D.W. (1987). The effect of myasthenic syndrome antibody on presynaptic calcium channels in the mouse. *J. Physiol. Lond.* **390**: 257–270.

Lang, B., Newsom-Davis, J., Prior, C., and Wray, D. (1983). Antibodies to motor nerve terminals: an electrophysiological study of a human myasthenic syndrome transferred to mouse. *J. Physiol. Lond.* **344**: 335–345.

Lang, B., Newsom-Davis, J., Wray, D., Vincent, A., and Murray, N.M.F. (1981). Autoimmune aetiology for myasthenic (Eaton–Lambert) syndrome. *Lancet* **ii**: 224–226.

Lang, B., Vincent, A., Murray, N.M., and Newsom-Davis, J. (1989). Lambert–Eaton myasthenic syndrome: immunoglobulin G inhibition of Ca^{2+} flux in tumor cells correlates with disease severity. *Ann. Neurol.* **25**: 265–271.

Lennon, V.A., Lambert, E.H., Whittingham, S., and Fairbanks, V. (1982). Autoimmunity in the Lambert–Eaton myasthenic syndrome. *Muscle Nerve* **5**: S21–S25.

Leveque, C., Hoshino, T., David, P., Shoji-Kasai, Y., Leys, K., Omori, A., Lang, B., El Far, O., Sato, K., Martin-Moutot, N., Newsom-Davis, J., Takahashi, M., and Seagar, M.J. (1992). The synaptic vesicle protein synaptotagmin associates with calcium channels and is a putative Lambert–Eaton myasthenic syndrome antigen. *Proc. Natl Acad. Sci. USA* **89**: 3625–3629.

Leys, K., Lang, B., Johnston, I., and Newsom-Davis, J. (1991). Calcium channel autoantibodies in the Lambert–Eaton myasthenic syndrome. *Ann. Neurol.* **29**: 307–314.

McEvoy, K.M., Windebank, A.J., Daube, J.R., and Low, P.A. (1989). 3,4-Diaminopyridine in the treatment of Lambert–Eaton myasthenic syndrome. *N. Engl. J. Med.* **321**: 1567–1571.

Mertens, H.G. and Zschocke, S. (1965). Neuromyotonie. *Klin. Wochenschr.* **43**: 917–925.

Molenaar, P.C., Newsom-Davis, J., Polak, R.L., and Vincent, A. (1982). Eaton–Lambert syndrome: acetylcholine and choline acetyltransferase in skeletal muscle. *Neurology* **32**: 1062–1065.

Morris, C.S., Esiri, M.M., Marx, A., and Newsom-Davis, J. (1992). Immunocytochemical characteristics of small-cell lung carcinoma associated with the Lambert–Eaton myasthenic syndrome. *Am. J. Pathol.* **140**: 839–845.

Motomura, M., Johnston, I., Lang, B., Vincent, A., and Newsom-Davis, J. (1995). An improved diagnostic assay for Lambert–Eaton myasthenic syndrome. *J. Neurol. Neurosurg. Psychiatry* **58**: 85–87.

Morvan, A. (1890). De la chorée fibrillaire. *Gaz. Hebd. Med. Chir.* **27**: 173–200.

Newsom-Davis, J. and Mills, K.R. (1993). Immunological associations of acquired neuromyotonia (Isaacs' syndrome): report of 5 cases and literature review. *Brain* **116**: 453–469.

Newsom-Davis, J. and Murray, N.M. (1984). Plasma exchange and immunosuppressive drug treatment in the Lambert–Eaton myasthenic syndrome. *Neurology* **34**: 480–485.

O'Neill, J.H., Murray, N.M., and Newsom-Davis, J. (1988). The Lambert–Eaton myasthenic syndrome. A review of 50 cases. *Brain* **111**: 577–596.

Peers, C., Lang, B., Newsom-Davis, J., and Wray, D.W. (1990). Selective action of myasthenic syndrome antibodies on calcium channels in a rodent neuroblastoma×glioma cell line. *J. Physiol. (Lond.)* **421**: 293–308.

Roberts, A., Perera, S., Lang, B., Vincent, A., and Newsom-Davis, J. (1985). Paraneoplastic myasthenic syndrome IgG inhibits $^{45}Ca^{2+}$ flux in a human small cell carcinoma line. *Nature* **317**: 737–739.

Roberts, M., Willison, H., Vincent, A., and Newsom-Davis, J. (1994). Serum factor in Miller–Fisher variant of Guillain-Barré syndrome and neurotransmitter release. *Lancet* **343**: 454–455.

Rosenfeld, M.R., Wong, E., Dalmau, J., Manley, G., Posner, J.B., Sher, E., and Furneaux, H.M. (1993). Cloning and characterization of a Lambert-Eaton myasthenic syndrome antigen. *Ann. Neurol.* **33**: 113–120.

Sher, E., Canal, N., Piccolo, G., Gotti, C., Scoppetta, C., Evoli, A., and Clementi, F. (1989). Specificity of calcium channel autoantibodies in Lambert–Eaton myasthenic syndrome. *Lancet* **ii**: 640–643.

Shillito, P., Lang, B., Newsom-Davis, J., Bady, B., and Chauplannaz, G. 1992. Evidence for an autoantibody mediated mechanism in acquired neuromyotonia. *J. Neurol. Neurosurg. Psychiatry* **55**: 1214.

Sinha, S., Newsom-Davis, J., Mills, K., Byrne, N., Lang, B., and Vincent, A. (1991). Autoimmune aetiology for acquired neuromyotonia (Isaacs' syndrome). *Lancet* **338**: 75–77.

Squier, M., Chalk, C., Hilton-Jones, D., and Newsom-Davis, J. (1991). Type 2 fiber predominance in Lambert–Eaton myasthenic syndrome. *Muscle Nerve* **14**: 625–632.

Tahmoush, A.J., Alonso, R.J., Tahmoush, G.P., and Heiman-Patterson, T.D. (1991). Cramp-fasciculation syndrome: a treatable hyperexcitable peripheral nerve disorder. *Neurology* **41**: 1021–1024.

Takamori, M., Hamada, T., Komai, K., Takahashi, M., and Yoshida, A. (1994). Synaptotagmin can cause an immune-mediated model of Lambert–Eaton myasthenic syndrome in rats. *Ann. Neurol.* **35**: 74–80.

Trontelj, J.V. and Stålberg, E. (1990). Single motor end-plates in myasthenia gravis and LEMS at different firing rates. *Muscle Nerve* **14**: 226–232.

Uchitel, O.D., Protti, D.A., Sanchez, V., Cherskey, B.D., Sugimori, M., and Llinas, R. (1992). P-type voltage-dependent calcium channel mediates presynaptic calcium influx and transmitter release in mammalian synapses. *Proc. Natl Acad. Sci. USA* **89**: 3330–3333.

Willcox, N., Demaine, A.G., Newsom-Davis, J., Welsh, K.I., Robb, S.A., and Spiro, S.G. (1985). Increased frequency of IgG heavy chain marker Glm(2) and of HLA-B8 in Lambert–Eaton myasthenic syndrome with and without associated lung carcinoma. *Hum. Immunol.* **14**: 29–36.

Willison, H.J. (1994). Antiglycolipid antibodies in peripheral neuropathy: fact or fiction? *J. Neurol. Neurosurg. Psychiatry* **57**: 1303–1307.

Willison, H.J., Roberts, M., O'Hanlon, G., Paterson, G., Vincent, A., and Newsom-Davis, J. (1994). Human monoclonal anti-GM1 ganglioside antibodies interfere with neuromuscular transmission. *Ann. Neurol.* **36**: 289.

18 Toxin- and drug-induced immune neuropathies

N.L. Rosenberg

Introduction

Although there are several toxins known to produce peripheral neuropathy, the mechanisms are primarily related to direct toxic effects on the nerve, typically resulting in a distal axonopathy (Rosenberg 1992). Toxin-induced immune dysfunction resulting in peripheral neuropathy is extremely uncommon.

The field of immunology has undergone tremendous growth over the past decade, spurred both by technical developments and by research focused on the acquired immune deficiency syndrome (AIDS) epidemic. The spector of AIDS has also influenced the public's perception of the immune system as a target for environmental exposures. This concern has developed increasing interest in the field of immunotoxicology. Immunotoxicology is the study of adverse effects on the immune system resulting from any xenobiotic agent, defined as any environmental chemical, prescription drug, biological material, or physical agent such as radiation, noise, or vibration (Luster et al. 1990). The three broad categories of immune dysfunction relevant to immunotoxicology are:

1. Hypersensitivity
2. Immune suppression
3. Autoimmune phenomena/disease

In this chapter, the focus will be on autoimmune phenomena as this would be the most likely explanation of a neuropathy that would occur from an immunotoxic exposure. It needs to be kept in mind, however, that toxin-induced immune neuropathies are rare, as are toxin-induced autoimmune disorders in general. It is also critical for physicians to realize that the general principles of neurotoxicology still apply when dealing with immunological disorders and need to be considered when evaluating potential toxin-induced disorders (Rosenberg 1992).

This chapter will discuss two epidemic toxin-induced autoimmune disorders, eosinophilia-myalgia syndrome and toxic oil syndrome, both having peripheral neuropathy as a prominent part of the clinical picture. Parenteral ganglioside associated Guillian-Barré syndrome (GBS) is discussed as a possible iatrogenic-induced peripheral neuropathy. An intentionally-induced toxic sympathetic neuropathy caused by guanethidine for the treatment of reflex sympathetic dystrophy will also be discussed. Finally, a recent concern of peripheral neuropathy associated with silicone breast implants will be presented as an example of a situation not supported by scientific evidence, but is typical of how public misperceptions can fuel the current hysteria in this country over chemicals and their possible effects on the immune system.

Neuropathies associated with toxin-induced systemic immune disorders

Eosinophilia-myalgia syndrome

Introduction and epidemiology

In October 1989, the State Health Department of New Mexico had been notified of an unexplained acute illness in three patients characterized by incapacitating myalgias, eosinophilia and no identifiable cause (Centers for Disease Control 1989). All three patients had been consuming L-tryptophan (LT)-containing products for treatment of insomnia. Eosinophilia-myalgia syndrome (EMS) was soon recognized nationwide, and subsequent epidemiological studies confirmed as association between EMS and the consumption of LT-containing products (Slutzger et al. 1990; Swygert et al. 1990). Over 1500 individuals were determined to have EMS based on surveillance criteria, and over 30 deaths occurred in those individuals.

EMS is a disorder that has been well studied as far as the pathophysiology (Belongia et al. 1990; Flannery et al. 1990; Mayeno et al. 1990; Varga et al. 1993). It constitutes a tragedy not only for the people who have been stricken by the disease, but also for the manufacturers of tryptophan, who could not possibly have foreseen such devastating effects arising from a harmless, supposedly beneficial product.

The total number of people affected by EMS was small in relation to the total number of individuals consuming LT-containing products, but it has often been the case in medical research that a rare disease in a small patient group can provide critical insights into common pathological processes which affect the entire population. The similarities of EMS to other autoimmune diseases such as scleroderma, fasciitis, eosinophilic fasciitis, idiopathic myositis and the toxic oil syndrome, suggest that these disorders are all interrelated and have some similarities in pathophysiology (Sternberg et al. 1980; Tabuenca 1981; Kilbourne et al. 1988; Silver et al. 1990; Kaufman and Seidman 1991; Martin and Duffy 1991). In addition, abnormalities of tryptophan metabolism have long been associated with autoimmune disease states (Brown 1981), and EMS research may provide the missing link between the biochemical pathways of tryptophan metabolism and the immune system.

Most of the victims of the EMS epidemic have recovered, and few new cases have been reported since tryptophan was removed from the market. Many patients are suffering from the residual effects of their disease, and there is significant morbidity associated with these residual effects from peripheral neuropathy (Draznin and Rosenberg 1993). The epidemiology for peripheral neuropathy in EMS is not known, but the frequency in a large series has been reported as high as 27% (Swygert et al. 1990).

Clinical features

Peripheral neuropathy (PN) is a common problem in patients with EMS and a common cause of morbidity and mortality (Heiman-Patterson et al. 1990; Selwa et al. 1990; Smith and Dyck 1990; Herrick et al. 1991; Kirkpatrick 1991; Rosenberg 1991; Schaumburg 1991; Seidman et al. 1991; Verity et al. 1991; Draznin and Rosenberg 1993). Many of the deaths associated with EMS were in individuals who developed progressive respiratory failure, at least in part due to progressive weakness due to the PN. Currently, many survivors of EMS have significant functional problems associated with residual PN. Many are severely disabled from the PN and have had prolonged and costly attempts at rehabilitation with some limited success (Draznin and Rosenberg 1993).

One study was of ten patients with EMS in whom PN was a prominent or only presenting feature (Smith and Dyck 1990). Two of these patients had severe PN requiring mechanical ventilation, and one died. Pathological changes included epineural inflammation, which was occasionally marked, and was often accompanied by vasculopathy and angiogenesis. Other pathological changes in the nerve biopsy specimens have included axonal degeneration (Smith and Dyck 1990; Heiman-Patterson et al. 1990; Herrick et al. 1991) and demyelination and remyelination (Smith and

Dyck 1990). Clinically, most patients presented with subacute progressive (predominantly motor) neuropathies (Heiman-Patterson 1990; Selwa et al. 1990; Smith and Dyck 1990; Draznin and Rosenberg 1993) and occasionally with a picture of a mononeuropathy multiplex (Selwa et al. 1990). Most cases of PN have had features of axonal degeneration, but some cases of EMS with neuropathy have presented with features of chronic inflammatory demyelinating polyneuropathy (CIDP) (Donofrio et al. 1992).

In some cases, severe neuropathy may occur, become quiescent, but leave the affected individual with severe residual effects, which may respond to intensive rehabilitation (Draznin and Rosenberg 1993). PN has been noted to be a common long-term sequelae of EMS, in addition to arthralgia, muscle-cramping, and thickened skin (Sack and Criswell 1992).

Most neuromuscular pathology studies of EMS have looked only or predominantly at muscle (Herrick et al. 1991; Kirkpatrick 1991; Seidman et al. 1991; Verity et al. 1991). In these studies, often there was noted to be prominent inflammation surrounding intramuscular nerve twigs (Herrick et al. 1991; Kirkpatrick 1991; Seidman et al. 1991; Verity et al. 1991). This latter finding has been suggested to be the source of the neurogenic changes seen both on electrodiagnostic (i.e. electromyography; EMG) studies and on muscle biopsy, particularly in those cases where nerve conduction studies and nerve biopsy are normal.

Experimental data

Animal models of EMS have been recently described in both rats (Crofford et al. 1990; Love et al. 1993) and in mice (Weller et al. 1993; Silver et al. 1994). Studies have utilized either parenteral injections of 1,1′-ethylidenebis (L-tryptophan) (EBT) (Silver et al. 1994), gavaged implicated-LT (Crofford et al. 1990) or EBT (Love et al. 1993), while one utilized oral feedings (with LT or implicated-LT placed in drinking water) to more closely mimic the human situation (Weller et al. 1993). While most studies found that only implicated-LT or EBT were able to induce a disorder similar to EMS (Crofford et al. 1990; Love et al. 1993; Silver et al. 1994), one study found that reagent-grade LT was also capable of causing an EMS-like disorder in SJL/J mice, of equal severity to that produced by implicated-LT (Weller et al. 1993).

While all studies reported inflammation affecting multiple tissues, the peripheral nervous system (PNS) was not evaluated. Two studies, however, did reveal inflammation surrounding intramuscular nerve fibers (Crofford et al. 1990; Weller et al. 1993), similar to that seen in human EMS (Herrick et al. 1991; Kirkpatrick 1991; Seidman et al. 1991; Verity et al. 1991).

Therapy

Therapy for EMS has been disappointing both for the general systemic problems and for the PN. Treatment with corticosteroids, other immunosuppressive agents (e.g. cyclophosphamide, cyclosporin), and plasmapheresis have not been found to be of benefit, either for EMS in general or with the PN, even in those cases where a demyelinating neuropathy was found (Donofrio et al. 1992; Draznin and Rosenberg 1993). Some reports suggest that EMS may respond to methotrexate (Martinez-Osuna et al. 1991) or the mast cell stabilizing agent, ketotifen (Kaufman 1992), but neither agent has been studied in the treatment of the PN associated with EMS.

The neuropathy in some patients, even when severe, may stabilize, at which time intensive rehabilitation may afford some functional improvement (Draznin and Rosenberg 1993).

Future developments

The EMS epidemic is over. Subsequent studies have revealed that cases of EMS were present prior to the epidemic beginning in 1989, and was even present in the USA prior to the commercial availability of LT (Swygert et al. 1990). In addition, not all cases of EMS can be related to the consumption of LT-containing products. All of these facts raise the fear that a similar problem, potentially of epidemic proportions, can occur in the future. Therefore, trying to better understand the pathogenetic mechanisms of EMS may help to divert, or allow us to more rapidly respond to, a future epidemic. Supplies of EMS patient tissues and sera are limited, creating a great need for a good animal model. The unique situation of knowing exactly the disease trigger offers the excellent chance of working out the pathogenic mechanisms of the disease in an animal model. As noted above, there are currently three viable animal models that may provide clues to understanding the pathogenesis of EMS. Development of a reliable animal model will also allow treatments to be first tested in animals to see if they are to be potentially useful in survivors of EMS.

Further study of the association of EMS with L-tryptophan may provide important clues to understanding other autoimmune phenomena that may be induced by other drugs or chemicals.

Conclusions

PNS involvement can occur in both the extramuscular portion of the peripheral nerve (and be associated with slowing of conduction velocity) and/or in the intramuscular portion of the peripheral nerves (and be associated with normal nerve conduction studies, but neurogenic changes on EMG and muscle biopsy).

Toxic oil syndrome

Introduction and epidemiology

Beginning early in May of 1981, a previously unknown disease appeared in Spain. It was a severe multisystem disease, with prominent neuromuscular features, and became known as the toxic oil syndrome (TOS) (Kilbourne et al. 1983, 1991; Ortega-Benito 1992; Alonzo-Ruiz et al. 1993). The epidemic is over, but over 20 000 individuals were affected and there were over 350 deaths between the onset of the epidemic in May 1981 and the end of 1982. Although exact numbers are not known, hundreds or perhaps thousands still suffer from the residual effects of this disease.

An exact cause is not known, and early in the epidemic, an infectious cause was suspected as patients presented with non-productive cough, dyspnea, pleuritic pain, and fever associated with bilateral pulmonary infiltrates. No infectious agent was identified, and within a month of onset of the epidemic, it was suggested that ingestion of contaminated rapeseed oil was the cause of the disease. It was found that food oils sold as olive oil contained a high percentage of rapeseed oil. This identification was first suspected by Dr Juan Manuel Tabuenca-Oliver, who noticed that young individuals (under 6 months of age) were unaffected, suggesting that perhaps dietary ingestion may be the link with the disease (Kilbourne et al. 1983, 1991; Vazquez Roncero et al. 1983). The suspect oils were sold by itinerant salesmen and were found to be contaminated with industrial rapeseed oil. The rapeseed oil was produced in France, denatured by the addition of aniline, treated by a refining process in Madrid and Seville and then supplied to the distributing company, which supplied it to the salesmen. On 10 June 1981, the Spanish government issued a warning against consumption of the suspect oil, and a rapid reduction of new cases of TOS ensued.

There are many clinical and pathological similarities between TOS and EMS, and a recent study suggests a possible biochemical link between these two disorders (Mayeno et al. 1992). In this study, peak UV-5 of implicated L-tryptophan lots is 3-(Phenylamino)alanine (PAA). PAA is chemically similar to 3-phenylamino-1,2-propanediol, an aniline derivative found in the oil consumed by individuals who developed TOS. This intriguing chemical similarity suggests a possible biochemical link between these two epidemic disorders, neither of which have known specific etiologies.

The epidemiological data seem rather convincing that TOS developed in individuals who ingested oil mixtures containing rapeseed oil denatured with aniline; however, the precise agent has not been determined, but is not aniline. There is no suspect agent, with perhaps the exception of 3-phenylamino-1,2-propanediol, but only because of its similarity to PAA, a 'suspect' agent for EMS. It is likely that aniline reacting with some other oil product or products in the ingested mixture caused TOS.

The clinical epidemiology is the primary evidence linking ingestion of the contaminated oil to TOS, as no toxicological evidence is available, and no reliable animal model exists. So much of what we know of the association is based on this epidemiological evidence, and a recent study critically analysed this data (Ortega-Benito 1992). This analysis found a high statistical association (odds ratio=30) between ingestion of adulterated oil and the development of TOS. The association was not felt to be related to effects of bias or other confounding factors. The association was also found to be highly specific and, additionally, a dose–response relationship was seen.

Clinical features

The clinical features of TOS have been well described, including different clinical features appearing in different phases of the evolution of the disease (Kilbourne et al. 1983; Olmedo Garzon et al. 1983; Cruz Martinez et al. 1984; Gilsanz et al. 1984; Alonzo-Ruiz et al. 1986, 1993; Phelps and Fleischmajer 1988; dePablos et al. 1989; Martin Escribano et al. 1991; James et al. 1991; Kilbourne et al. 1991; Martinez-Tello and Tellez 1991). Most authors agree that there exists a fairly well-defined acute phase with less clearly defined intermediate and chronic phases (Kilbourne et al. 1983, 1991; Alonzo-Ruiz et al. 1993).

The acute/early phase (generally felt to be the first 2 months) is characterized by pulmonary involvement (cough, hypoxemia, interstitial pulmonary infiltrates, pulmonary edema), low grade fever, skin rash, myalgias, and a marked peripheral eosinophilia. Interestingly, respiratory problems have been documented to persist even 4 years after the onset of TOS (Martin Escribano et al. 1991).

The intermediate phase was defined as incomplete resolution of acute phase involvement and before the onset of chronic or late phase complications. It occurred 1–4 four months after the onset of illness and was characterized by severe myalgias, eosinophilia, subcutaneous edema, and thromboembolic complications (Kilbourne et al. 1991). These thromboembolic problems were uncommon, but have included strokes, mesenteric thromboses, and coronary artery changes (James et al. 1991). A pathological study found cardiac abnormalities affecting coronary arteries and neural structures in all individuals studied (James et al. 1991).

Chronic or late phase complications (generally, from the fourth month through the second year) include scleroderma-like changes, other connective tissue manifestations, and prominent neuromuscular complications (Kilbourne et al. 1983, 1991; Olmedo Garzon et al. 1983; Cruz Martinez 1984; Gilsanz et al. 1984; Alonzo-Ruiz et al. 1986, 1993; Phelps and Fleischmajer 1988; dePablos et al. 1989; Martinez-Tello and Tellez 1991).

A neuromuscular component of TOS was identified early in the course of the epidemic (Kilbourne et al. 1983). An early study reported on the clinical epidemiology of TOS. Twenty-eight of 116 (23%) individuals whose records were thoroughly reviewed were found to have 'neuromuscular illness' defined as having at least one of the following: incapacitating myalgias severe enough to restrict movement (n=21), atrophy of major muscle groups (n=10), motor weakness on physical examination (n=14), or extremity contractures (n=8) (Kilbourne et al. 1983). Other neuromuscular features included sensory abnormalities in 16.8%, hyporeflexia in 8.4%, and muscle cramps in 10.9%. No specific neuromuscular diagnoses were made in this study. Another study of the clinical, pathological, and immunological manifestations of TOS in 14 individuals revealed that seven of seven individuals studied in the chronic phase of the illness had the 'neuromuscular syndrome', but with no other details of these cases given beyond designating that diagnostic category (Phelps and Fleischmajer 1988).

The most detailed analysis of the 'neuromuscular syndrome' was of 145 patients who underwent electrophysiological studies in addition to clinical examination (Cruz Martinez et al. 1984). Muscle biopsies were performed in 31 patients and sural nerve biopsy was performed in 73. Of the 145 patients studied 68 were normal or with mild neuromuscular impairment (group A), 52 had mild to moderate impairment (group B), and 25 had severe impairment (group C). There were increasingly more common and more severe signs in those groups (least in group A and most in group C) including muscle cramps, muscle weakness and atrophy (generalized, focal distal, and focal proximal), generalized areflexia, weight loss, and sensory loss (characterized as either predominantly distal bilaterally, patchy, or mononeuropathic). Electrophysiological studies revealed a mixed motor and sensory axonal polyneuropathy, sometimes beginning asymmetrically, involving distal and proximal (including paraspinal and respiratory) muscles. Muscle biopsies (details were not reported) revealed inflammation in perimysial and fascial regions, particularly in earlier phases of the disease and in those with severe myalgias. In later stages of TOS, perimysial inflammation was much less commonly seen, and was less prominent. In later stages of TOS, the muscle biopsy revealed signs of denervation and endomysial and perimysial fibrosis. Sural nerve biopsies (details were not reported) revealed early prominent lymphocytic infiltration in the epineural and perineural regions. In the later stages, inflammation was primarily confined to the perineurium and was associated with fibrosis of the perineurium as well. These clinical and pathological features have also been reported in other studies (Alonzo-Ruiz et al. 1986; Martinez-Tello and Tellez 1991) and the 'neuromuscular syndrome' has been felt to be the primary cause of functional disability in patients with TOS (Alonzo-Ruiz et al. 1986). In one study of 32 patients with TOS, 31 (96.8%) were diagnosed as having a PN, though only seven had electrophysiological studies performed, which showed a predominantly axonal mixed polyneuropathy (Alonzo-Ruiz et al. 1986).

Similar to the neuropathy associated with EMS, the neuropathy of TOS is clinically predominantly motor, perhaps reflecting the predilection of inflammation of the intramuscular nerve fibers (Cruz Martinez et al. 1984). This motor neuropathy is associated with significant morbidity and mortality in both early and chronic phases of TOS (Gilsanz et al. 1984). In a study of 317 patients with TOS, 3.2% of survivors at 12 months had a 'severe' motor neuropathy, 52.9% were asymptomatic, and 39.4% were found to have residual myalgia (Gilsanz et al. 1984). Five patients who died in the later phases of TOS in this study had a severe motor neuropathy affecting the respiratory muscles.

In an 8-year follow-up study of 332 patients with TOS, 229 (68.9%) were initially found to have a PN (based on symptoms and clinical findings on examination), but at 8 years only 42 (13.1%) had clinical evidence of neuropathy (Alonzo-Ruiz et al. 1993). PN was seen in a higher percentage of patients with scleroderma-like changes than those without (102 of 112 compared with 127 of 220).

Carpal tunnel syndrome (CTS) has also been reported in the late stages of TOS (Olmedo Garzon et al. 1983). Of 214 patients diagnosed with TOS in a town near Madrid, 31 developed a clinical picture that suggested CTS. Only 11 had electrophysiological confirmation of CTS, and in spite of the author's claim that this frequency of CTS is higher than in any other disease associated with CTS, the data are not convincing. It is possible that some of the individuals who were diagnosed as having CTS, actually had a PN or some other aspect of the 'neuromuscular syndrome', and secondarily developed CTS. This possible predisposition to develop CTS or a worse neuropathy was not seen in a report of three patients who had hereditary motor and sensory neuropathy type I and developed TOS with neuromuscular manifestations (dePablos et al. 1989).

Experimental data

As noted above, an animal model displaying most of TOS has not been developed, and none had found clinical or pathological involvement of a neuromuscular disorder or PN. Some experimental studies in humans have revealed some interesting neurological changes (del Ser et al. 1986; Tellez et al. 1987; Silver et al. 1992; Gomez-Reino et al. 1993). Of these studies, the only one with any potential relationship to PN is one which looked at mRNA expression of collagen types I, III, and IV in fibrotic skin and nerve lesions of TOS patients (Gomez-Reino et al. 1993). It was found that there was increased mRNA expression of type IV collagen within the fibrotic areas of peripheral nerves.

Therapy

As with EMS, there is no particularly effective therapy for the systemic features of TOS, and no effective treatment has been seen for the PN. Many with PN will improve spontaneously (Alonzo-Ruiz et al. 1993). Of those who do not improve, most are left with some type of permanent residual effect, some severe.

Future developments

Most of the future developments in TOS are likely to come from developments in EMS. Increasing evidence suggests that these two disorders, if not identical, are clinically very similar with similar pathophysiologies. Collaborative research may show that similar agents may cause both disorders (Mayeno et al. 1992). Identification of causative agents may avert future epidemics.

Conclusions

PN was a common complication of TOS. It was primarily axonal, with mixed sensory and motor features, and associated with early and prominent perineural inflammation. It was not seen in isolation, but rather as a component of a systemic immune disorder.

Toxin-induced immune neuropathies

Guanethidine-induced immune sympathetic neuropathy

Introduction

Guanethidine, a guanedyl derivative developed in 1959 (Plummer and DeStevens 1973), was used as an antihypertensive agent for refractory hypertension for many years. It was used for its ability to produce a 'chemical sympathectomy' at the level of postganglionic sympathetic nerve terminals. Though now replaced by other antihypertensive agents with fewer side-effects, guanethidine has found a role in the treatment of painful conditions which appear to be modulated by the sympathetic nervous system, such as causalgia and reflex sympathetic dystrophy (RSD) (Hannington-Kiff 1974).

Systemic drugs have been used for many years that interrupt sympathetic function to treat painful disorders, but since 1974, guanethidine has been used to treat such disorders with a technique which minimizes the side-effects (Hannington-Kiff 1974). This technique is now known as intravenous regional sympathetic blockade (IRSB), and can produce a prolonged improvement in RSD in some individuals (Schwartzman and McLellan 1987). More recent findings implicate the proinflammatory contributions of the sympathetic nervous system (Levine et al. 1984). It has been suggested that the mechanism of improvement of signs and symptoms with guanethidine treatment in RSD, a disorder which includes inflammation of the synovium, is by reduction of proinflammatory factors of the sympathetic nervous system, particularly substance P. IRSB with guanethidine has also been shown to improve signs and symptoms of rheumatoid arthritis, a systemic inflammatory disorder with inflammation of the synovium (Levine et al. 1986).

Because of the clinical effects of regional intravenous guanethidine on painful neuropathic states, and its potential use in autoimmune and other inflammatory disorders, guanethidine will have an expanded role in the future in the treatment of these disorders. It produces a sympathetic neuropathy which is therefore therapeutic rather than pathological, and the desired outcome of its 'toxicity'.

This 'positive toxicity' produced in the clinical setting has been shown in animal studies (primarily rats) to be due to chromatolysis and nerve cell death of the neurons in the sympathetic ganglia associated with a mononuclear cell inflammatory infiltrate (Jensen-Holm and Juul 1968; Manning et al. 1982), which suggests an immune mechanism of destruction of these cells.

Clinical features

IRSB with guanethidine is given via the technique of a Bier block as follows: a tourniquette cuff is carefully applied and secured proximal to the area on the affected extremity. The limb is raised above the heart level for approximately 1 minute (to drain venous blood) and then the tourniquette is inflated to 50 mmHg above systolic (100 mmHg in the lower extremity). Guanethidine is then injected. Due to the release of norepinephrine, one then sees patchy areas of pallor due to arteriolar vasoconstriction. If the tourniquette is left on for 20 minutes, systemic effects are rarely seen. The positive effects seen from IRSB with guanethidine include increased blood flow and skin temperature, pain relief in RSD and peripheral vascular disease (Bonica and Buckley 1990). Sweating is not affected because it is mediated by cholinergic postganglionic sympathetics, which are not affected by guanethidine.

Experimental data

Guanethidine-induced selective degeneration of the postganglionic sympathetic neurons has been well documented in the rat (Jensen-Holm and Juul 1968; Burnstock et al. 1971; Manning et al. 1982; Johnson and Manning 1984). These earlier studies focused on the degeneration of the nerve cell bodies and unmyelinated axons, while more recent studies have addressed the degeneration of the myelinated fibers (Kidd et al. 1986) and myelin sheath survival in adult animals, where double myelination is found in adult sympathetic nerves (Kidd et al. 1992). Several mechanisms for this injury have been tested experimentally, but most of the experimental evidence supports the hypothesis that guanethidine exerts its cytotoxic effects by an immune-mediated mechanism (Zochodne et al. 1988; Juul et al. 1989; Thygesen et al. 1990, 1992; Schmidt et al. 1990; Hickey et al. 1992; Hougen et al. 1992).

Mononuclear cellular infiltration of the ganglia has been noted since the earliest studies, but more recent studies have begun to dissect the specific immune effector mechanisms which may be involved. Additional early evidence of immune system involvement includes the prevention of the inflammatory response and subsequent neuronal death by irradiation and immunosuppressive drugs (Manning et al. 1982), though a subsequent study of immunosuppressive agents failed to prevent reduction of sympathetic neurons (Hougen et al. 1992). In addition, guanethidine is unable to kill sympathetic neurons in vitro (Johnson and Aloe 1974), which suggests that some other type of in vivo mechanisms are necessary other than pure toxic effects of guanethidine. The natural killer (NK) cell is felt to be the most likely immune cell mediating destruction of the sympathetic neurons for several reasons:

1. Guanethidine can still induce its effect in athymic nude rats (animals with essentially no T lymphocytes) to the same degree as in euthymic rats (Juul et al. 1989; Thygesen et al. 1990; Hougen et al. 1992).
2. Immunohistochemical identification of NK cells in the sympathetic ganglia of rats (Schmidt et al. 1990; Thygesen et al. 1990, 1992; Hougen et al. 1992).
3. Prevention of sympathetic neuron destruction in rats by treatment with an antibody (anti-asialo GM1) which binds to the glycolipid asialo GM1, and which is expressed on rodent NK cells (Thygesen et al. 1992).

Conclusions

Guanethidine, no longer used as an antihypertensive agent, is primarily used now to treat painful neuropathic conditions, such as RSD. Its ability to induce a specific autoimmune (mediated by NK cells in the rat) destruction of peripheral sympathetic neurons has essentially pioneered guanethidine as a treatment for disorders felt to be related to proinflammatory substances produced by these cells. Guanethidine has also enabled us to better understand the effects of the sympathetic nervous system in the modulation of inflammation. It is an excellent example how a 'toxic effect' (and probably, 'immunotoxic') of a drug may be targeted for therapeutic purposes. Newer substances are now becoming available which will more selectively block these proinflammatory substances, and allow us to treat these same disorders perhaps without having to destroy neurons in the process, or at least to more selectively target specific neuronal populations.

Parenteral ganglioside-associated Guillain-Barré syndrome

Introduction

GBS, discussed in detail in Chapter 6, is felt to result from an immunological reaction directed against some myelin antigen(s), triggered by exposure to some type of xenobiotic agent or concomitant disease. As antibodies to various gangliosides can be found in GBS (Gregson et al. 1993; Willison and Kennedy 1993), these peripheral nerve antigens may be important in the pathogenesis of this disorder.

The report of a possible association between parenteral ganglioside therapy and a motor neuron-like disorder was reported from Japan (Yuki et al. 1991). This case was of an individual with diabetic neuropathy, being treated with parenteral gangliosides, who then developed a motor neuron-like disorder. There were also noted to be high antibody titers to certain gangliosides and improvement from immunosuppressive therapy correlated with reduction of these titers. This was felt most likely to be GBS by other investigators (Latov et al. 1991), and though the association had been previously noted (Schonhofer 1991), this case lead to further reports of this probably rare association (Latov et al. 1991; Schonhofer 1992).

Epidemiology

Two cohort studies have been performed in Italy to investigate the association between ganglioside therapy and the risk of developing GBS (Granieri et al. 1991; Raschetti et al. 1992). One study from Ferrara, Italy (Granieri et al. 1991), failed to find an association when evaluating a cohort of 13 373 subjects receiving ganglioside therapy (no cases). Small numbers were limiting to the power of this study. A second study performed in Rome province, Italy (3 700 000 inhabitants), looked at ganglioside prescriptions and cases of GBS in patients being prescribed gangliosides. Eight cases of GBS inpatients receiving gangliosides were reported between 1989 and 1991. It was estimated that 151 393 individuals (4.1% of the population) received at least one prescription for gangliosides in 1989, and no conclusions could be reached regarding the possible association with GBS.

Clinical features

Clinical features are identical to those of GBS in patients not taking gangliosides, with the possibility that some individuals may develop features that suggest a motor neuron-like disorder. The diagnosis is suggested in an individual taking gangliosides who develops GBS with high titers to various gangliosides (Latov et al. 1991; Yuki et al. 1991).

Therapy

Immunosuppressive therapy may result in clinical improvement with a subsequent lowering of the antibody titers to gangliosides (Yuki et al. 1991).

Future developments

Further epidemiologic studies are necessary to accurately assess risk for the development of GBS from ganglioside therapy.

Conclusions

If there is a risk for the development of GBS from parenteral ganglioside therapy, the risk is very small.

Silicone neurotoxicity and the myth of immune-mediated neuropathy

Introduction

Over the past few years, there has been a great deal of interest in possible toxic, particularly immunotoxic and neurotoxic, effects of silicone. Although silicone is contained in a large number of medical devices, the focus of interest and discussion has been in the one to two million American women who have undergone breast augmentation or reconstruction procedures with silicone gel-filled elastomer envelope breast prostheses, procedures that have occurred over approximately the past three decades.

This issue has primarily been discussed in the political and legal arenas, with the medical and scientific communities only being secondarily involved. This has created the scenario of the presentation of 'junk science' in the courtroom setting, and leaving the judicial process to attempt to analyse the merits of the medical and scientific publications. This has lead to an advocacy approach and a lessened ability to judge in a non-biased fashion the available information. The primary fault lies in the lack of utilization of a scientific method to assess causation in this setting.

The scientific method in assessing causation

There exists a formalised process with principles and methods which have been refined with the advancements of scientific knowledge for the assessment of causation (Evans 1976, 1993). Any physician or scientist assessing causation from exposure to a chemical and some clinical situation must follow a general methodology that is scientifically rigorous and defensible. Causation analysis is not simply a matter for one's personal experience or opinion to the exclusion of utilization of such a defined scientific methodology. Thus, one needs to consider such factors as the qualitative toxicology of the chemical in question, the individual's opportunity for exposure, the degree and duration of exposure, the dose of the chemical received, the clinical condition of the individual (including a differential diagnosis), and the biological plausibility of the association.

The available medical and scientific literature regarding toxicity of silicone does not suggest a cause and effect relationship with any disease, and certainly not with neurological disorders of any kind, including peripheral neuropathy. This is based on the utilization of criteria which have been proposed as the scientific basis for establishing causation (based on review of the data, including critical analysis of the literature) and include the strength and consistency of the association, specificity, time course, dose–response, biological plausibility, experimental association, confounders, and the coherence of evidence. Utilizing these criteria, it is clear that those who advocate the position that a silicone breast implant causes neurological disease have not utilized these methods, and admittedly so (Ostermeyer et al. 1994). These individuals have relied on the legal standard, the 'preponderance of evidence', rather than the scientific standard, to present their positions. The 'preponderance of evidence' in the legal setting is based on being 'medically probable' (i.e. more likely than not), and is a judgmental decision the jury must make on the basis of often conflicting evidence presented by medical experts on both sides in a case.

The opinion of the scientific community is that 'experts' that do not follow the established scientific approach to causation analysis engage in nothing more than speculation (Black 1988; Muscat and Huncharek 1989; Foster et al. 1993). It has been suggested that certain criteria need to be applied in the assessment of expert witnesses in order to improve the quality of testimony, particularly in toxic tort situation (Brent 1982, 1988).

Most of the problems involved in 'experts' assigning causation of a disorder to an exposure is reasoning by the use of *post hoc, ergo propter hoc* (after the fact, therefore, because of the fact). This circular 'logic' has been particularly evident in the issue of silicone and adverse neurological effects: it has been argued that the neurological symptoms (or subtle findings if present), or actual neurological disorder (such as multiple sclerosis, peripheral neuropathy, or motor neuron disease) 'prove' that exposure to silicone (i.e. presence of silicone breast implants) caused the problem. Then, it is argued that as there is proof of exposure, the exposure is the likely cause of the neurological symptoms or condition. In essence, the symptoms become the basis for explaining themselves. Such 'logic' is not accepted by the scientific and medical communities and should be guarded against. When all data needed to make such a scientific analysis are not available, they either need to be obtained by doing additional studies or one must admit the limits of the analysis. Scientific speculation should be avoided at all costs.

When the Council of Scientific Affairs of the American Medical Association addressed these issues of causation of breast implants and disease, they concluded that 'sufficient data do not exist to establish a statistically valid relationship between silicone gel breast implants and systemic disease' (Council on Scientific Affairs, American Medical Association 1993). The Council's analysis, not surprisingly, was criticized (Kessler et al. 1993); however, politics and not a scientific causation analysis was the basis of the criticism.

Epidemiology

There has been only one published epidemiological study to date looking at the association of human disease to silicone breast implants (Gabriel et al. 1994), and this study did not address neurological diagnoses. After analysing 749 women who had received breast implants, and comparing them with 1498 community controls, no association was found between breast implants and connective tissue diseases (scleroderma, systemic lupus erythematosus, rheumatoid arthritis, polymyositis, dermatomyositis, Sjögren's syndrome, Hashimoto's thyroiditis, keratoconjunctivitis sicca), lymphoproliferative disorders, cancer (other than breast cancer), primary biliary cirrhosis, and other symptoms and signs. Like any epidemiological study, there has been criticism of this study, both published and non-published, but it has been accepted as a 'meticulous' if not 'definitive' study by the medical and scientific community (Angell 1994). Although it did not address neurological diagnoses, it seems unlikely that there will prove to be an association when further epidemiological studies are analysed.

Epidemiological studies have lead both to over-estimating and underestimating risk, based on different interpretations of the data (Muscat and Huncharet 1989; Foster et al. 1993). Even in those situations where epidemiological studies have found an increased association between a toxic exposure and a disease the weakness of the association is not sufficient to reliably assume that the exposure caused the disease (Hill 1965; Black and Lilienfield 1984). Unfortunately, the uncertainties in epidemiological studies are frequently large enough to be significant in the legal arena, where the standards for scientific causation are not stringently adhered to (Black 1988). The apparent correlations or associations produced in epidemiological studies do not by themselves establish the existence of a cause and effect relationship between a chemical exposure and a particular health condition for a given individual.

Clinical features

The entirety of the clinical publications of neurological problems related to silicone are three (Gomez and Little 1989; Sanger et al. 1992b; Ostermeyer-Shoaib et al. 1994). One deals with silicone-coated dacron dural grafts and not silicone breast implants, which were associated with cervical cord compression in two individuals (Gomez and Little 1989). In both cases extensive scar tissue formation was seen at the site of compression, and two factors were felt to possibly play a role in the formation of the scar tissue: the introduction of the grafts and repeated motion at the graft site.

There is a case report of a woman who developed constrictive neuropathies related to silicone gel which had migrated down fascial planes from a ruptured breast implant into the right arm (Sanger et al. 1992b). Migration down the arm was demonstrated radiographically, and pathologically, patchy areas of inflammation and fibrosis were seen along the course of the median nerve as well as within certain muscle groups. There was no evidence of a generalized disorder of the peripheral nerves.

Recently, a series of 100 cases of what the authors called 'adjuvant breast disease' was published in a Japanese medical journal (Ostermeyer-Shoaib et al. 1994). In this article the authors summarized symptoms, findings on neurological examination, and findings on certain laboratory studies. A large number of studies were performed on these patients, but complete analysis was not performed on all individuals. In addition, no control data were presented, and no specific neurological diagnoses were reported, although the authors offer the diagnosis of 'adjuvant breast disease' (ABD) in all patients. Based on this report, ABD is a heterogeneous collection of symptoms and findings (both clinical and laboratory) in patients with silicone breast implants. Clinical features are so non-specific and vague that their value is virtually worthless in making a diagnosis in an individual or in creating a syndrome (i.e. ABD). The only discriminating aspect of ABD from numerous other similar non-specific 'syndromes' is the presence of silicone implants (or having had silicone injections). This is a clear example of the circular reasoning of *post hoc, ergo propter hoc* described above.

In regard to peripheral nerve disease, certain aspects of this manuscript should be addressed. Symptoms which may indicate peripheral nerve disease included 'numbness' (77%), 'tingling' (72%), and 'weakness' (95%). Many patients also had complaints of 'fatigue' (95%) and 'muscle aches and pain' (91%). Most of these complaints are seen in high frequency in other common disorders, including fibromyalgia, chronic fatigue syndrome, and certain psychiatric disorders, which are also common diagnoses in this patient population. Neurological findings included 'weakness' (94%), 'loss of vibration' (78%), 'loss of pin-prick' (72%), 'increased DTR' (14%), 'decreased DTR' (11%), 'facial weakness' (19%), and muscle atrophy (4%).

Of 93 individuals who underwent electromyography/nerve conduction studies, 44 were entirely normal, 24 had 'myopathic potentials' (although the distribution was not reported), 23 had 'polyphasia, giant motor units, fibrillations, or decreased recruitment' (again, the distribution was not reported), 11 had findings of carpal tunnel syndrome, four had 'findings of an axonal neuropathy', and two patients had myasthenia gravis. No details of these electrophysiological studies were given, nor were any specific diagnoses based on these studies, and one is left to ponder what actually is occurring neurologically, if anything.

Finally, 66 patients had sural nerve biopsies. The nerve specimens were frozen and prepared for light microscopy only. It was reported that 80% had abnormal sural nerve biopsies. The only abnormal finding reported was a loss of myelinated fibers (79%), with 'moderate loss' (estimated at '35–45'% loss). How this estimated loss was determined is not clear, nor is there any attempt to correlate the symptoms, signs, and other laboratory findings with the nerve or muscle biopsy abnormalities, and whether any individuals had a specific diagnosis of peripheral neuropathy.

In contrast to their manuscript, which is merely a compilation of anecdotal 'data', without a synthesis of the 'data' into a format which is analysable, these same authors have published a few abstracts which appear to give at least some idea of a synthesis of their findings, and certain specific neurological diagnoses which they feel are related to silicone breast implants (Ostermeyer-Shoaib et al. 1992; Ostermeyer-Shoaib and Patten 1992, 1994). Disorders which they link as associated to silicone include motor neuron disease (Ostermeyer-Shoaib et al. 1992; Ostermeyer-Shoaib and Patten 1992), a 'multiple sclerosis-like' disorder (Ostermeyer-Shoaib and Patten 1992, 1994), multiple sclerosis (Ostermeyer-Shoaib and Patten 1992), a mixed sensory-motor neuropathy (Ostermeyer-Shoaib and Patten 1992), and myasthenia gravis (Ostermeyer-Shoaib and Patten 1992). These abstract data appear to be similar to the 'data' in their full manuscript, in that they are a compilation of findings of only multiple case reports, with no control population ever studied or a *coherence* (see section on

Epidemiology above) to suggest any kind of association of any neurologic disorder with silicone. A personal review of 45 of their cases not only failed to find evidence of neurologic disease in the population of women with silicone breast implants (including peripheral neuropathy), but also suggested that they failed to follow accepted standards in making their diagnoses (Rosenberg 1995). This was most evident in their diagnoses in 30 individuals of having CIDP, where not a single criterion necessary to make the diagnosis of CIDP was seen in any of the 30 cases (American Academy of Neurology 1991).

Experimental data

A single experimental study has addressed the possible effects of silicone gel on peripheral nerve (Sanger et al. 1992a). In this study, silicone gel was placed either extraneurally adjacent to or injected directly into the sciatic nerve of Sprague-Dawley rats. The neuropathological changes were then assessed every 2 weeks during a 20 week period. The silicone gel which was placed extraneurally, elicited an intense inflammatory response which peaked at about 4 weeks after which time collagen deposition increased and inflammation decreased. Perineural fibrosis was marked by 20 weeks, but there was no penetration of the epineurium by the gel. Silicone gel which was injected intraneurally caused a similar response. The intraneural gel did not migrate. The significance of this study in relationship to the claims in women with implants is that there was neither any direct toxicity to peripheral nerve demonstrated nor a generalized disorder of the peripheral nerves. This study demonstrated similar findings to the single case report where migration of gel resulted in focal constrictive neuropathy, but not a generalized disorder of the peripheral nerves (Sanger et al. 1992b).

Future developments

Because of the problems related to litigation, it is unlikely that future clinical studies will be able to be performed which will not have significant bias. Additional epidemiological studies are currently underway which will address the neurological issues. Further animal studies may help to elucidate any possible mechanisms that could be involved in possible issues of neurological significance.

Conclusions

Utilizing a scientific approach to causation, there is no evidence that silicone gel filled breast implants are associated with peripheral neuropathy, or any neurological disorder. Physicians evaluating these patients should exercise caution when evaluating neurological claims of causation.

References

Alonso-Ruiz, A., Calabozo, M., Perez-Ruiz, F., and Mancebo, L. (1993). Toxic oil syndrome: a long-term follow-up of a cohort of 332 patients. *Medicine* **72**: 285–295.

Alonso-Ruiz, A., Zea-Mendoza, A.C., Salazar-Vallinas, J.M., Rocamora-Ripoll, A., and Beltran-Gutierrez, J. (1986). Toxic oil syndrome: a syndrome with features overlapping those of various forms of scleroderma. *Semin. Arthritis Rheum.* **15**: 200–212.

American Academy of Neurology. (1991). Criteria for diagnosis of chronic inflammatory demyelinating polyneuropathy. *Neurology* **41**: 617–618.

Angell, M. (1994). Do breast implants cause systemic disease? Science in the courtroom. *N. Engl. J. Med.* **330**: 1748–1749.

Belongia, E.A., Hedberg, C.W., Gleich, G.J., White, K.E., Mayeno, A.N., Loegering, D.A., Dunnette, S.L., Pirie, P.L., MacDonald, K.L., and Osterholm, M.T. (1990). An investigation of the cause of eosinophilia-myalgia syndrome associated with tryptophan use. *N. Engl. J. Med.* **323**: 357–365.

Black, B. (1988). Evolving legal standards for the admissibility of scientific evidence. *Science* **239**: 1508–1512.

Black, B. and Lilienfeld, D.E. (1984). Epidemiological proof in toxic tort litigation. *Fordham Law Rev.* **52**: 723–785.

Bonica, J.J. and Buckley, F.P. (1990). Regional analgesia with local anesthetics. In *The Management of Pain*, 2nd edn, vol. II, ed. J.J. Bonica, pp. 1883–1966. Philadelphia: Lea & Febiger.

Brent, R.L. (1982). The irresponsible expert witness: a failure of biomedical graduate education and professional accountability. *Pediatrics* **70**: 754–762.

Brent, R.L. (1988). Improving the quality of expert witness testimony. *Pediatrics* **82**: 511–513.

Brown, R.R. (1981). The tryptophan load test as an index of vitamin B6 nutrition. In *Methods in Vitamin B-6 Nutrition: Analysis and Status Assessment*, ed. J.E. Leklem, and R.D. Reynolds, pp. 321–340. New York: Plenum Press.

Burnstock, G., Evans, G., Gannon, B.J., Heath, J.W., and James, V. (1971). A new method of destroying adrenergic nerves in adult animals using guanethidine. *Br. J. Pharmacol.* **43**: 295–301.

Centers for Disease Control. (1989). Eosinophilia-myalgia syndrome: New Mexico. *Morbid. Mortal. Weekly Rep.* **38**: 765–767.

Council on Scientific Affairs, American Medical Association (1993). Silicone gel breast implants. *JAMA* **270**: 2602–2606.

Crofford, L.J., Rader, J.I., Dalakas, M.C., Hill, R.H.Jr., Page, S.W., Needham, L.L., Brady, L.S., Heyes, M.P., Wilder, R.L., Gold, P.W., Illa, I., Smith, C., and Sternberg, E.M. (1990). L-tryptophan implicated in human eosinophilia-myalgia syndrome causes fasciitis and perimyositis in the Lewis rat. *J. Clin. Invest.* **86**: 1757–1763.

Cruz Martinez, A., Perez Conde, M.C., Ferrer, M.T., Canton, R., and Tellez, I. (1984). Neuromuscular disorders in a new toxic syndrome: electrophysiological study: a preliminary report. *Muscle Nerve* **7**: 12–22.

Del Ser, T., Franch, O., Portera, A., Muradas, V., and Yebenes, J.G. (1986). Neurotransmitter changes in cerebrospinal fluid in the Spanish toxic oil syndrome: human clinical findings and experimental results in mice. *Neurosci. Lett.* **67**: 135–140.

DePablos, C., Calleja, J., Combarros, O., and Berciano, J. (1989). Spanish toxic oil syndrome neuropathy in three patients with hereditary motor and sensory neuropathy type I. *Arch. Neurol.* **46**: 202–204.

Donofrio, P.D., Stanton, C., Miller, V.S., Oestreich, L., Lefkowitz, D.S., Walker, F.O., and Ely, E.W. (1992). Demyelinating polyneuropathy in eosinophilia-myalgia syndrome. *Muscle Nerve* **15**: 796–805.

Draznin, E. and Rosenberg, N.L. (1993). Intensive rehabilitation approach to eosinophilia myalgia syndrome associated with severe polyneuropathy. *Arch. Phys. Med. Rehab.* **74**: 774–776.

Evans, A.S. (1976). Causation and disease: the Henle-Koch postulates revisited. *Yale J. Biol. Med.* **49**: 175–195.

Evans, A.S. (1993). *Causation and Disease: A Chronological Journey.* New York: plenum Medical Book Company.

Flannery, M.T., Wallach, P.M., Espinoza, L.R., Dohrenwend, M.P., and Moscinski, L.C. (1990). A case of the eosinophilia-myalgia syndrome associated with use of an L-tryptophan product. *Ann. Intern. Med.* **112**: 300–301.

Foster, K.R., Bernstein, D.E., and Huber, P.W. (1993). *Phantom Risk: Scientific Inference and the Law.* Cambridge, MA: MIT Press.

Gabriel, S.E., O'Fallon, W.M., Kurland, L.T., Beard, C.M., Woods, J.E., and Melton III, L.J. (1994). Risk of connective-tissue diseases and other disorders after breast implantation. *N. Engl. J. Med.* **330**: 1697–1702.

Gilsanz, V., Lopez Alvarez, J., Serrano, S., and Simon, J. (1984). Evolution of the alimentary toxic oil syndrome due to ingestion of denatured rapeseed oil. *Arch. Intern. Med.* **144**: 254–256.

Gomez, H. and Little, J.R. (1989). Spinal cord compression: a complication of silicone-coated dacron dural grafts. Report of two cases. *Neurosurgery* **24**: 115–118.

Gomez-Reino, J.J., Sandberg, M., Carreira, P.E., and Vuorio, E. (1993). Expression of types I, III and IV collagen genes in fibrotic skin and nerve lesions of toxic oil syndrome patients. *Clin. Exp. Immunol.* **93**: 103–107.

Granieri, E., Casetta, I., Govoni, V., Tola, M.R., Paolino, E., and Rocca, W.A. (1991). Ganglioside therapy and Guillain-Barré syndrome: a historical cohort study in Ferrara, Italy, fails to demonstrate an association. *Neuroepidemiology* **10**: 161–169.

Gregson, N.A., Koblar, S., and Hughes, R.A. (1993). Antibodies to gangliosides in Guillain-Barré syndrome: specificity and relationship to clinical features. *Q. J. Med.* **86**: 111–117.

Hannington-Kiff, J.G. (1974). Intravenous regional sympathetic block with guanethidine. *Lancet* **1**: 1019–1020.

Heiman-Patterson, T.D., Bird, S.J., Parry, G.J., Varga, J., Shy, M.E., Culligan, N.W., Edelsohn, L., Tatarian, G.T., Heyes, M.P., Garcia, C.A., and Tahmoush, A.J. (1990). Peripheral neuropathy associated with eosinophilia-myalgia syndrome. *Ann. Neurol.* **28**: 522–528.

Herrick, M.K., Chang, Y., Horoupian, D.S., Lombard, C.M., and Adornato, B.T. (1991). L-tryptophan and the eosinophilia-myalgia syndrome. *Hum. Pathol.* **22**: 12–21.

Hickey, W.F., Ueno, K., Hiserodt, J.C., and Schmidt, R.E. (1992). Exogenously-induced, natural killer cell-mediated neuronal killing: a novel pathogenetic mechanism. *J. Exp. Med.* **176**: 811–817.

Hill, A.B. (1965). The environment and disease: association or causation? *Proc. R. Soc. Med.* **58**: 295–300.

Hougen, H.P., Thygesen, P., Christensen, H.B., Rygaard, J., Svendsen, O., and Juul, P. (1992). Effect of immunosuppressive agents on the guanethidine-induced sympathectomy in athymic and euthymic rats. *Int. J. Immunopharmacol.* **14**: 1113–1123.

James, T.N., Gomez-Sanchez, M.A., Martinez-Tello, F.J., Posada-de la Paz, M., Abaitua-Borda, I., and Soldevilla, L.B. (1991). Cardiac abnormalities in the toxic oil syndrome, with comparative observations on the eosinophilia-myalgia syndrome. *J. Am. Coll. Cardiol.* **18**: 1367–1379.

Jensen-Holm, J. and Juul, P. (1968). Changes of the rat superior cervical ganglion induced by guanethidine (histology and cholinesterase histochemistry). *Br. J. Pharmacol.* **34**: 211P.

Johnson, E.M. and Aloe, L. (1974). Suppression of the in vitro and in vivo cytotoxic effects of guanethidine in sympathetic neurons by nerve growth factor. *Brain Res.* **81**: 519–532.

Johnson, E.M. and Manning, P.T. (1984). Guanethidine induced destruction of sympathetic neurons. *Int. Rev. Neurobiol.* **25**: 1–37.

Juul, A., Juul, P., and Christensen, H.B. (1989). Guanethidine-induced sympathectomy in the nude rat. *Pharmacol. Toxicol.* **64**: 20–22.

Kaufman, L.D. (1992). The eosinophilia-myalgia syndrome: current concepts and future directions. *Clin. Exp. Rheum.* **10**: 87–91.

Kaufman, L.D. and Seidman, R.J. (1991). L-tryptophan-associated eosinophilia-myalgia syndrome: perspective of a new illness. *Rheum. Dis. Clin. N. Am.* **17**: 427–441.

Kessler, D.A., Merkatz, R.B., and Schapiro, R. (1993). A call for higher standards for breast implants. *JAMA* **270**: 2607–2608.

Kidd, G.J., Heath, J.W., and Dunkley, P.R. (1986). Degeneration of myelinated sympathetic fibers following treatment with guanethidine. *J. Neurocytol.* **15**: 561–572.

Kidd, G.J., Heath, J.W., Trapp, B.D., and Dunkley, P.R. (1992). Myelin sheath survival after guanethidine-induced axonal degeneration. *J. Cell Biol.* **116**: 395–403.

Kilbourne, E., Bernert, J.T.Jr., de la Paz, M.P., Hill, R.H.Jr., Abaitua Borda, I., Kilbourne, B.W., and Zack, M.M. (1988). Chemical correlates of pathogenicity of oils related to the toxic oil syndrome epidemic in Spain. *Am. J. Epidemiol.* **127**: 1210–1227.

Kilbourne, E.M., Posada de la Paz, M., Abaitua Borda, I., Ruiz-Navarro, M.D., Philen, R.M., and Falk, H. (1991). Toxic oil syndrome: a current clinical and epidemiological summary, including comparisons with the eosinophilia-myalgia syndrome. *J. Am. Coll. Cardiol.* **18**: 711–717.

Kilbourne, E.M., Rigau-Perez, J.G., Heath, C.W., Zack, M.M., Falk, H., Martin-Marcos, M., and de Carlos, A. (1983). Clinical epidemiology of toxic-oil syndrome: manifestations of a new illness. *N. Engl. J. Med.* **309**: 1408–1414.

Kirkpatrick J.B. (1991). Eosinophilia myalgia (editorial). *Hum. Pathol.* **22**: 1–2.

Latov, N., Koski, C.L., and Walicke, P.A. (1991). Guillain-Barré syndrome and parenteral gangliosides. *Lancet* **338**: 757.

Levine, J.C., Clark, R., Devor, M., Helms, C., Moskowitz, M.A., and Basbaum, A.I. (1984). Intraneuronal substance P contributes to the severity of experimental arthritis. *Science* **226**: 547–549.

Levine, J.D., Fye, K., Heller, P., Basbaum, A.I., and Whiting-O'Keefe, Q. (1986). Clinical response to regional intravenous guanethidine in patients with rheumatoid arthritis. *J. Rheumatol.* **13**: 1040–1043.

Love, L.A., Rader, J.I., Crofford, L.J., Raybourne, R.B., Principato, M.A., Page, S.W., Trucksess, M.W., Smith, M.J., Dugan, E.M., Turner, M.L., Zelazowski, E., Zelazowski, P., and Sternberg, E.M. (1993). Pathological and immunological effects of ingesting L-tryptophan and 1,1′-ethylidenebis (L-tryptophan) in Lewis rats. *J. Clin. Invest.* **91**: 804–811.

Luster, M.I., Wierda, D., and Rosenthal, G.J. (1990). Environmentally related disorders of the hematologic and immune systems. *Med. Clin. N. Am.* **74**: 425–440.

Manning, P.T., Russell, J.H., and Johnson, E.M. (1982). Immunosuppressive agents prevent guanethidine-induced destruction of rat sympathetic neurons. *Brain Res.* **241**: 131–143.

Martin, R.W. and Duffy, J. (1991). Eosinophilic fasciitis associated with use of L-tryptophan: a case-control study and comparison of clinical and histopathologic features. *Mayo Clin. Proc.* **66**: 892–898.

Martin Escribano, P., Diaz de Atauri, M.J., and Gomez Sanchez, M.A. (1991). Persistence of respiratory abnormalities four years after the onset of toxic oil syndrome. *Chest* **100**: 336–339.

Martinez-Osuna, P., Wallach, P.M., Seleznick, M.J., Levin, R.W., Silveira, L.H., and Espinoza, L.R. (1991). Treatment of the eosinophilia myalgia syndrome. *Semin. Arthritis Rheum.* **21**: 110–121.

Martinez-Tello, F.J. and Tellez, J. (1991). Extracardiac vascular and neural lesions in the toxic oil syndrome. *J. Am. Coll. Cardiol.* **18**: 1043–1047.

Mayeno, A.N., Belongia, E.A., Lin, F., Lundy, S.K., and Gleich, G.J. (1992). 3-(Phenylamino)alanine, a novel aniline-derived amino acid associated with the eosinophilia-myalgia syndrome: a link to the toxic oil syndrome? *Mayo Clin. Proc.* **67**: 1134–1139.

Mayeno, A.N., Lin, F., Foote, C.S., Loegering, D.A., Ames, M.M., Hedberg, C.W., and Gleich, G.J. (1990). Characterization of 'Peak E', a novel amino acid associated with eosinophilia-myalgia syndrome. *Science* **250**: 1701–1708.

Muscat, J.E. and Huncharek, M.S. (1989). Causation and disease: biomedical science in toxic tort litigation. *J. Occup. Med.* **31**: 997–1002.

Olmedo Garzon, F.J., Leiva Santana, C., Alonso Ruiz, A., and Riva Meana, C. (1983). The toxic-oil syndrome: a new cause of the carpal-tunnel syndrome. *N. Engl. J. Med.* **309**: 1455.

Ortega-Benito, J.M. (1992). Spanish toxic oil syndrome: ten years after the disaster. *Public Health* **106**: 3–9.

Ostermeyer-Shoaib, B. and Patten, B.M. (1992). Silicone adjuvant breast disease: more neurological cases. *Ann. Neurol.* **32**: 254.

Ostermeyer-Shoaib, B. and Patten, B.M. (1994). A multiple sclerosis-like syndrome in women with breast implants or silicone fluid injections into breasts. *Neurology* **44** (suppl. 2): A158.

Ostermeyer-Shoaib, B., Patten, B.M., and Ashizawa, T. (1992). Motor neuron disease after silicone breast implants and silicone injections into the face. *Ann. Neurol.* **32**: 254.

Ostermeyer-Shoaib, B., Patten, B.M., and Calkins, D.S. (1994). Adjuvant breast disease: an evaluation of 100 symptomatic women with breast implants or silicone fluid injections. *Keio J. Med.* **43**: 79–87.

Phelps, R.G. and Fleischmajer, R. (1988). Clinical, pathologic, and immunopathologic manifestations of the toxic oil syndrome. Analysis of fourteen cases. *J. Am. Acad. Dermatol.* **18**: 313–324.

Plummer, A.J. and DeStevens, F. (1973). Chemical transmitters and the control of blood pressure. In *How Modern Medicines are Discovered*, ed. F.H. Clark, pp. 107–31. New York, NY: Futura Publishers.

Raschetti, R., Maggini, M., and Popoli, P. (1992). Guillain-Barré syndrome and ganglioside therapy in Italy. *Lancet* **340**: 60.

Rosenberg, N.L. (1991). Toxic myopathies. *Curr. Opin. Neurol. Neurosurg.* **4**: 433–437.

Rosenberg, N.L. (1992). Neurotoxicology. In *Medical Toxicology of Hazardous Materials*, ed. J.B. Sullivan and G.R. Krieger, pp. 145–153. Baltimore: Williams and Wilkins.

Rosenberg, N.L. (1995). The neuromythology of silicone breast implants (abstract). *Neurology.*

Sack, K.E. and Criswell, L.A. (1992). Eosinophilia-myalgia syndrome: the aftermath. *S. Med. J.* **85**: 878–882.

Sanger, J.R., Kolachalam, R., Komorowski, R.A., Yousif, N.J., and Matloub, H.S. (1992a). Short-term effect of silicone gel on peripheral nerves: a histologic study. *Plastic Reconstruct. Surg.* **89**: 931–940.

Sanger, J.R., Matloub, H.S., Yousif, N.J., and Komorowski, R. (1992b). Silicone gel infiltration of a peripheral nerve and constrictive neuropathy following rupture of a breast prosthesis. *Plastic Reconstruct. Surg.* **89**: 949–952.

Schaumburg, H.H. (1991). Toxic and metabolic neuropathies. *Curr. Opin. Neurol. Neurosurg.* **4**: 438–441.

Schmidt, R.E., Summerfield, A.L., and Hickey, W.F. (1990). Ultrastructural and immunohistologic characterization of guanethidine-induced destruction of peripheral sympathetic neurons. *J. Neuropathol. Exp. Neurol.* **49**: 150–167.

Schonhofer, P.S. (1991). Guillain-Barré syndrome and parenteral gangliosides. *Lancet* **338**: 757.

Schonhofer, P.S. (1992). GM-1 ganglioside for spinal-cord injury. *N. Engl. J. Med.* **326**: 493.

Schwartzman, R.J. and McLellan, T.L. (1987). Reflex sympathetic dystrophy: a review. *Arch. Neurol.* **44**: 555–561.

Seidman, R.J., Kaufman, L.D., Sokoloff, L., Miller, F., Iliya, A, and Peress, N.S. (1991). The neuromuscular pathology of the eosinophilia-myalgia syndrome. *J. Neuropathol. Exp. Neurol.* **50**: 49–62.

Selwa, J.F., Feldman, E.L., and Blaivas, M. (1990). Mononeuropathy multiplex in tryptophan-associated eosinophilia-myalgia syndrome. *Neurology* **40**: 1632–1633.

Silver, R.M., Heyes, M.P., Maize, J.C., Quearry, B., Vionnet-Fuasset, M., and Sternberg, E.M. (1990). Scleroderma, fasciitis, and eosinophilia associated with the ingestion of tryptophan. *N. Engl. J. Med.* **322**: 874–881.

Silver, R.M., Ludwicka, A., Hampton, M., Ohba, T., Bingel, S.A., Smith, T., Harley, R.A., Maize, J., and Heyes, M.P. (1994). A murine model of the eosinophilia-myalgia syndrome induced by 1,1′-ethylidenebis (L-tryptophan). *J. Clin Invest.* **93**: 1473–1480.

Silver, R.M., Sutherland, S.E., Carreira, P., and Heyes, M.P. (1992). Alterations in tryptophan metabolism in the toxic oil syndrome and in the eosinophilia-myalgia syndrome. *J. Rheumatol.* **19**: 69–73.

Slutzger, L., Hoesley, F.C., Miller, L., Williams, L.P., Watson, J.C., and Fleming, D.W. (1990). Eosinophilia-myalgia syndrome associated with exposure to tryptophan from a single manufacturer. *JAMA* **264**: 213–217.

Smith, B.E. and Dyck, P.J. (1990). Peripheral neuropathy in the eosinophilia-myalgia syndrome associated with L-tryptophan ingestion. *Neurology* **40**: 1035–1040.

Sternberg, E.M., van Woert, M.H., Young, S.N., Magnussen, I., Baker, H., Gauthier, S., and Osterland, C.K. (1980). Development of a scleroderma-like illness during therapy with L-5-hydroxytryptophan and carbidopa. *N. Engl. J. Med.* **303**: 782–787.

Swygert, L.A., Maes, E.F., Sewell, L.E., Miller, L.M., Falk, H., and Kilbourne, E.M. (1990). Eosinophilia-myalgia syndrome: results of national surveillance. *JAMA* **264**: 1698–1703.

Tabuenca, J.M. (1981). Toxic-allergic syndrome caused by ingestion of rapeseed oil denatured with aniline. *Lancet* **2**: 567–568.

Tellez, I., Cabello, A., Franch, O., and Ricoy, J.R. (1987). Chromatolytic changes in the central nervous system of patients with the toxic oil syndrome. *Acta Neuropathol.* **74**: 354–361.

Thygesen, P., Hougen, H.P., Christensen, H.B., Rygaard, J., Svendson, O., and Juul, P. (1990). Identification of the mononuclear cell infiltrate in the superior cervical ganglion of the athymic nude and euthymic rats after guanethidine-induced sympathectomy. *Int. J. Immunopharmacol.* **12**: 327–330.

Thygesen, P., Hougen, H.P., Christensen, H.B., Rygaard, J., Svendsen, O., and Juul, P. (1992). Anti-asialo GM1 antibodies prevents guanethidine-induced sympathectomy in athymic rats. *Immunopharmacol. Immunotoxicol.* **14**: 219–232.

Varga, J., Jimenez, S.A., and Uitto, J. (1993). L-tryptophan and the eosinophilia-myalgia syndrome: current understanding of the etiology and pathogenesis. *J. Invest. Dermatol.* **100**: 97S–105S.

Vazquez Roncero, A., Janer del Valle, C., Maestro Duran, R., and Graciani Constante, E. (1983). New aniline derivatives in cooking oils associated with the toxic oil syndrome. *Lancet* **2**(8357): 1024–1025.

Verity, M.A., Bulpitt, K.J., and Paulus, H.E. (1991). Neuromuscular manifestations of L-tryptophan-associated eosinophilia-myalgia syndrome. *Hum. Pathol.* **22**: 3–11.

Weller, A., Rosenberg, N., Schlitz, P., Giorno, R., and Claman, H. (1993). Tryptophan causes EMS-like skin changes and induction of ICAM and LFA in SJL/J mice. *J. Immunol.* **150** (8, Part II): 172A.

Willison, H.J. and Kennedy, P.G. (1993). Gangliosides and bacterial toxins in Guillain-Barré syndrome. *J. Neuroimmunol.* **46**: 105–112.

Yuki, N., Sato, S., Miyatake, T., Sugiyama, K., Katagiri, T., and Sasaki, H. (1991). Motoneuron-disease-like disorder after ganglioside therapy. *Lancet* **337**: 1109–1110.

Zochodne, D.W., Ward, K.K., and Low, P.A. (1988). Guanethidine adrenergic neuropathy: an animal model of selective autonomic neuropathy. *Brain Res.* **461**: 10–16.

PART IV Neuropathies caused by infection

19 The post-polio syndrome

M.C. Dalakas

Introduction

Post-polio syndrome (PPS) defines the development of new muscle weakness and fatigue in skeletal or bulbar muscles that begin 25–30 years after an acute attack of paralytic poliomyelitis (Mulder et al. 1972; Dalakas 1987b, 1994; Halstead & Wiechers 1987; Jubelt & Cashman 1987; Dalakas & Hallet 1988; Munsat 1990; Dalakas & Illa 1991; Dalakas et al. 1995d).

PPS has evolved into a distinct clinical entity causing new disabilities and anxieties among polio survivors. More than 300 000 polio survivors in the United States are now experiencing new symptoms, making PPS the most commonly acquired motor neuron disease in which postviral, autoimmune, degenerative, or accelerated aging processes may be involved. Although the cause of PPS is still unknown, significant progress has been made regarding the behavior of the reinnervating motor neurons and the motor unit remodeling. The possibility of persistence of the poliovirus in a mutated form and its potential to trigger a smoldering immune response has generated additional interest regarding the role of autoimmunity in other motor neuronopathies. We will review here the current symptoms, diagnostic criteria, etiopathogenesis, autoimmune phenomena and therapeutic interventions in patients with PPS.

Clinical signs and diagnosis

For the diagnosis of PPS the patients need to have: (1) a history of documented acute paralytic poliomyelitis in childhood or adolescence; (2) partial recovery of motor function and functional stability or recovery for at least 15 years; (3) residual asymmetric muscle atrophy with weakness, areflexia and normal sensation, in at least one limb; and (4) normal sphincteric function (Mulder et al. 1972; Dalakas 1987b, 1994; Halstead & Wiechers 1987; Jubelt & Cashman 1987; Dalakas & Hallett 1988; Munsat 1990; Dalakas & Illa 1991; Dalakas et al. 1995d). As virological confirmation before the 1950s was not available, a well-documented acute febrile paralytic attack during polio epidemics that resulted in residual lower motor neuron weakness is a sine qua non inclusion criterion for the diagnosis of PPS.

PPS still remains a clinical diagnosis requiring the need to exclude any other known medical, neurologic, orthopedic or psychiatric illness that could explain the development of such symptoms (Mulder et al. 1972; Dalakas 1987b, 1994; Halstead & Wiechers 1987; Jubelt & Cashman 1987; Dalakas & Hallett 1988; Munsat 1990; Dalakas & Illa 1991; Dalakas et al. 1995d). Some commonly encountered unrelated problems, mislabeled as PPS or contributing to the severity of PPS, include: radiculopathies, degenerative arthritis, or compression neuropathies (i.e. carpal tunnel syndrome, ulnar neuropathies) as the result of a long-term use of wheelchairs, crutches, braces or poor posture. In addition, a variety of psychosocial concerns, anxieties, depression, and non-specific diffuse pains are not uncommon among post-polio patients. Such symptoms, if mild and proportional to those expected in patients with long-term disability, are not of diagnostic concern. If they dominate the clinical picture and overshadow the new somatic symptomatology, secondary or psychogenic causes should be excluded. Patients with bonefide PPS who fulfill the above criteria do not experience an increased incidence of neuropsychiatric or cognitive dysfunction on detailed neuropsychological and cognitive testing (Clark et al. 1994; Grafman et al. 1995).

The symptoms and signs of PPS include the combination of: (1) musculoskeletal symptoms; and (2) the postpoliomyelitis progressive muscular atrophy (PPMA).

Musculoskeletal symptoms

These include the combination of diminished endurance, fatigue, joint pains in biomechanically deformed or marginally stable joints, worsening mobility owing to long standing scoliosis or poor posture, increasing difficulties due to unnatural or unusual mechanics imposed by tendon transfers or uneven size of limbs and recent increase in body weight that further reduces endurance and increases fatigue (Mulder et al. 1972; Dalakas 1986b, 1987b, 1994; Halstead & Wiechers 1987; Jubelt & Cashman 1987; Dalakas & Hallet 1988; Munsat 1990; Dalakas & Illa 1991; Dalakas et al. 1984a, 1986a,b, 1995d; Halstead & Rossi 1987). Some of these patients describe their symptoms rather vaguely and often with a frustrating degree of variability. Although they feel 'weak', it is often difficult to determine if they have any new muscle weakness because the overwhelming fatigue, diminished endurance, various emotional difficulties, and the frequent presence of a fibromyalgia-like syndrome may complicate the clinical picture. Such symptoms have been noted in post-polio patients since 1972 (Anderson et al. 1972). In our experience, these symptoms are not necessarily progressive and in many patients stabilize.

Post-poliomyelitis progressive muscular atrophy (PPMA)

This term is used to describe the new slowly progressive muscle weakness with or without muscle pain and atrophy that affects certain muscle groups of post-polio patients (Mulder et al. 1972; Dalakas, 1986b, 1987b, 1994; Halstead & Wiechers 1987; Jubelt & Cashman 1987; Dalakas & Hallett 1988; Munsat 1990; Dalakas & Illa 1991; Dalakas et al. 1984a,b, 1986b, 1995; Halstead & Rossi 1987). Patients with PPMA have objective signs and symptoms that reflect new lower motor neuron deterioration that, in contrast to patients in the previous group, have a slowly progressive disease. The symptoms of PPMA include:

New muscular weakness and atrophy

This involves either previously affected muscles that have fully or partially recovered or, less often, muscles clinically unaffected by the original disease. The new weakness is asymmetrical affecting one or two extremities or certain muscles of one or two limbs and can be associated with new focal atrophy. The asymmetry and random distribution of new weakness even among muscle groups of the same limb is so striking that post-polio patients need to be examined and followed on a 'muscle-by-muscle basis' (Dalakas 1995a). Patients with new weakness have increasing difficulties in daily activities such as walking, standing, climbing stairs, ambulating for the same distances as before, transferring from bed to chair, driving, dressing, combing their hair or shaving. As a result of the very asymmetrical nature of their motor weakness even among muscles of the same limb, disabled post-polio patients have demonstrated a unique ability to maintain for years a high level of performance with an unconventional or improvised use of the remaining healthy muscles in any given limb (Mulder et al. 1972; Dalakas 1986b, 1987b, 1994; Halstead & Wiechers 1987; Jubelt & Cashman 1987; Dalakas & Hallett 1988; Munsat 1990;

Dalakas & Illa 1991; Dalakas et al. 1984a,b, 1986b, 1995; Halstead and Rossi 1987). For this reason, a new weakness, affecting even a single muscle, if critical for a specific movement, often leads to a disturbance of motor balance with a disproportionate loss of functional skill.

Fatigue

This is a universal phenomenon in post-polio patients that probably precedes muscle weakness. Although fatigue is difficult to define and it often means 'different things to different patients', the majority of the PPS patients define it as lack of energy and stamina that improves after a brief period of 1–2 hours of rest, usually at midday. They feel 'pooped-out' after they try to maintain or perform a task they used to do, not only with their previously weak extremities but also with their healthier muscles. In contrast to the fatigue of patients with chronic fatigue syndrome, the post-polio fatigue is prominent at the early hours of the afternoon, and improves after brief periods of rest. Although frustrating and distressing, post-polio fatigue does not usually keep the patients out of work and it is not due to psychogenic or depressive causes.

Myalgia

This is often mixed with arthralgias but at times it presents as a peculiar deep ache or as an intrinsic muscle pain often like a muscle cramp similar to the one we see in patients with other neurogenic conditions (Glasberg et al. 1978). Although myalgia is a recognizable symptom, it should raise suspicion of co-existing psychogenic causes if its severity is disproportionate to the rest of the clinical picture or requires narcotics. In such cases, it may not be different from the rubric of myofascial pain syndrome or fibromyalgia.

Fasciculations

Although infrequent, they can be seen in all the muscles, stable or weakening, if one waits and watches carefully, especially by needle EMG (Mulder et al. 1972; Fetell et al. 1982; Dalakas 1986b, 1987b, 1994; Halstead & Wiechers 1987; Jubelt & Cashman 1987; Dalakas & Hallett 1988; Munsat 1990; Dalakas & Illa 1991; Dalakas et al. 1995; Dalakas et al. 1984a,b, 1986b; Halstead & Rossi 1987; Ravits et al. 1990). The fasciculations in PPMA are less frequent than those seen in ALS (Dalakas 1987a, 1990c) and they are not as fine or rippling but more coarse, giving the impression that more fascicles are involved.

Weakness of bulbar muscles

New weakness in the bulbar muscles is clinically manifested predominantly in patients who have had residual bulbar muscle weakness. Subclinical asymmetrical weakness in the pharyngeal constrictor muscles is almost always present in all PPMA patients including those who do not complain of new swallowing difficulties (Sonies & Dalakas 1991, 1995; Dalakas 1991a). Of the 32 patients we examined for clinical or subclinical signs of oropharyngeal dysfunction, 14 had symptoms of new swallowing difficulties and 18 were asymptomatic in this respect (Sonies & Dalakas 1991) even though only 12 of them had a history of bulbar poliomyelitis. Swallowing function, assessed objectively by ultrasonography, videofluoroscopy, and an oral motor index score for ten components of oral function, demonstrated abnormal mean oral index score (a quantitative measure of oral sensorimotor function), compared with age-matched normal subjects ($p<0.001$). Videofluoroscopic examination has also shown varying degree of abnormalities including unilateral bolus transport through the pharynx, pooling in the valleculae or piriform sinuses, delayed pharyngeal constriction and impaired tongue movements. Ultrasound swallowing confirmed that PPS patients have a longer mean duration of wet swallows compared with age-matched controls (Sonies & Dalakas 1991, 1995). These findings indicate that in the bulbar neurons of post-polio patients there is a slowly progressive deterioration similar to that occurring in the muscles of the limbs.

New respiratory difficulties

These are more likely to occur in patients left with some degree of residual respiratory muscle weakness from the original illness. They are very rare in patients left with adequate or normal respiratory muscle function. The reserves of the respiratory muscles of such patients are already diminished, and as new neuronal dysfunction occurs later in life, additional respiratory muscle weakness develops. At times, this can be severe requiring some mechanical support at night (Fisher 1984; Bach et al. 1987). The new respiratory difficulties in

PPMA patients are not only related to the new muscle weakness of the respiratory muscles, but also to other factors such as increasing scoliosis, pulmonary emphysema, cardiovascular insufficiency and, in the wheelchair-bound patients, poor posture (Mulder et al. 1972; Dalakas 1987b, 1994; Halstead & Wiechers 1987; Jubelt & Cashman 1987; Dalakas & Hallet 1988; Munsat 1990; Dalakas & Illa 1991; Dalakas et al. 1995). A central component may also co-exist as the acute bulbar polio was often affecting the medullary structures, including the reticular formation system and the sleep regulatory centers (Plum & Swanson 1959; Lane et al. 1974).

Sleep apnea

It is not an uncommon phemonenon in patients left with residual bulbar dysfunction or severe respiratory compromise (Guilleminault & Motta 1978; Fisher 1987;). It appears to be due to a combination of (1) central apnea, probably due to a residual dysfunction of the surviving bulbar reticular neurons, (2) obstructive apnea due to pharyngeal weakness and increasing musculoskeletal deformities from scoliosis or emphysema, and (3) PPMA resulting in diminished muscle strength of the respiratory, intercostal and abdominal muscle groups (Mulder et al. 1972; Dalakas 1987b, 1994; Halstead & Wiechers 1987; Jubelt & Cashman 1987; Dalakas & Hallett 1988; Munsat 1990; Dalakas & Illa 1991; Dalakas et al. 1995).

Risk factors

Well-proved risk factors responsible for the development of PPS are unknown. Based on repeated clinical observations and epidemiological surveys (Mulder et al. 1972; Halstead 1984; Dalakas 1987, 1994; Halstead & Wiechers 1987; Jubelt & Cashman 1987; Dalakas & Hallett 1988; Munsat 1990; Dalakas & Illa 1991; Dalakas et al. 1995; Halstead & Rossi 1987), however, the following factors appear associated with an earlier onset of PPS: (1) new symptoms appear first in the weakest limbs and in patients with the most severe residual paralysis, (2) earlier bulbar or respiratory difficulties occur in patients with residual bulbar and respiratory weakness, and (3) symptoms occur earlier in the patients who had the acute poliomyelitis at an older age.

A common clinical diagnostic dilemma is faced with patients who present with some symptoms of PPS and give a history of acute paralytic or non-paralytic illness labeled as poliomyelitis, but who do not demonstrate residual signs of an atrophic or weak limb and do not have any available records to document the cause of the original illness. We are aided in our evaluation of a polio-like illness in these circumstances, if the electromyography and the muscle biopsy show signs of diffuse denervation and reinnervation (Mulder et al. 1972; Dalakas 1987b, 1988, 1994; Halstead & Wiechers 1987; Jubelt & Cashman 1987; Dalakas & Hallett 1988; Munsat 1990; Dalakas & Illa 1991; Dalakas et al. 1995d) that cannot be explained by another disease process.

Progression and outcome

The rate of progression of patients with PPMA and the risk of developing ALS were examined in our original follow-up evaluation of patients we followed during an average period of 8.2 years (range 4.5–20 years) (Dalakas 1986a; Dalakas et al. 1984a, 1986b). The new post-polio symptoms appear to begin after a mean period of 28.8 years (range 15–54 years), after the original attack of acute paralytic poliomyelitis. Using the MRC scale (Medical Research Council 1981) we have found that the pace of worsening differs from patient to patient, being generally slow and variable even within the same patient. Long periods (up to 10 years) of stability are not uncommon; however, on a cumulative 10-year-period, the average progression was estimated as 1% per year. We have now confirmed this observation using more sensitive quantitative measurements of muscle strength, the Maximum Voluntary Isometric Contraction (MVIC) (Andres et al. 1986). With the MVIC scores performed in ten patients, first in 1990 and then in 1993, we found that during a 3-year period there were no signs of worsening (Dalakas et al. 1995). The patients have not only remained stable but some of them have noted improvement. Similar findings were noted by Windebank et al. 1995. These data, using objective measurements, support our initial view that PPS patients can remain stable for long periods and that progression has to be viewed on periods longer than 3 years. Whether these scores in skeletal muscles also reflect or correspond to similar changes in the bulbar muscles is unclear. Using a different quantitative method of strength in the tongue and swallowing muscles, we have demonstrated a mild worsening in these muscles during the same period (Sonies & Dalakas 1995). This suggests either insensitivity and variability of the methods used to evaluate strength in the skeletal muscles, or differences in the degree of progression between bulbar and skeletal muscles.

Neither the age of onset of new symptoms, the patient's sex nor the degree and type of physical activities preceding the development of new weakness appear to be significant factors in contributing to the rate of progression (Dalakas & Hallett 1988; Dalakas et al. 1986b). The impact of the new weakness on the patient's functional capabilities is variable but it appears to depend mostly on the residual deficit the patients were left with, at the outset of PPMA. The more severe the residual poliomyelitis deficit, the greater the functional impact of PPMA on the patient's neuromuscular functions.

Incidence and prevalence

The incidence and prevalence of new weakness in post-polio patients is unknown. The best available data are Codd et al. performed in Olmstead County Minnesota (Codd et al. 1984), as reviewed by Kurland (Okumura et al. 1995). The incidence can vary according to how narrow the definition of PPS is. Codd et al. in a well executed epidemiological study performed early in the recognition of PPS, found that 22% of the polio survivors had new symptoms (Codd et al. 1984). The increased awareness of PPS by the public over the next few years, however, raised the incidence to 68% when the same population was interviewed 3 years later (Windebank et al. 1987). Our own impression is that post-polio patients left with very minimal residual symptoms have minimal chances to develop PPS and, if they do, it is limited to fatigue and new weakness in the muscles with the residual weakness. In contrast, patients with significant residual deficit are left with minimal neuronal reserves and their chances to develop PPS after 25–30 years are high. Munsat has suggested that 100% of polio survivors, if followed for a long period, can develop some symptoms of PPS (Munsat 1991).

The number of polio survivors is also not clear. A study from the Center for Health Statistics points to approximately 1.4 million survivors in the USA. Although some studies suggest an increase incidence of ALS in areas prevalent for acute polio (Martyn et al. 1988), there is clearly no evidence to indicate that post-polio patients are at risk of developing ALS as stressed by Kurland (Okumura et al. 1995). We have seen only two post-polio patients that developed ALS among hundreds of PPS patients we have followed. We feel that these two cases fall within the expected frequency of ALS among the general population (Dalakas 1987a).

Pathogenesis

Process of recovery from the acute polio attack

The clinical symptoms, histological signs and electrophysiological findings of PPS are directly related to the new motor neuron deterioration of the previously affected motor neurons and the effectiveness of the remaining motor neuron pool to maintain large motor units for many years. To place the pathogenetic mechanisms of the PPS and generally the post-polio state in perspective, it is helpful to review pertinent observations, regarding the motor neuron injury during the acute poliomyelitis infection and combine these morphological observations with data obtained from the study of muscle biopsy specimens, electromyography, immunology and the molecular virology in the serum, lymphocytes, muscle and spinal cord of PPS patients.

Acute phase of motor neuron injury: necrosis and apoptosis

Based on the original studies of Bodian (Bodian 1949, 1982), during the second or third day of the acute polio infection, there is a striking scarcity of normal-appearing neurons even in cases of very mild paralysis. This indicates that acute paralytic polio was a generalized neuronal disease. Further, the distribution of the pathological changes within CNS were not limited to motor neurons but also involved the intermediate, intermediolateral, posterior horn and dorsal root ganglionic neurons, as well as neurons in the hypothalamus, thalamus, cerebellum and brainstem. The average proportion of injured neurons that were destroyed, the 'case fatality rate', was almost 50% with a 30% probability that an invaded motor neuron would be destroyed by the poliomyelitis virus (Bodian 1949, 1982). Up to 20% of neurons corresponding to normal limbs or to limbs with minimal weakness died. Furthermore, the distribution of the destroyed neurons was scattered, sparing at times muscle groups innervated by two or three contiguous levels of the spinal cord, an observation consistent with the clinically obvious focal sparing of one muscle in a weak or paralyzed limb.

Bodian had provided impressive details of the acute neuronal damage in relationship to the inflammation (Bodian 1949, 1982). The earliest cellular changes in the motor neurons were dissolution of the cytoplasmic Nissl substance (chromatolysis) followed by nuclear invagination and perinuclear chromatin aggregation, in the absence of inflammation. Bodian had remarked that neuronal destruction can be independent of inflammation and inflammation could be mild in areas of extensive neuronal loss. Intense inflammation, associated with neuronophagia followed completion of the neuronal destruction and was a sign of poor recovery (Bodian 1949, 1982).

With this in mind, we reviewed the spinal cords of children that died of acute poliomyelitis diagnosed and studied by Drs Albert Sabin and Ramos Alvarez. In these blocks (courtesy of Drs Sabin and Alvarez), we noted neurons undergoing chromatolysis with fragmentation of the nuclear chromatin without signs of inflammation. With today's knowledge, these signs are suggestive of apoptotic neuronal cell death. Using molecular techniques we have now shown that the poliovirus causes cell death by apoptosis not only within the spinal cord motor neurons during the acute polio but also in tissue cultures infected with the poliovirus (Leon-Monzon and Dalakas 1995b).

Early recovery phase

In his classic studies, Bodian had noted that up to 50% of neurons corresponding to paralyzed limbs can recover histologically. In general, infected neurons exhibiting only mild degree of diffuse chromatolysis, survive and can support motor units; in contrast, the permanent loss of function in muscle groups appears to correlate only with severe cytoplasmic and nuclear changes within the neurons. When paralysis was not complete, many motor neurons affected by the virus were able to recover (Bodian 1949, 1982). The reversibility of the damage in the infected neurons was predictable in those neurons that had intranuclear inclusions but lacked signs of inflammation by the first month of the acute infection. Neuronal recovery was proceeding from the periphery inwards, when Nissl substance began to regenerate. We interpret this observation as suggesting that some of the infected neurons that recovered from non-inflammatory chromatolytic apoptotic changes may potentially be able to retain segments of the viral RNA. Accordingly, there is a possibility for viral persistence as discussed later and elsewhere (Leon-Monzon & Dalakas 1995a).

Late recovery phase

After the acute polio attack, patients experienced a dramatic degree of full or partial recovery even of completely paralyzed limbs. This was first due to recovery of neurons which, as discussed above, were in a state of neuronal nonfunction rather than cell death, and second due to the extensive axonal branching of the surviving motor neurons that began as early as the first month of the infection (Bodian 1949, 1982). In this phase, the terminal axons of the surviving motor neurons sprout in an attempt to reinnervate the muscle fibers deprived by the death of their parent motor neurons (Wiechers and Hubbell 1981; Wiechers 1987). During this process, the uninvolved or recovered anterior horn cells adopt in their motor unit territories additional muscle fibers that could extend up to four or five new muscle fibers for every muscle fiber innervated originally, increasing the number of muscle fibers innervated by a single motor neuron by four to five times above normal (Dalakas et al. 1986b). This process produces large motor units and is so effective that despite the loss of up to 50% of the original number of motor neurons, the muscle can retain clinically normal strength. Consequently, after full recovery and apparent clinical stability, the post-polio spinal cord is left with (1) less than the normal number of normal neurons which had been either unimpaired or fully recovered, (2) neurons with extensive axonal branching necessary to support reinnervation, and (3) an increased number of abnormal, partially recovered or dying neurons, which have limited reserves for axonal sprouting or cannot support all the axonal branches to maintain large motor units for a lengthy period.

Changes in the motor neuron, the motor unit and the muscle in PPS

PPS represents the decompensation of the chronic, ongoing denervation and reinnervation process that occurs effectively in the asymptomatic post-polio state. New weakness (the PPS) occurs when the remaining motor neurons can no longer maintain all the distal sprouts and the degree of denervation exceeds that of reinnervation. In that case, there is loss of some distal nerve terminals resulting in atrophy of individual muscle fibers and reduction in the size of the motor unit that correspond to new weakness and increased muscle atrophy (Dalakas 1990b). These changes are based on the following electrophysiological and morphological observations.

Electrophysiological and muscle biopsy correlations

Conventional electromyographic observations have shown that the motor units in post-polio patients have large amplitude and increased duration in almost all the muscles including those that appear to be clinically normal or historically not affected (Lutschg and Ludin 1981; Wiechers, and Hubbell 1981; Cruz-Martinez et al. 1983, 1984; Kimura 1983; Cashman et al. 1987b; Sanders et al. 1987; Wiechers 1987; Ravits et al. 1990). This is not surprising when one considers the generalized nature of the acute illness. The size of the voluntary motor unit action potentials, the fiber density and the macro EMG amplitude are also increased due to a very successful reinnervating process that results in giant-size motor units (Lange et al. 1989; Luciano et al. 1996). A histological correlate of such electrophysiological finding is the presence in the muscle biopsy of groups with a large number (up to 200) of muscle fibers of normal size (Dalakas 1995c).

Single fiber EMG has repeatedly shown, since the remarkable observation of Wiechers (Wiechers and Hubbell 1981), increased jitter and blocking in both the stable and the newly weakening muscles (Lutschg & Ludin 1981; Cruz-Martinez et al. 1983, 1984; Kimura 1983; Dalakas et al. 1986b; Cashman et al. 1987b; Sanders et al. 1987; Ravits et al. 1990; Maselli et al. 1992). Jitter measures the time difference of the generation of the muscle action potentials in two or more muscle fibers in successive firings and represents the variation of the time of action potential propagation into the two (or more) branches of an axon at the axonal branching point (Stalberg 1982). In normal muscle, the depolarizations of two muscle fiber potentials within the same motor unit run almost together upon activation. In acute denervation with ongoing reinnervation, the jitter increases because of the variability of impulse conduction due to immature synapses which are not capable of supporting normal neuromuscular transmission. When reinnervation becomes complete, however, the jitter decreases. In post-polio patients the jitter is increased and persists indefinitely after the acute poliomyelitis infection, suggestive of an ongoing denervation and reinnervation (Lutschg & Ludin 1981; Wiechers & Hubbell 1981; Cruz-Martinez et al. 1983; Kimura 1983; Cashman et al. 1987b; Sanders et al. 1987; Ravits et al. 1990; Trojan et al. 1993). The jitter in PPS is unrelated to recent deterioration and can be so unstable that it may be difficult to quantify because of the high number of clusters (Ravits et al. 1990). Blocking, which is due to failure of impulse propagation at one of the neuromuscular junctions or one of the axonal branch points (Dalakas et al. 1986b) is also frequently present in post-polio patients. Although jitter is abnormal in post-polio muscles, there is no 'neurogenic jitter', the jitter ascribed to the axonal branch points (Dalakas et al. 1986b). Neurogenic jitter is characterized by two or more potentials that move together with respect to a third potential and cannot be due to a process at a single end plate. As neurogenic jitter develops in ALS patients, we interprete its absence in post-polio muscle as an abnormality at the individual axonal twigs rather than the whole nerve.

The histological correlates of the abnormal jitter and the absence of neurogenic jitter are denoted by the presence of normal-in-size muscle fibers, which are positive for Neural Cell Adhesion Molecular (N-CAM) (Cashman and Trojan 1995; Dalakas & Illa 1991; Illa et al. 1995a; Dalakas 1995c), and the lack of atrophic fibers in groups. N-CAM is not expressed in normal muscle fibers; however, when muscle fiber loses its nerve supply it expresses N-CAM, as early as 2 days (Covault & Sanes 1985; Covault et al. 1986; Cashman et al. 1987a). N-CAM expression, therefore, is a sign of a very recent denervation. Immunocytochemically, using anti-CD56 monoclonal antibodies that identify muscle-specific N-CAM molecules (Illa et al. 1992), we found that N-CAM is expressed by normal-size muscle fibers which are scattered or in small groups within the large groups of reinnervated fibers (Dalakas & Illa 1991; Illa et al. 1992; Dalakas 1995c). These fibers represent failure of re-innervation and can be potentially rescued if the collateral sprouts from the surviving motor neurons (that also have N-CAM) will make contact and form a new effective synapse. There is also recent evidence suggesting that some of the re-reinnervated fibers may not be forming effective synapses (Maselli et al. 1992). These observations supplement the electrophysiological findings of increased jitter and conclude that the muscles in post-polio patients remain unstable because at a given time there are more denervated fibers that could possibly be reinnervated. If the denervated fibers cannot be rescued and make an effective synapse with a distal sprout, they lose their N-CAM expression and become atrophic. The presence of small, atrophic, esterase-positive angulated fibers which are scattered among normal-size fibers suggest recent but permanent denervation and represent the histological hallmark of the newly weakened muscles. As PPMA progresses, more adjacent fibers may become atrophic eventually producing small grouped atrophy either due to degeration of terminal sprouts and major axonal branches that belong to a large motor unit, or due to death of an entire small motor unit that emanated from a previously scarred neuron that has marginal reserves and limited capacity to reinnervate. The loss of muscle fibers from a motor unit, corresponds electrophysiologically to the reduction of the macro EMG amplitude that drops in sequential studies as the weakness progresses (Lange et al. 1989; Luciano et al. 1996).

Although the new weakness can be explained on the basis of the reduced size of the motor unit when the reinnervation cannot keep pace with the ongoing denervation, the cause of fatigue, the earliest symptom in PPS, is unclear. It has been proposed by Cashman and Trojan that this may be due to impaired neuromuscular transmission which, based on single fiber electromyographic studies, can improve with anticholinesterases (Cashman & Trojan 1995). As such an impaired neuromuscular transmission can occur in all muscles even in asymptomatic patients and it is unrelated to the manifestation of new symptoms, we have offered another potential explanation for the fatigue in PPS muscles. As early as 1984, we had shown that muscles originally affected and partially recovered demonstrate a variable degree of neurogenic grouped atrophy combined with myopathic features characterized by increased connective tissue, occasional necrotic or phagocytosed fibers, variation of fiber size with big and small rounded fibers, fiber splitting, internal nuclei and a surprisingly large number of moth-eaten fibers with oxidative enzyme stains (Dalakas 1986a,b, 1987b, 1988, 1992; Dalakas et al. 1984a,b; Sivakumar et al. 1994). Study of these muscles in vivo with ^{31}P MRS spectroscopy, shows a greater depletion of phosphocreatine during a steady-state exercise indicating abnormal energy metabolism due to impaired oxidative phosphorylation (Sivakumar et al. 1995). We have proposed, therefore, a metabolic basis for the post-polio fatigue related to impaired energy metabolism within the individual muscle fibers that emanated from their long-standing denervation and reinnervation. Similar metabolic changes were recently shown by others with MRS spectroscopy techniques (Sharma et al. 1994).

All the above described histological, clinicopathological electrophysiological correlations are graphically summarized in Figure 19.1

Causes of motor neuron degeneration and distal motor unit disintegration

The cause for the loss of the distal axonal sprouts and neuronal deterioration described above that results in new muscle weakness and fatigue are currently unclear. There are several etiologic considerations derived either from well proven studies, or unconfirmed observations.

Attrition

This is the theory we favor. PPMA appears to express itself clinically after approximately 30 years from the original polio attack when the remaining motor neurons have overbranched and overstressed to maintain function (Dalakas 1995c). As discussed earlier, even after maximum recovery from the acute polio-attack, the reinnervated motor units have not matured or stabilized as expected. To the contrary, the

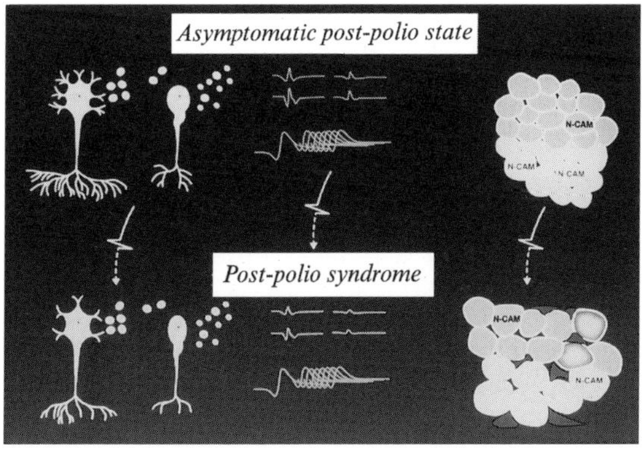

Figure 19.1 *Diagrammatic summary on the mechanism of post-polio syndrome (PPS) from the asymptomatic post-polio state to development of post-polio syndrome. In the asymptomatic post-polio state there is mild inflammation in the spinal cord motor neurons, oversprouting of the distal axons resulting in effective reinnervation, enlarged motor units with high amplitude macro EMG potentials, and very large-size fiber type grouping histochemically. In addition, there is ongoing denervation with effective reinnervation resulting in abnormal jitter and N-CAM-positive, normal size, muscle fibers. The post-polio syndrome occurs when the remaining motor neurons can no longer maintain all the distal sprouts and the degree of denervation exceeds that of reinnervation. In that case, there is loss of some distal nerve terminals resulting in atrophy of individual muscle fibers (seen in the biopsy as small angulated fibers (arrows)) and reduction in the size of the motor unit represented by the fall of macro-EMG amplitude. Many of the chronically denervated/reinnervated and often hypertrophic muscle fibers appear 'moth-eaten' with enzyme histochemical staining due to impaired oxidative staining (arrowheads) (D1), that correspond to impaired oxidative metabolism with MRS spectroscopy.*

motor units are unstable because not all of the excessive distal sprouts can form effective synapses resulting in failure to re-reinnervate all the newly denervated fibers. This ongoing denervating and re-reinnervating process is stressing the neuronal cell bodies which after a number of years are left with diminished reserves and reduced ability to maintain the metabolic demands for all their sprouts. Consequently, there is slow deterioration of some nerve terminals. As each terminal dies, muscle fibers drop out because they can no longer be reinnervated and weakness develops.

Normal aging

Although post-polio neurons may succumb earlier than normal to the aging process or may even have a shorter life span if previously scarred and survived, aging alone cannot be the cause of PPMA. Motor neuron loss does not occur in persons younger than age 60 (Tomlinson & Irving 1977) and muscle biopsy specimens from normal persons younger than 60 years old rarely show small angulated fibers indicative of denervation (unpublished results). Furthermore, epidemiological observations indicate that it is the length of the interval between onset of acute polio and the appearance of new symptoms that is a determining variable for PPMA and not chronological age (Halstead & Wiechers 1987).

Immune dysregulation

Although PPMA is not an immune disease, the following primary or secondary immunological abnormalities should not be ignored.

INFLAMMATION IN THE SPINAL CORD. Our study, 10 years ago (Pezeshkpour & Dalakas 1987, 1988), of the spinal cord sections in seven patients with prior polio, (three with PPMA and four with stable post-polio but without new symptoms) that died from unrelated causes 9 months to 44 years after the original polio attack, revealed mild but definite perivascular inflammation in the parenchyma of the gray matter as well as active gliosis disproportional to the neuronal loss. Neuronal atrophy and chromatolysis were also noted. In three PPMA patients we found axonal spheroids. Several surviving neurons were present throughout the

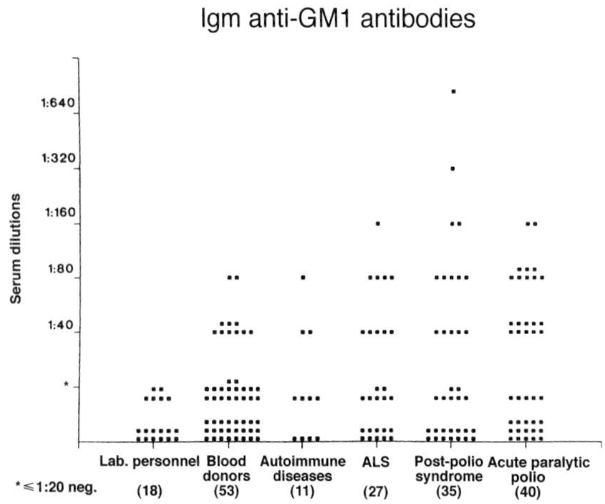

Figure 19.2 *Serum IgM anti-GM1 antibody titers in post-polio syndrome and various diseases.*

gray matter but some of them had abnormal configuration of their somata consisting of atrophy, accumulation of lipofuscin and loss of Nissl substance. These findings were unrelated to new weakness or the time of death after the original illness and suggest some degree of ongoing activity in the post-polio spinal cord, the site of the original viral infection. Similar findings have been noted recently by two other groups (Miller 1995; Kamiski et al. 1995).

ENDOMYSIAL INFLAMMATION. Mild inflammation is present in the muscle biopsies consisting of $CD8^+$ and $CD4^+$ cells surrounding healthy muscle fibers that express MHC-I class antigen on their surface, in a pattern similar to that seen in some immune-mediated inflammatory myopathies (Dalakas 1991b). Furthermore, the MHC-I class expression can be in small groups and it is analogous to the larger groups of MHC-I-positive fibers we noted in the acute polio (Illa et al. 1995). Although the significance of these observations is unclear, we have proposed that neuronally-regulated lymphokines or cytokines released anterogradely by those motor neurons surrounded by inflammatory cells (see above), can trigger a smoldering, low grade, upregulation of self antigens.

ABNORMAL PERIPHERAL BLOOD LYMPHOCYTE SUBSETS. In our early studies we noted abnormal phenotypic expression of peripheral blood lymphocyte subsets (Dalakas et al. 1984a,b; Dalakas 1986b). As these changes were not internally consistent, their significance was unclear. Ginsberg et al. (1989), however, found depletion of native T cells suggestive of a chronic activation of T cells only in patients with new symptoms but not in those with stable polio.

HIGH GM_1 ANTIBODIES. We have found increased IgM, but not IgG, GM_1 antiganglioside antibodies in patients with PPS and acute polio (Illa et al. 1995b) (Figure 19.2). Although the significance of such antibodies in neurological diseases has been questioned, the correlation with the acute polio was of interest. Sequential determinations in the acute polio showed that the antibodies correlate with the neuronal damage because they appear early in the disease and normalize by the third month. Whether in PPS GM_1 antibodies represent a primary or a secondary response to a neuronal surface antigen is unknown.

HIGH INTERLEUKIN 2 (IL-2), IL-2 RECEPTORS (IL-2R) AND THE PRESENCE OF OLIGOCLONAL BANDS IN THE SPINAL FLUID. Oligoclonal IgG bands in the spinal fluid have been noted in some PPS patients (Dalakas et al. 1984a,b, 1986b; Dalakas 1986b, 1990a). We interpreted this observation as implying an antibody response to an unknown antigenic stimulation. In 1991, Sharief et al. found increased levels of IL-2 and IL-2R along with high poliovirus-specific IgM bands (Sharief et al. 1991). They suggested that in some PPS patients there is a possibility of an active viral infection and an ongoing antibody response.

POSSIBLE ASSOCIATION WITH HLA-DQ17 HAPLOTYPE. Preliminary data from our laboratory in 40 PPS patients demonstrated an increased association with HLA-DQ17 haplotype (Dinsmore & Dalakas 1992). If confirmed with larger number of patients, these data would suggest a genetic susceptibility to the acute polio infection.

Response to poliovirus RNA and the possibility of persistent viral mutants

Recent findings from several laboratories using molecular techniques provide evidence that the possibility of residual viral genomes in the remaining motor neurons of post-polio patients is not remote.

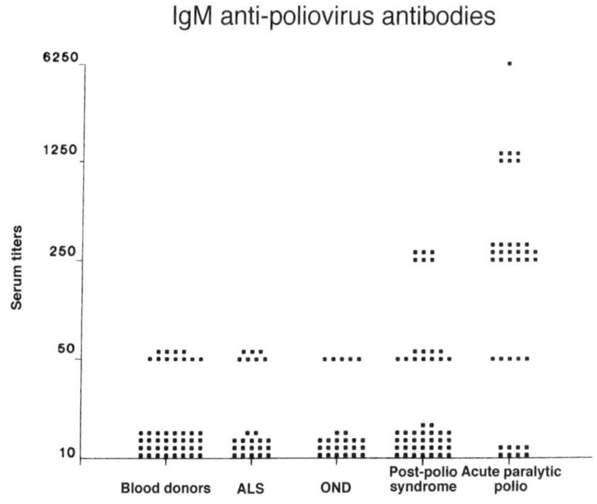

Figure 19.3 *Serum IgM anti-poliovirus antibodies in post-polio syndrome and other diseases including acute polio. ALS: amyotrophic lateral sclerosis; OND: other neurological diseases.*

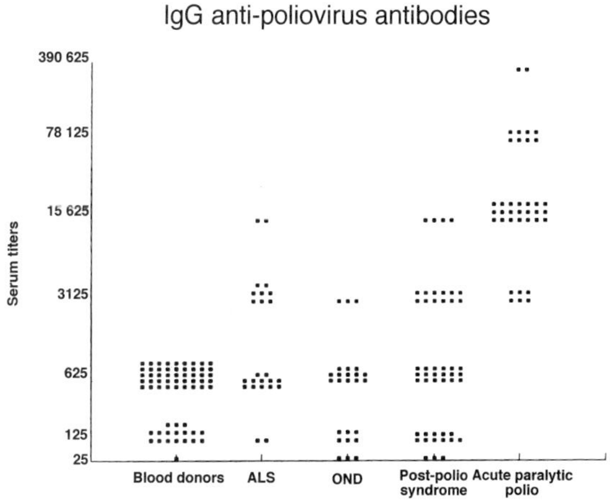

Figure 19.4 *Serum IgG anti-poliovirus antibodies in post-polio syndrome and other diseases including acute polio. ALS: amyotrophic lateral sclerosis; OND: other neurological diseases.*

POLIOVIRUS-SPECIFIC IgG ANTIBODY SYNTHESIS. One out of six patients we reported in 1984 (Dalakas et al. 1984b), had increased intrathecal synthesis of IgG that was poliovirus-specific, but not specific for other viruses.

INTRATHECAL SYNTHESIS OF POLIOVIRUS-SPECIFIC IgM ANTIBODIES. Oligoclonal IgM bands specific for polioviruses were detected by Sharief et al. (1991) in the CSF of 21 of 36 patients with PPS and intrathecal synthesis of IgM antibodies against poliovirus was noted among their symptomatic post-polio patients. These abnormalities, if confirmed, point towards an ongoing intrathecal immune response to the poliovirus.

HIGH SERUM, IgM POLIOVIRUS-SPECIFIC, ANTIBODIES. We have found high IgM antibody titers to poliovirus in the serum of six of 25 post-polio patients using a sensitive ELISA assay (Leon-Monzon & Dalakus 1995a) (Figure 19.3). This was very carefully done and included for the first time IgM-positive controls. We have not, however, tested the CSF. IgG antipoliovirus antibodies were seen in some patients and controls (Figure 19.4), as expected for patients exposed to a prior poliovirus infection.

STUDIES WITH POLYMERASE CHAIN REACTION (PCR). Under stringent conditions and numerous positive and negative controls, we have been able to amplify polioviral RNA using three different pairs of specific primers of the picornavirus genome in the spinal fluid from four of 40 patients with PPS and from the lymphocytes of seven of 37 PPS patients (Leon-Monzon & Dalakas 1995b). The amplified product was sequenced and preliminary findings suggest the presence of a truncated mutated poliovirus type I. Similar findings have been seen by two other groups (Leparc et al. 1995; Muir et al. 1995). Using similar techniques we were unable to amplify virus from the muscle biopsies (Leon-Monzon & Dalakas 1992). Work on the PPS spinal cord using in situ/PCR has not yet been completed. In the spinal cord from patients with acute polio, we were able to localize with in situ/PCR the virus within motor neurons and their axon hillock (Isaacson et al. 1995).

Can poliovirus persist and play a role in the cause of post-polio syndrome?

Acute poliomyelitis is a monophasic disease (Sabin 1980; Johnson 1982). As the virus in culture is very lytic, the possibility of persistence was considered impossible. Furthermore, recurrent poliomyelitis is not known to occur; however, the poliovirus can cause a persistent infection in animals or immunosuppressed humans (Johnson 1982, 1995; Miller 1981). In addition, persistent poliovirus infection has been shown to correlate with a selection of highly mutated viral strains that were capable of producing a cytopathic effect in neuroblastoma cell lines even over a nine month period (Colbere-Garopin et al. 1989).

The poliovirus can theoretically persist years later in the motor neurons of surviving PPS patients if (1) the immune system did not clear completely the initial infection and the virus escaped immunologic surveillance (Dalakas 1995b). In this case, some of the infected neurons with the abnormal nuclei and cytoplasmic inclusions described earlier, can recover and potentially harbor viral genome, and (2) during the initial infection the generated defective interfering particles or possibly mutant polioviruses were trapped in a few motor neurons that were not lysed but survived. A subsequent change of the biological properties of the virus could result in restrained RNA synthesis that allows persistence without replication. During periods of repair, division, stress of the cell or metabolic alterations in responses to cytokines, the virus can again mutate and express new epitopes shared by host cell proteins that may trigger a slow, smoldering, inflammatory response. This scenerio would explain the inflammation we noted in the spinal cord and muscle and support the hypothesis that the MHC-I class expression seen in groups of muscle fibers could have been neuronally regulated due to cytokines secreted by the dysfunctioning neurons. Similarly, it can explain the high titer of antibodies directed against GM1, a cell-surface motor neuron glycoprotein, the abnormal lymphocyte subsets, the oligoclonal IgG bands and the high IL-2 and soluble IL-2R receptors in the CSF. It can also explain the viral RNA product found in the CSF. The CSF RNA product could have been derived from the few dying neurons that shed the truncated form of the polioviruses genome that they were potentially harboring. As neurons with such viral products are expected to be only a few, it is not surprising that the virological and immunological abnormalities we described are not ubiquitous or consistently present in all the patients and vary even from patient to patient.

Although these observations can explain some of the immunopathological and laboratory findings, we have no evidence at present that they contribute to the clinical manifestations of PPS. They open, however, a new era in exploring the persistence of poliovirus and other enteroviruses. In acute polio, the virus appears to cause neuronal cell death through apoptosis. If the apoptotic cell death is inhibited, via the expression of specific genes as occurs in other models (Johnson 1995), the poliovirus persistence should not be a surprise to a virologist or a neurobiologist. The patients with PPS offer the only human model to explore this phenomenon with the modern tools of molecular virology.

Treatment trials

The following trials (Dalakas 1995a) have been conducted in PPS patients.

Interferon

An uncontrolled trial using alpha 2 recombinant interferon in two patients that we have conducted was ineffective (Dalakas et al. 1986a). Other interferons in large scale studies have not been tried.

Prednisone

In the first double-blind study that we performed, high-dose (1 mg/kg), prednisone had mild benefit with a trend towards improvement (Dinsmore et al. 1995). The degree of improvement in the 17 patients we enrolled did not, however, reach statistical significance. Considering the side-effects of the drug, we do not recommend immunosuppressive doses of prednisone for the treatment of PPS. Whether low-dose prednisone has an effect in fatigue and endurance of some PPS patients, without causing long-term side-effects, is unclear.

Anticholinesterases (Mestinon)

This drug has been tried on and off for several years to improve the fatigue in PPS patients with variable results. A recent, well-designed, but uncontrolled study showed that low doses of Mestinon can improve the fatigue of some patients with a concomitant improvement of the electrophysiological decrement (Trojan & Cashman 1995). A multi-center controlled study has now been completed; the results are pending.

Amantadine

In a double-blind placebo-controlled study that we conducted, Amantadine was not superior to placebo in improving the fatigue of PPS patients (Stein et al. 1995). Although some patients felt better, overall there was no statistical significance between the placebo and the amantadine-treated patients.

Deprenyl

In an uncontrolled trial, deprenyl was found to improve strength in PPS patients. Whether this drug has any effect on PPS is unclear without a carefully controlled study. The scientific basis for such a study is still unclear.

Exercise

This is a highly controversial issue because of the belief by some that too much exercise can worsen the patients, whereas rest can preserve energy; however, there is no documented evidence that exercise is deleterious to PPS patients. Until this is established, we recommend 'common sense' physical activities and advise the patients to stay active. We consider the level of 'tolerance' as the limit at which excessive physical activities should stop or slow down. The tolerance is defined as the level of acceptable discomfort. When fatigue or muscle pain develops, we recommend termination and rest. We do not feel that rest conserves energy. To the contrary, we have evidence that during periods of inactivity strength can decline. We have witnessed a number of patients who had to immobilize a post-polio limb in a cast because of a joint injury. Some of these patients could not regain the strength they had in the same limb prior to injury, in spite of intense rehabilitation after the cast was removed (unpublished results).

The issue of exercise needs to be systematically addressed not only with regards to whether it is beneficial, deleterious or ineffective, but also in reference to the type of exercise, i.e. isotonic, isometric, isokinetic or repetitive. We began to study this phenomenon by applying a controlled, 8 week, exercise program to investigate its efficacy by (1) measuring the strength before and after completion of exercise using the MVIC and Cybex method, (2) screening for changes in the fatigue using validated fatigue scales before and after completion of exercise, (3) examining the muscle biopsies before and after completion of the exercise for changes in the size and diameter of muscle fibers, expression of cytokines or lymphokines, induction of inflammation or muscle fiber injury, changes in the size of the fiber-type grouping and conversion of one fiber type to another, (4) measuring parameters of muscle injury in the serum, i.e. CK level before, during and after completion of the exercise program, and (5) examining the effect and levels of cytokines or lymphokines in the circulation. Our preliminary results are encouraging because they suggest that exercise is not only non-damaging, but it could be beneficial by increasing muscle endurance and enhancing the ability to perform activities of daily living (Spector et al. 1996).

Nerve growth factors

Based on their biological properties, these factors, such as the insulin-like growth-factor (IGF-1) can enhance the ability of the motor neurons to sprout new branches, or maintain the existing branches and make more effective synapses. As the problem in PPS is degeneration of some distal sprouts due to the weakness of their neuronal soma, growth factors could target the very heart of the problem. A pilot study using IGF-1 has just been completed.

References

Anderson, A.D., Levine, S.A., and Gellert, H. (1972). Loss of ambulatory ability in patients with old anterior poliomyelitis. *Lancet* **ii**: 1061–1063.

Andres, P., Hedlund, W., Finison, L., et al. (1986). Quantitative motor assessment in amyotropic lateral sclerosis. *Neurology* **36**: 937–941.

Bach, J.R., Alba, A.S., Bodofsky, E., Curran, F.J., and Schulthless, M. (1987). Glossopharyngeal breathing and non-invasive aids in the management of post-polio respiratory insufficiency. In: *Ann. N.Y. Acad. Sci.* **23**: 99–113.

Bodian, D. (1949). Histopathologic basis of clinical findings. In: Poliomyelitis. *Am. J. Med.* **6**: 563–578.

Bodian, D. (1982). Poliomyelitis. In: *Pathology of the Nervous System*, vol 3, ed. J. Minckler, pp. 2323–2364. McGraw-Hill, New York.

Cashman, N.R., Covault, J., Wollman, R.L., and Sonies. J.R. (1987a). Neural cell adhesion molecule in normal, denervated and myopathic human muscle. *Ann. Neurol.* **21**: 481–489.

Cashman, N.R., Maselli, R., Wollman, R.L., Roos, R., Simon, R., and Antel, J.P. (1987b). Late denervation in patients with antecedent paralytic poliomyelitis. *N. Engl. J. Med.* **317**: 7–12.

Cashman, N.R. and Trojan, D.A. (1995). Correlation of electrophysiology with pathology, pathogenesis, and anticholinesterase therapy in post-polio syndrome. In: *The Post-Polio Syndrome: Advances in the Pathogenesis and Treatment*, ed. M.C. Dalakas, H. Bartfeld, L.T. Kurland. *Ann. N.Y. Acad. Sci.* **753**: 138–150.

Clark, K., Dinsmore, S., Grafman, J., and Dalakas, M.C. (1994). A personality profile of patients diagnosed with post-polio syndrome. *Neurology* **44**: 1809–1811.

Codd, M.B., Mulder, D.W., Kurland, L.T., Beard, C.H., and O'Fallon, W.M. (1984). Poliomyelitis in Rochester Minnesota 1935–1955. Epidemiology and long-term sequelae: a preliminary report. In: *Late Effects of Poliomyelitis.* ed. L.S. Halstead and D.O. Wiechers, pp. 121–134. Symposia Foundation.

Colbere-Garopin, F., Christodoulou, C., Crainic, R., and Pelletier, T. (1989). Persistent poliovirus infection of human neuroblastoma cells. *Proc. Natl. Acad. Sci. USA* **86**: 354–359.

Covault, J., Merlie, J.P., Goudis, C., and Sanes, J.R. (1986). Molecular forms of N-CAM and its mRNA in developing and denervated skeletal muscle. *J. Cell Biol.* **102**: 731–739.

Covault, J. and Sanes, J.R. (1985). Neural cell adhesion molecule (N-CAM) accumulates in denervated and paralyzed skeletal muscles. *Proc. Natl. Acad. Sci. USA* **82**: 4544–4548.

Cruz-Martinez, A., Ferrer, M.T., and Perez Conde, M.C. (1984). Electrophysiological features in patients with non-progressive and late progressive weakness after paralytic poliomyelitis. Conventional EMG, automatic analysis of the electromyogram and single fiber electromyography study. *Electromyorgr. Clin. Neurophysiol.* **24**: 469–479.

Cruz-Martinez, A., Perez Conde, M.C., and Ferrer, M.T. (1983). Chronic partial denervation is more widespread than is suspected clinically in paralytic poliomyelitis: electrophysiological study. *Eur. Neurol.* **22**: 312–321.

Dalakas, M.C. (1986a). Morphological changes in the muscles of patients with post-poliomyelitis new weakness. A histochemical study of 39 muscle biopsies. *Muscle Nerve* **9**: 117.

Dalakas, M.C. (1986b). New neuromuscular symptoms in patients with old poliomyelitis: a three year follow-up study. *Eur. Neurol.* **25**: 381–387.

Dalakas, M.C. (1987a). ALS and post-polio: differences and similarities. *Ann. N.Y. Acad. Sci.* **23**: 63–81.

Dalakas, M.C. (1987b). New neuromuscular symptoms after polio (The post-polio syndrome): clinical studies and pathogenetic mechanisms. *Ann. N.Y. Acad. Sci.* **23**: 241–264.

Dalakas, M.C. (1988). Morphological changes in the muscles of patients with post-poliomyelitis neuromuscular symptoms. *Neurology* **38**: 99–104.

Dalakas, M.C. (1990a). Oligoclonal bands in postpoliomyelitis muscular atrophy. *Ann. Neurol.* **28**: 196–197.

Dalakas, M.C. (1990b). Pathogenesis of post-polio syndrome: clues from muscle and CNS studies. In *The Post-Polio Syndrome*, ed. T. Munsat, pp. 39–65. Butterworths, Stoneham.

Dalakas, M.C. (1990c). Post-poliomyelitis motor neuron diseases: what did we learn in reference to amyotrophic lateral sclerosis? In *Amyotrophic Lateral Sclerosis: Concepts in Pathogenesis and Etiology*, ed. A.J. Hudson pp. 326–356.

Dalakas, M.C. (1991a). Dysphagia in the post-polio syndrome. *N. Engl. J. Med.* **325**: 1107–1109.

Dalakas, M.C. (1991b). Polymyositis, dermatomyositis and inclusion-body myositis. *N. Engl. J. Med.* **325**: 1487–1498.

Dalakas, M.C. (1992). Elevated creatine kinase levels in post-polio syndrome. *JAMA* **268**: 3248.

Dalakas, M.C. (1994). Post-polio motor neuron diseases. In: *Motor Neuron Diseases*, ed. A.C. Williams, pp. 83–107. London, Chapman and Hall.

Dalakas, M.C. (1995a). How to design an experimental therapeutic study in patients with post-polio syndrome. In: *The Post-Polio Syndrome: Advances in the Pathogenesis and Treatment*, ed. M.C., Dalakas, H. Bartfeld and L.T. Kurland *Ann. N.Y. Acad. Sci.* **753**: 314–320.

Dalakas, M.C. (1995b). Infection of human muscle, nerve and motor neurons with polioviruses and other enteroviruses. In: *Human Enterovirus Infections*, ed. H.A. Rotbard (in press).

Dalakas, M.C. (1995c). Pathogenetic mechanisms of postpolio syndrome: morphological, electrophysiological, virological and immunopathological correlations. *Ann. N.Y. Acad. Sci.* **753**: 167–185.

Dalakas, M.C., Aksamit, A.J., Madden, D.L., and Sever, J.L. (1986a). Recombinant α_2 interferon in a pilot trial of patients with amyotrophic lateral sclerosis. *Arch. Neurol.* **43**: 933–935.

Dalakas, M.C., Bartfeld, H., and Kurland, L.T. (eds). (1995d). *The Post Polio Syndrome: Advances in the Pathogenesis and Treatment. Ann. N.Y. Acad. Sci.* **753**: 411.

Dalakas, M.C., Elder, G., Hallett, M., et al. (1986b). A long-term follow-up study of patients with postpoliomyelitis neuromuscular symptoms. *N. Engl. J. Med.* **314**: 959–963.

Dalakas, M.C. and Hallett, M. (1988). The post-polio syndrome. In: *Advances in Contemporary Neurology*, ed. F. Plum pp. 51–94.

Dalakas, M.C. and Illa, I. (1991). The post-polio syndrome: concepts in pathogenesis and etiologies. In: *Advances in Neurology*, vol. 56, *Amyotrophic Laterial Sclerosis*, ed. L.P. Rowland, pp. 495–511. Raven Press, New York.

Dalakas, M.C., Sever, J.L., Fletcher, M., Madden, D.L., Papadopoulos, N., Shekarchi, I., and Albrecht, P. (1984a). Neuromuscular symptoms in patients with old poliomyelitis: clinical, virological, and immunological studies. In: *Late Effects of Poliomyelitis*, ed. L.S. Halstead and D.O. Wiechers, pp. 73–90. Symposia Foundation, Miami.

Dalakas, M.C., Sever, J.L., Madden, D.L., Papadopoulos, N.M., Shekarchi, I.C., Albrecht, P., and Krezlewecz, A. (1984b). Late post-poliomyelitis muscular atrophy: clinical, virological and immunological studies. *Rev. Infect. Dis.* **6**: S562–S567.

Dinsmore, S.T. and Dalakas, M.C. (1992). Immunogenetic and immunoregulatory factors in patients with the post-polio syndrome (PPS). *Neurology* **42(S)**: 314.

Dinsmore, S., Dambrosia, J., and Dalakas, M.C. (1995). A double-blind, placebo-controlled trial of high-dose prednisone for the treatment of post-poliomyelitis syndrome. In: *The Post-Polio Syndrome: Advances in the Pathogenesis and Treatment*, ed. M.C. Bartfeld and L.T. Kurland, *Ann. N.Y. Acad. Sci.* **753**: 303–313.

Fetell, M.R., Smallberg, G., Lewis, L.D., Lovelace, R.E., Hays, A.P., and Rowland, L.P. (1982). A benign motor neuron disorder: delayed cramps and fasciculation after poliomyelitis or myelitis. *Ann. Neurol.* **11**: 423–427.

Fisher, D.A. (1984). Poliomyelitis: late pulmonary complications and management. In *Late Effects of Poliomyelitis*, ed. L.S. Halstead and D.O. Wiechers, pp. 185–192. Symposia Foundation, Miami.

Fisher, D.A. (1987). Sleep disordered breathing as a late effect of poliomyelitis. In: *Research and Clinical Aspects of the Late Effects of Poliomyelitis*, ed. L.S. Halstead and D.O. Wiechers *Ann. N.Y. Acad. Sci.* **23**: 115–120.

Ginsberg, A.H., Gale, M.J., Rose, L.M., and Clark, E.A. (1989). T-cell alteration in late post-poliomyelitis. *Arch. Neurol.* **46**: 497–501.

Guilleminault, C. and Motta, J. (1978). Sleep apnea syndrome as a long-term sequela of poliomyelitis. In: *Sleep Apnea Syndromes*, vol 2, ed. C. Guilleminault, pp. 309–315. Kroc Foundation, New York.

Glasberg, M., Dalakas, M.C., and Engel, W.K. (1978). Muscle cramps and pains: histochemical analysis of muscle biopsies in 63 patients. *Neurology* **28**: 387.

Grafman, J., Clark, K., Richardson, D., Dinsmore, S., and Dalakas, M.C. (1995). Neuropsychology of post-polio syndrome. In: *The Post-Polio Syndrome: Advances in the Pathogenesis and Treatment*, ed. M.C. Dalakas, H. Bartfeld and L.T. Kurland. *Ann. N.Y. Acad. Sci.* **753**: 103–110.

Halstead, L.S. (1984). In: *Late Effects of Poliomyelitis*, ed. L.S. Halstead and D.O. Weichers. Symposia Foundation, Miami.

Halstead, L.S. and Rossi, D.C. (1987). Postpolio syndrome: clinical experience with 132 consecutive outpatients. In: *Ann. N.Y. Acad. Sci.* **23**: 13–26.

Halstead, L.S. and Wiechers, D.O. (eds.) (1987). Research and clinical aspects of the late effects of poliomyelitis. *Ann. N.Y. Acad. Sci.* vol. 23.

Illa, I., Leon-Monzon, M., Agboatwalla, M., Dure-Samin, A., and Dalakas, M.C. (1995a). The role of muscle in acute poliomyelitis infection. In: *The Post-Polio Syndrome: Advances in the Pathogenesis and Treatment*, ed. M.C. Dalakas, H. Bartfeld and L.T. Kurland, *Ann. N.Y. Acad. Sci.* **753**: 58–67.

Illa, I., Leon-Monzon, M., and Dalakas, M.C. (1992). Regenerating and denervated human muscle fibers and satellite cells express N-CAM recognized by monoclonal antibodies to NK cells. *Ann. Neurol.* **31**: 46–52.

Illa, I., Monzon, M., Ilyas, A., Latov, N. and Dalakas, M.C. (1995b). Antiganglioside antibodies in patients with acute polio and post-polio syndrome. In: *The Post-Polio Syndrome: Advances in the Pathogenesis and Treatment*, ed. M.C. Dalakas, H. Bartfeld and L.T. Kurland. *Ann. N.Y. Acad. Sci.* **753**: 374–377.

Isaacson, S.H., Sivakumar, K., Pomeroy, K., Asher, D.M., Alvarez, R., Gibbs, C.J. Jr, Gajdusek, D.C. and Dalakas, M.C. (1995). Cellular localization of poliovirus RNA in the spinal cord during acute paralytic poliomyelitis. In: *The Post-Polio Syndrome: Advances in the Pathogenesis and Treatment*, ed. M.C. Dalakas, H. Bartfeld and L.T. Kurland. *Ann. N.Y. Acad. Sci.* **753**: 194–200.

Johnson, R.T. (1982). *Viral Infections of the Nervous System*. Raven Press, New York.

Johnson, R.T. (1995). Pathogenesis of poliovirus infections. In: *The Post-Polio Syndrome: Advances in the Pathogenesis and Treatment*, ed. M.C. Dalakas, H. Bartfeld and L.T. Kurland. *Ann N.Y. Acad. Sci.* **753**: 361–365.

Jubelt, B. and Cashman, N.R. (1987). Neurologic manifestations of the postpolio syndrome. *Crit. Rev. Neurobiol.* **3**: 199–220.

Kamiski, H.J., Tresser, N., Hogan, R.E., and Martin, E. (1995). Pathological analysis of spinal cords from survivors of poliomyelitis. In: *The Post-Polio Syndrome: Advances in the Pathogenesis and Treatment*, ed. M.C. Dalakas, H. Bartfeld and L.T. Kurland. *Ann. N.Y. Acad. Sci.* **753**: 390–393.

Kimura, J. (1983). *Electrodiagnosis in Diseases of Nerve and Muscle*. F.A. David, Philadelphia.

Lane, D.J., Haselman, B., and Nichols, P.J.R. (1974). Late onset respiratory failure in patients with previous poliomyelitis. *Q. J. Med.* **43**: 551–568.

Lange, D.J., Smith, T., and Lovelace, R.E. (1989). Postpolio muscular atrophy. Diagnostic utility of macroelectro-myography. *Arch. Neurol.* **46**: 502–506.

Leon-Monzon, M.E. and Dalakas, M.C. (1995a). Detection of poliovirus antibodies and poliovirus genome in patients with the post-polio syndrome. *Ann. N.Y. Acad. Sci.* **753**: 208–218.

Leon-Monzon, M.E. and Dalakas, M.C. (1995b). Poliovirus causes lysis of infected cells by apoptosis. *Neurology* **45(S)**: 305–306.

Leparc, I., Kopeka, H., Fuchs, F., Janatova, I., Aymard, M., and Julien, J. (1995). Search for poliovirus in specimens from patients with the post-polio syndrome. In: *The Post-Polio Syndrome: Advances in the Pathogenesis and Treatment*, ed. M.C. Dalakas, H. Bartfeld and L.T. Kurland. *Ann. N.Y. Acad. Sci.* **753**: 233–236.

Luciano, C.A., Sivakumar, K., Spector, S., and Dalakas, M.C. (1996). Electrophysiologic and histologic studies in clinically unaffected muscles of patients with prior paralytic poliomyelitis. *Muscle Nerve* **19**: 1413–1420.

Lutschg, J. and Ludin, H.P. (1981). Electromyographic findings in patients after recovery from peripheral nerve lesions and poliomyelitis. *J. Neurol.* **225**: 25–32.

Martyn, C.N., Barker, D.J.P., and Osmond, C. (1988). Motor neuron disease and postpoliomyelitis in England and Wales. *Lancet* **i**: 1319–1322.

Maselli, R.A., Cashman, N.R., Wallman, R.L., Salazar-Gouesso, E.F., and Roos, R. (1992). Neuromuscular transmission as a function of motor unit size in patients with prior poliomyelitis. *Muscle Nerve* **15**: 648–655.

Medical Research Council. (1981). *Aids to the Examination of the Peripheral Nervous System*. Her Majesty's Stationary Office, London.

Miller, D.C. (1995). Post-polio syndrome spinal cord pathology: case report with immunopathology. In: *The Post-Polio Syndrome: Advances in the Pathogenesis and Treatment*, ed. M.C. Dalakas, H. Bartfeld and L.T. Kurland. *Ann. N.Y. Acad. Sci.* **753**: 186–193.

Miller, J.R. (1981). Prolonged intracerebral infection with poliovirus in asymptomatic mice. *Ann. Neurol.* **9**: 590–596.

Muir, P., Nicholson, F., Sharief, M.K., Thompson, E.J., Cairns, N.J., Lantos, P., Spencer, G.T., Kaminski, H.J., and Banatvala, J.E. (1995). Evidence for persistent enterovirus infection of the central nervous system in patients with previous paralytic poliomyelitis. In: *The Post-Polio Syndrome: Advances in the Pathogenesis and Treatment*, ed. M.C. Dalakas, H. Bartfeld and L.T. Kurland. *Ann. N.Y. Acad. Sci.* 753: 219–232.

Mulder, D.W., Rosenbaum, R.A. and Layton, D.O. Jr. (1972). Late progression of poliomyelitis or forme fruste amyotrophic lateral sclerosis. *Mayo Clin. Proc.* 47: 756–761.

Munsat, T. (ed.). (1990). *The Post-Polio Syndrome.* Butterworths, Stoneham.

Munsat, T.L. (1991). Postpoliomyelitis, new symptoms with an old disease. *N. Engl. J. Med.* 324: 1206–1207.

Okumura, H., Kurland, L.T., and Waring, S.C. (1995). Amyotrophic lateral sclerosis and polio: is there an association? In: *The Post-Polio Syndrome: Advances in the Pathogenesis and Treatment*, ed. M.C. Dalakas, H. Bartfeld and L.T. Kurland. *Ann. N.Y. Acad. Sci.* 753: 245–256.

Pezeshkpour, G.H. and Dalakas, M.C. (1987). Pathology of the spinal cord in post-poliomyelitis muscular atrophy. *Ann. N.Y. Acad. Sci.* **23**: 229–236.

Pezeshkpour, G.H. and Dalakas, M.C. (1988). Long-term changes in the spinal cord of patients with old poliomyelitis: signs of continuous disease activity. *Arch. Neurol.* 45: 505–508.

Plum, F. and Swanson, A.G. (1959). Central neruogenic hypoventilation in man. *Arch. Neurol. Psychiatry* 81: 531–560.

Ravits, J., Hallett, M., Baker, M., Nilsson, J., and Dalakas, M.C. (1990). Clinical and electromyographic studies of post-poliomyelitis muscular atrophy. *Muscle Nerve* 13: 667–674.

Sabin, A.B. (1980). Poliomyelitis. In: *Viral and Rickettsial Infections of Man*, vol. 5, ed. F.L. Horsfall Jr and I. Tamm, pp. 1348–1381. J.B. Lippincott, Philadelphia.

Sanders, D.B., Massey, J.M., and Nandedkar, S.D. (1987). Quantitative electromyography after poliomyelitis. *Ann. N.Y. Acad. Sci.* **23**: 189–200.

Sharma, K.R., Fraum-Kent, J., Mynhier, M.A., Weiner, M.W., and Miller, R.G. (1994). Excessive muscular fatigue in the postpoliomyelitis syndrome. *Neurology* 44: 642–646.

Sharief, M.K., Hentges, R., and Ciardi, M. (1991). Intrathecal immune response in patients with the post-polio syndrome. *N. Engl. J. Med.* 325: 748–755.

Sivakumar, K., Sinnwell, T., McLaughlin, A., Frank, J., and Dalakas, M.C. (1994). Abnormal energy metabolism in the fatiguing muscles of patients with the post-polio syndrome (PPS) using ^{31}P magnetic resonance spectroscopy (MRS). *Neurology* 44(S): 411.

Sivakumar, K., Sinnwell, T., Yildiz, E., McLaughlin, A., and Dalakas, M.C. (1995). Study of fatigue in muscles of patients with post-polio syndrome by in vivo ^{31}P magnetic resonance spectroscopy: a metabolic cause for fatigue. In: *The Post-Polio Syndrome: Advances in the Pathogenesis and Treatment*, ed. M.C. Dalakas, H. Barfeld and L.T. Kurland. *Ann. N.Y. Acad. Sci.* 753: 397–401.

Sonies, B.C. and Dalakas, M.C. (1991). Dysphagia in patients with the post-polio syndrome. *N. Engl. J. Med.* 324: 1162–1167.

Sonies, B.C. and Dalakas, M.C. (1995). Progression of oral-motor and swallowing symptoms in the post-polio syndrome. *Ann. N.Y. Acad. Sci.* 753: 87–95.

Spector, S.A., Gordon, P.L., Feuerstein, I.M., Sivakumar, K., Hurley, B.F., Dalakas, M.C. (1996). Strength gains without muscle injury after strength training in patients with post-polio muscle atrophy. *Muscle Nerve* 19: 1282–1290.

Stalberg, E. (1982). Electrophysiological studies of reinnervation in amyotrophic lateral sclerosis: In: *Human Motor Neuron Diseases*, ed. L.P. Rowland, pp. 47–59. Raven Press, New York.

Stein, D.P., Dambrosia, J.M., and Dalakas, M.C. (1995). In: *The Post-Polio Syndrome: Advances in the Pathogenesis and Treatment*, ed. M.C. Dalakas, H. Bartfeld and L.T. Kurland. *Ann. N.Y. Acad. Sci.* 753: 296–302.

Tomlinson, B.E. and Irving, D. (1977). The numbers of limb motor neurons in the human lumbosacral cord throughout life. *J. Neurol. Sci.* 34: 213–219.

Trojan, D.A. and Cashman, N.R. (1995). Anticholinesterases in post-poliomyelitis syndrome. In: *The Post-Polio Syndrome: Advances in the Pathogenesis and Treatment*, ed. M.C. Dalakas, H. Bartfeld and L.T. Kurland. *Ann. N.Y. Acad. Sci.* 753: 285–295.

Trojan, D.A., Gendron, D., and Cashman, N.R. (1993). Stimulation frequency-dependent neuromuscular transmission defects in patients with prior poliomyelitis. *J. Neurol. Sci.* **118**: 150–157.

Wiechers, D.O. (1987). Reinnervation after acute poliomyelitis. *Ann. N.Y. Acad. Sci.* **23**: 213–221.

Wiechers, D.O. and Hubbell, S.L. (1981). Late changes in the motor unit after acute poliomyelitis. *Muscle Nerve* 4: 524–528.

Windebank, A.J., Daube, J.R., Litchy, W.J., et al. (1987). Late sequelae of paralytic poliomyelitis in Olmstead County, Minnesota. *Ann. N.Y. Acad. Sci.* **23**: 27–38.

Windebank, A.J., Litchy, W.J., and Daube, J.R. (1995). Prospective Cohort Study of Polio Survivors in Olmsted County, Minnesota. In: *The Post Polio Syndrome: Advances in the Pathogenesis and Treatment.* eds. M.C. Dalakas, H. Bartfeld and L.T. Kurland. *Ann. N.Y. Acad. Sci.* 753: 81–86.

20 Peripheral neuropathy in HIV-1 infection

T.H. Brannagan III, T. McAlarney and N. Latov

Introduction

The acquired immune deficiency syndrome (AIDS), which is caused by the human immunodeficiency virus (HIV), is characterized by progressive failure of the immune system resulting in an inability to fight opportunistic infection and cancer. The neurological manifestations of AIDS were first reported in 1982 (Britton et al. 1982; Horowitz et al. 1982; Miller et al. 1982), and the entire neuroaxis may be affected. Neurological disease usually occurs as a consequence of opportunistic infection or lymphoma, but neurodegenerative syndromes such as dementia, myelopathy, or peripheral neuropathy may also occur in the absence of other infections or tumor, by as yet unknown mechanisms (Pitlik et al. 1983; Snider et al. 1983).

Peripheral neuropathy is one of the more common neurological complications of HIV infection. Most patients develop a predominantly sensory axonal neuropathy, but other neuropathic syndromes such as acute or chronic demyelinating neuropathies, mononeuritis or mononeuritis multiplex, autonomic neuropathy, or mono or polyradiculopathy may also occur (Table 20.1). This chapter will describe the different neuropathic syndromes which are associated with HIV-1 infection, review their epidemiology and pathogenesis, and discuss their clinical management and therapy.

Epidemiology

Classification and staging of HIV infection

Several classification schemes for staging HIV infections have been developed since AIDS was first described in keeping with our growing understanding of the disease and its mechanisms. Initially, patients with HIV infection were classified as having AIDS when they developed a defined opportunistic infection. Prior to HIV testing, the lymphadenopathy syndrome (LAS) described patients with lymphadenopathy, fevers, malaise, weight loss and night sweats (Abrams et al. 1984). Later, with the advent of HIV antibody testing, those with HIV infection but without AIDS-defining opportunistic infections were classified as having either AIDS related complex (ARC) or asymptomatic. ARC was characterized by fever, weight loss, diarrhea, fatigue, night sweats, lymphadenopathy and minor infections (Fauci and Lane 1987). In 1986, the Centers for Disease

Table 20.1 *Peripheral neuropathy syndromes in HIV infection*

1. *Predominantly sensory axonal neuropathy*
2. *Mononeuropathy or mononeuropathy multiplex*
   a. Vasculitis
   b. CMV infection
   c. Tumor – lymphoma or Kaposi's sarcoma
   d. Diffuse lymphocytic infiltrative syndrome
3. *Demyelinating neuropathy*
   a. GBS
   b. CIDP
4. *Polyradiculopathy*
   a. CMV infection
5. *Herpes zoster radiculitis*
6. *Drug toxicity*
   a. zalcitabine (ddC)
   b. didanosine (ddI)
   c. stavudine (D4T)
   d. isoniazid
   e. dapsone
   f. vincristine
7. *Autonomic neuropathy*

Note:
CIDP: chronic inflammatory demyelinating neuropathies; CMV: cytomegalovirus; GBS: Guillain-Barré syndrome.

Table 20.2 *Classification of HIV-1 infection*

1986 CDC Classification
Group I. Acute infection
Group II. Asymptomatic infection
Group III. Persistent generalized lymphadenopathy
Group IV. Other disease
- Subgroup A. Constitutional disease
- Subgroup B. Neurologic disease
- Subgroup C. Secondary infectious diseases
  - Category C-1. Specified secondary infections in the CDC definition for AIDS
  - Category C-2. Other specified secondary infections
- Subgroup D. Secondary cancers
- Subgroup E. Other conditions

1993 CDC Classification
$CD4^+$ lymphocyte categories
Category 1: ≥500 cells/μL
Category 2: 200–499 cells/μL
Category 3: <200 cells/μL

Clinical categories
Category A: asymptomatic HIV infection, persistent generalized lymphadenopathy, acute HIV infection
Category B: symptomatic conditions not included among Category C, that are related to cell-mediated immunity or requires management complicated by HIV infection (thrush, persistent fever or diarrhea, recurrent or multiple dermatome herpes zoster, peripheral neuropathy, etc.)
Category C: presence of any of 25 clinical conditions listed in the AIDS surveillance case definition

Sources: 1986 CDC Classification from Centers for Disease Control and Prevention. (1986). *MMWR* **35**:334–339; 1993 CDC Classification adapted from Centers for Disease Control and Prevention (1992). *MMWR* **41**(No. RR-17):1–19.

control (CDC) proposed a classification system (Table 20.2) which then became widely used (CDC 1986). In 1992, the CDC revised their classification system and included patients with fewer than 200 CD4 cells in their definition of AIDS (CDC 1992).

Prevalence of peripheral neuropathy in HIV-1 infection

Estimates of the prevalence of peripheral neuropathy in the AIDS or HIV-1 infected population is largely derived from institutional clinical and pathological studies. In the first large study of the neurological complications of AIDS, Snider et al. (1983) found that 50 of 160 patients with clinically defined AIDS, had neurological complications, and eight (10%) had a progressive neuropathy characterized by painful dysesthesias and distal symmetrical large and small fiber sensory loss. In 1985, Lipkin et al. reported 12 HIV-1 positive homosexual men with LAS who were referred for evaluation of sensory symptoms; six were part of a 200 patient study cohort of homosexual men with diffuse lymphadenopathy. Nine of the 12 had mononeuritis multiplex and three had distal symmetrical neuropathy (DSN). In a retrospective analysis of 352 patients with AIDS or generalized lymphadenopathy followed at the University of California San Francisco between 1979 and 1984, Levy et al. (1985) found 124 of 318 patients with neurological symptoms, and 33 (10%) had peripheral neuropathy syndromes including multiple cranial neuropathies, Bell's palsy, chronic inflammatory polyneuropathy, distal symmetrical neuropathy, and herpes zoster radiculitis.

In prospective studies, a larger percentage of patients had peripheral neuropathy. So et al. (1988) evaluated 40 hospitalized patients with AIDS and found 17 (40%) with clinical and electrophysiological evidence of distal symmetric polyneuropathy. The neuropathy occurred only in those with systemic illness of greater than 5 months duration. Janssen et al. (1988) evaluated 39 HIV-positive homosexual males with LAS. Nine patients had distal symmetrical polyneuropathy, nine had herpes zoster radiculitis, and six had mononeuropathy (two Bell's palsies, two bilateral carpal tunnel syndromes, and two ulnar neuropathies). All together, 15 of 39 (38%) of patients with LAS had neuropathy. Hall et al. (1991) reported that 34% of 94 patients with HIV-1 infection had clinical (19%) or electrophysiological (23%) evidence of a peripheral neuropathy, increasing to 45% in patients with AIDS. Six of those patients had other possible causes of neuropathy (diabetes mellitus, alcohol abuse, dapsone, isoniazid).

The multicenter AIDS cohort study is an ongoing longitudinal study of the natural history of HIV infection in over 5000 homosexual men without AIDS using the 1987 CDC definition in five USA cities (Baltimore, Washington, Pittsburgh, Chicago, and Los Angeles). The incidence of six neurological disorders (toxoplasmosis, cryptococcal meningitis, primary central nervous system (CNS) lymphoma, progressive multifocal leukoencephalopathy, dementia, and sensory neuropathy) was examined in 2641 homosexual men who were HIV positive. Sensory neuropathy was detected in 139 (5%) and had the highest yearly rate of increased incidence, when compared with the other neurological disorders. The incidence was less than 1 per 100 person-years for CD4 cell counts greater than 200, but increased to 3.43 per 100 with a CD4 count of 101–200 and 7.75 per 100 for CD4 cell counts of less than 100. The authors also examined the potential neurotoxic antiretrovirals didanosine (ddI), zalcitabine (ddC) and stavudine (d4T). Those taking ddI, ddC and d4T had an increased risk of developing sensory neuropathy, but the association did not reach statistical significance (Bacellar et al. 1994). A later report of the multicenter AIDS cohort study noted sensory neuropathy in 8% of those with CD4 counts of less than 200 without an AIDS-defining illness, 14% in those meeting the 1987 CDC definition of AIDS without dementia and 69% in those with HIV dementia (Selnes et al. 1995). All of these patients would meet 1993 CDC criteria for AIDS and in total 23% had sensory neuropathy.

Electrophysiological studies often revealed the presence of subclinical neuropathy in asymptomatic patients. Comi et al. (1986) found electrophysiological abnormalities in 11 of 15 patients with AIDS. Gastaut et al. (1989) found clinical or electrophysiological evidence of peripheral neuropathy in 50 of 56 patients infected with HIV-1. Fuller et al. (1991) found electrophysiological evidence for neuropathy in four of 30 patients with AIDS who did not have signs or symptoms of peripheral neuropathy. Chavanet et al. in 1989 prospectively studied peripheral nerve conduction in 57 HIV infected individuals. Forty patients were classified to stages CDC II–III, and 17 were in CDC stage IV. None of these patients had neurological signs or symptoms of neuropathy, but 20 (35%) had a decrease in at least one electrophysiologic measurement (H-reflex, sural or sciatic nerve conduction velocities, or sural nerve amplitude). Ten of the 40 patients in CDC stages II–III (25%), and 10 of 17 patients in CDC stage IV (60%), were affected, indicating that neuropathy occurs more commonly in the more advanced disease. In another prospective study, Husstedt et al. (1993) evaluated the development of distal symmetric neuropathy in 41 patients with HIV infection by clinical examination and electrophysiologic studies; 14 patients (33%) had peripheral neuropathy at study entry and 27 patients (64.3%) had neuropathy at the end of the 13±6 month follow up. $CD4^+$ T-helper cells declined from 274.3 to 203.9 during the study period. A study of 35 AIDS and five ARC patients, noted 15 with symptoms of neuropathy, 17 with signs of symmetrical polyneuropathy and 27 (68%) with signs of peripheral neuropathy on nerve conduction studies (Vishnubhakat and Beresford 1988). In two other studies, clinical and electrophysiological signs of peripheral neuropathy in the asymptomatic stage of HIV infection with high CD4 counts was uncommon (Ronchi et al. 1992; Barohn et al. 1993;

Connolly et al. 1995). Intravenous drug users, however, appeared to have peripheral neuropathy more commonly than homosexuals (Greenberg et al. 1992).

Pathological studies of the peripheral nerves in patients with HIV-1 infection revealed an even higher incidence of neuropathy. De la Monte et al. (1988) analysed 21 patients with AIDS (n=18) or ARC (n=3). Eleven of 21 (52%) had a clinically evident peripheral neuropathy; nine with DSN and two with CIDP. Two had symptoms of autonomic neuropathy. On pathological examination, 19 of 20 (95%) had evidence of neuropathy including demyelination (95%), axonal degeneration (74%), and mononuclear cell inflammation (84%). Mah et al. (1988) analysed sural nerve specimens obtained at autopsy from 25 HIV infected patients (24 with AIDS and one with ARC); 12 patients (48%) had a loss of myelinated fibers, and in 13 there was no abnormality. In a series of 24 patients who died with AIDS, eight of whom had clinically detectable neuropathies, all patients had evidence of Wallerian degeneration (Griffin et al. in press a).

The autonomic nervous system (ANS) may also be affected in HIV-1 infection. Cohen and Laudensloager (1989) examined 10 HIV positive patients. Five of the 10 patients had abnormalities on clinical ANS testing; four had AIDS and one LAS. None of the patients had presented with ANS dysfunction as an initial complaint. Similarly, Freeman et al. (1990) found significant abnormalities in autonomic function in HIV infected patients, especially those with AIDS, when compared with controls.

Peripheral neuropathy is rare in children with HIV-1 infection (Koch et al. 1989). Belman (1990) described two children who developed peripheral neuropathy; both had lymphoid interstitial pneumonia. One child had disseminated CMV infection and a symmetrical neuropathy of the lower extremities and the other had renal failure and a sensory neuropathy. A 5-year-old boy with symptomatic HIV infection developed an acute demyelinating neuropathy and recovered significantly over 8 months (Raphael et al. 1991).

Relative incidence of the different neuropathy syndromes

The relative incidence of the different types of neuropathy associated with ARC and AIDS was investigated by several authors, Miller et al. (1988) studied 30 homosexual men with peripheral neuropathy; 21 had ARC and nine had AIDS. Eighteen of the 30 had distal symmetrical polyneuropathy, ten had chronic inflammatory demyelinating polyneuropathy, two had mononeuropathy multiplex, and three additional patients had a progressive lumbosacral polyradiculopathy. Leger et al. (1989) also reported on the spectrum of peripheral neuropathy in 25 patients with neuropathy at different stages of HIV infection. Six patients with asymptomatic HIV infection had an inflammatory demyelinating polyneuropathy. Of five patients with ARC, three had DSN, one had CIDP, and one a mixed neuropathy. Fourteen patients had AIDS; 13 had DSN and one mononeuropathy multiplex.

Fuller et al. (1993) examined the incidence of neuropathy in a population of 1500 HIV positive patients, among those who were referred to the neurology service for evaluation over a 15 month period. Patients were excluded if they had been exposed to neurotoxins, or had diabetes, uremia or a family history of neuropathy and patients not referred for neurological evaluation would not be included. Of 331 patients with AIDS, 11.5% had distal sensory polyneuropathy, 0.6% had mononeuritis multiplex, 0.6% had lumbosacral polyradiculopathy and 3% had mononeuropathy. Of 763 ARC patients 0.1 % had mononeuritis multiplex (necrotizing vasculitis) and 3% had mononeuropathy. No patients had demyelinating neuropathies and none of the 565 HIV positive asymptomatic patients had peripheral neuropathy.

Though several larger series of demyelinating neuropathies including some with ten to 16 patients were reported (Cornblath et al. 1987; Miller et al. 1988; Thornton et al. 1991), most prospective studies have not encountered many cases. No cases were identified by So et al. (1988), McArthur et al. (1989), or Fuller et al. (1993). In a cohort study of 798 HIV positive patients detected by the US Air Force HIV screening program, which included many in the early phases of the HIV infection including 454 with greater than 600 CD4 cells, only the case of chronic inflammatory demyelinating polyneuropathies (CIDP) was found, which occurred in a patient with AIDS. No cases of Guillain-Barré syndrome (GBS) were identified in this series.

Summary of epidemiologic studies

It appears that peripheral neuropathy is common in HIV infection. In clinical series, 11.5–43% of patients with AIDS have a detectable clinical neuropathy (So et al. 1988; Vishnubhakat and Beresford 1988; Fuller et al. 1993). Electrophysiological studies may add some patients with a subclinical neuropathy (Comi et al. 1986, Vishnubhakat and Beresford 1988). This figure increases to between 48 and 100% in pathological studies (Mah et al. 1988; de la Monte et al. 1988; Griffin et al. in press a). Most patients have a sensory axonal neuropathy. There appears to be a stage-specific pattern of neuropathy with inflammatory demyelinating polyneuropathies (IDP) occurring early on, predominantly sensory axonal polyneuropathy, progressive polyradiculopathy, and autonomic neuropathy occurring during full-blown AIDS and mononeuritis multiplex occurring in all stages. Recognition of these distinct neuropathic syndromes is important because therapeutic strategies differ with the type of neuropathy.

Peripheral neuropathy syndromes in HIV-1 infection

Predominantly sensory axonal polyneuropathy

Distal symmetrical polyneuropathy (DSP) is the most common type of peripheral neuropathy seen in HIV-1 infection and occurs predominantly during the later stages of disease. Snider et al. (1983), first described this syndrome in eight patients with AIDS that developed neuropathy, seven had painful dysesthesias; six had symmetrical large and small fiber sensory loss in a stocking and glove distribution; six had depressed or absent ankle jerks, and four had distal weakness and wasting. In a study of 26 patients with AIDS and DSN (Cornblath and McArthur 1988), the most common complaint was pain in the soles of the feet (62%) and many of the patients walked on their heels to lessen the pain. Paresthesias involving the entire foot were noted in 38% of patients. The sensory symptoms were generally symmetrical, limited to the feet, and rarely occurred above the ankles. In 85% of patients there was elevated threshold to pain or vibration, and 95% had absent or reduced ankle reflexes. None of the patients complained of focal weakness but, on examination, 37% had weakness of intrinsic foot muscles. Serial examination revealed progression of the neuropathy in all the patients except one, with progressive decrease in the ankle reflexes. So et al. reported 13 patients with AIDS and DSN, symptoms and signs of peripheral neuropathy were generally mild and only three of the patients complained of pain. Weakness and atrophy was mild or absent and confined to the feet. At 6 months follow-up, six of the 13 patients had died of complications of AIDS and the remaining seven had no progression of their neuropathy. Bailey et al. (1988) reported six patients with DSN. Weakness and sensory changes were also present in the hands, but this was less marked than in the feet.

In the study by Snider et al. (1983), electromyography (EMG) and nerve conduction velocity studies in five of the patients were interpreted to indicate a predominantly demyelinating type of sensorimotor neuropathy. Subsequent detailed studies from several centers, however (Bailey et al. 1988; Cornblath and McArthur 1988; So et al. 1988) described axonal loss with a lesser degree of demyelination. Cornblath and McArthur (1988) found a pattern consistent with dying-back axonopathy, with denervation potentials in distal leg muscles. Bailey et al. (1988) found mild generalized slowing of nerve conduction velocities, with reduction in amplitudes of distal and proximal evoked responses, consistent with an axonopathy. So et al. (1988) detected amplitude reduction of sural nerve action potentials with normal or mildly decreased sensory and motor nerve conduction velocities, providing evidence of distal axonal degeneration.

Laboratory analysis of blood and urine for metabolic, infectious, toxic or nutritional causes of DSN were usually normal (Bailey et al. 1988; Cornblath and McArthur 1988; So et al. 1988; Winer et al. 1992). In Bailey's study of six patients, serological testing for cytomegalovirus (CMV), Epstein–Barr virus, herpes simplex virus, *Toxoplasma gondii* and *Cryptococcus neoformans* were negative. Fuller et al. (1989) noted a temporal association with clinical cytomegalovirus (CMV) infection in nine of 12 patients with painful peripheral neuropathy; however, immunocytochemical studies failed to reveal CMV in sural nerves from six of the nine patients obtained by biopsy or at necropsy. Direct CMV infection of peripheral nerve has not been demonstrated in any patient with distal symmetrical polyneuropathy associated with AIDS.

Analysis of cerebrospinal fluid (CSF) from patients with AIDS and DSN typically reveals acellular fluid with normal or moderately elevated protein concentrations of up to 1050 mg L^{-1} (Bailey et al. 1988; Cornblath and McArthur 1988). HIV may be cultured from the CSF of infected individuals with or without clinically evident neurological abnormalities including neuropathy (Hollander and Levy 1987).

The pathological changes in peripheral nerves were described by several investigators. Bailey et al. (1988) examined sural nerve biopsies from six patients with AIDS and DSN, and found axonal loss and segmental demyelination in all of the nerves, with perivascular mononuclear cell infiltrates in the epineurium of two specimens, and mononuclear cell infiltrates in the endoneurium of one. Complement or immunoglobulin deposition was not detected by direct immunofluorescence microscopy. Dalakas and Pereshkpour (1988) found axonal degeneration without inflammation in a sural nerve biopsy of a patient with AIDS and painful neuropathy. In a histoimmunopathologic study of 21 patients with AIDS or ARC, 11 of whom had DSN or chronic inflammatory demyelinating polyneuropathy (CIDP), de la Monte et al. (1988) found moderate to severe demyelination in 79%, axonal degeneration in 36% and mononuclear cellular inflammation in 37% of the cases. Symptomatic DSN patients had a mixed axonal and demyelinating neuropathy with only slight inflammation while patients with CIDP had moderate or severe inflammation and demyelination with a variable degree of axonal degeneration. Immunohistochemical staining of the inflammatory cells identified them as macrophages or T lymphocytes, predominantly of the $CD8^+$ cytotoxic/suppressor cell type. MHC class I antigens were expressed in the vasa nervorum endothelium, on mononuclear cells, and occasionally on nerve fibers. MHC class II antigens were expressed by endothelial cells, mononuclear inflammatory cells, and variable nerve fibers, including on Schwann cells. In a postmortem study of 24 patients who died with AIDS (Griffin in press a,b) eight of whom had clinical neuropathy, all 24 cases exhibited Wallerian degeneration of distal long cutaneous nerves. In two-thirds of the cases, activated macrophages were present in nerve and less so in dorsal root ganglia. Degeneration of unmyelinated pain fibers was observed in several patients, including in two patients who died shortly after the development of pain in their feet. Regeneration was virtually absent in both myelinated and unmyelinated fibers. Electron microscopic studies of nerves from affected patients usually reveal tubular reticular inclusions in endomysial or endoneurial vessels (Dalakas and Pezeshkpour 1988; Mezin et al. 1991), which can also seen in systemic lupus erythematosus (SLE) and dermatomyositis.

The spinal cord and dorsal root ganglia were also examined by several investigators. Rance et al. (1988) studied the spinal cord of four patients with DSN who died with AIDS, and found degeneration of both axons and myelin sheaths confined to the fasciculus gracilus, most severe in the upper thoracic and cervical segments. No perivascular inflammatory cells or opportunistic organisms were observed except for two inclusions 'consistent with CMV' in a single section. Examination of lumbar dorsal root ganglia (DRG) in one patient revealed a mild reduction in the number of sensory neurons, proliferation of satellite cells (residual nodules of Nageotte), and infrequent giant axonal swelling. A lymphocytic infiltration was seen in association with some of the nodules. This study suggested that DSN in AIDS may result from primary involvement of the dorsal root ganglia neurons, with subsequent central-peripheral distal axonal degeneration. Scaravilli et al. (1992) examined the spinal cord, and thoracic and lumbar DRG of 14 patients with AIDS and found pathological changes in the DRGs in seven of the 14 cases including neuronal loss and an increased number of nodules of Nageotte. Six of the seven cases with DRG neuronal loss also had gracile tract pallor. In two of the cases with gracile tract pallor, the pallor involved only the cranial gracile fasciculus, the region which contains the most distal segments of the longest axons of the DRG sensory neurons.

Other types of sensory neuropathy have also been described in HIV-1 infected patients. Several patients with a sensory ataxia or large fiber sensory neuropathy have been reported (Elder et al. 1986, So et al. 1990). One patient who developed numbness and ataxia at the time of seroconversion, died 2 years later and at autopsy, there was loss of neurons and inflammation in the sensory ganglia (Elder et al. 1986). Another patient with AIDS had migrant sensory neuritis of Wartenberg (Pavesi et al. 1994). The patient developed paresthesias, hypoesthesia and intermittent pain in the territories of eight non-contiguous cutaneous nerves at different times lasting a few days to 2 months over a period of a year. Nerve conduction studies and upper extremity somatosensory evoked potentials were normal. Though no nerve biopsy was obtained, previously described cases of this syndrome have had perineurial inflammation and fibrosis.

The syndrome of symmetric distal neuropathy can also be caused in HIV-1 infected patients by drug toxicity, necrotizing vasculitis, cryoglobulinemia and the diffuse infiltrative lymphocytosis syndrome (DILS). These are discussed separately in later sections. In addition, coexisting conditions, not related to HIV infection, such as diabetes mellitus, renal failure, alcoholism or B12 deficiency, can also cause a predominantly sensory axonal neuropathy as in patients without HIV infection.

Mononeuritis and mononeuritis multiplex

Mononeuritis and mononeuritis multiplex can occur early or late in the course of HIV infection (So 1992). The differential diagnosis includes vasculitis (Said et al. 1988), cryoglobulinemia (Lange et al. 1988, Stricker et al. 1992), lymphoma (Gold et al. 1988), and CMV infection (Said et al. 1991). It is an uncommon complication of HIV infection; it occurs in 0.1–3% of patients with ARC or AIDS (Levy et al. 1985; Fuller et al. 1993) and occasionally in a seropositive asymptomatic patient (Lange et al. 1988).

So and Olney (1991) and So (1992) noted the distinction between patients with mononeuritis multiplex early in the course of HIV infection (CD4 cells more than 180) and those late in the course of infection (CD4 less than 122). Eleven patients with $CD4^+$ T cell counts of 180–850 (mean 359), resolved spontaneously without treatment, though no mention of histology is provided. Patients with $CD4^+$ T cell counts of 2–122 (mean 30) had evidence of systemic CMV infection. In seven patients treated with gancyclovir, the neuropathy stabilized, whereas two untreated patients died within 3 months.

Mononeuritis multiplex with vasculitis or perivasculitis

Mononeuritis and mononeuritis multiplex can be a manifestation of necrotizing vasculitis, or polyarteritis nodosa, which affects medium size vessels. It can occur at any stage of HIV infection, and be the first sign of the disease. The predominant manifestation of vasculitic neuropathy is often a distal and symmetric polyneuropathy with weight loss, myalgias, weakness, and leg tenderness (Lange et al. 1988; Said et al. 1988; Gherardi et al. 1993). In most patients the vasculitis is non-systemic (Gherardi et al. 1993), although in some it is associated with systemic manifestations such as skin rash, arthritis, or hypertension. The clinical and laboratory features of reported cases of necrotizing vasculitis and HIV infection are summarized in Table 20.3. Patients generally had a monophasic course, without relapses and remissions. The inflammation was characterized by $CD8^+$ T cells and macrophages, with some studies showing HIV antigens in perivascular macrophages. Pathological studies showed inflammation and fibrinoid necrosis of arteries which were smaller than those typically affected in polyarteritis nodosa with systemic disease, with marked involvement of the microcirculation. The erythrocyte sedimentation rate (ESR) was usually elevated, and several patients were positive for hepatitis B surface antigen (Lange et al. 1988; Fuller et al. 1993). Hepatitis C antibodies were generally not tested. ANCA antibodies, which are associated with microscopic vasculitis (Jennette et al. 1994) were absent in two patients tested (Gherardi et al. 1993; Younger et al. 1996); however, ANCA antibodies may be non-specific in HIV infected patients as they are frequently elevated without clinical symptoms (Koderisch et al. 1990; Klaassen et al. 1992).

Mononeuritis multiplex has also been described in patients with HIV-1 infection in association with unspecified vasculitis (Gherardi et al. 1993). This type of vasculitis is defined by 1990 American College of Rheumatology criteria as involving small (less than 70 μm) vessels, with neutrophilic inflammatory vascular disease, mononuclear inflammatory vascular disease or other forms of transmural inflammation without associated necrosis, karyolysis, thrombosis or erythrocyte extravasation.

A milder form of mononeuritis or mononeuritis multiplex is associated with a pathological picture of perivasculitis, in which there are perivascular inflammatory cells but without vasonecrosis or fibrosis. Nine such patients were described by Lipkin et al. (1985). All

Table 20.3 *Necrotizing vasculitis with neuropathy in HIV infection*

Author	Age/risk Stage/CD4	Pattern	ESR │ cryo hepatitis serology	Cerebrospinal fluid	Biopsy	Treatment/ course
Bardin et al. (1987)	72 CDC II	Symm	│ B−	17W, P61	Necrotizing vasculitis (muscle)	Rapidly progressive
Bardin et al. (1987)	75 CDC II	Asymm	│ + B−	19W, P69	Necrotizing vasculitis (muscle)	
Calabrese et al. (1989)	42 AIDS/81	Symm	88 │ + B−			
Chamouard et al. (1993)	33 homosexual 480 480	Asymm	│ B+			
Conri et al. (1991)	62 BT CDC III/209	Symm	65 │ − B, C 62 │		Necrotizing vasculitis, vasculitis, angio-aneurysms	Steroids, PE-improved
Cornblath et al. (1993)	43 homosexual CDC III	Mononeuritis multiplex	62 │		Necrotizing vasculitis	Slow progression over 1 year
Cornblath (1988)						Prednisone/cyclophosphamide Developed AIDS and died in 4 months
Dalakas and Pezeshkpour (1988)		Mononeuritis multiplex⇒ symm			Necrotizing vasculitis (sural)	
Fuller et al. (1993)	57 ARC	Mononeuritis multiplex	│ B+		Large vessel vasculitis	Rapid deterioration died
Gherardi et al. (1989)	33 homosexual CDC 3 or 4	Symm	│ B−	Moderate pleocytosis increased protein		
Gherardi et al. (1989)	63 homosexual AIDS	Symm	│ B−	Moderate pleocytosis increased protein	HIV in vessel wall	
Gherardi et al. (1989)	74 homosexual AIDS	Symm	│ B−	Moderate pleocytosis		

Gherardi et al. (1989)	74 homosexual AIDS	Symm	B−	Moderate pleocytosis increased protein		
Lafeuillade et al. (1988)	65 BT	Symm	115 | +	Normal	Epineural fibrinoid necrosis	Improved with Melphalan, prednisone, died – stroke
Lange et al. (1988)	homosexual CDC II	Mononeuritis multiplex	| + B+	0 cells P 330	Necrotizing vasculitis (muscle)	No response to prednisone and cyclophosphamide, LTF after 6 months
Monteagudo et al. (1991)	32 IVDU CDC IV		B−		Necrotizing vasculitis	
Said et al. (1988)						Persisting (1 year) improvement with steroids
Said et al. (1988)						Persisting (1 year) improvement with steroids
Said et al. (1988)						Persisting (1 year) improvement with steroids
Valeriano-Marcet et al. (1990)	36 IVDU CDC III	Asymm	132 | − B−		Fibrinoid necrosis medium vessel (rectal)	Improved with prednisone
Weber et al. (1987)	37 CDC III	Asymm	117 | B+		Fibrinoid necrosis, PMN in vessel wall of sural	
Younger et al. (1996)	45 homosexual CDC III/361	Symm	77 | B, C−	6L P 41	Fibrinoid necrosis, thrombosis	Stabilized-steroids, cyclophosphamide

Note:
Asymm: asymmetrical; BT: blood transfusion; CDC: Center for Disease Control class; cryo: cryoglobulins; IVDU: intravenous drug user; L: lymphocyte; LTF: lost to follow-up; P: protein; PE: plasmapheresis; PMN: polymorphonuclear leukocyte; symm: symmetrical.

had sensory symptoms and focal weakness, some with cranial nerve involvement (CN IV, V, VII) or Babinski signs. All had a reduced CD4/CD8 ratio, but none had AIDS-defining opportunistic infections. The neuropathy appeared to follow a rather benign course; most patients resolved spontaneously or stabilized within 2 weeks to 4 months.

Cryoglobulinemia, which may be a cause of vasculitis, has also been described in several patients with HIV infection and mononeuritis multiplex (Lafeuillade et al 1988; Lange et al. 1988; Bardin et al. 1989; Stricker et al. 1992; le Lostic et al. 1994). One of the patients was positive for hepatitis B (Lange et al. 1988) and two tested negative for hepatitis C (Stricker and Kiprov 1993; le Lostic et al. 1994), which may be associated with cryoglobulinemia in the absence of HIV infection (Phillips and Dougherty 1991). Cryoglobulinemia has also reported to be associated with symmetric sensorimotor neuropathy and HIV infection (Calabrese et al. 1989).

Other causes of vasculitis, such as Lyme disease, can also cause neuropathy, as in patients without HIV infection, and should be routinely tested for in patients with mononeuritis multiplex.

Mononeuritis multiplex with CMV infection

CMV infection of the peripheral nerves is associated with a rapidly progressive multifocal neuropathy in the late stage of HIV infection. Most patients have fewer than 50 T4 cells. CMV infection, in general, appears to be more common in HIV infected homosexuals than intravenous drug users, although CMV neuropathy specifically was not examined (Greenberg et al. 1992). Nerve biopsies typically reveal multiple foci of endoneurial necrosis with inflammatory infiltrates of mononuclear and polymorphonuclear cells. CMV itself may be seen in endothelial cells of endoneurial capillaries, with surrounding inflammation (Said et al. 1991). This contrasts with necrotizing vasculitis, in which inflammatory cells and neutrophils cells are present around necrotizing epineurial arteries, but not in the endoneurium (Said et al. 1988). Cells with intranuclear and intracytoplasmic inclusions characteristic of CMV infection, which are also recognized by monoclonal antibodies to CMV may be present, but were found in only two of eight specimens in one series (Roullet et al. 1994). The characteristic pathological finding is therefore multifocal endoneurial neutrophilic inflammatory lesions without CMV inclusions.

Roullet et al. (1994) identified 15 consecutive cases of CMV multifocal neuropathy, based on markedly asymmetric neuropathy, CD4 count less than 100, exclusion of other causes of neuropathy, characteristic CMV cytopathic changes on nerve biopsy (two of eight), positive CSF culture (two of 13) or clinical improvement on anti-CMV therapy. Eleven of the patients did not have pathological or culture confirmation of the diagnosis, but 14 of the 15 had neurological improvement with gancyclovir or foscarnet. Patients typically presented with multifocal neuropathy, but isolated nerves can also be affected. In one case, hoarseness developed following CMV invasion of the laryngeal nerve (Small et al. 1989).

CSF findings are variable. Of 14 patients, CSF was normal in six, and four showed only an elevated protein of up to 1320 mg L^{-1}. Four patients had a CSF pleocytosis of 6–310/mm^3, usually with a polymorphonuclear predominance and protein elevation from 460 to 8200 mg L^{-1}. CSF culture was positive for CMV in two of 13. CSF PCR for CMV was positive in nine of ten patients.

Because of the difficulty of making a diagnosis of CMV infection in some cases, empiric treatment with ganciclovir or foscarnet, has been advocated in the setting of mononeuritis multiplex, CD4 count of less than 50/mm^3, and the exclusion of other causes of neuropathy.

Mononeuritis multiplex and lymphoma or Kaposi's sarcoma

Neuropathy can also be associated with lymphoma in HIV infected patients, and be the presenting symptom in the disease. It is usually manifest as a mononeuritis multiplex and results from lymphomatous invasion of the peripheral nerves (Gold et al. 1988; Fuller et al. 1993). Gold et al. (1988) reported four patients with HIV-associated lymphoma, in whom three had peripheral neuropathy as the presenting symptom. An additional patient diagnosed with Hodgkin's lymphoma developed ankle numbness and asymmetric facial weakness, but refused nerve biopsy. Cranial nerve involvement of the optic, oculomotor or facial nerves was relatively common. CSF examination revealed seven lymphocytes with normal protein concentration in one patient, 20 white blood cells, predominantly lymphocytes in another, and one had normal CSF. An elevated lactate dehydrogenase (LDH), may alert the physician to the presence of lymphoma (Gold et al. 1988).

Invasion of the peripheral nerves by Kaposi's sarcoma can also cause peripheral neuropathy. Levy et al. (1985) reported a case of brachial plexopathy and Kaposi's sarcoma, in which there was sarcomatous invasion of the peripheral nerves.

Facial palsies

Facial nerve palsies including bilateral facial palsy (Wechsler and Ho 1989) have been reported in HIV infection. They are most commonly seen at the time of seroconversion, but also occur at the ARC or AIDS stage of the disease (Belic et al. 1988; Murr and Benecke 1991). We have seen a patient with bilateral facial palsy as the presenting symptom of AIDS, at which time he had 28 $CD4^+$ T cells.

Unilateral or bilateral facial nerve involvement is also common in DILS. It is associated with parotid gland enlargement, sicca symptoms, low or absent autoantibodies (SS-A,SS-B, RF, ANA), $CD8^+$ lymphocytosis, diffuse visceral lymphocytic infiltration and low rate of progression or opportunistic infections (Itescu and Winchester 1992). It appears to be genetically restricted, occurring with HLA-DR5,6 in Afro-Americans and with HLA-DR6 in Caucasians. Symmetrical sensorimotor neuropathy (Guillon et al. 1987; Chaunu et al. 1989; Malbec et al. 1994) and motor neuropathy (Itescu et al. 1990) have also been reported in a few patients. In some cases the facial nerve palsies appear to be caused by local pressure by the parotid gland; AZT treatment often results in shrinkage of the parotid gland, with improvement of the facial palsy (Itescu and Winchester 1992). CNS manifestations of DILS have responded dramatically to AZT (Bachmeyer et al. 1995), but the effect on peripheral neuropathy has not been described.

Other mononeuropathies

Mononeuropathies in HIV infection may precede the development of mononeuritis multiplex, or occur as isolated events. In one study of 80 HIV infected patients (Winer et al. 1992), five had meralgia paresthetica, and two went on to develop generalized neuropathy. Bilateral brachial neuritis has been described at seroconversion with pain, weakness, winging of the scapula and muscle atrophy (Calabrese et al. 1987). One patient developed atrophy of the C5 muscles attributed to neuralgic amyotrophy. Two cases of intraneural hemorrhage into the ulnar nerve were reported (Ciccarese et al. 1991; Poppi et al. 1991).

Demyelinating neuropathy

Both acute and chronic demyelinating diseases have been reported to occur in HIV infection. They are characterized by weakness, absent reflexes, elevated CSF protein and improvement spontaneously or with immunosuppression (Cornblath et al. 1987; Riggs et al. 1987). Painful dysesthesias are unusual (Miller et al. 1988).

GBS may occur in otherwise asymptomatic HIV positive patients (Cornblath et al. 1987) or at the time of seroconversion, 1–5 months prior to appearance of HIV antibodies (Hagberg et al. 1986; Piette et al. 1986; Vendrell et al. 1987). GBS has rarely been reported in patients with full-blown AIDS (Mishra et al. 1985). Clinical presentation is usually similar in HIV-infected and non-infected patients (Winer et al. 1992; Thornton et al. 1991), although CSF pleocytosis is sometimes present (Cornblath et al. 1987; Miller et al. 1988). In one study of 29 patients with GBS in Zimbabwe, 55% of whom were HIV positive, those with HIV infection were more likely to have generalized lymphadenopathy, CSF pleocytosis, coexistent CNS disturbance, or history of other sexually transmitted diseases. In that study, there was no significant difference in the history of antecedant infection, age, cranial nerve involvement, need for mechanical ventilation, onset to maximal weakness or onset to improvement (Thornton et al. 1991). In another study, however, HIV infected patients had a worse outcome and none was walking at 6 months, despite the favorable prognostic factors of young age, normal CMAP amplitudes and treatment with plasmapheresis (Cornblath 1988).

Most patients developing CIDP are also in the early stages of HIV infection, although patients in the late stages of the disease have also been reported (Miller et al. 1988; Przedborski et al. 1988).

In some cases, patients suspected of having CIDP are found to have CMV neuropathy at autopsy. Morgello and Simpson (1995) reported a patient with multifocal weakness, CD4 count of 10, CSF cytoalbuminological dissociation (protein 1290 mg L^{-1}, WBC 2/mm^3), and conduction block, who had evidence of a multifocal CMV polyradiculopathy at autopsy. Said et al. (1991), also described segmental demyelination and remyelination in some nerves from patients with CMV multifocal neuropathy. The electrophysiology was more consistent with a multifocal axonal neuropathy, but conduction block was seen in the peroneal nerve of one patient.

Polyradiculopathy

Another syndrome associated with HIV-1 infection is polyradiculopathy, which is characterized by flaccid lower extremity weakness, sacral and lower extremity sensory loss, sphincter disturbances and CSF abnormalities. The most common cause is CMV infection (Eidelberg et al. 1986), but it may occur in the absence of CMV infection (So and Olney 1994), or be associated with syphilis (Lanska et al. 1988), lymphoma (Leger et al. 1992; Fuller et al. 1993), vasculitis (Oberlin et al 1989), toxoplasmosis (Kayser et al. 1990), tuberculosis (Bötzel 1993) or primary CNS lymphoma with lymphomatous meningitis (Klein et al. 1990).

In CMV polyradiculopathy, weakness is typically more prominent than sensory loss (Miller et al. 1990). One patient presented with an ALS-like syndrome, although with abnormal CSF (Behar et al. 1987). Polyradiculopathy is distinguished from CIDP by the presence of urinary retention, sensory loss in a saddle distribution and occasionally a sensory level. Cranial nerve and arm weakness are uncommon but may occur later in the course of the disease. WBC in the CSF is usually markedly elevated (mean 449) with a polymorphonuclear predominance and hypoglycorrhachia. The classical electrophysiological signs of polyradiculopathy are denervation in lower extremity and paraspinal muscles, with normal nerve conduction velocity and normal sensory potentials. In CMV infection these may be absent or masked by coexisting polyneuropathy (Beydoun 1991).

In one study (So and Olney 1994), 15 of 23 patients with AIDS and acute lumbosacral polyradiculopathy had CMV infection, and treatment with ganciclovir was followed by stabilization. Of the remaining eight patients, two had lymphoma and six had no identifiable cause with a relatively benign course. The CSF was the most useful diagnostic tool. Nine of the 15 (60%) patients with CMV infection had a positive CSF CMV culture, and 14 had a polymorphonuclear (PMN) pleocytosis. Nine of the 23 patients had a mononuclear pleocytosis, and only one had CMV infection. Magnetic resonance imaging (MRI) may show enhancement of the cauda equina (Bazan et al. 1991; Talpos et al. 1991).

Herpes zoster radiculitis

Herpes zoster radiculitis is a common manifestation of HIV infection, occurring early as well as in the symptomatic phases of the infection in about 10% of patients (Levy et al. 1985; Friedman-Kien et al. 1986; Janssen et al. 1988). Pain typically precedes the rash which develops in a dermatomal distribution on the face or trunk. Motor involvement and weakness can also occur in more severe cases (McArthur 1987). Oral treatment with acyclovir is usually effective (Sawyer 1988).

Toxic neuropathies

Several drugs used in the treatment of HIV or opportunistic infections can cause a distal symmetrical polyneuropathy. These include the nucleoside analogues, didanosine or dideoxinosine (ddI) (Lambert et al. 1990), dideoxycytidine or zalcitabine (ddC) (Dubinsky et al. 1989), and 2′,3′-didehydro-2′,3′-dideoxythymidine or stavudine (D4T), all which cause an axonal peripheral neuropathy. The toxicity of the nucleoside analog drugs is thought to be caused by their interference with mitochondrial DNA replication (Lewis and Dalakas 1995). ddC is a more common cause of neuropathy than ddI, and neuropathy is a major dose-limiting factor for both drugs. Lamivudine or 2′-deoxy-3′-thiacytidine (3-TC), is relatively non-neurotoxic, and is the least toxic to mitochondria. It has, however, been associated with exacerbation of a pre-existing neuropathy (Cupler and Dalakas 1995). Zidovudine (AZT) has not been associated with neuropathy (Bozzette et al. 1991), but is associated with myopathy. Predisposing factors for the development of toxic neuropathy include pre-existing neuropathy, low B12 and heavy alcohol use (Fichtenbaum et al. 1995).

In a phase I trial of ddI given twice daily (Lambert et al. 1990), 17 patients with AIDS and 20 patients with ARC were given ddI for up to 44 weeks. In eight patients, the major dose limiting factor was peripheral neuropathy characterized principally by pain in the legs, especially the soles of the feet, and beginning 55–201 days after the initiation of therapy. Neuropathy developed in nine of 19 patients whose total dose exceeded 12 mg kg^{-1} per day, but in only one of 18 patients who received a total dose of less than 2 mg kg^{-1} per day. Pain resolved spontaneously or significantly subsided 4–8 weeks after discontinuance in seven of the eight patients and persisted in one. The neurological examinations were unremarkable except for occasional decreased vibratory sensation or decreased ankle reflexes. Nerve conduction velocities were normal in six patients studied. Three patients were rechallenged at doses of 10 mg kg^{-1} per day without reccurrence of symptoms after 4–12 weeks. Another phase I study, Cooley et al. (1990) suggested that once daily dosing allowed higher daily doses of ddI, with a lower incidence of neuropathy.

In a phase I study of ddC (Yarchoan et al. 1988a), symptoms of neuropathy developed 9–12 weeks after initiation of therapy and were characterized initially by aching in the feet followed 2–3 weeks later by burning dysesthesias. Examination revealed decreased vibratory, pain and temperature threshold to the midcalf level with absent ankle jerks. Improvement in the neuropathy usually occurs 3–6 weeks after discontinuance of the ddC (Yarchoan et al. 1988a, Dubinsky et al. 1989).

Differentiating nucleoside-associated neuropathy from distal predominantly sensory neuropathy may be difficult. Discontinuing the drug should alleviate the symptoms, but there may be a 2-week worsening or 'coasting period', before improvement occurs (Berger et al. 1993). Children do not appear to develop neuropathy from nucleoside analogues (Dalakas et al. 1994).

Medication used in the treatment of opportunistic infections and tumors may also cause peripheral neuropathy. These include isoniazid for the treatment of tuberculosis, if supplemental pyridoxine is not taken (Figg 1991), vincristine used in the treatment of AIDS related Kaposi's sarcoma (Mintzer et al. 1985; Gill et al. 1990), and dapsone which can cause a predominantly motor peripheral neuropathy (Koller et al. 1977).

Autonomic neuropathy

Lin-Greenberger and Taneja-Uppal (1987) first reported a patient with AIDS and dysautonomia and severe orthostatic hypotension, intermittent diarrhea, impotence and decreased sweating. Craddock et al. (1987) described four of five patients with AIDS, who had syncopal reactions during fine-needle aspiration of the lung. One of these patients and four subsequent patients with AIDS or HIV infection had abnormal autonomic functions on formal testing. In another study comparing HIV-infected patients and normal subjects (Freeman et al. 1990), the HIV patients had abnormalities detected in multiple tests of autonomic function, and autonomic dysfunction occurred more frequently and with greater severity as the disease progressed from ARC to AIDS. There was no correlation between autonomic dysfunction and specific neurological signs, but the three patients with the most severe abnormalities had dementia, myelopathy and distal sensory neuropathy. Another study, however, did not find frequent autonomic involvement in HIV-infected patients (Lohmöller et al. 1987).

Autonomic failure could be due to pathology at multiple levels of the neuroaxis, including the brain, spinal cord or peripheral nerves (Freeman and Cohen 1993). Pathological abnormalities are detected at autopsy in sympathetic ganglia (Chimelli and Scaravilli 1991) and there is evidence of depletion of autonomic nerves in jejunal mucosa of HIV-infected patients (Batman et al. 1991). In addition, medications such as antidepressants, pentamidine or vincristine may cause autonomic dysfunction.

Pathogenesis

Identifiable causes of peripheral neuropathy in patients with HIV infection include CMV or herpes zoster infections, drug toxicity, or direct invasion by tumor cells, but these are only present in a minority of patients. In patients with GBS or CIDP, the mechanisms by which HIV infection might trigger the neuropathy are unknown. Some cases of vasculitis might be caused by vascular deposition of immune complexes, which are commonly found in HIV-infected patients (Gupta and Licorish 1984; Aguilar et al. 1988; McDougal et al. 1985), and most nerve biopsies exhibit deposits of IgM and complement in the blood vessel walls (Gherardi et al. 1993). In most patients, however, and in particular in those with the distal sensory neuropathy which is most commonly associated with HIV infection, the cause of the neuropathy is unknown. It is not known whether the nerve cell body or processes are primarily affected, or whether DRG neurons die by apoptotic cell death, which has been observed in DRG neurons (Shapshak et al. 1995), as well as in cortical neurons in HIV dementia (Adle-Biassette et al. 1995; Gelbard et al. 1995; Petito and Roberts 1995). Proposed mechanisms for the neuropathy include direct infection of neural cells by HIV or other opportunistic viruses, toxic effects of gp120 or other HIV proteins, injury by macrophages either directly or via release of cytokines or other toxic factors, autoimmune mechanisms, interference with growth factors, or metabolic effects. To date, however, none of these mechanisms has been proven to be responsible.

HIV is a member of the lentivirinae group of the retrovirus family. Other lentiviruses include the Visna/Maedi virus, caprine arthritis-encephalitis virus (CAEV), equine infectious anemia virus (EIAV), feline immunodeficiency virus (FIV), simian immunodeficiency virus (SIV), and human immunodeficiency virus (HIV-1 and 2). All lentoviruses are known to cause chronic neurological and/or immunological diseases. HIV-1 infects T helper cells and cells of the monocyte/macrophage lineage through interaction of its gp120 envelope glycoprotein with CD4 on the cells' surface, and becomes integrated into the cells' DNA by reverse transcription of the viral RNA. HIV-2, a related virus, also causes an immmunodeficiency syndrome, and is present primarily in Western Africa (Kanki et al. 1986). Following infection there is a period of clinical latency typically lasting several years, but during this time there is constant and rapid viral production with production of 10^9 virions per day, and with almost complete replacement of wild-type virus in 14 days (Ho et al. 1995; Wei et al. 1995).

Whether HIV-1 infects DRG neurons in vivo is controversial. In a study of dorsal root and sympathetic ganglia from patients with HIV-1 infection, Esiri et al. (1993) detected HIV-1 antigens (p24 or gp41) in macrophages in 58% of those with HIV infection and 71% of those with AIDS. No HIV-1 antigen was detected in neurons. There was a mild inflammatory response with increased T lymphocytes, macrophages and MHC II expression, beyond the usual resident macrophages present in normal ganglia was noted. Yoshioka et al. (1994) detected HIV-1 RNA in a few perivascular cells, but not neurons, in five of 16 cases by in situ hybridization using ^{35}S-labeled RNA probes specific for the pol region of the HIV genome, and in four of five cases by PCR using HIV-1 gag primers. HIV-1 can non-productively infect DRGs in vitro (Kunsch and Wigdahl 1991), and Brannagan et al. (1997) recently reported identifying HIV-1 DNA and RNA gag sequences in DRG neurons from patients with neuropathy using PCR amplified in situ hybridization and RT-PCR. HIV-1 DNA and RNA have also been recently identified in brain neurons of HIV-1 infected patients by similar techniques (Nuovo et al. 1994). In peripheral nerve, HIV-1 has also sometimes been found in rare macrophages (Gherardi et al. 1989; Wessenleigh et al. 1994). Viral tropism might be a factor in HIV-1 infection of the nervous system as distinct V3 sequences of the HIV envelope were found in the brains of patients with dementia compared with non-demented AIDS patients (Power et al. 1994), which suggests a role for gp120 or viral tropism in the development of dementia.

Fuller et al. (1989, 1993) reported an association between sensory neuropathy and CMV infection, which suggests that CMV infection of DRG neurons might be responsible. Others, however, have not been able to confirm a higher incidence of CMV infection in this type of neuropathy (Winer 1992), and examination of the DRGs in affected patients has not shown the presence of CMV in the majority of cases (Scaravilli et al 1992; Esiri et al. 1993; Yoshioka et al. 1994; Griffin et al. in press a,b). In the study by Esiri et al. (1993), no evidence of CMV infection of the ganglia was noted despite one patient having CMV encephalitis and another with systemic CMV infection. In an epidemiological study of intravenous drug users, with and without HIV infection, infection with HTLV-II was independently associated with the development of neuropathy, but this would not explain the neuropathy in most patients with HIV-1 infection (Dooneief et al. 1996).

HIV infected or activated macrophages, which can release cytokines or other neurotoxic factors have been implicated in the pathogenesis of AIDS dementia (Giulian et al. 1990, 1993; Lipton and Gendelman 1995), and might similarly have a role in the development of peripheral neuropathy. The number of HIV-1 infected macrophages in brain or peripheral nerves is relatively small, but gp120 alone appears to be able to activate macrophages to secrete neurotoxic factors (Lipton 1992; Giulian et al. 1993). The activation process might be enhanced by the loss of $CD4^+$ $TH2^+$ T cells which normally counteract macrophage activation by elaborating IL-4 and IL-10 (Choa et al. 1993; Wessenleigh et al. 1994, Tyor et al. 1995). Tardieu et al. (1992) reported that HIV-1 infected macrophages can damage neurons by direct contact, but cell to cell contact in the nervous system may in addition enhance macrophage activation (Gendleman et al. 1994). Several products of activated macrophages, including TNF-alpha, neural proteases, plasmin and urokinase have been shown to induce lesions when injected into peripheral nerve (Said and Hontebeyrie-Joskowicz 1992), and TNF-alpha has been shown to induce apoptosis in neuronal cells (Talley et al. 1995). Arachidonic acid, another substance released by activated macrophages, can activate neuronal *N*-methyl-D-aspartate (NMDA) receptors, resulting in influx of calcium ions, and stimulation of nitric oxide synthase. Accordingly, the neurotoxic effects are lessened by nitric oxide synthase inhibitors (Dawson et al. 1993), NMDA antagonists, and in some cases calcium channel blockers (Lipton and Gendelman 1995). Additionally, in peripheral nerve, macrophage-derived factors such as prostaglandin E2 and leukotrienes may sensitize C polymodal nociceptors, and contribute to the neuropathic pain and hyperpathia which is commonly seen in HIV-1 neuropathy (Griffin et al. in press b).

The gp120 glycoprotein itself has been implicated in the development of both HIV-1 associated dementia and neuropathy. It has been reported to activate brain macrophages (see above), induce apoptosis in neuroectodermal cells (Muller et al. 1992), and to bind to DRG neurons and damage the cells by activating the complement cascade (Apostolski et al. 1993, 1994). Its binding to DRG neurons appears to be mediated through an as yet unidentified glycoprotein receptor, and the interaction is blocked by antibodies to galactocerebroside, which also inhibit HIV-1 infection of neurons in vitro. Soluble gp120 can be found in the serum or CSF of HIV infected individuals (Buzy et al. 1992; Oh et al. 1992) and may be released by HIV infected macrophages in the nervous system.

Nutritional factors or interference with neurotrophic factors, has also been proposed as a mechanism of HIV-1 dementia or neuropathy. Nutritional deficiencies might result from a number of causes including anorexia, diarrhea, malabsorption, or continued hypermetabolism (Grunfield et al. 1992), and a deficiency in vitamin B12 was reported in some studies (Harriman et al. 1989; Kieburtz et al. 1991), but not confirmed by others (Robertson et al. 1993; Trimble et al. 1993; Veilleux et al. 1995). Impairment in the production of nerve growth factor (NGF), indirectly resulting from depletion of $CD4^+$ T cells, has also been proposed as a possible mechanism for HIV-1 neuropathy. Both IL-4 and IL-1, which stimulate NGF production in glial cells (Awatsuji et al. 1993; Brodie and Goldreich 1994), or fibroblasts (Heumann et al. 1987; Lindholm et al. 1988), respectively, are secreted by $CD4^+$ T cells and are decreased in late stages of HIV infection; however, demonstration of a decrease of NGF in HIV-1 neuropathy is lacking. In other studies involving neurotrophic factors, gp120 induced neuronal cell death in vitro was reportedly prevented by vasoactive intestinal peptide (VIP) (Brenneman et al. 1988; Pert et al. 1988), and gp120 appeared to block the neurotrophic effect of neuroleukin on culture (Apatoff et al. 1987; Lee et al. 1987). In both cases, sequence homology between the putative trophic factors and gp120 was given as an explanation for the observed effects; however, these findings were not confirmed by other laboratories, and neuroleukin was later shown to be identical to phosphoglucoisomerase, questioning its significance (Rogers et al. 1990).

Autoantibodies to peripheral nerve antigens have also been implicated in the development of some cases of HIV-1 associated peripheral neuropathy. Patients with HIV-1 infection frequently have hyperglobulinemia and increased autoantibody activity (Silvestria et al. 1995), and antibodies to brain antigens have been reported in HIV encephalopathy (Kumar et al. 1989). In preliminary studies of 20 HIV-infected patients with neuropathy, four patients (20%) had antibodies against peripheral nerve antigens; three patients with sensory neuropathy had increased titers of IgM anti-sulfatide antibodies, and one with a demyelinating neuropathy had increased IgM anti-MAG antibodies (Briani et al. 1996). Antibodies with the same specificities have been implicated in the development of neuropathy in non-HIV infected patients (Latov 1995). An increase in IgM autoantibodies might result from absence or dysfunction of regulatory T cells in combination with chronic stimulation by infectious agents bearing crossreactive antigens. Further studies are needed to determine the significance of these observations.

Therapy

Therapy of the demyelinating neuropathies, GBS and CIDP, is the same as for non-HIV-1 infected patients. Both conditions respond to plasmapheresis (Cornblath and McArthur 1988; Kiprov et al. 1988), or IVIG (Chimowitz et al. 1989; Malamut et al. 1992), and corticosteroids are useful in the treatment of CIDP.

Treatment of vasculitis presents a particular problem because cytotoxic agents, normally used in the treatment of arteritis, are contraindicated in significantly immunocompromised patients. Furthermore, Winchester et al. (1987) reported the development of full-blown AIDS shortly after the use of methotrexate in two patients with Reiter's syndrome. Dramatic improvements following corticosteroid therapy alone have been reported by several investigators (Said et al. 1988; Valeriano-Marcet et al. 1990, Chaumouard et al. 1993), and IVIG may be effective (Libman et al. 1995). Mononeuritis multiplex in the early stages of HIV infection, with perivasculitis, may be self-limiting and not requiring therapy (Lipkin et al. 1985).

Mononeuritis multiplex or polyradiculopathy associated with CMV infection is effectively treated with ganciclovir or foscarnet. The average time of survival in untreated patients with CMV polyradiculopathy is 3 weeks, with a 100% mortality rate (Kim and Hollander 1993). Because of the rapid progression, difficulty in diagnosis, and prompt response to treatment, some investigators advocate empiric treatment for presumed CMV infection in patients with mononeuritis multiplex or polyradiculopathy with fewer than 50 or 100 $CD4^+$ T cells or with endoneurial polymorphonuclear cells, even in the absence of definitive evidence of CMV infection. CMV strains resistant to ganciclovir have been reported (Tokumoto and Hollander 1993), and some patients who no longer respond to foscarnet or ganciclovir, may respond to the other drug (Miller et al. 1990; Roullet et al. 1994). There may be continued deterioration during the first 1–4 weeks of treatment (Roullet et al. 1994; So and Olney 1994), and recovery may continue for months. Lifelong maintenance therapy for CMV is usually required (Kim and Hollander 1993).

Several patients with polyradiculopathy or multifocal neuropathy improved following therapy with AZT (Yarchoan et al. 1987, 1988b; Dalakas et al. 1988; Fiala et al. 1988). The HIV-1 associated sensory axonal neuropathy, however, has not responded to any therapies including AZT (Cornblath and McArthur 1988; Smith et al. 1990), plasmapheresis (Kiprov et al. 1988), or a trial of peptide-T, an analogue of VIP (Simpson et al. 1994). Treatment in these patients is largely symptomatic, with the use of tricyclic antidepressants, anticonvulsants, salicylates, narcotic analgesics, or topical capsaicin (Cornblath and McArthur 1988; Simpson and Wolfe 1991).

References

Abrams, D.I., Lewis, B.J., Beckstead, J.H., Casavant, C.A., and Drew, W.L. (1984). Persistent diffuse lymphadenopathy in homosexual men: endpoint or prodrome? *Ann. Intern. Med.* **100**: 801–808.

Adle-Biassette, H., Levy, Y., Colombel, M., Pron, F., Natchev, S., Keohane, C., and Gray, F. (1995). Neuronal apoptosis in HIV infection in adults. *Neuropathol. Appl. Neurobiol.* **21**: 218–227.

Aguilar, J.L., Berman, A., Espinoza, L.R., Blitz, O., and Lockey, R. (1988). Autoimmune phenomena in human immuno-deficiency virus infection. *Am. J. Med.* **85**: 283–284.

Apatoff, B.R., Lee, M.R., and Gurney, M.E. (1987). HIV envelope protein antagonizes trophic effects of neuroleukin on central neurons. *Ann. Neurol.* **22**: 156.

Apostolski, S., McAlarney, T., Hays, A.P., and Latov, N. (1994). Complement dependent cytotoxicity of sensory ganglion neurons mediated by the gp120 glycoprotein of HIV-1. *Immunol. Invest.* **23**: 47–52.

Apostolski, S., McAlarney, T., Quattrini, A., Levison, S.W., Rosoklija, G., Lugaressi, A., Corbo, M., Sadiq, S.A., Lederman, S., Hays, A.P., and Latov, N. (1993). The gp120 glycoprotein of human immunodeficiency virus type 1 binds to sensory ganglion neurons. *Ann. Neurol.* **34**: 855–863.

Awatsuji, H., Furukawa, Y., Hirota, M., Murakami, Y., Nii, S., Furukawa, S., and Hayashi, K. (1993). Interleukin-4 and -5 as modulators of nerve growth factor synthesis/secretion in astrocytes. *J. Neurosci. Res.* **34**: 539–545.

Bacellar, H., Munoz, A., Miller, E.N., Cohen, B.A., Besley, D., Selnes, O.S., Becker, J.T., and McArthur, J.C. (1994). Temporal trends in the incidence of HIV-1 related neurologic disease: Multicenter AIDS cohort study, 1985–1992. *Neurology* **44**: 1892–1900.

Bachmeyer, C., Dhôte, R., Blanche, P., Tulliez, M., Sicard, D., and Christoforov, B. (1995). Diffuse infiltrative CD8 lymphocytosis syndrome with predominant neurologic manifestations in two HIV-infected patients responding to zidovudine. *AIDS* **9**: 1101–1102.

Bailey, R.O., Baltch, A.L., Venkatesh, R., Singh, J.K., and Bishop, M.B. (1988). Sensory motor neuropathy associated with AIDS. *Neurology* **38**: 886–891.

Bardin, T., Gaudouen, C., Kuntz, D., Dryll, A., Leibowitch, J., Lacroix, C., and Said, G. (1987). Necrotizing vasculitis in human immunodeficiency virus infection. *Arthritis Rheum.* **30**(suppl. 4): S105.

Barohn, R.J., Gronseth, G.S., LeForce, B.R., McVey, A.R., McGuire, S.A., Butzin, C.A., and King, R.B. (1993). Peripheral nervous system involvement in a large cohort of human immunodeficiency virus-infected individuals. *Arch. Neurol.* **50**: 167–171.

Batman, P.A., Miller, A.R.O., Sedgwick, P.M., and Griffin, G.E. (1991). Autonomic denervation in jejunal mucosa of homosexual men infected with HIV. *AIDS* **5**: 1247–1252.

Bazan, C., Jackson, C., Jinkins, J.R., and Barohn, R.J. (1991). Gadolinium-enhanced MRI in a case of cytomegalovirus polyradiculopathy. *Neurology* **41**: 1522–1523.

Behar, R., Wiley, C., and McCutchan, J.A. (1987). Cytomegalovirus polyradiculoneuropathy in acquired immune deficiency syndrome. *Neurology* **37**: 557–561.

Belic, L., Georges, A.J., Vuillecard, E. et al. (1988). Peripheral facial paralysis indicating HIV infection. *Lancet* **ii**: 1421–1422.

Belman, A.L. (1990). AIDS and pediatric neurology. *Neurol. Clin.* **8**: 571–603.

Berger, A.R., Arezzo, J.C., Schaumburg, H.H., Skowron, G., Merigan, T., Bozzette, S., Richman, D., and Soo, W. (1993). 2′,3′-Dideoxycytidine (ddC) toxic neuropathy: a study of 52 patients. *Neurology* **43**: 358–362.

Beydoun, S.R. (1991). Misdiagnosis of cytomegalovirus polyradiculopathy, coexisting with HIV neruopathy. *Muscle Nerve* **14**: 575–576.

Bötzel, K. (1993). Tuberkulöse Radikulomyelitis-gut therapierbar nur bei frühem Erkennen. *Der Nervenar.* **64**: 282–283.

Bozette, S.A., Santangelo, J., Villasana, D., Fraser, A., Wright, B., Jacobsen, C., Hayden, E., Schnack, J., Spector, S.A., and Richman, D.D. (1991). Peripheral nerve function in persons with asymptomatic or minimally symptomatic HIV disease: absence of zidovudine neurotoxicity. *J. Acq. Im. Def. Syn.* **4**: 851–855.

Brannagan, T.H., Nuovo, G.J., Hays, A.P., and Latov, N. (1997). HIV infection of dorsal root ganglion neurons detected by PCR in situ hybridization. *Ann. Neurol.* (in press).

Brenneman, D.E., Westbrook, G.L., Fitzgerald, S.P., Ennist, D.L., Elkins, K.L., Ruff, M.R., and Pert, C.B. (1988)., Neuronal cell killing by the envelope protein of HIV and its prevention by vasoactive intestinal peptide. *Nature* **353**: 639–642.

Briani, C., Dalakas, M., Zakir, R., Revesz, K., Berger, J., Sivac, M., Brannagan, T., Britton, C., and Latov, N. (1996). AIDS neuropathy: presence of autoantibodies to peripheral nerve antigens (Abstract). *Neurology* **46**: A236.

Britton, C.B., Marruardt, M.D., Koppel, B., Garvey, G., and Miller, J.R. (1982). Neurological complications of the gay immunosuppressed syndrome: clinical and pathological features. *Ann. Neurol.* **12**: 80.

Brodie, C. and Goldreich, N. (1994). Interleukin-4 modulates the proliferation and differentiation of glial cells. *J. Neuroimmunol.* **55**: 91–97.

Buzy, J., Brenneman, D.E., Pert, C.B., Martin, A., Salazar, A., and Ruff, M.R. (1992). Potent gp120-like neurotoxic activity in the cerebrospinal fluid of HIV-infected individuals is blocked by peptide T. *Brain Res.* **598**: 10–18.

Calabrese, L.H., Estes, M., Yen-Lieberman, B., Proffitt, M.R., Tubbs, R., Fishleder, A.J., and Levin, K.H. (1989). Systemic vasculitis in association with human immunodeficiency virus infection. *Arthritis Rheum.* **32**: 569–576.

Calabrese, L.H., Proffitt, M.R., Levin, K.H., Yen-Lieberman, B., and Starkey, C. (1987). Acute infection with the human immunodeficiency virus associated with acute brachial neuritis and exanthematous rash. *Ann. Intern. Med.* **107**: 849–851.

Centers for Disease Control. (1986)., Classification system for human T lymphocyte virus type III/lymphadenopathy-associated virus infections. *MMWR* **35**: 334–339.

Centers for Disease Control and Prevention. (1992). 1993 revised classification system for HIV infection and expanded surveillance case definition for AIDS among adolescents and adults. *MMWR* **41**(No. RR-17) 1–19.

Chamouard, J.M., Smadja, D., Chaunu, M.P., and Bouche, P. (1993). Neuropathie par vasculite nécrosante au cours de l'infection par le vih1. *Rev. Neurol.* **149**: 358–361.

Chaunu, M.P., Ratinahirana, H., Raphael, M., Henin, D., Leport, C., Brun-Vezinet, F., Leger, J.-M., Brunet, P., and Hauw, J.-J. (1989). The spectrum of changes on 20 nerve biopsies in patients with HIV infection. *Muscle Nerve* **12**: 452–459.

Chavanet, P., Solary, E., Giroud, M., Waldner, A., Beuriat, P., Nordman, P., and Portier, H. (1989). Infraclinical neuropathies related to immunodeficiency virus infection associated with higher T-helper cell count. *J. Acq. Immune Def. Synd.* **2**: 564–569.

Chimmelli, L. and Scaravilli, F. (1991). Morphological changes in the autonomic nervous system of patients with AIDS. In *Proceedings of the Seventh International Conference on Neuroscience of HIV Infection*. Padova, Italy, p. 89.

Chimowitz, M.I., Audet, A.M.J., Hallet, A., and Kelly, J.J. (1989). HIV-associated CIDP. *Muscle Nerve* **12**: 695–696.

Choa, C.C., Molitor, T.W., and Hu, S. (1993). Neuroprotective role of IL4 against activated microglia. *J. Immunol.* **151**: 1473.

Ciccarese, E., Staffa, G., Brusori, S., Acciarri, N., and Gambari, P.I. (1991). A rare case of spontaneous intraneural hemorrhage in a patient with AIDS. *Radiol. Med.* **81**: 169–171.

Cohen, J.A. and Laudensloager, M. (1989). Autonomic nervous system involvement in patients with human immunodeficiency virus infection. *Neurology* **29**: 1111–1112

Comi, G., Medaglini, S., Galardi, G., Comola, M., Corbo, M., Nemmi, R., Lazzarin, A., Irato, L., and Moroni, M. (1986). Subclinical neuromuscular involvement in acquired immune deficiency syndrome. *Muscle Nerve* **9**: 665.

Connolly, S., Manji, H., McAllister, R.H., Griffin, G.B., Loveday, C., Kirkis, C., Sweeney, B., Sartawi, O., Durrance, P., Fell, M., Boland, M., Fowler, C.J., Newman, S.P., Weller, I.V.D., and Harrison, M.J.G. (1995). Neurophysiological assessment of peripheral nerve and spinal cord function in asymptomatic HIV-1 infection: results from the UCMSM/Medical Research Council neurology cohort. *J. Neurol.* **242**: 406–414.

Conri, C., Mestre, C., Constans, J., and Vital, C. (1991). Vascularite type périartérite noueuse et infection par le virus de l'immunodéficience humaine. *Red. Med. Intern* **12**: 47–51.

Cooley, T.P., Kunches, L.M., Saunders, C.A., Ritter, J.K., Perkins, C.J., McLaren, C., McCaffrey, R.P., and Liebman, H.A. (1990). Once-daily administration of 2′,3′-dideoxyinsosine (ddI) in patients with the acquired immunodeficiency syndrome or AIDS-related complex. *N. Engl. J. Med.* **322**; 1340–1345.

Cornblath, D.R. (1988). Treatment of the neuromuscular complications of human immunodeficiency virus infection. *Ann. Neurol.* **23**(suppl.): S88–S91.

Cornblath, D.R. and McArthur, J.C. (1988). Predominantly sensory neuropathy in patients with AIDS and AIDS-related complex. *Neurology* **38**: 794–796.

Cornblath, D.R., McArthur, J.C., Kennedy, P.G.E., Witte, A.S., and Griffin, J.W. (1987). Inflammatory demyelinating peripheral neuropathies associated with human T-cell lymphotropic virus type III infection. *Ann. Neurol.* **21**: 32–40.

Cornblath, D.R., McArthur, J.C., Parry, G.J.G., and Griffin, J.W. (1993). Peripheral neuropathies in human immunodeficiency virus infection. In *Peripheral Neuropathy*, 3rd edn, ed. P.J. Dyck, P.K. Thomas et al., pp. 1343–1353. Philadelphia: W.B. Saunders.

Craddock, C., Pasvol, G., Bull, R., Protheroe, A., and Hopkin, J. (1987). Cardiorespiratory arrest and autonomic neuropathy in AIDS. *Lancet* **2**: 16–18.

Cupler, E.J. and Dalakas, M.C. (1995). Exacerbation of peripheral neuropathy by lamivudine. *Lancet* (letter) **345**: 460–461.

Dalakas, M.C., Illa, I., and Monzon, M. (1994). Retrovirus-related neuromuscular diseases. In *Immunology of Neuromuscular Disease*, ed. H. Hohlfeld, pp. 256–288. Boston: Kluwar Publishing.

Dalakas, M.C. and Pezeshkpour, G.H. (1988). Neuromuscular diseases associated with human immunodeficiency virus infection. *Ann. Neurol.* **23**(suppl.): S38–48.

Dalakas, M.C., Yarchoan, R., Spitzer, R., Elder, G., and Sever, J.L. (1988). Treatment of human immunodeficiency virus-related polyneuropathy with 3′azido-2′,3′-dideoxythymidine. *Ann. Neurol.* **23**(suppl.): S92–94.

Dawson, V.L., Dawson, T.M., Uhl, G.R., and Synder, S.H. (1993). Human immunodeficiency virus type 1 coat protein neurotoxicity mediated by nitric oxide in primary cortical cultures. *Proc. Natl Acad. Sci. USA* **90**: 3256–3259.

De la Monte, S.M., Gabuzda, D.H., Ho, D.D., Brown, R.H., Hedley-Whyte, E.T., Schooley, R.T., Hirsh, M.S., and Bhan, A.K. (1988). Peripheral neuropathy in the acquired immunodeficiency syndrome. *Ann. Neurol.* **23**: 485–492.

Dooneief, G., Marlink, R., Bell, K., Marder, K., Renjifo, B., Stern, Y., and Mayeux, R. (1996). Neurologic consequences of HTLV-II infection in injection drug users. *Neurology* **46**: 1556–1560.

Dubinsky, R.M., Yarchoan, R., Dalakas, M., and Broder, S. (1989). Reversible axonal neuropathy from the treatment of AIDS and related disorders with 2′,3′-dideoxycytidine (ddC). *Muscle Nerve* **12**: 856–860.

Eidelberg, D., Sotrel, A., Vogel, H., Walker, P., Kleefield, J., and Crumpacker, C.S. (1986). Progressive polyradiculopathy in acquired immune deficiency syndrome. *Neurology* **36**: 912–916.

Elder, G., Dalakas, M., Pezeshkpour, G., and Sever, J. (1986). Ataxic neuropathy due to ganglioneuronitis after probable acute human immunodeficiency virus infection. *Lancet* **ii**: 1275–1276.

Esiri, M.M., Morris, C.S., and Millard, P.R. (1993). Sensory and sympathetic ganglia in HIV-1 infection: immunocytochemical demonstration of HIV-1 viral antigens, increased MHC class II antigen expression and mild reactive inflammation. *J. Neurol. Sci.* **114**: 178–187.

Fauci, A.S., and Lane, H.C. (1987). The acquired immunodeficiency syndrome. In *Harrison's Principles of Internal Medicine*, 11th edn, ed. E. Braunwald et al., pp. 1392–1396. New York: McGraw-Hill.

Fiala, M., Cone, L.A., Cohen, N., Patel, D., Williams, K., Casareale, D., Shapshak, P., and Tourtelotte, W. (1988). Responses of neurologic complications of AIDS to 3′-azido-3′-deoxythymidine and 9-(1,3-dihydroxy-2-propoxymethyl) guanine. I. Clinical features. *Rev. Infect. Dis.* **10**: 250–256.

Fichtenbaum, C.J., Clifford, D.B., and Powderly, W.G. (1995). Risk factors for Dideoxynucleoside-induced toxic neuropathy in patients with the human immunodeficiency virus infection. *J. Acq. Immune Def. Synd. Hum. Retrovir.* **10**: 169–174.

Figg, W.D. (1991). Peripheral neuropathy in HIV patient after isoniazid therapy initiated. DICP, *Ann. Pharmacother.* **25**: 100–101.

Freeman, R. and Cohen, J.A. (1993). Autonomic Failure and AIDS. In *Clinical Autonomic Disorders: Evaluation and Management*, ed. P.A. Low. Boston: Little, Brown and Company.

Freeman, R., Roberts, M.S., Friedman, L.S., and Broadbridge, C. (1990). Autonomic function and human immunodeficiency virus infection. *Neurology* **40**: 575–580.

Friedman-Kien, A.E., Lafleur, F.L., Gendler, E., Hennessey, N.P., Montagna, R., Halbert, S., Rubinstein, P., Krasinski, K., Zang, E., and Poiesz, B. (1986). Herpes zoster: a possible early clinical sign for development of acquired immunodeficiency syndrome in high-risk individuals. *J. Am. Acad. Dermatol.* **14**: 1023–1028.

Fuller, G.N., Jacobs, J.M., and Guiloff, R.J. (1989). Association of painful neuropathy in AIDS with cytomegalovirus infection. *Lancet* **2**: 937–941.

Fuller, G.N., Jacobs, J.M., and Guiloff, R.J. (1991). Subclinical peripheral nerve involvement in AIDS: an electrophysiological and pathological study. *J. Neurol. Neurosurg Pyschiatry* **54**: 318–324.

Fuller, G.N., Jacobs, J.M., and Guiloff, R.J. (1993). Nature and incidence of peripheral nerve syndromes in HIV infection. *J. Neurol. Neurosurg. Psychiatry* **56**: 372–381.

Gastaut, J.L., Gastaut, J.A., Pellissier, J.F., Tapko, J.B., and Weill, O. (1989). Neuropathies Peripheriques au cours de l'infection par le virus de l'immunod fience humaine. *Rev. Neurol.* **145**: 451–459.

Gelbard, H.A., James, H.J., Sharer, L.R., Perry, S.W., Saito, Y., Kazee, A.M., Blumberg, B.M., and Epstein, L.G. (1995). Apoptotic neurons in brains from paediatric patients with HIV-1 encephalitis and progressive encephalopathy. *Neuropathol. Appl. Neurobiol.* **21**: 208–217.

Gendelman, H.E., Lipton, S.A., Tardieu, M., Bukrinsky, M.I., and Nottet, H.S.L.M. (1994). The neuropathogenesis of HIV-1 infection. *J. Leuk. Biol.* **56**: 389–398.

Gherardi, R., Belec, L., Mhiri, C., Gray, F., Lescs, M.C., Sobel, A., Guillevin, L., and Wechsler, J. (1993). The spectrum of vasculitis in human immunodeficiency virus-infected patients. *Arthritis Rheum.* **36**: 1164–1174.

Gherardi, R., Lebargy, F., Gaulard, P., Mhiri, C., Bernaudin, J.F., and Gray, F. (1989). Necrotizing vasculitis and HIV replication in peripheral nerves. *N. Engl. J. Med.* **321**: 685–686.

Gill, P., Rarick, M., Bernstein-Singer, M., Harb, M., Espina, B., Shaw, V., and Levine, A. (1990). Treatment of advanced Kaposi's sarcoma using a combination of bleomycin and vincristine. *Am. J. Clin. Oncol.* **13**: 315–319.

Giulian, D., Wendt, E., Vaca, K., and Noonan, C.A. (1993). The envelope glycoprotein of human immunodeficiency virus type 1 stimulates release of neurotoxins from monocytes. *Proc. Natl Acad. Sci. USA* **90**: 2769–2773.

Giulian, D., Vaca, K., and Noonan, C.A. (1990). Secretion of neurotoxins by mononuclear phagocytes infected with HIV-1. *Science* **250**: 1593–1596.

Gold, J.E., Jimenez, E., and Zalusky, R. (1988). Human immunodeficiency virus-related lymphoreticular malignancies and peripheral neurologic disease. *Cancer* **61**: 2318–2324.

Greenberg, A.E., Thomas, P.A., Landesman, S.H., Mildvan, D., Seidlin, M., Friedland, G.H., Holzman, R., Starreett, B., Braun, J., Bruan, E.L., and Evans, R.F. (1992). The spectrum of HIV-1–related disease among outpatients in New York City. *AIDS* **6**: 849–859.

Griffin, J.W., Crawford, T.O., Tyor, W.R., Glass, J.D., Price, D.L., Cornblath, D.R., and McArthur, J.C., Sensory neuropathy in AIDS. I. Neuropathology. *Brain* (in press a).

Griffin, J.W., Tyor, W.R., Glass, J.D., Li, C.Y., Crawford, T.O., Lobato, C., Wesselingh, S.L., Griffin, D.E., and McArthur, J.C., Sensory neuropathy in AIDS. II. Immunopathology. *Brain* (in press b).

Grunfield, C., Pange, M., Shimizu, L., Sigenaga, J.K., Jensen, P., and Feingold, K.R. (1992). Resting energy expenditure, caloric intake and short-term weight change in human immunodeficiency virus infection and the acquired immunodeficiency syndrome. *Am. J. Clin. Nutr.* **55**: 455–460.

Guillon, J.M., Fouret, P., Mayaud, C., Picard, F., Raphael, M., Touboul, J.L., Chaunu, M.P., Hauw, J.J., and Akoun, G. (1987). Extensive t8–positive lympocytic visceral infiltration in a homosexual man. *Am. J. Med.* **82**: 655–661.

Gupta, S. and Licorish, K. (1984). Circulating immune complexes in AIDS. *N. Engl. J. Med.* **310**: 1510–1531.

Hagberg, L., Malmvall, B.-E., Svennerholm, L. et al. (1986). Guillain-Barré syndrome as an early manifestation of HIV central nervous system infection. *Scand. J. Infect. Dis.* **18**: 591–592.

Hall, C.D., Sunder, C.R., Messenheimer, J.A., Wilkins, J.W., Robertson, W.T., Whaley, R.A., and Robertson, K.R. (1991). Peripheral neuropathy in a cohort of human immunodeficiency virus-infected patients. Incidence and relationship to other nervous system dysfunction. *Arch. Neurol.* **48**: 1273–1274.

Harriman, G.R., Smith, P.D., Horne, M.K., Fox, C.H., Koenig, S., Lack, E.E., Lane, H.C., and Fauci, A.S. (1989). Vitamin B12 malabsorption in patients with acquired immunodeficiency syndrome. *Arch. Intern. Med.* **149**: 2039–2041.

Heumann, R., Lindholm, D., Bandtlow, C., Meyer, M., Radeke, M., Misko, T.P., Shooter, E., and Thoenen., H. (1987). Differential regulation of mRNA encoding nerve growth factor and its receptor in rat sciatic nerve during development, degeneration, and regeneration: Role of macrophages. *Proc. Natl Acad. Sci. USA* **84**: 8735–8739.

Ho, D.D., Neumann, A.U., Perelson, A.S., Chen, W., Leonard, J.M., and Markowitz, M. (1995). Rapid turnover of plasma virions and CD4 lymphocytes in HIV-1 infection. *Nature* **373**: 123–126.

Hollander, H. and Levy, J.A. (1987). Neurologic abnormalities and recovery of human immunodeficiency virus from cerebrospinal fluid. *Ann. Intern. Med.* **106**: 692–695.

Horowitz, S.L., Benson, D.F., Gottlieb, M.S., Davos, I., and Bentson, J.R. (1982). Neurological complications of gay-related immunodeficiency disorder. *Ann. Neurol.* **12**: 80.

Husstedt, I.W., Grotemeyer, K.H., Busch, H., and Zidek, W. (1993). Progression of distal-symmetric polyneuropathy in HIV infection: a prospective study. *AIDS* **7**: 1069–1073.

Itescu, S., Brancato, L.J., Buxbaum, J., Gregersen, P.K., Rizk, C.C., Croxson, T.S., Solomon, G.E., and Winchester, R. (1990). A diffuse infiltrative CD8 lymphocytosis syndrome in human immunodeficiency virus (HIV) infection: a host immune response associated with HLA-DR5. *Ann. Intern. Med.* **112**: 3–10.

Itescu, S. and Winchester, R. (1992). Diffuse infiltrative lymphocytosis syndrome: a disorder occurring in human immunodeficiency virus-1 infection that may present as a sicca syndrome. *Rheum. Dis. Clin. N. Am.* **18**: 683–697.

Janssen, R.S., Saykin, A.J., Kaplan, J.E., Spira, T.J., Pinsky, P.F., Sprehn, G.C., Hoffman, J.C., Mayer, W.B., and Schonberger, L.B. (1988). Neurological complications of human immunodeficiency virus infection in patients with lymphadenopathy syndrome. *Ann. Neurol.* **23**: 49–55.

Jennette, J.C., Falk, R.J., Andrassy, K., Bacon, P.A., Churg, J., Gross, W.L., Hagen, E.C., Hoffman, G.S., Hunder, G.G., Kallenberg, C.G.M., McCluskey, R.T., Sinico, R.A., Rees, A.J., van, Es, L.A., Waldherr, R., and Wiik, A. (1994). Nomenclature of systemic vasculitides. *Arthritis Rheum.* **37**: 187–192.

Kanki, P.J., Barin, F., M'Boup, S., Allan, J.S., Romet-Lemonne, J.L., Marlink, R., McLane, M.F., Lee, T.H., Arbeille, B., Denis, F., and Essex, M. (1986). New human T-lymphotropic retrovirus related to simian T-lymphotropic virus type III (STLV-IIIAGM). *Science* **232**: 238–243.

Kayser, C., Campbell, R., Sartorious, C., and Bartlett, M. (1990). Toxoplasmosis of the conus medullaris in a patient with hemophilia A-associated AIDS. Case report. *J. Neurosurg.* **73**: 951–953.

Kieburtz, K.D., Giang, D.W., Schiffer, R.B., and Vakil, N. (1991). Abnormal vitamin B12 metabolism in human immunodeficiency virus infection. Association with neurological dysfunction. *Arch. Neurol.* **48**: 312–314.

Kim, Y.S. and Hollander, H. (1993). Polyradiculopathy due to cytomegalovirus: report of two cases in which improvement occurred after prolonged therapy and review of the literature. *Clin. Infect. Dis.* **17**: 32–37.

Kiprov, D., Pfaeffl, W., Parry, G., Lippert, R., Lang, W., and Miller, R. (1988). Antibody-mediated peripheral neuropathies associated with ARC and AIDS: successful treatment with plasmapheresis. *J. Clin. Apheresis* **4**: 3–7.

Klaassen, R.J.L., Goldschmeding, R., Dolman, K.M., Vlekke, A.B.J., Weigel, H.M., Eeftinck Schattenkerk, J.K.M., Mulder, J.W., Westedt, M.L., and Von Dem, A.E.G.K.R. (1992). Anti-neutrophil cytoplasmic autoantibodies in patients with symptomatic HIV infection. *Clin. Exp. Immunol.* **87**: 24–30.

Klein, P., Zientek., VandenBerg, S.R., and Lothman, E. (1990). Primary CNS lymphoma: lymphomatous meningitis presenting as a cauda equina lesion in an AIDS patient. *Can. J. Neurol. Sci.* **17**: 329–331.

Koch, T.K., Koerper, M.A., Wesley, A.M., Lewis, E.M., Weintrub, P.S., and Bredesen, D.E. (1989). Absence of an AIDS-related neuropathy in children and young adult hemophiliacs. *Ann. Neurol.* **26**: 476–477.

Koderisch, J., Andrassy, K., Rasmussen, N., Hartmann, M., and Tilgen, W. (1990). 'False-positive' anti-neutrophil cytoplasmic antibodies in HIV infection. *Lancet* **ii**: 1227–1228.

Koller, W.C., Gehlmann, L.K., Malkinson, F.D., and Davis, F.A. (1977). Dapsone-induced peripheral neuropathy. *Arch. Neurol.* **34**: 644–646.

Kumar, M., Resnick, L., Loenstein, D., Lowenstein, D.A., Berger, J., and Eisdorfer, C. (1989). Brain reactive antibodies and the AIDS dementia complex. *J. Acq. Immune Defic. Syn.* **2**: 469–471.

Kunsch, C. and Wigdahl, B. (1991). Maintenance of human immunodeficiency virus type-1 proviral DNA in human fetal dorsal root ganglia neural cells following a nonproductive infection. *J. Leuko. Biol.* **49**: 505–510.

Lafeuillade, A., Aubert, L., Detolle, P., Chaffanjon., and Quilichini, R. (1988). Dysglobulinémie monoclonale et vascularite systémique nécrosante associées au sida. *Sem. Hôp. Paris* **64**: 1477–1480.

Lambert, J.S., Seidlin, M., Reichman, R.C., Plank, C.S., Laverty, M., Morse, G.D., Knupp, C., McLaren, C., Pettinelli, C., Valentine, F.T., and Dolin, R. (1990). 2',3'-dideoxyinosine (ddI) in patients with the acquired immunodeficiency syndrome or AIDS-related complex: a phase I trial. *N. Engl. J. Med.* **322**: 1333–1340.

Lange, D.J., Britton, C.B., Younger, D.S., and Hays, A.P. (1988). The neuromuscular manifestations of human immunodeficiency virus infection. *Arch. Neurol.* **45**: 1084–1088.

Lanska, M.J., Lanska, D.J., and Schmidley, J.W. (1988). Syphilitic polyradiculopathy in an HIV-positive man. *Neurology* **38**: 1297–1301.

Latov, N. (1995). Pathogenesis and therapy of neuropathies associated with monoclonal gammopathies. *Ann. Neurol.* **37**(suppl. 1): S32–S42.

Lee, M.R., Ho, D.D., and Gurney, M.E. (1987). Function interaction and partial homology between human immunodeficiency virus and neuroleukin. *Science* **237**: 1047–1051.

Leger, J.M., Bouche, P., Bolgert, F., Chaunu, M.P., Rosenheim, M., Cathala, H.P., Gentilini, M., Hauw, J.J., and Brunet, P. (1989). The spectrum of polyneuropathies in patients infected with HIV. *J. Neurol. Neurosurg. Pyschiatry* **52**: 1369–1374.

Leger, J.M., Hénin, D., Bélec, L., Mercier, B., Cohen, L., Bouche, P., Hauw., J.J., and Brunet, P. (1992). Lymphoma-induced polyradiculopathy in AIDS: two cases. *J. Neurol.* **239**: 132–134.

Le, Lostic, Z., Fegueux, S., Vitale, C., Geoffroy, O., Bleton, F., and Mornet, P. (1994). Peripheral neuropathy associated with cryoglobulinaemia but not related to hepatitis C virus in an HIV infected patient. *AIDS* **8**: 1351–1352.

Levy, R.M., Bredesen, D.E., and Rosenblum, M.L. (1985). Neurological manifestations of the acquired immunodeficiency syndrome: experience at UCSF and review of the literature. *J. Neurosurg.* **62**: 475–495.

Lewis, W. and Dalakas, M.C. (1995). Mitochondrial toxicity of antiviral drugs. *Nature Med.* **1**: 417–422.

Libman, B.S., Quismorio, F.P., and Stimmler, M.M. (1995). Polyarteritis nodosa-like vasculitis in human immunodeficiency virus infection. *J. Rheumatol.* **22**: 351–355.

Lindholm, D., Heumann, R., Hengere, B., and Thoenen, H. (1988). Interleukin 1 increases stability and transcription of mRNA encoding nerve growth factor in culture rat fibroblasts. *J. Biol. Chem.* **263**: 16348–16351.

Lin-Greenberger, A., and Taneja-Uppal, N. (1987). Dysautonomia and infection with the human immunodeficiency virus. *Ann. Intern. Med.* **106**: 167.

Lipkin, W.I., Parry, G., Kiprov, D., and Abrams, D. (1985). Inflammatory neuropathy in homosexual men with lymphadenopathy. *Neurology* **35**: 1479–1483.

Lipton, S.A. (1992). Requirement for macrophages in neuronal injury induced by HIV envelope glycoprotein gp120. *Neuroreport* **3**: 913–915.

Lipton, S.A. and Gendelman, H.E. (1995). Dementia associated with acquired immunodeficiency syndrome. *New Engl. J. Med.* **332**: 934–940.

Lipton, S.A., Dafni, U., Simpson, D., Yu, B.H., Slasor, P., and Navia, B.A. (1995). Double-blinded, randomized, placebo-controlled trial of the calcium channel antagonist nimodipine for the neurological manifestations of acquired immunodeficiency syndrome, including dementia and painful neuropathy. *Ann. Neurol.* 38: 347.

Lohmöller, G., Matuschke, A., and Goebel, F.D. (1987). Testing for neurological involvement in HIV infection. *Lancet* **ii**: 1532.

Mah, V., Vartavarian, L.M., Akers, M., and Vinters, H.V. (1988). Abnormalities of peripheral nerve in patients with human immunodeficiency infection. *Ann. Neurol.* **24**: 713–717.

Malamut, R.I., Leopald., N., and Parry, G.J. (1992). The treatment of HIV-associated chronic inflammatory demyelinating polyneuropathy (HIV-CIDP) with intravenous immunoglobulin (IVIG). *Neurology* **42**(suppl. 3): 335.

Malbec, D., Pinès, E., Boudon, P., Lusina, D., and Choudat, L. (1994). Syndrome d'hyperlymphocytose CD8 et infection par le virus de l'immunodéficience humaine: cinq observations. *Rev. Méd. Interne* **15**: 630–633.

McArthur, J.C. (1987). Neurologic manifestations of AIDS. *Medicine* **66**: 407–408.

McArthur, J.C., Cohen, B.A., Selnes, O.A., Kumar, A.J., Cooper, K., McArthur, J.H., Soucy, G., Cornblath, D.R., Chmiel, J.S., Wang, M., Starkey, D.L., Ginzburg, H., Ostrow, D.G., Johnson, R.T., Phair, J.P., and Polk, B.F. (1989). Low prevalence of neurological and neuropsychological abnormalities in otherwise healthy HIV-1 infected individuals: results from the multicenter AIDS cohort study. *Ann. Neurol.* **26**: 601–611.

McDougal, J.S., Hubbard, M., Nicholson, J.K.A., Jones, B.M., Holman, R.C., Roberts, J., Fishbein, D.B. et al. (1985). Immune complexes in the acquired immunodeficiency syndrome (AIDS); relationship to disease manifestation, risk group, and immunologic defect. *J. Clin. Immunol.* **5**: 130–138.

Mezin, P., Brion, J.P., Vermont, J., Micoud, M., and Stoebner, P. (1991). Ultrastructural changes associated with peripheral neuropathy in HIV/AIDS. *Ultrastr. Pathol.* **15**: 593–602.

Miller, J.R., Barrett, R.E., Britton, C.B., Tapper, M.L., Bahr, G.S., Bruno, P.J., Marquardt, M.D. (1982). Progressive multifocal leukoencephalopathy in a male homosexual with T-cell immune deficiency. *N. Engl. J. Med.* **307**: 1436–1438.

Miller, R.G., Parry, G.J., Pfaeffl, W., Lang, W., Lippert, R., and Kiprov, D. (1988). The spectrum of peripheral neuropathy associated with ARC and AIDS. *Muscle Nerve* **11**: 857–863.

Miller, R.G., Storey, J.R., and Greco, C.M. (1990). Ganciclovir in the treatment of progressive AIDS-related polyradiculopathy. *Neurology* **40**: 569–574.

Mintzer, D.M., Real, F.X., Jovino, L., and Krown, S.E. (1985). Treatment of Kaposi's sarcoma and thrombocytopenia with vincristine in patients with the acquired immunodeficiency syndrome. *Ann. Intern. Med.* **102**: 200–202.

Mishra, B.B., Sommers, W., Koski, C.L. et al. (1985). Acute inflammatory demyelinating polyneuropathy in the acquired immune deficiency syndrome. *Ann. Neurol.* **18**: 131–132.

Monteagudo, I., Rivera, J., Lopez-Longo, J., Cosin, J., Garcia-Monforte, A., and Carreño, L. (1991). AIDS and rheumatic manifestations in patients addicted to drugs. An analysis of 106 cases. *J. Rheumatol.* **18**: 1038–1041.

Morgello, S., and Simpson, D.M. (1995). Multifocal cytomegalovirus demyelinative polyneuropathy associated with AIDS. *Muscle Nerve* **17**: 176–182.

Muller, W.E., Schroder, H.C., Ushijima, H., Dapper, J., and Barmann, J. (1992). Gp 120 of HIV-1 induces apoptosis in rat cortical cell cultures: prevention by memantine. *Eur. J. Pharmacol.* **226**: 209–214.

Murr, A.H. and Benecke, J.E. (1991). Association of facial paralysis with HIV positivity. *Am. J. Otol.* **12**: 450–451.

Nuovo, G.J., Gallery, F., MacConnell, P., and Braun, A. (1994). In situ detection of polymerase chain reaction-amplified HIV-1 nucleic acids and tumor necrosis factor-α RNA in the central nervous system. *Am. J. Pathol.* **144**: 659–666.

Oberlin, F., Alcaix, A., Rosenheim, M., Follezou, J.Y., Artru, L., and Camus, J.P. (1989). Aspects rhumatologiques des infections par le virus de l'immunodéficience humaine. *Semin. Hôp. Paris* **65**: 144–150.

Oh, S.K., Cruikshank, W.W., Raina, J., Blanchard, G.C., Adler, W.H., Walker, J., and Kornfeld, H. (1992). Identification of HIV-1 envelope glycoprotein in the serum of AIDS and ARC patients. *J. Acq. Immune Def. Synd.* **5**: 251–256.

Pavesi, G., Medici, D., Lusvardi, M., Gemignani, F., Macaluso, G.M., Magnani, G., and Mancia, D. (1994). Migrant sensory neuritis associated with AIDS: case report. *Ital. J. Neurol. Sci.* **15**: 433–436.

Pert, C.B., Smith, C.C., Ruff, M.R., and Hill, J.M. (1988). AIDS and its dementia as a neuropeptide disorder: role of VIP receptor blockade by human immunodeficiency virus envelope. *Ann. Neurol.* **23**(suppl.): S71–S73.

Petito, C.K. and Roberts, B. (1995). Evidence of apoptotic cell death in HIV encephalitis. *Am. J. Pathol.* **146**: 1121–1130.

Phillips, P.E. and Dougherty, R.M. (1991). Hepatitis C virus and mixed cryoglobulinemia. *Clin. Exp. Rheumatol.* **9**: 551–555.

Piette, A.M., Tusseau, F., Vignon, D., Chapman, A., Parrot, G., Leibowitch., and Montagnier, L. (1986). Acute neuropathy coincident with seroconversion for anti-LAV/HTLV-III. *Lancet* **1**: 852.

Pitlik, S.D., Fainstein, V., Bolivar, R., Guarda, L., Rios, A., Mansell, P.A., and Gyorkey, F. (1983). Spectrum of central nervous system complications in homosexual men with acquired immune deficiency syndrome. *J. Infect. Dis.* **148**: 771–772.

Poppi, M., Staffa, G., Martinelli, P., Fabrizi, A.P., and Guiliani, G. (1991). Neuropathy caused by spontaneous intraneural hemorrhage: Case report. *Neurosurgery* **28**: 292–295.

Power, C., McArthur, J.C., Johnson, R.T., Griffin, D.E., Glass, J.D., Perryman, S., and Chesebro, B. (1994). Demented and non-demented patients with AIDS differ in brain-derived human immunodeficiency virus type 1 envelope sequences. *J. Virol.* **68**: 4643–4649.

Przedborski, S., Liesnard, C., Voordecker, P., Gerard, J.M., Taelman, H., Spreches, S., Goldman, M., and Hildebrand, J. (1988). Inflammatory demyelinating polyradiculoneuropathy associated with human immunodeficiency virus infection. *J. Neurol.* **235**: 359–361.

Raphael, S.A., Price, M.L., Lischner, H.W., Griffin, J.W., Grover, W.D., and Bagasra, O. (1991). Inflammatory demyelinating polyneuropathy in a child with symptomatic human immunodeficiency virus infection. *J. Pediatr.* **118**: 242–245.

Rance, N.E., McArthur, J.C., Cornblath, D.R., Landstrom, D.L., Griffin, J.W., and Price, D.L. (1988). Gracile tract degeneration in patients with sensory neuropathy and AIDS. *Neurology* **38**: 265–271.

Riggs, J.E., Rogers, J.S., Schochet, S.S., and Gutmann, L. (1987). AIDS-related neuropathy. *W. Virg. Med. J.* **83**: 167–169.

Robertson, K.R., Stern, R.A., Hall, C.D., Perkins, D.O., Wilkens, J.W., Gortner, J.J., Donovan, M.K. et al. (1993). Vitamin B12 deficiency and nervous system disease in HIV infection. *Arch. Neurol.* **50**: 807–811.

Rogers, A.T., Harrison, R., Lunt, G.G., and Bramble, C. (1990). Phosphoglucoisomerase (neuroleukin), fibroblast growth factor, and catalase: lack of neuronotrophic activity for cultured rat spinal neurons. *Biochem. Soc. Trans.* **18**: 1012–1013.

Ronchi, O., Grippo, A., Ghidini, P., Lolli, F., Lorenzo, M., Di, Pietro, M., and Mazzotta, F. (1992). Electrophysiologic study of HIV-1+patients without signs of peripheral neuropathy. *J. Neurol. Sci.* **113**: 209–213.

Roullet, E., Assuerus, V., Gozlan, J., Ropert, A., Said, G., Baudrimont, M., El, Amrani, M., Jacomet, C., Duvivier, C., Gonzales-Canali, G., Kirstetter, M., Meyohas, M.-C., Picard, O., and Rozenbaum, W. (1994). Cytomegalovirus multifocal neuropathy in AIDS: analysis of 15 consecutive cases. *Neurology* **44**: 2174–2182.

Said, G. and Hontebeyrie-Joskowicz, M. (1992). Nerve lesions induced by macrophage activation. *Res. Immunol.* **143**: 589–599.

Said, G., Lacroix, C., Andrieu, J.M., Gaudouen, C., and Leibowitch, J. (1987). Necrotizing arteritis in patients with inflammatory neuropathy and human immunodeficiency virus infection. *Neurology* **37**(suppl. 1): 176.

Said, G., Lacroix, C., Chemouilli, P., Goulon-Goeau, C., Roullet, E., Penaud, D., de, Broucker, T., Meduri, G., Vincent, D., Torchet, M., Vittcoq., Leport, C., and Vilde, J.L. (1991). Cytomegalovirus neuropathy in acquired immunodeficiency syndrome: a clinical and pathological study. *Ann. Neurol.* **29**: 136–146.

Said, G., Lacroix-Ciaudo, C., Fujimura, H., Blas, C., and Faux, N. (1988). The peripheral neuropathy of necrotizing arteritis: a clinicopathological study. *Ann. Neurol.* **23**: 461–465.

Sawyer, M.H. (1988). Treatment and prevention of varicella-zoster virus infections, pp. 229–234. In Straus SE, moderator. Varicella-zoster virus infections: biology, natural history, treatment and prevention. *Ann. Intern. Med.* **1008**: 221–237.

Scaravilli, F., Sinclair, E., Arango, J.-C., Manji, H., Lucas, S., and Harrison, M.J.G. (1992). The pathology of the posterior root ganglia in AIDS and its relationship to the pallor of the gracile tract. *Acta Neuropath.* **84**: 163–170.

Selnes, O.A., Galai, N., Bacellar, H., Miller, E.N., Becker, J.T., Wesch, J., van Gorp, W., and McArthur, J.C. (1995). Cognitive performance after progression to AIDS: a longitudinal study from the multicenter AIDS cohort study. *Neurology* **45**: 267–275.

Shapshak, P., Nagano, I., Xin, K., Bradley, W., McCoy, C.B., Sun, N.C., Stewart, R.V., Yoshioka, M., Petito, C., Goodkin, K. et al. (1995). HIV-1 heterogeneity and cytokines. Neuropathogenesis. *Adv. Exp. Med. Biol.* **373**: 225–238.

Silvestria, F., Williams Jr, R.C., and Dammacco, F. (1995). Autoreactivity in HIV-1 infection, the role of molecular mimickry. *Clin. Immunol. Immunopath.* **75**: 197–205.

Simpson, D.M. and Wolfe, D.E. (1991). Neuromuscular complications of HIV infection and its treatment. *AIDS* **5**: 917–926.

Simpson, D.M., Olney, R.K., McKinley, G., Dobkin, J., So, Y., Berger, J., Fordon, M.B., and Friedman, B. (1994). Peptide in the treatment of painful distal neuropathy associated with AIDS. *Neurology* **47**: 1254–1259.

Small, P.M., McPhaul, L.W., Sooy, C.D., Wofsy, C.B., and Jacobson, M.A. (1989). Cytomegalovirus infection of the laryngeal nerve presenting as hoarseness in patients with acquired immunodeficiency syndrome. *Am. J. Med.* **86**: 108–110.

Smith, T., Jakobsen, J., Gaub, J., and Trojaborg, W. (1990). Symptomatic polyneuropathy in human immunodeficiency virus antibody seropositive men with and without immune deficiency: a comparative electrophysiological study. *J. Neurol. Neurosurg. Psychiatry* **53**: 1056–1059.

Snider, W.D., Simpson, D.M., Nielsen, S., Gold, J.W.M., Metroka, C.E., and Posner, J.B. (1983). Neurological complications of acquired immune deficiency syndrome: analysis of 50 patients. *Ann. Neurol.* **14**: 403–418.

So, Y.T. (1992). Clinical subdivision of mononeuropathy multiplex in patients with HIV infection. *Neurology* **42**(suppl. 3): 409 (abstract).

So, Y.T. and Olney, R.K. (1991). The natural history of mononeuropathy multiplex and simplex in patients with HIV infection. *Neurology* **41**(suppl. 1): 375 (abstract).

So, Y.T. and Olney, R.K. (1994). Acute lumbosacral polyradiculopathy in acquired immunodeficiency syndrome: Experience in 23 patients. *Ann. Neurol.* **35**: 53–58.

So, Y.T., Holtzman, D.M., Abrams, D.I., and Olney, R.K. (1988). Peripheral neuropathy associated with acquired immunodeficiency syndrome. Prevalence and clinical features from a population-based survey. *Arch. Neurol.* **45**: 945–948.

So., Y.T., Holtzman, D.M., and Miller, R.G. (1990). Sensory myeloneuropathy in patients with human immunodeficiency virus infection. *Neurology* **40**(suppl. 1)429.

Stricker, R.B. and Kiprov, D.D. (1993). Mononeuritis and cryoglobulins. *Neurology* **43**: 2159 (letter).

Stricker, R.B., Sanders, K.A., Owen, W.F., Kiprov, D.D., and Miller, R.G. (1992). Mononeuritis multiplex associated with cryoglobulinemia in HIV infection. *Neurology* **42**: 2103–2105.

Talley, A.K., Dewhurst, S., Perry, S.W., Dollard, S.C., Gummuluru, S., Fine, S.M., New, D., Epstein, L.G., Gendelman, H.E., and Gelbard, H.A. (1995). Tumor necrosis factor alpha-induced apoptosis in human neuronal cells: protection by the antioxidant n-acetylcysteine and the genes bcl 2 and crmA. *Mol. Cell. Biol.* **15**: 2359–2366.

Talpos, D., Tien, R., and Hesselink, J.R. (1991). Magnetic resonance imaging of AIDS-related polyradiculopathy. *Neurology* **41**: 1996–1997.

Tardieu, M., Hery, C., Peudenier, S., Boespflug, O., and Montagnier, L. (1992). Human immunodeficiency virus type 1–infected monocytic cells can destroy human neural cells after cell to cell adhesion. *Ann. Neurol.* **32**: 11–17.

Thornton, C.A., Latif, A.S., and Emmanuel, J.C. (1991). Guillain-Barré syndrome associated with human immunodeficiency virus infection in Zimbabwe. *Neurology* **41**: 812–815.

Tokumoto, J.I.N. and Hollander, H. (1993). Cytomegalovirus polyradiculopathy caused by a ganciclovir-resistant strain. *Clin. Infect. Dis.* **17**: 854–856.

Trimble, K.C., Goggins, M.G., Molloy, A.M., Mulcahy, F., Scott, J.M., and Weir, D.G. (1993). Vitamin B12 deficiency is not a cause of HIV-associated neuropathy. *AIDS* **7**: 1132–1133.

Tyor, W.R., Wesselingh, S.L., Griffin, J.W., McArthur, J.C., and Griffin, D.E. (1995). Unifying hypothesis for the pathogenesis of HIV-associated dementia complex, vacuolar myelopathy, and sensory neuropathy. *J. AIDS Hum. Retrovir.* **9**: 379–388.

Valeriano-Marcet, J., Ravichandran, L., and Kerr, L.D. (1990). HIV associated systemic necrotizing vasculitis. *J. Rheum.* **17**: 1091–1093.

Veilleux, M., Paltiel, O., and Falutz, J. (1995). Sensorimotor neuropathy and abnormal vitamin b12 metabolism in early hiv infection. *Can. J. Neurol. Sci.* **22**: 43–46.

Vendrell, J., Heredia, C., Pujol, M., Vidal, J., Blesa, R., and Graus, F. (1987). Guillian-Barré syndrome associated with seroconversion for HTLV-III. *Neurology* 37;544.

Vishnubhakat, S.M. and Beresford, H.R. (1980). Prevalence of peripheral neuropathy in HIV disease: prospective study of 40 patients. *Neurology* **38**(suppl. 1): 350.

Weber, C.A., Figueroa, J.P., Calabro, J.J., Marcus, E.M., and Gleckman, R.A. (1987). Co-occurrence of the Reiter syndrome and acquired immunodeficiency. *Ann. Intern. Med.* (letter). **107**: 112–113.

Wechsler, A.F. and Ho, D. (1989). Bilateral Bell's palsy at the time of HIV seroconversion. *Neurology* **39**: 747–784.

Wei, X., Ghosh, S.K., Taylor, M.E., Johnson, V.A., Emini, E.A., Deutsch, P., Lifson, J.D., Bonhoeffer, S., Nowak, M.A., Hahn, B.H., Saag, M.S., and Shaw, G.M. (1995). Viral dynamics in human immunodeficiency virus type 1 infection. *Nature* **373**: 117–122.

Wessenlei, S.L., Glass, J., McArthur, J.C., Griffin, J.W., and Griffin, D.E. (1994). Cytokine dysregulation in HIV-associated neurological disease. *Adv. Neuroimmunol.* **4**: 199–206.

Winchester, R., Bernstein, D.H., Fischer, H.D., Enlow, R., and Solomon, G. (1987). The co-occurrence of Reiter's syndrome and acquired immunodeficiency. *Ann. Intern. Med.* **106**: 19–26.

Winer, J.B. (1993). Neuropathies and HIV infection. *J. Neurol. Neurosurg. Psychiatry* **56**: 739–741.

Winer, J.B., Bang, B., Clarke, J.R., Knox, K., Cook, T.J., Gompels, M., Hughes, R.A.C., Hall, S.M., Pinching, A.J., Harris, J.W.R., Kitchens, V., Jeffries, D.J., Leibowitz, S., Smith, S., Cockbain, Z., Ekong, T., and Hughes, C. (1992). A study of neuropathy in HIV infection. *Q. J. Med.* **83**: 473–488.

Yarchoan, R., Berg, G., Brouwers, P., Fischl, M.A., Spitzer, A.R., Wichman, A., Grafman, J., Thomas, R.V., Safai, B., Brunetti, A., Perno, C.F., Schmidt, P.J., Larson, S.M., Myers, C.E., and Broder, S. (1987). Response of human-immunodeficiency-virus-associated neurological disease to 3′azido-3′deoxoythymidine. *Lancet* **1**: 132–135.

Yarchoan, R., Perno, C.F., Thomas, R.V., Klecker, R.W., Allain, J.P., Wills, R.J., McAtee, N., Fischl, M., Dubinsky, R., McNeely, M.C., Mitsuya, H., Pluda, J.M., Lawley, T.J., Leuther, M.,Safai, B., Collins, J.M., Myers, C.E., and Broder, S. (1988a). Phase I studies of 2′,3′-dideoxycytidine in severe human immunodeficiency virus infection as a single agent and alternating with zidovudine (AZT). *Lancet* **i**: 76–80.

Yarchoan, R., Thomas, R.V., Grafman, J., Wichman, A., Dalakas, M., McAtee, N., Berg, G., Fischl, M., Perno, C.F., Klecker, R.W., Buchbinder, A., Tay, S., Larson, S.M., Myers, C.E., and Broder, S. (1988b). Long-term administration of 3′azido-2′3′-dideoxythymidine to patients with AIDS-related neurological disease. *Ann. Neurol.* **23**(suppl.): S82–S87.

Yoshioka, M., Shapshak, P., Srivastava, A.K., Stewart, R.V., Nelson, S.J., Bradley, W.G., Berger, J.R., Rhodes, R.H., Sun, N.C.J., and Nakamura, S. (1994). Expression of HIV-1 and interleukin-6 in lumbosacral dorsal root ganglia of patients with AIDS. *Neurology* **44**: 1120–1130.

Younger, D.S., Rosoklija, G., Hays, A.P., Nienstedt, L.J., Latov, N., Jaffe, I.A., and Hayo, A.P. (1996). HIV-1 Associated sensory neuropathy: a patient with peripheral nerve vasculitis. *Muscle Nerve* **19**: 1364–1366 (letter).

21 Lyme neuropathy

P.K. Coyle and M.A. Kaufman

Introduction

Definition

Lyme disease (also called Lyme borreliosis) is a systemic bacterial infection due to a tick-borne spirochete, *Borrelia burgdorferi* (Steere 1989). This infection targets specific body organs to cause disease manifestations of the skin, joint, heart, eye, and both the central (CNS) and peripheral (PNS) nervous systems. Lyme disease is now recognized worldwide, with endemic foci throughout North America, Europe, and northern Asia (Dennis 1993). Additional cases have been reported from Africa, Australia, and South America.

Historical aspects

The skin and neurological syndromes of Lyme disease were first recognized in Europe (Burgdorfer 1993). The earliest clinical case report dates to 1883, when the German physician Buchwald described a patient with idiopathic skin atrophy. This lesion, which was subsequently named acrodermatitis chronica atrophicans (ACA), is now known to be a late skin manifestation of Lyme disease. In 1909 the Swedish dermatologist Afzelius reported a patient with an expanding ring-like skin lesion following a tick bite, which he called erythema migrans (EM). In 1922 the French neurologists Garin and Bujadoux described a patient with a red skin lesion and painful meningoradiculitis following a tick bite. By 1930 the Swedish dermatologist Hellerström had associated EM with neurological involvement. The painful meningoradiculitis related to EM was subsequently called Bannwarth's syndrome. By 1951 it was appreciated that EM responded to penicillin, but the causal infectious agent remained unknown.

The first case of EM in the USA was reported in 1969, and involved a Wisconsin physician who had been bitten by a tick while hunting (Burgdorfer 1993). In 1975 a cluster of four EM cases was described from southeast Connecticut. By October 1975 Allen Steere had begun a study of children living near Old Lyme, Connecticut, who had developed what appeared to be juvenile rheumatoid arthritis. In 1977 he reported this new clinical entity, Lyme arthritis, which was subsequently renamed Lyme disease. Willy Burgdorfer, working at the Rocky Mountain laboratories in 1981, isolated a new spirochete from Ixodid ticks collected on Shelter Island. Identical spirochetes were soon shown to be present in European Ixodid ticks. In 1983 two separate groups cultured this new spirochete, *B. burgdorferi*, from patients with Lyme disease (Benach et al. 1983; Steere et al. 1983).

Epidemiological aspects

Lyme disease now accounts for 91% of vector-borne infections in the USA (Dennis 1993). Over 70 000 cases have been reported to the Centers for Disease Control and Prevention (CDC) since surveillance began in 1982. Cases cluster in the coastal northeast and mid-Atlantic, north central, and Pacific coastal regions. In 1993 over 85% of cases were reported from eight states (New York, Connecticut, Pennsylvania, New Jersey, Wisconsin, Rhode Island, Maryland, Massachusetts).

The incidence rate of Lyme disease in the USA is 3.3 per 100 000, but in hyperendemic regions is as high as 150 per 100 000. The disease directly maps to locations of the hard body Ixodid tick vector. This tick is not only spreading to new geographical areas, but there is an increasing tick infection rate within original endemic areas (White et al. 1991). In most parts of the USA, the specific Ixodid vector is *Ixodes scapularis*. In hyperendemic regions *I. scapularis* infection rates can approach 30–60%. In striking contrast, the western vector, *I. pacificus*, shows infection rates of only 1–6%. All Ixodes ticks have a 2-year life cycle of larval, nymphal, and adult stages (Steere 1989). Each stage involves a single blood feed. Although ticks feed on dozens of different mammals and birds, the most important host is the white-footed wild mouse. Humans are accidental hosts, and are most likely to be bitten by questing nymphs in the spring. To transmit infection, experimental studies indicate the tick has to remain attached for a prolonged period of at least 24 hours.

Almost all Lyme infections occur through the tick bite. Congenital cases are rare; there is only a single case of possible blood transfusion infection, and there have been no well-documented infections associated with other ticks or blood-sucking insects (fleas, mosquitoes, horseflies).

Lyme disease affects men and women equally, with a bimodal age distribution. Children (aged 5–14 years) and young adults (aged 30–49 years) are particular targets. Lyme cases peak during summer but can occur year-round, with seasonality least marked in the west. The only consistent risk factor is occupational or recreational time spent out of doors.

Table 21.1. *Clinical stages of Lyme disease*

Early local infection
Erythema migrans (EM)
Early disseminated infection
Multifocal EM
Lymphocytoma (Europe)
Cardiac
Arthritis
Hepatitis
Conjunctivitis
Neurological
Late disseminated infection
Acrodermatitis chronica atrophicans (ACA) (Europe)
Cardiac
Arthritis
Keratitis, uveitis
Neurological

Clinical aspects

Natural history

Infection with *B. burgdorferi* is asymptomatic in up to 50% of cases (Hanrahan et al. 1984; Steere et al. 1986). Similar to other human spirochetal infections, symptomatic illness can occur early or late in the infection. Clinical problems tend to be episodic, punctuated by asymptomatic periods (Table 21.1). There are discrete syndromes associated with early local (generally within 1 month of infection), early disseminated (within 3 months), and late disseminated infection; however, a patient may present with illness in one stage without manifesting features of other stages.

Local infection

Early local infection refers to the EM skin lesion, which is noted by 60–80% of Lyme disease patients (Malane et al. 1991). This is an expanding red lesion that occurs at the tick bite site an average of 8–9 days (range 1–30 days) after infection. The lesion is generally painless, although sometimes it itches or burns. The key feature of EM is expansion over time. The lesion begins as a macule which evolves into a papule and then an annular erythematous plaque which can enlarge to 42 cm. The center may be clear, vesicular, crusted, or edematous, and may form a bull's eye lesion. Spirochetes are detected in the EM lesion, particularly at the expanding edge, in as high as 60–86% of patients by culture, polymerase chain reaction detection of Borrelial DNA, or immunohistochemical staining of a punch biopsy (Malane et al. 1991; Berger et al. 1992). This early skin lesion is the only high-yield biopsy or culture site in Lyme disease. Perhaps half of EM cases are associated with mild flu-like symptoms (fever, headache, fatigue, myalgia, arthralgia).

Disseminated infection

After a brief period of time, spirochetes disseminate to various body organs. Early dissemination may be associated with multifocal EM, joint, cardiac, or ocular problems. Elevated liver transaminases may be seen, consistent with mild hepatitis. Lymphocytoma, involving lymphocytic infiltration of earlobe or areola, is a skin lesion associated with dissemination which occurs in 1% of European patients (Malane et al. 1991). Neurological syndromes of early dissemination are an 'aseptic' meningitis or meningoencephalitis, cranial neuropathy, and radiculoneuritis (see below) (Pachner and Steere 1985; Reik 1991; Coyle 1993).

Once spirochetes sequester within discrete body organs, they can cause late disease months to years after infection. ACA is a late atrophic skin lesion. It is regularly seen as a feature of European Lyme disease, but only a handful of cases have been reported from North America (Malane et al. 1991). Joint, cardiac, and ocular disease may be seen. Neurological syndromes associated with late infection are encephalopathy, polyradiculoneuropathy, and encephalomyelitis (see below) (Logigian et al. 1990; Krupp et al. 1991; Reik 1991; Logigian and Steere 1992; Coyle 1993).

The most characteristic joint problem of Lyme disease is an oligoarticular arthritis, with intermittent painless swelling. The knee is most often involved, and there may be a Baker's cyst. Lyme disease frequently causes migratory arthralgias, with large joints involved more commonly than small joints. This may begin shortly after the organism disseminates. There may also be migratory muscle, tendon, bone or bursa pain. Jaw pain is an early suggestive feature. Arthritis in a minority of patients can even present as a septic joint, or as a chronic process. The most characteristic cardiac manifestation is atrioventricular conduction block. Other problems include sinus node problems, infra-His block, pericarditis, myocarditis, cardiomyopathy, congestive heart failure, and atrial or ventricular arrythmias. Ocular manifestations include conjunctivitis, photophobia, periorbital edema, keratitis, and uveitis.

Table 21.2 *Neurological syndromes associated with Lyme disease*

CNS
meningitis, meningoencephalitis
encephalopathy
encephalomyelitis, meningoencephalomyelitis
PNS
cranial neuropathy
radiculoneuritis
plexopathy
mononeuritis multiplex
polyradiculoneuropathy
with ACA
with or without encephalopathy
Guillain-Barré syndrome
carpal tunnel syndrome
myositis

Neurological involvement

Neurological involvement occurs in up to 40% of symptomatic infections, and includes discrete CNS and PNS syndromes (Table 21.2).

CNS manifestations

Shortly after *B. burgdorferi* disseminates from its skin entry site, it can seed the CNS to produce a meningitis that mimics an aseptic viral process (Pachner and Steere 1985). Meningitis is usually acute, but in rare instances has taken a relapsing or chronic course. The meningitis is most often subtle, but occasionally is associated with severe headache with prostration. Clues to the etiology include concurrent prominent facial nerve or spinal nerve root involvement, prominent associated fatigue, joint pain, or cardiac features, and an atypical lymphocytosis or plasma cell component to the cerebrospinal fluid (CSF) pleocytosis. The most common late CNS involvement is encephalopathy characterized by difficulty in word retrieval, slowed reaction time, and memory and attention problems (Krupp et al. 1991; Kaplan et al. 1992). The encephalopathy is generally mild enough that the patient is not demented, and is able to continue to work. Usually there is associated prominent fatigue and malaise. A rare late CNS manifestation is encephalomyelitis with frank parenchymal involvement of brain or spinal cord (Pachner et al. 1989). Patients may develop movement disorders, hemiparesis, cerebellar syndromes, psychiatric syndromes, transverse myelitis, or other problems. The symptoms can mimic brain tumor or demyelinating disease.

Cranial neuropathy

Cranial nerve palsy is the most frequent neurological abnormality noted in Lyme patients (Reik 1991; Belman et al. 1993). Cranial neuropathy is considered an early dissemination syndrome, but rare cases have been reported preceding the occurrence of EM (Clark et al. 1985). It can be the initial presentation of Lyme disease. The facial nerve accounts for 80–90% of cranial neuropathies. Much less common is involvement of the optic nerve (optic neuritis, papilledema, ischemic optic neuropathy) (Jacobson et al. 1991); cranial nerves VI, III or IV; cranial nerves V or VIII; and rarely cranial nerves IX or X (Reik 1991). Cranial nerve involvement can be unilateral, bilateral, or multiple.

Facial neuropathy occurs in 11–14% of Lyme disease patients, and is bilateral in 23–37% (Clark et al. 1985; Pachner and Steere 1985; Belman et al. 1993). Most cases occur during summer. It has been estimated that in endemic regions Lyme disease can account for up to 25% of patients who present with peripheral facial weakness (Halperin and Golightly 1992). Lyme related facial neuropathy can be an isolated syndrome, or can occur in the setting of associated meningitis or radiculoneuritis (Smouha et al. 1997). Bilateral facial nerve palsy is highly suggestive for Lyme disease, although other conditions (acute viral infections, neurosarcoidosis, acute polyradiculoneuropathy, Melkersson's syndrome) can also cause bilateral neuropathy. The facial neuropathy is often accompanied by other features, such as headache, fever, or marked fatigue. Many patients show an elevated (erythrocyte sedimentation rate (ESR), increased quantitative serum IgM, and serum cryoglobulins. CSF typically shows mononuclear pleocytosis and elevated protein when the facial palsy coincides with meningitis or radiculoneuritis, but may be entirely normal with isolated facial involvement. Experimental studies have detected Borrelial antigen and DNA in otherwise normal CSF obtained from patients with acute cranial neuropathy (Luft et al. 1992; Coyle et al. 1993). Contrast magnetic resonance imaging (MRI) has shown enhancement of cranial nerves and meninges which may even be asymptomatic (Nelson et al. 1992). MRI may also be normal. From a prognostic point of view, Lyme facial nerve palsy does not differ from idiopathic Bell's palsy. Complete recovery occurs within weeks to months in 86% of patients (Clark et al. 1985), and will occur even without antibiotic treatment.

Radiculoneuritis

The most common neurological manifestation of Lyme disease in Europe is painful lymphocytic meningoradiculoneuritis, referred to as Bannwarth's syndrome (Hansen and Lebech 1992). This is an early dissemination syndrome which occurs within 3 months of infection. Adults are much more likely to be affected than children, and pain tends to be worse in older individuals. Patients note severe radicular, burning, deep or superficial pain worse at night. Pain often migrates, but is most typical in the upper or lower back and between the scapulae. There are often associated patchy areas of skin dysesthesia. Objective sensory findings tend to be subtle. Sensory symptoms may be associated with focal motor weakness, depressed reflexes, and rarely with evidence of associated myelitis. Patients generally show inflammatory CSF changes (mononuclear pleocytosis, increased protein, intrathecal specific antibody production). Electromyography (EMG) may show loss of motor units, fibrillations and positive sharp waves, increased duration of motor unit potentials, and increased polyphasic potentials. Studies overall suggest a predominantly axonal process.

Painful radiculoneuritis is much less common in North American Lyme disease. It may be associated with facial nerve palsy or symptomatic meningitis (Pachner and Steere 1985). There has been a single case report of a patient with thoracic involvement who presented with increasing abdominal girth and only subtle dysesthesias rather than frank pain (Daffner et al. 1990). As part of the spectrum of this early dissemination syndrome, some patients show evidence of plexopathy (brachial, lumbosacral) or a mononeuritis multiplex (Pachner and Steere 1985; Garcia-Monco et al. 1993).

Even without therapy, Lyme radiculoneuritis will improve or clear within 2–16 weeks. Antibiotics result in rapid improvement in pain. Paresthesias may persist for months, and in a minority of patients there is permanent mild weakness.

Polyradiculoneuropathy

Mild chronic neuropathy and radiculopathy syndromes have been described as complications of late Lyme disease, distinct from the painful radiculoneuritis which occurs within a few weeks to months after *B. burgdorferi* infection. These late PNS syndromes may occur in association with late skin involvement (ACA), in isolation, or in association with late encephalopathy.

ACA develops in about 10% of European Lyme cases. It is more common in the elderly, and occurs 6 months to 8 years after initial infection (Malane et al. 1991). Spirochetes have been identified within the chronic skin lesion by culture and staining, even in a lesion present over 10 years. Approximately 40–60% of ACA patients show clinical or laboratory evidence of mild, chronic PNS disease (Hopf 1975; Kristoferitsch et al. 1988). This takes the form of a predominantly distal sensory neuropathy. Variations include subclinical neuropathy, sensory cutaneous neuropathy, and asymmetric or symmetric polyneuropathy. Subjective complaints involve pain or paresthesias, and much less commonly weakness, muscle cramps, or restless legs. Objective deficits (generally sensory loss) are most marked in the region affected with ACA, but can also be found elsewhere. Nerve biopsy shows perivascular mononuclear cell infiltration around small and medium sized epineural blood vessels, with occasional involvement of the vessel wall. Nerve fiber damage corresponds with inflammation.

A similar rather mild late peripheral nerve involvement has been noted in up to 40% of North American Lyme patients (Halperin et al. 1987, 1990; Logigian and Steere 1992). These patients do not have ACA, but may have an associated late CNS syndrome (encephalopathy). Typically patients have been infected months to years earlier. The neuropathy may be so subtle as to be subclinical, but most patients note nonpainful distal paresthesias or radicular pains. Paresthesias tend to be intermittent, may be symmetrical or asymmetrical, and involve legs more than arms (and rarely face). Radicular pains are also intermittent, and generally asymmetric. Unlike the early radiculoneuritis syndrome, these patients have no associated meningitis or facial neuropathy. Objective abnormalities are also subtle, and include distal light touch and vibration sensory loss (most commonly in the toes) or stocking/glove sensory loss. Weakness, depressed reflexes, or muscle tenderness are uncommon.

Neurophysiological testing generally shows abnormalities suggestive of a rather diffuse neuropathy, even in clinically uninvolved limb and trunk regions. Nerve conduction abnormalities are particularly common in patients with paresthesias, and include mildly prolonged distal motor or sensory latencies, and mild slowing of distal motor conduction velocities. Abnormalities suggestive of marked demyelination are exceedingly rare. EMG changes indicate minor motor nerve fiber abnormalities, with mild to moderate denervation of distal muscles, paraspinal muscles, and proximal limb muscles. Both active denervation changes, and chronic denervation-reinnervation changes (with prolonged, polyphasic motor potentials) are noted. Based on electrophysiological criteria, this neuropathy has been divided into a chronic axonal polyradiculoneuropathy syndrome (56%), with evidence of root and distal nerve involvement; a chronic axonal polyradiculopathy syndrome (24%), with evidence of root involvement only; a distal sensory polyneuropathy (8%); and a distal sensorimotor polyneuropathy (4%). CSF changes are unusual unless there is an associated Lyme encephalopathy.

Unlike radiculoneuritis, chronic neuropathy does not spontaneously remit. With antibiotic treatment symptoms and neurophysiological abnormalities improve, but recovery occurs typically over weeks to months after treatment.

Guillain-Barré syndrome

The acute radiculoneuritis syndrome which occurs during early dissemination may rarely mimic Guillian-Barré syndrome (GBS). Patients can show loss of reflexes with predominant motor involvement (Sterman et al. 1982; Halperin et al. 1990). An important clue that this is not typical GBS is the finding of CSF pleocytosis. A second clue is that careful neurophysiological studies will be more consistent with a polyradiculopathy and distal axonal damage, rather than a primary demyelinating process. In addition to this mimicking syndrome, true GBS may occur as a post-infectious complication following *B. burgdorferi* exposure. Such patients do show cytoalbuminologic dissociation and a demyelinating pattern on neurophysiological testing. As is true for all the early dissemination syndromes, patients will spontaneously improve even without antibiotic treatment.

Carpal tunnel syndrome

Entrapment neuropathy is reported to be increased in patients with late Lyme disease. In a prospective evaluation of 68 patients with late infection, neurophysiological evidence of median nerve entrapment was noted in 25% (Halperin et al. 1989). Although patients presented for rheumatological or systemic complaints, most who had objective entrapment also complained of intermittent hand paresthesias, particularly at night or with use. Only one patient had an associated wrist tenosynovitis. Median nerve entrapment was more common in men. Although paresthesias were often noted in both hands, objective deficits were bilateral in only 35%. Neurophysiological abnormalities included slowed sensory conduction, prolonged motor distal latency, and decreased sensory potential amplitude. Median nerve entrapment could occur in isolation, as well as in the setting of a more diffuse late Lyme neuropathy. Following antibiotic treatment, 60% noted improvement in paresthesias and 30% had objective improvement in neurophysiological parameters. Entrapment neuropathy appears to be limited to adults, and is not common in pediatric Lyme disease (Belman et al. 1993).

Myositis

Although primary muscle involvement is unusual in Lyme disease, there are at least a dozen well-studied cases of myositis associated with *B. burgdorferi* infection in the literature, including a recent patient who developed dermatomyositis in the setting of multifocal EM (Horowitz et al. 1994). Myositis may complicate early or late infection, and may be acute or gradual in onset. Most patients have had preceding skin manifestations of Lyme disease. Symptoms include weakness, muscle pain, and muscle swelling or atrophy. Oropharyngeal and orbital muscles may be involved, to give dysphagia, dysphonia, proptosis, or diplopia. Multiple muscle groups may be affected.

Creatine kinase may be normal, or mild to moderately elevated. EMG may show myopathic features, may be normal, or may show spontaneous activity (perhaps due to accompanying neuropathy). Muscle biopsy has shown focal nodular, interstitial, or a necrotizing myositis. In rare cases a few spirochetes have been visualized within affected muscle by silver and immunogold-silver staining (Atlas et al. 1988; Reimers et al. 1993). Mononuclear cells (predominantly B cells, CD4 cells, macrophages and scattered plasma cells) infiltrate the perimysium and muscle fascicles, around small blood vessels. Sometimes there is an associated panniculitis and fasciitis. The myositis is antibiotic-responsive, with improvement (partial or complete) noted within weeks to months following treatment.

Diagnosis

Neurological Lyme disease is a clinical diagnosis which should be supported by appropriate laboratory data. EM is the only pathognomonic clinical marker of infection. The CDC surveillance case definition requires EM (more than 5 cm) diagnosed by a physician, or a specific late manifestation (arthritis; high degree heart block; meningitis, cranial neuropathy, radiculoneuritis, or encephalomyelitis with intrathecal antibody production) accompanied by seropositivity. The clinical diagnosis of neurological Lyme disease is supported when there is a prior history of EM, exposure to an endemic region, prior tick bite or constitutional syndrome, suggestive accompanying extraneural features, or occurrence of a characteristic neurological syndrome.

Laboratory investigation

Unlike most bacterial infections, in Lyme disease routine culture or staining of body fluids for the etiologic agent, *B. burgdorferi*, has negligible yield. Detection of serum antibodies to *B. burgdorferi* is the most commonly utilized laboratory test for Lyme disease. Seropositivity confirms prior exposure to *B. burgdorferi*, although not active infection. ELISA antibody assays have had a number of problems, and the CDC now recommends Western blot confirmation of all borderline or positive ELISAs. In the Western blot assay *B. burgdorferi* proteins are first separated on a gel by molecular weight, and then transferred to nitrocellulose paper. The paper is overlayed with the patient's serum. Antibody reactivity to specific proteins is detected as discrete bands on the nitrocellulose paper. Criteria for positive Western blots are now standardized (for IgM, two of the following three bands: p23,39,41; for IgG, 5 of the following ten bands: 18, 23, 28, 30, 39, 41, 45, 58, 66, 93); however, not all patients develop detectable antibodies. There is at least a 7% seronegativity rate (Berardi et al. 1988; Dattwyler et al. 1988b). Most well characterized seronegative patients have received early antibiotics which aborted the typical humoral response. Sometimes seronegative patients can be shown to have complexed antibodies (Schutzer et al. 1990), or to have lymphocytes sensitized to *B. burgdorferi* (Dattwyler et al. 1988b). Blood tests are also useful to exclude other diagnostic possibilities, including infections (such as babesiosis and ehrlichiosis) due to other tick-borne agents. Non-specific abnormalities which have been seen in Lyme disease include elevations in ESR, quantitative IgM, liver enzymes, and circulating immune complexes, and detectable cryoglobulins and IgM anticardiolipin antibodies.

CSF studies are very helpful to support a diagnosis of neurological Lyme disease, but North American patients tend not to show the marked inflammatory changes reported in European Lyme cases. In fact, normal CSF does not exclude neurological *B. burgdorferi* infection. CSF is most apt to be abnormal in patients with CNS or radicular syndromes. Mononuclear pleocytosis, atypical plasma cells, and elevated protein are non-specific abnormalities which can be seen in Lyme disease patients. Much more supportive of the diagnosis are specific CSF abnormalities, including intrathecal Borrelial antibody production, detection of Borrelial antigens or DNA, and detection of Borrelial immune complexes or specific IgM (Coyle et al. 1990, 1993, 1995; Luft et al. 1992). Neuroimaging (MRI is superior to CT) is abnormal in about 25% of neurological Lyme cases (Belman et al. 1992). There is no specific pattern, and abnormalities range from small scattered white matter lesions suggestive of a vasculitis, to deeper basal ganglia lesions, to large white matter lesions, and even single large granulomatous lesions. Functional neuroimaging (SPECT) may be helpful in late CNS infections with encephalopathy (Logigian et al. 1994). Cognitive function testing and angiography or MR angiography are appropriate in selected cases. Neurophysiological studies are helpful to detect PNS involvement, typically with a multifocal axonal radiculoneuropathy pattern. Nerve biopsy can be suggestive for Lyme disease, but has not been diagnostic. Biopsy findings are discussed below.

Case histories

Case 1

A 26-year-old left-handed law student presented in late August with right facial nerve palsy. An active outdoors person, he recalled a tick bite 10 weeks ago. Six weeks ago he developed fever to 104°F, chills, headache, and profound malaise, associated with a bull's eye rash on his leg. His illness resolved with oral antibiotics (Cefzil). Three weeks ago he developed severe bilateral shoulder and shoulder muscle pain. This resolved within a week, but he had continued to note left arm tightness.

Examination showed almost no movement of the right face, winging of the left scapula, and very limited left shoulder movement. Blood studies were unremarkable. CSF studies showed 243 mononuclear cells and 27 red blood cells, protein of 196, glucose of 44 (peripheral glucose 98), positive oligoclonal bands, IgG index 0.82, VDRL negative, and Lyme antibody reactive at 0.488 (reactive cutoff 0.128). Paired serum Lyme antibody was also reactive at 0.271. Spinal fluid culture and antigen studies for *B. burgdorferi* was negative.

Nerve conduction velocity studies were remarkable for a reduced compound muscle action potential amplitude recorded over the left flexor pollicis longus muscle following stimulation of the anterior interosseous nerve in the forearm. The identical study was normal on the right side. Routine left median and ulnar sensory and motor nerve conduction velocity studies were normal. Needle EMG abnormalities were restricted to specific muscles not in a pattern consistent with nerve root or plexus disease. Profound signs of denervation with fibrillations and positive sharp waves were seen in the left deltoid and supraspinatus muscles, while the cervical paraspinal, biceps brachii, and triceps muscles were electrically silent at rest. The left serratus anterior muscle was atrophic and fibrotic. Similar severe features of denervation were found in the left flexor pollicis longus muscle. Ulnar and median nerve innervated musculature was electro-physiologically normal. Markedly reduced numbers of motor units, some of markedly increased amplitude, duration and polyphasia, were noted in all the abnormal muscles except for the atrophic serratus anterior.

The patient received intravenous ceftriaxone, 2 g daily, for 3 weeks. Over the course of the next 2 months his facial weakness cleared completely. At 12 months he still had weakness of the shoulder, and difficulty writing with the left hand for any length of time.

Discussion: This young man had a meningoradiculitis syndrome associated with early dissemination. Following a tick bite, he had an EM lesion with a severe flu-like illness. His occult meningitis was associated with facial nerve palsy and radicular features. CSF showed marked inflammatory changes, despite negative culture and antigen studies; however CSF was obtained weeks after the CNS was likely invaded. Neurophysiological studies supported a mononeuritis multiplex of the long thoracic, suprascapular, axillary, and anterior interosseous nerves. Unfortunately, nerve damage was severe enough to preclude a complete recovery.

Case 2

This 31-year-old nurse developed burning and numbness in the lower back and hips following epidural anesthesia for childbirth. Past medical history was positive only for Gilbert's syndrome, and a 1 year history of intermittent temporomandibular joint problems. Neurological evaluation was entirely negative, and the patient was followed with no specific therapy. Over the next 4 months her pain worsened, with new burning sensation radiating to her right hip. Neurophysiological studies demonstrated normal sural sensory as well as posterior tibial and peroneal motor nerve conduction velocity studies in the lower extremities. Long latency potentials including H reflexes and F waves were symmetric and normal. Needle EMG abnormalities were found in lumbar sacral paraspinal muscles. On the right side, fibrillations and positive sharp waves as well as complex repetitive discharges were identified from the L2 through S1 levels. Less significant findings were noted adjacent to the L2 and L4 spinous processes on the left side. Lower extremity muscle studies were normal, except for minor amounts of sharp waves at rest along with mildly increased amplitude motor units found in the right tibialis anterior muscle. An MRI of the lumbosacral spine was unremarkable. An extensive workup for radiculoneuropathy revealed only a positive Lyme serology (0.168, reactive cutoff 0.112) confirmed by Western blot. The patient's only risk factor was that she lived in a high endemic area for Lyme disease. CSF studies were entirely negative except for Borrelial antigen.

The patient received 3 weeks of intravenous ceftriaxone. Her symptoms gradually cleared over the next 6 months.

Discussion: This woman had an axonal lumbosacral polyradiculopathy. It is unclear how long she had been infected, but this syndrome is associated with late infection. She had no prior history to suggest Lyme disease, except for the unexplained jaw pain. Lyme serology should be included in the workup of patients from endemic areas who present with PNS syndromes that can be seen in Lyme disease.

Pathogenesis

It is unclear how *B. burgdorferi* produces nerve damage. The limited neuropathological studies on Lyme patients have not been terribly revealing.

Peripheral nerve biopsies show random collections of epineural and perineural perivascular mononuclear cells, limited axonal damage or loss, and no detectable spirochetes or bound antibody or complement (Halperin et al. 1987; Vallat et al. 1987; Meier et al. 1989). Some biopsies have noted a focal vasculitis involving epineural blood vessels. This lack of striking neural tissue damage has led to the concept that the neuropathies associated with Lyme disease may be due to indirect immune or inflammatory effects of the spirochete, rather than damage from direct infection.

There is immunological crossreactivity between Borrelial and neural antigens. Flagellin, the p41 protein of *B. burgdorferi*, shares sequence homology with myelin basic protein (Weigelt et al. 1992). Certain monoclonal antibodies direct against spirochetal epitopes have been shown to crossreact with CNS and PNS axons, Schwann cells, myelin, and other autoantigens (Aberer et al. 1989; Sigal 1993). *B. burgdorferi* infection can result in detectable autoantibodies to axonal proteins, gangliosides, neurons, myelin components, and cardiolipin (Garcia-Monco et al. 1988; Sigal and Tatum 1988; Ryberg et al. 1991), and can result in T cells sensitized to myelin, galactocerebroside, and cardiolipin (Martin et al. 1988). It appears likely that the neuropathies of Lyme disease are mediated by indirect mechanisms, such as inflammatory vasculitic or immune-mediated changes. This hypothesis is supported by recent studies in a rhesus monkey model (England et al. 1997).

Therapy

Lyme disease is a bacterial infection and typically responds well to antibiotic therapy. Unfortunately, therapeutic trials to examine drug treatment of Lyme disease have been rather limited. In fact the optimal antibiotic, duration of therapy, and route of drug delivery have not been established. It is a peculiarity of this infection that certain symptoms (fatigue, muscle and joint pain, headache, paresthesias, cognitive difficulties) may improve gradually weeks to months after treatment. The earlier in the infection the patient receives adequate antibiotics, the less likely they are to have prolonged symptoms or to develop a post-Lyme syndrome (defined as persistent complaints which are not improving more than 6 months after treatment).

Current treatment for neurological Lyme infection generally involves intravenous ceftriaxone, given as 2 g once a day (Dattwyler et al. 1988a; Steere 1989). Patients are treated for a minimum of 2 weeks, and often treated for 4 weeks in late disseminated infections or severe infections. When involvement is limited to the PNS without any evidence of CNS involvement (such as a mild polyneuropathy syndrome with negative CSF), oral therapy with amoxicillin (500–1000 mg three times daily) or doxycycline (300–400 mg) given for 1 month may be adequate. One of the difficulties in evaluating therapy of Lyme disease is the lack of an active infection assay. Patients who are treated and continue to have symptomatic complaints are sometimes subjected to months and years of chronic antibiotics. A reasonable approach to such patients is to re-evaluate them carefully for evidence of persistent infection or an alternative diagnosis, and then make a decision about the appropriateness of a self-limited repeat course of antibiotics.

Alternative intravenous therapies to ceftriaxone include cefotaxime, another third generation cephalosporin, as well as doxycycline. In a recent European study oral doxycycline (200 mg every fourth day) was as effective as intravenous pencillin for neurological Lyme disease (Karlsson et al. 1994). It is not known whether these results are generalizable to North American patients. Alternative oral therapies have included azalide agents such as azithromycin, but data are limited on their use in Lyme disease.

In addition to antibiotics, symptomatic therapies (such as tricyclic antidepressants) are appropriate to relieve nerve pain. In cases of GBS, plasmapheresis or intravenous gammaglobulin are used when appropriate in addition to antibiotic treatment. Physical and occupational therapy can be very helpful in the more severe radiculoneuritis cases.

Future developments

Current efforts in Lyme disease are particularly focused on improved diagnostic techniques, prevention strategies, and pathogenesis studies. New serological techniques are under development using recombinant proteins unique to *B. burgdorferi*. These will likely replace current ELISA and Western blot assays. In addition, assays to determine active infection by detection of Borrelial antigens or DNA in body fluids are being standardized. Better diagnostic techniques will allow us to define the accurate spectrum of neurological Lyme disease.

The ultimate prevention strategy is an effective vaccine. Several monovalent and multivalent vaccines, based on recombinant proteins, are now being evaluated. Studies to date indicate the vaccines are safe, and if efficacy is proven they are likely to be marketed.

Finally, it is still unclear how Lyme disease produces its neurological manifestations. Peripheral nerve damage occurs in the absence of detectable spirochetes. A better understanding of the pathogenesis of CNS and PNS syndromes in Lyme disease will permit focused therapeutic strategies, as well as providing a broader understanding of how an infectious agent can affect the nervous system.

In addition to the above targeted areas, there is growing interest in the issue of the post-Lyme syndrome and chronic Lyme disease. The therapeutic approach to such patients varies tremendously, without any established guidelines. It is very likely that therapeutic issues pertinent to this group will become a priority for future research efforts.

Conclusions

Lyme disease is a recognized infectious cause of peripheral neuropathy. It is an important diagnosis to consider in the appropriate setting, because it is very treatable. The pathogenesis of nerve injury in Lyme disease appears to be indirect, with suggestive evidence that immune or inflammatory processes are involved; however, these mechanisms remain to be worked out. Lyme disease provides an excellent paradigm to examine the indirect effects of infection on the nervous system that may be generalizable to a wider number of conditions.

References

Aberer, E., Brunner, C., Suchanek, G., Klade, H., Barbour, A., Stanek, G., and Lassmann, H. (1989). Molecular mimicry and Lyme borreliosis: shared antigenic determinants between *B. burgdorferi* and human tissue. *Ann. Neurol.* **26**: 732–737.

Atlas, E., Novak, S.N., Duray, P.H., and Steere, A.C. (1988). Lyme myositis: muscle invasion by *Borrelia burgdorferi. Ann. Intern. Med.* **109**: 245–246.

Belman, A.L., Coyle, P.K., Roque, C., and Cantos, E. (1992). MRI findings in children infected with *B. burgdorferi. Pediatr. Neurol.* **8**: 428–431.

Belman, A.L., Iyer, M., Coyle, P.K., and Dattwyler, R. (1993). Neurologic manifestations in children with North American Lyme disease. *Neurology* **43**: 2609–2614.

Benach, J.L., Bosler, E.M., Hanrahan, J.P., Coleman, J.L., Habicht, G.S., Bast, T.F., Cameron, D.J., Ziegler, J.L., Barbour, A.G., Burgdorfer, W., Edelman, R., and Kaslow, R.A. (1983). Spirochetes isolated from the blood of two patients with Lyme disease. *N. Engl. J. Med.* **308**: 740–742.

Berardi, V.P., Weeks, K.E., and Steere, A.C. (1988). Serodiagnosis of early Lyme disease: analysis of IgM and IgG antibody responses by using an antibody-capture enzyme immunoassay. *J. Infect. Dis.* **158**: 754–760.

Berger, B.W., Johnson, R.C., Kodner, C., and Coleman, L. (1992). Cultivation of *B. burgdorferi* from erythema migrans lesions and perilesional skin. *J. Clin. Microbiol.* **30**: 359–361.

Burgdorfer, W. (1993). Discovery of *Borrelia burgdorferi.* In *Lyme Disease*, ed. P.K. Coyle, pp. 3–7. St. Louis: Mosby Year Book.

Clark, J.R., Carlson, R.D., Sasaki, C.T., Pachner, A.R., and Steere, A.C. (1985). Facial paralysis in Lyme disease. *Laryngoscope* **95**: 1341–1345.

Coyle, P.K. (1993). Neurologic complications of Lyme disease. *Rheum. Dis. Clin. N. Am.* **19**: 993–1009.

Coyle, P.K., Deng, Z., Schutzer, S.E., Belman, A.L., Benach, J., Krupp, L.P., and Luft, B. (1993). Detection of *Borrelia burgdorferi* antigens in cerebrospinal fluid. *Neurology* **43**: 1093–1097.

Coyle, P.K., Schutzer, S.E., Belman, A.L., Krupp, L.B., and Golightly, M.G. (1990). Cerebrospinal fluid immune complexes in patients exposed to *B. burgdorferi*: detection of *Borrelia*-specific and non-specific complexes. *Ann. Neurol.* **28**: 739–744.

Coyle, P.K., Schutzer, S.E., Deng, Z., Krupp, L.B., Belman, A.L., Benach, J.L., and Luft, B.J. (1995). Detection of *Borrelia burgdorferi* specific antigen in antibody-negative cerebrospinal fluid in neurologic Lyme disease. *Neurology* **44**: 2010–2015.

Daffner, K.R., Saver, J.L., and Biber, M.P. (1990). Lyme polyradiculoneuropathy presenting as increased abdominal girth. *Neurology* **40**: 373–375.

Dattwyler, R.J., Halperin, J.J., Volkman, D.J., and Luft, B.J. (1988a). Treatment of late Lyme borreliosis-randomized comparison of ceftriaxone and penicillin. *Lancet* **2**: 1191–1194.

Dattwyler, R.J., Volkman, D.J., Luft, B.J., Halperin, J.J., Thomas, J., and Golightly, M.G. (1988b). Seronegative Lyme disease. *N. Engl. J. Med.* **319**: 1441–1446.

Dennis, D.T. (1993). Epidemology. In *Lyme Disease*, ed P.K. Coyle pp. 27–37. St. Louis: Mosby Year Book

England, J.D., Bohm Jr., R.P., Roberts, E.D., Philipp, M.T. (1997). *Ann. Neurol.* **41**: 375–384.

Garcia-Monco, J.C., Beldarrain, M.G., and Estrade, L. (1993). Painful lumbosacral plexitis with increased ESR and *Borrelia burgdorferi* infection. *Neurology* **43**: 1269.

Garcia-Monco, J.C., Coleman, J.L., and Benach, J.L. (1988). Antibodies to myelin basic protein in Lyme disease. *J. Infect. Dis.* **158**: 667–668.

Halperin, J.J. and Golightly, M. (1992). Long Island Neuroborreliosis Collaborative Study Group. *Neurology* **42**: 1268–1270.

Halperin, J.J., Little, B.W., Coyle, P.K., and Dattwyler, R.J. (1987). Lyme disease: cause of a treatable peripheral neuropathy. *Neurology* **37**: 1700–1706.

Halperin, J.J., Luft, B.J., Volkman, D.J., and Dattwyler, R.J. (1990). Lyme neuroborreliosis. *Brain* **113**: 1207–1221.

Halperin, J. J., Volkman, D.J., Luft, B.J., and Dattwyler, R.J. (1989). Carpal tunnel syndrome in Lyme borreliosis. *Muscle Nerve* **12**: 397–400.

Hanrahan, J.P., Benach, J.L., Coleman, J.L., Bosler, E.M., Morse, D.L., Cameron, D.J., Edelman, R., and Kaslow, R.A. (1984). Incidence and cumulative frequency of endemic Lyme disease in a community. *J. Infect. Dis.* **150**: 489–496.

Hansen, K. and Lebech, A.-M. (1992). The clinical and epidemiological profile of Lyme neuroborreliosis in Denmark 1985–1990. *Brain* **115**: 399–423.

Hopf, H.C. (1975). Peripheral neuropathy in acrodermatitis chronica atrophicans (Herxheimer). *J. Neurol. Neurosurg. Psychiatry* **38**: 452–458.

Horowitz, H.W., Sanghera, K., Goldberg, N., Pechman, D., Kamer, R., Duray, P., and Weinstein, A. (1994). Dermatomyositis associated with Lyme disease: case report and review of Lyme myositis. *Clin. Infect. Dis.* **18**: 166–171.

Jacobson, D.M., Marx, J.J., and Dlesk, A. (1991). Frequency and clinical significance of Lyme seropositivity in patients with isolated optic neuritis. *Neurology* **41**: 706–711.

Kaplan, R.F., Meadows, M.-E., Vincent, L.C., Logigian, E.L., and Steere, A.C. (1992). Memory impairment and depression in patients with Lyme encephalopathy. *Neurology* **42**: 1263–1267.

Karlsson, M., Hammers-Berggren, S., Lindquist, L., Stiernstedt, G. and Svenungsson, B. (1994). Comparison of intravenous penicillin G and oral doxycycline for treatment of Lyme neuroborreliosis. *Neurology* **44**: 1203–1207.

Kristoferitsch, W., Sluga, E., Graf, M., Partsch, H., Neumann, R., Stanek, G., and Budka, H. (1988). Neuropathy associated with acrodermatitis chronica atrophicans. *Ann. N.Y. Acad. Sci.* **539**: 35–45.

Krupp, L.B.,Masur, D., Schwartz, J., Coyle, P.K., Langenbach, L.J., Fernquist, S.K., Jandorf, L., and Halperin, J.J. (1991). Cognitive functioning in late Lyme borreliosis. *Arch. Neurol.* **48**: 1125–1129.

Logigian, E.L. and Steere, A.C. (1992). Clinical and electrophysiological findings in chronic neuropathy of Lyme disease. *Neurology* **42**: 303–311.

Logigian, E.L., Johnson, K.A., Becker, J.A., Kijewski, M.F., Kaplan, R.F., Holman, B.L., and Steere, A.C. (1994). Cerebral hypoperfusion in Lyme encephalopathy: a quantitative SPECT study. *Neurology* **44**: A186.

Logigian, E.L., Kaplan, R.F., and Steere, A.C. (1990). Chronic neurologic manifestations of Lyme disease. *N. Engl. J. Med.* **323**: 1438–1444.

Luft, B.J., Steinman, C.R., Neimark, H.C., Mupralidhar, B., Rush, T., Finkel, M.F., Kunkel, M., and Dattwyler, R.J. (1992). Invasion of the central nervous system by *Borrelia burgdorferi* in acute disseminated infection. *JAMA* **267**: 1364–1367.

Malane, M.S., Grant-Kels, J.M., Feder Jr, H.M. and Luger, S.W. (1991). Diagnosis of Lyme disease based on dermatologic manifestations. *Ann. Intern. Med.* **114**: 490–498.

Martin, R., Ortlauf, J., Sticht-Groh, V., Bogdahn, U., Goldmann, S.F., and Mertens, H.G. (1988). *B. burgdorferi* specific and autoreactive T cell lines from CSF in Lyme radiculomyelitis. *Ann. Neurol.* **24**: 509–516.

Meier, C., Grahmann, F., Engelhardt, A., and Dumas, M. (1989). Peripheral nerve disorders in Lyme borreliosis: nerve biopsy studies from 8 cases. *Acta Neuropath.* **79**: 271–278.

Nelson, J.A., Wolf, M.D., Yuh, W.T.C., and Peeples, M.E. (1992). Cranial nerve involvement with Lyme borreliosis by magnetic resonance imaging. *Neurology* **42**: 671–673.

Pachner, A.R., Duray, P., and Steere, A.C. (1989). CNS manifestations of Lyme disease. *Arch. Neurol.* **46**: 790–795.

Pachner, A.R. and Steere, A.C. (1985). The triad of neurologic manifestations of Lyme disease. *Neurology* **35**: 47–53.

Reik Jr, L.R. (1991). *Lyme Disease and the Nervous System.* New York: Thieme.

Reimers, C.D., De Koning, J., Neubert, U., Preac-Mursic, V., Koster, J.G., Muller-Felber, W., Pongratz, D.E., and Duray, P.H. (1993). Borrelia burgdorferi myositis; report of eight patients. *J. Neurol.* **240**: 278–283.

Ryberg, B., Hindfelt, B., Nilsson, B., and Olsson, J.E. (1991). Antineural antibodies in Guillain-Barré syndrome and lymphocyte meningoradiculitis (Bannwarth's syndrome). *Arch. Neurol.* **41**: 1277–1281.

Schutzer, S.E., Coyle, P.K., Belman, A.L., Golightly, M.G., and Drulle, J. (1990). Sequestration of antibody to *B. burgdorferi* in immune complexes in seronegative Lyme disease. *Lancet* **1**: 312–315.

Sigal, L.H. (1993). Cross reactivity between *Borrelia burgdorferi* flagellin and a human axonal 64 000 molecular weight protein. *J. Infect. Dis.* **167**: 1372–1378.

Sigal, L.H. and Tatum, A.H. (1988). Lyme disease patients' serum contains IgM antibodies to B. burgdorferi that cross react with neuronal antigens. *Neurology* **38**: 1439–1442.

Smouha, E.E., Coyle, P.K., and Shukri, S. (1997). *Am. J. Otol.* **18**: 257–261.

Steere, A.C. (1989). Lyme disease. *N. Engl. J. Med.* **321**: 586–596.

Steere, A.C., Grodzicki, R.L., Kornblatt, A.N., Craft, J.E., Barbour, A.G., Burgdorfer, W., Schmid, G.P., Johnson, E., and Malawista, S.E. (1983). The spirochetal etiology of Lyme disease. *N. Engl. J. Med.* **308**: 733–740.

Steere, A.C., Taylor, E., Wilson, M.L., Levine, J.L., and Spielman, A. (1986). Longitudinal assessment of the clinical and epidemiological features of Lyme disease in a defined population. *J. Infect. Dis.* **154**: 295–300.

Sterman, A.B., Nelson, S., and Barclay, P. (1982). Demyelinating neuropathy accompanying Lyme disease. *Neurology* **32**: 1302–1305.

Vallat, J.M., Hugon, J., Lubeau, M., Leboutet, M.J., Dumas, M., and Desproges-Gotteron, R. (1987). Tick bite meningoradiculoneuritis: clinical, electrophysiologic, and histologic findings in 10 cases. *Neurology* **37**: 749–753.

Weigelt, W., Schneider, T., and Lange, R. (1992). Sequence homology between spirochete flagellin and human myelin basic protein. *Immunol Today* **13**: 279–280.

White, D.J., Chang, H.-G., Benach, J.L., Bosler, E.M., Meldrum, S.C., Means, R.G., Debbie, J.G., Birkhead, G.S., and Morse, D.L. (1991). The geographic spread and temporal increase of the Lyme disease epidemic. *JAMA* **266**: 1230–1236.

22 Neuropathy in leprosy

F.G.I. Jennekens and W.H. van Brakel

Introduction

Leprosy is a chronic disease predominantly of skin and nerves; it is caused by an infection with *Mycobacterium leprae.* 'Were it not for the progressive destruction of peripheral nerve trunks and the consequences of this, leprosy would largely remain a cutaneous condition of cosmetically unsightly hypopigmented or erythematous areas and aggregations of nodular thickenings' (Browne 1975). The loss of sensibility is the primary cause of most of the ulcerations and mutilations for which leprosy is widely known and feared. Often there is also weakness of one or several limbs or of the face. *M. leprae* not only invade macrophages but also Schwann cells and occasionally myelinated and non-myelinated axons (Hirata and Harada 1994; Job 1994) and differs in these respects from other bacteria. Leprosy may be considered as a model immunological disease. Patients differ in response to infection and either develop very local manifestations (tuberculoid leprosy or TL), widespread lesions (lepromatous leprosy or LL), or anything in between these extremes.

Despite all these remarkable features, the discipline 'neurology' has never demonstrated much interest in this disorder. Physicians in leprosy hospitals apparently do not need special training in neurology, leprosy congresses are not attended by neurologists, publications on leprosy in the large international neurology journals are rare and neurologists rarely contribute to multiauthor handbooks on leprosy. The explanation for this curious situation is in part related to the histories of the disease and of neurology. In the Middle Ages, leprosy was endemic in Europe but almost disappeared thereafter, for reasons unknown. It only remained in Scandinavia, and more specifically in Norway, until late in the nineteenth, and even the twentieth, century. When an interest in neurological disorders developed in Western Europe, the leading clinical scientists did not encounter leprosy, with the exception of course, of those in Norway. It is thus not surprising that it was a Norwegian investigator, Gerhard Henrick Armhauer Hansen, who in 1873, discovered the bacillus responsible for the disease. Neurological research during subsequent decades was (and still is) mainly concentrated in Europe, Japan and North America, in areas with no or only few cases of leprosy. Another possible reason for the lack of 'neurological' interest is that, in the first instance, leprosy usually presents with skin lesions. If the skin is unaffected, which happens occasionally, it is not always easy to demonstrate that the asymmetrical neuropathy with weakness and sensory changes is leprotic in origin.

We describe in this chapter the complex clinical picture of neuropathy in leprosy, the pathological changes and immunological mechanisms, and the different forms of therapy. We shall first, however, provide some information on the causative pathogen and present data on the epidemiology of the disease. For extensive and excellent reviews on nearly all aspects of leprosy the reader is referred to the recently published second edition of *Leprosy*, edited by Hastings (1994) and for a thorough discussion of the neurological aspects to the chapter on leprosy by Sabin, Swift and Jacobson in *Peripheral Neuropathy*, volume 2, third edition, edited by Dyck, Thomas and others (1993).

Mycobacterium leprae

Structure and biochemistry

M. leprae is a Gram positive, rod-like structure up to 8 μm in length and 0.3 μm in width. Morphologically it cannot be distinguished from other mycobacteria. *M. leprae* are surrounded by a lipid capsule enclosing a 20 nm cell wall and a plasma membrane.

The lipid capsule helps to protect the bacteria from lysosomal enzymes and oxygen radicals and allows the mycobacteria to survive inside cells (Rees and Young 1994). The capsule contains phenolic glycolipid-I (PGL-I) which binds to complement 3b. This in turn binds to complement receptors on mononuclear phagocytes. The latter plays a role in phagocytosis of *M. leprae* (Brennan 1994). Several heat shock proteins (70, 65, 18, and 10 kDa) and a 28 kDa superoxide dismutase have been discovered in the cytoplasm (Table 22.1). Strain differences in *M. leprae* have not been found.

Replication, preferred temperature and viability

M. leprae is an obligate intracellular parasite and divides by binary fission (for a review see Rees and Young 1994). Attempts to cultivate it have been unsuccessful. It does, however, survive and multiply in mouse footpads and leprosy can be transmitted to armadillos (seven-, eight- and nine-banded) and non-human primates (chimpanzees, sooty mangabey monkeys, rhesus monkeys, African green monkeys) (for a review see Meyers et al. 1994). The preferred temperature for maximum growth is surprisingly low: ranging from 27 to 30°C. This explains why *M. leprae* grow in mouse footpads and not elsewhere in the animal. Naturally-acquired leprosy has been discovered in the nine-banded armadillo and in a few sooty mangabey monkeys and chimpanzees. Clinical evidence of leprosy was found in up to 5% of the nine-banded armadillos in Louisiana. The armadillo has a core temperature of 30–36°C which is sufficiently low to allow growth of *M. leprae* in internal organs such as the liver and spleen: a single animal may harbor up to 10^{11} viable organisms. This curious animal generates the bacteria required for experimental investigations. The captive sooty mangabey monkey is advocated as another good model for experimental investigations (Gormus et al. 1995).

Demonstration of M. leprae: *skin smears and other techniques*

M. leprae are demonstrable in biopsy material from skin or nerve and in smears from skin and nasal secretions. So-called 'slit skin smears' are widely used for diagnostic purposes and to evaluate the effect of therapy. Skin smears are decisive for the classification of leprosy as 'multibacillary' or 'paucibacillary' and this in turn determines the choice of therapy. Briefly, the technique is as follows. A cut is made in the skin, 2–3 mm in depth. The side of the cut is scraped with the scalpel and the material obtained in this fashion is smeared out on a glass slide, air-dried and fixed by heating. Overheating affects acid-fastness of the bacteria. The material is flooded with freshly filtered carbol-fuchsin and then destained with a 1% HCl solution. Only mycobacteria maintain their red color. The number of acid-fast bacilli (AFB) is assessed under the microscope and scored, from 0+ (no bacilli) to 6+ (more than 1000 per field) (Table 22.2). Several skin smears are prepared from different sites in each patient (both earlobes and up to four other representative sites). The mean score is calculated by adding the scores of the individual sites and dividing the total by the number of sites examined. The figure thus obtained is the bacterial index (BI) of the

Table 22.1 *Chemistry of* Mycobacterium leprae

	Lipids and carbohydrates	Role	Major proteins (kDa)	Role
Secreted substances	LAMs	Immunosuppression	30–31	Responsible for protective immunity?
Capsule	PGL-I PDIM	Phagocytosis; anti-bactericidal; B-cell immunogen		
Wall	Peptidoglycans		10	GroES hsp
	Arabinogalactan		17	
			65	GroEL hsp
	Mycolic acids			
	LAMs	replication		
Membrane	PIMs		35	
			22	Bacterioferritin
Cytoplasm			10	GroES hsp
			18	hsp
			28	Superoxide dismutase
			36	
			65	GroEL hsp
			70	DnaK hsp

Note:
LAMs: lipoarabinomannan; PGL-I: phenolic glycolipid-I; PDIM: phthiocerol dimycocerosate; PIMs: phosphatidylinositol mannosides; hsp: heatshock proteins; GroEL: equivalent of the GroEL gene product of *E. coli;* GroES: equivalent of GroES gene product in *E. coli*; GroEL and GroES type proteins are chaperones and involved in protein folding and translocation; DnaK: the homologue of DnaK hsp in *E. coli.*
Source: Booth and Watson 1994; Brennan 1994; Rees and Young 1994.

Table 22.2 *Scoring for the bacterial index of a patient*

Bacterial index of one site	Estimated number of bacilli per microscopic field(s) at one site
6+	>1000 per field
5+	100–1000 per field
4+	10–100 per field
3+	1–10 per field
2+	1–10 per 10 fields
1+	1–10 per 100 fields
0+	0 per 100 fields

Note:
The mean bacterial index of the patient is the total of all sites divided by the number of sites.

patient. Patients without bacilli in their skin smears (BI: 0+) are paucibacillary, all others (1+ to 6+) multibacillary. Evenly stained bacilli are viable; irregular staining points to loss of cytoplasm after cell death.

There are a few limitations to these skin smear stainings. The staining method may sound simple, but it is not so easy under field conditions. Adequate staining may fail due to impurity of the chemicals or to overheating. An important point in this context is that the prescriptions in handbooks do not provide an easy method for quality control of the staining technique. Assessment of the stained slides offers few difficulties when there are many bacilli, but the distinction between few bacilli or none and between evenly and irregularly stained bacilli is not so easy and requires expertise.

Another point is that the resolution limit of microscopic examination of carbol-fuchsin stainings is 10^4 bacilli per 50 mg tissue; the method cannot therefore be considered very sensitive. In spite of the limitations of skin smears, the leprosy control programs are extremely successful, as will become clear in the epidemiology section.

For classification of the type of leprosy, the laboratory technique has been replaced in some areas by a clinical investigation (few localized lesions point to PB leprosy and many widespread lesions to MB leprosy). Staining of *M. leprae* might in the near future be improved by the development of a simple immunohistochemical technique. Several groups have reported that the polymerase chain reaction can be used as a sensitive technique to demonstrate organism-specific DNA or RNA sequences. This technique cannot, however, be considered 'simple' and on its own is insufficient to allow a decision about whether the bacteria are dead or alive. It would seem that the current technique is not yet suitable for routine clinical practice and not for field conditions (Mistry and Antia 1993).

Lepromin tests

Lepromin is comparable to tuberculin and may induce a comparable reaction when used in skin tests. Lepromin was initially prepared from autoclaved *M. leprae* obtained from the skin of patients with lepromatous leprosy. Nowadays it is prepared from armadillo-derived *M. leprae.* The lepromin reaction is, in contrast to the tuberculin reaction, biphasic: there is a first response after 3–4 days with the features of a delayed-type hypersensitivity reaction (DTH) (the Fernandez reaction) and a second reaction after 3–4 weeks (Mitsuda reaction) when a nodule develops. The two reactions are positive in tuberculoid leprosy (TT) and borderline tuberculoid (BT) patients and provide evidence of a functioning cell-mediated immune reponse to *M. leprae* antigens in the host. Neither the early nor the late response is diagnostic for leprosy.

Epidemiology

Transmission of the disease

Humans are the main natural source of *M. leprae.* According to Davey and Rees (1974) nasal discharges from lepromatous patients contain up to 10 million viable organisms per day. The bacteria in dried nasal discharge retain their viability for approximately a week when kept at temperatures between 20 and 35°C in a humid atmosphere, and in warm moist soil viability is maintained even up to 46 days (Desikan and Sreevatsa 1979). Lepromatous patients do not appear to have any *M. leprae* on their skin. There is, however, the possibility that the organisms are released if the skin is damaged.

It is still a matter of debate how *M. leprae* enters the human body. The most likely route is via the upper respiratory tract. Transmission via defects in the skin is another possibility. Close or intimate contact between an infected and non-infected individual favors transmission but is not a definite requirement. The problem is that in so many cases of registered leprosy no contact with another patient has been established. In this respect, it is of interest that leprosy-specific PGL-I (see Table 22.1) has been demonstrated in soil (Blake et al. 1987). If skin would be covered by *M. leprae* from the soil, a sufficient number of organisms might enter the body via a thorn-prick (Job et al. 1994). In countries where it is common to walk barefoot, and where children are not always fully clothed, the exposed skin is often injured. If leprosy is endemic in such countries, large numbers of bacilli might be shed by multibacillary patients into the environment and might adhere to the damaged skin of other indivuduals. In addition, it would seem reasonable to speculate whether at least in some cases the infection could be of non-human origin. It is basically feasible for *M. leprae* to be transmitted by biting insects. Several authors have suggested that leprosy in humans might be derived from the armadillo (Lumpkin et al. 1983; Thomas et al. 1987). The nine-banded armadillo (called 'tatoe' in Brazil) is a bizarre, primitive South American mammal that has spread during the last century through Mexico to the southern states of the USA. It does not occur elsewhere in the world. Thorough surveys to find out whether leprosy is endemic in non-human primates in Asia, Africa and South America have not been carried out (Meyers et al. 1994).

Exposure to *M. leprae* is in itself not sufficient for the disease to develop. In fact, infection is probably contained in most individuals. Experience shows that in the affluent countries 'imported leprosy cases' do not trans-

Table 22.3 *Clinical presentations of leprosy*

	Clinical presentation
1.	Indeterminate
2.	Tuberculoid
3.	Borderline tuberculoid
4.	Borderline borderline
5.	Borderline lepromatous
6.	Lepromatous leprosy
7.	Pure neuritic
8.	1–7, complicated by Type 1 reaction
9.	5 or 6, complicated by Type 2 reaction
10.	Bacteriologically cured; Type 1 reaction
11.	Bacteriologically cured; Type 2 reaction

mit the disease. Apparently, factors such as nutrition, hygiene and household crowding play an important but not yet sufficiently defined role. The available figures indicate that in most countries the disease occurs more often in adult males than in females. It has been both suggested and denied that this difference is due to difficulties of ascertainment of the disease in females (Jakeman et al. 1995). In some African countries, however, there are more affected females than males (Pönnighaus et al. 1994). It is of interest that there is a male preponderance among patients with the lepromatous (multibacillary) type of leprosy and a female excess in paucibacillary leprosy.

The incubation period of leprosy is extremely variable, ranging from several months to decades. This has been concluded mainly on the basis of chance observations and not by systematic investigation. The latter is still not possible because suitable tools are lacking. The onset of the disease can occur at any age: in an infant of a few months or in an elderly individual. The proportion of multibacillary leprosy is low in children and increases with age.

Prevalence and distribution

In 1988, the World Health Organization (WHO) recommended that patients who had adequately completed standard multidrug therapy as proposed by WHO should be considered bacteriologically cured and should no longer be counted as a case of leprosy (see section on Treatment of infection). Using this definition the estimated number of leprosy cases worldwide has decreased to 2.4 million (December 1993) and the registered number of treated patients (mid-1993) to approximately 1.7 million (Noordeen 1995). In most countries, the sharp decrease in registered prevalence has not yet been matched by a concurrent drop in case detection rates (incidence). There is, therefore, still insufficient evidence that transmission of the disease has been interrupted by the current control strategies. The sharp decrease in prevalence implies that there must be millions of patients who are 'cured' of the infection but who still suffer from residual impairments.

Clinical description of leprosy

Classification of different types

The clinical manifestations of leprosy differ in nature and degree (Table 22.3). The differences in nature are not due to the leprosy bacilli but to the response of the host to the infection. A vigorous cell-mediated response (see section on Immunology) leads either to containment of the infection or to local manifestations with a tendency to spontaneous healing. The lepromin reaction is positive. A humoral response with little, if any, cell-mediated immunological reaction and no reaction to lepromin is typical for the more generalized forms of leprosy. In the first type of response, few if any leprosy bacilli are found in skin smears and biopsies. In the second type, leprosy bacilli are present in the dermis and the nasal mucosa, often in astounding numbers. These differences in responses form the basis for the classification of leprosy on a five-point scale, introduced by Ridley and Jopling (1966). The two extremes are tuberculoid leprosy or TT (vigorous cell-mediated immune response, positive reaction to lepromin, local manifestations, tendency to spontaneous healing) and lepromatous leprosy or LL (humoral response, no reaction to lepromin, tendency to generalize). The three other forms are different mixtures of the two extremes (borderline tuberculoid or BT, borderline lepromatous or BL and borderline borderline or BB). TT and BT are 'paucibacillary': the absence of bacilli in slit skin smears suggests a small total bacterial load. Patients with positive smears are called 'multibacillary'. At the very onset, allocation of leprosy to one of the five types is not yet possible; this is the stage at which leprosy is still 'indeterminate'.

Two other clinical forms of leprosy are not distinguished in the Ridley-Jopling classification which is based primarily on immunological criteria: the pure neuritic form without any skin lesions and the initial manifestation of leprosy which cannot yet be definitely classified. Histologically, the affected nerves in the pure neuritic type usually show the features of a borderline form of leprosy. Thus, from the clinical viewpoint, there are seven different presentations of leprosy: five of the Ridley-Jopling classification, indeterminate leprosy and the pure neuritic form.

The clinical picture may be complicated by 'reactions'. These can be present in different forms and are classified as Type 1 and 2 reactions and the Lucio phenomenon. Impairment of large peripheral nerves is particularly prominent during periods of Type 1 or 2 reaction. While in a reactionary state, the response of the host towards the infection can change and the clinical manifestations may shift towards either the tuberculoid or lepromatous pole of the disease (so called upgrading of the disease or downgrading). Lucio phenomenon occurs in untreated LL leprosy and has mainly been observed in South American patients. It is characterized by pink or dark lesions of the skin which are associated with vascular lesions. A particular relation to neuropathy has not been reported (Job 1994).

Neurological manifestations

The neurological manifestations of leprosy are peculiar in two respects: the sensory changes concern predominantly the superficial qualities and there is often an astonishing degree of nerve thickening, unlike anything seen in other disorders of peripheral nerves.

It is suggested that the prominent involvement of the superficial sensory qualities is due to the fact that *M. leprae* prefer a relatively cool environment: they invade in the first instance, nerves in or directly below the skin, leaving the larger nerves in deeper parts of the limbs to another stage of the disease (Sabin et al. 1993). Histological investigations point, however, to a preference of the bacteria for Schwann cells of unmyelinated compared with myelinated fibers even in large nerves (Shetty et al. 1988; Jacobs et al. 1993) implying that there may be more than one reason why the loss of superficial sensory qualities is so prominent. The impairment of the cutaneous nerves causes decrease or loss of temperature sensation and pain, and of touch or pressure sensation. Complaints about paresthesia and burning sensations are common. Sweat secretion is also affected and is diminished or absent in areas with sensory changes. Position sense and vibration sense are not likely to be entirely spared; surprisingly, investigations into the extent to which these modalities are involved and at what stage, have so far been inadequate. There is general agreement that tendon reflexes are largely preserved. Hypoestesia or anesthesia of hypopigmented or erythematous macules or plaques is one of the distinguishing features of leprosy.

In Europe, enlargement of peripheral nerves is a rare phenomenon and often questionable. It is much less frequent and prominent in the Charcot-Marie-Tooth and Dejerine-Sottas neuropathies than previously stated and is not present in every patient with Refsum's disease, which is an extremely rare disorder. The suggestion by Pfaltzgraff and Ramu (1994) that nerve enlargement is a feature of amyloid neuropathy is not a generally held view. Marked thickening of peripheral nerves may, however, occur in some cases of neurofibromatosis. In this latter disease, the enlarged nerves are much softer than in leprosy and the characteristic dermatological abnormalities of neurofibromatosis ease the distinction from leprosy. Unequivocal enlargement of one or several peripheral nerves in patients without evidence of neurofibromatosis is therefore in itself a strong reason for considering leprosy as the most likely diagnosis.

The enlarged nerves (Figure 22.1) are firm and sometimes knotted. String-like subcutaneous nerves can sometimes be observed, even from a distance, immediately under the skin of the forearm (ramus superficialis nervi radialis,), the neck (n. auricularis major) or the forehead (n. supraorbitalis). Thickening of large peripheral nerves is more focal and fusiform and is most prominent at the ulnar nerve just above the elbow, the peroneal nerve at the level of the popliteal fossa, the median nerve just proximal to the carpal tunnel, the radial nerve at the extensor side of the upper arm, and the posterior tibial nerve at the medial side of the ankle. These are the so-called predilection sites of nerve damage (Table 22.4).

Table 22.4 *Predilection sites of damage of large limb nerves*

Limb nerves	Anatomical sites
Ulnar	Above elbow
Median	Immediately above wrist
Radial	Middle of upper arm
Peroneal	Proximal to neck of fibula
Tibia	At ankle level

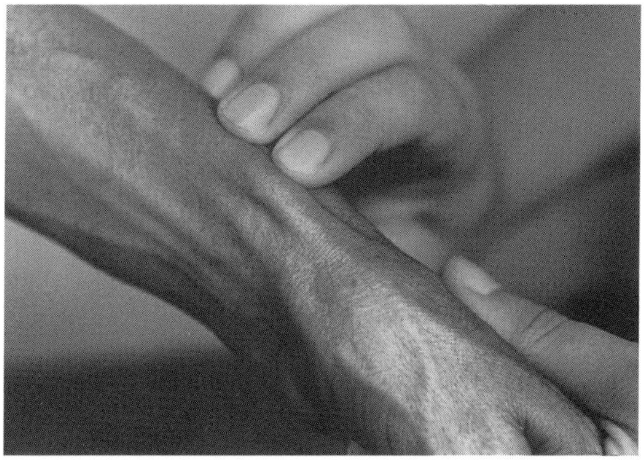

Figure 22.1 *A much enlarged ramus superficialis of the radial nerve. Nerve thickening of this degree and type is very rare in any other disease than leprosy.*

Motor and sensory loss often present with a characteristic distribution. As already stated, hypoesthesia is usually found, to a varying degree, at the site of skin lesions. It is not uncommon to find anesthesia on the footsoles and the hands. Weakness may be asymmetrical. The most frequent presentations are clawhand due to impairment of ulnar nerve function, footdrop due to involvement of the peroneal nerve or facial weakness with lagophthalmus due to facial nerve affliction.

Neurological examination of the leprotic patient in field conditions

Most of the world's leprosy patients are treated in peripheral health clinics in resource-poor countries. Methods of clinical examination therefore need to be simple and instruments readily available. A simple technique that has found widespread acceptance as a means to examine sensibility in the 'field' is the 'ballpen test': touching the skin with a ballpen. The result is scored as 'felt' or 'not felt'. Usually ten sites are tested on each handpalm and footsole. Touch/pressure is nowadays often tested with a standard set of 20 Semmes–Weinstein monofilaments, as described by Bell-Krotoski (1991). The nylon monofilaments are 38 mm in length and fit in lucid plastic rods that serve as handgrips. Each filament has a different standardized diameter and weight. When the filament is applied to the skin, at a straight angle, with enough force to make it bend, it will exert a constant pressure on the skin, irrespective of how much it bends. Usually only a few filaments are used. Gnostic sensibility and tendon reflexes are not routinely examined and pain sensation only occasionally. Muscle force is tested manually and scored according to a six point MRC scale. The neurological examination is often performed by medical technicians or physiotherapists.

Neurology of different types of leprosy

Indeterminate leprosy

One or a few ill-defined, hypopigmented maculae, no more than a few centimeters in diameter, appear most often on the extensor surfaces of the limbs, on the buttocks or on the face. The skin at the site of the maculae may be slightly hypoesthetic and somewhat dry but this is not always obvious. Histopathology is required for a definite diagnosis. Indeterminate leprosy heals spontaneously in most cases. In some cases, however, it may progress into one of the main forms of the disease.

Tuberculoid leprosy (TT)

There are only one or a few skin lesions, maculae or plaques, showing hypopigmentation or an erythematous aspect. They are larger than in indeterminate leprosy and well delineated. The skin at the site of the lesion is dry, scaly and hypo- or anesthetic. One or exceptionally two nearby subcutaneous nerves may be enlarged but this is not always very obvious. The large peripheral nerves are usually unaffected. The reaction to intracutaneously injected lepromin is positive and slit skin smears contain no AFB. Spontaneous recovery is the rule. Occasionally, however, the opposite occurs: the patient showing evidence of progression and downgrading.

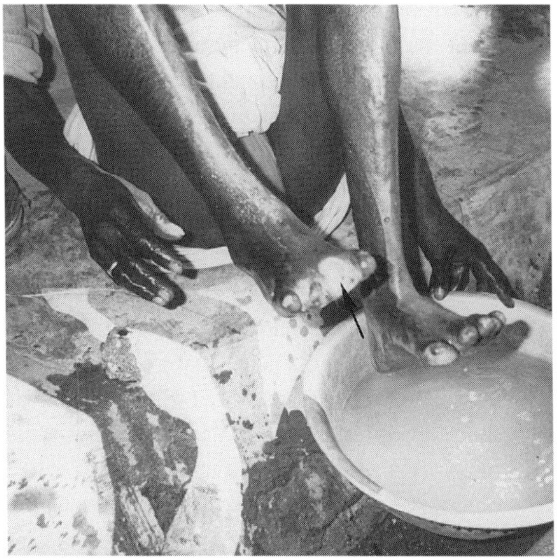

Figure 22.2 *Leprotic male washing his feet in disinfecting fluid in the Nepali sun. Notice ulcerations and missing toes of the right foot (arrow).*

Borderline tuberculoid leprosy (BT)

In BT, lesions are larger and more frequent than in TT and large peripheral nerves are involved. The skin lesions characteristically show hypo- or anhidrosis and hypo- or anesthesia. The distribution of the lesions is asymmetrical in contrast to the lesions in the lepromatous forms of leprosy. Nearby subcutaneous nerves are often enlarged and may be knotted, the latter pointing to the presence of abscesses. Abscess formation is often painful because of the pressure it exerts. One or several large peripheral nerves may also be involved as demonstrated by their enlargement, by abnormal sensation in non-lesioned parts of the skin and by asymmetrical weakness or paralysis. A strong cellular immune response to the infection can be demonstrated in the positive lepromin reaction and in the absence of bacilli in the skin smears of most patients. The cellular immune response is less effective than in TT leprosy and the disease is thus more widespread than in TT. The nerve lesions are due to this immune response.

The damage to the large peripheral nerves may progress 'silently', causing an increase in hypoesthesia and weakness (van Brakel Khawas 1994a). When the skin lesions are more widespread, 'silent' progression of involvement of large nerves is more frequent and more prominent. In addition, BT patients are prone to more obvious Type 1 reactions and, as will be explained below, neuritis forms an essential and ominous aspect of these reactions. Untreated BT patients become severely handicapped due to widespread involvement of the nerves. The disease evolves in some cases to the lepromatous pole of leprosy.

Anesthesia of the skin may allow for unperceived traumatic lesions, particularly on the footsoles and the fingers. The lesions may become infected, and ulceration, cellulitis and osteomyelitis often follow (Figure 22.2). When insufficiently treated, gross malformations of the distal parts of the limbs develop.

Lepromatous leprosy (LL)

The most astounding feature of this form of the disease is that manifestations do not become apparent before many millions of bacilli have been generated. This is exemplified by the skin smears which contain large numbers of bacilli. The striking absence of any cellular immune reaction to the bacilli is apparent when lepromin is injected: the Fernandez and Mitsuda reactions remain negative.

The initial skin lesions are not so easy to discern. Symmetrically distributed maculae or areas gradually appear, which are ill-defined, vague, somewhat shiny, slightly hypopigmented and which become hairless. These lesions spread over the dorsal aspects of the limbs and over the face and extend finally over almost the whole body with the exception of a few somewhat warmer areas: the axillae and the groins. The initial changes are dermatological, followed after some delay by neurological abnormalities: decrease of superficial sensibility and of sweating. The decrease is not very obvious and not easily established because the changes are symmetrically distributed over large parts of the body which precludes comparison of findings from one area to another. The large peripheral nerves are eventually also impaired at a relatively late stage, and at least initially, not to the same degree as in BT patients. The nerves become enlarged and partial loss of function is expressed in sensory changes, accompanied by some degree of muscle weakness. The main neurological features of LL are thus the symmetrical decrease of superficial sensibility and sweating over large areas of the body and the relatively minor degree (at least in early phases) of impairment of the large peripheral nerves.

LL leprosy is not restricted to the skin and nerves. The nasal mucosa is infiltrated and swollen, and secondary infections appear which eventually lead to collapse of the nose. The corneae and sclerae are also infiltrated and become anesthetic. Lagophthalmos allows for drying of the sclerae and corneae, traumatic lesioning and secondary infections and in the end ulceration, perforation and blindness. The fingers may shorten, ulcerations develop due to lesions of the anesthetic skin leading to osteomyelitis with destruction of the bones of the hands and feet. Other complications are acute orchitis or painless testicular atrophy, gynecomastia, and glomerulonephritis. Without treatment the disease runs a downhill course and may leave the patient severely deformed and disabled, or may be fatal.

Borderline lepromatous leprosy (BL)

BL differs from LL in that the lesions are less symmetrical and show more evidence of changes due to cellular immune reactions. Large peripheral nerves are involved at an earlier stage, and not as symmetrically as in LL. Skin smears show large numbers of bacilli; the lepromin reaction is negative. BL patients may have downgraded from untreated BT and are then likely to show evidence of asymmetrical lesioning of the large peripheral nerves. BL patients may in turn downgrade to LL or upgrade to BB or BT.

Mid-borderline leprosy (BB)

This is a stage of the disease in between BL and BT. Classification as BB occurs only in a small percentage of all cases.

Pure neuritic leprosy

The prevalence of so-called pure neuritic cases may have been underestimated. In a retrospective study of a cohort of 396 patients in Western Nepal, pure neuritic leprosy was diagnosed in ten cases (between 2 and 3%) (van Brakel Khawas 1994b). Patients present with clinical evidence of neuritis or neuropathy usually of one nerve, but on palpation other nerves may appear enlarged. Histology usually shows changes compatible with BT, or more rarely BL leprosy. The question raised by this form of leprosy is, of course, why the skin and the unmyelinated nerve fibers in the skin are spared. There is as yet no explanation.

Type 1 and 2 reactions

Type 1, or reversal, or upgrading reactions are episodes of increased inflammatory activity in the skin and/or nerves, with mild fever and malaise in some patients (for reviews see Rose and Waters 1991; Lienhardt and Fine 1994). Type 1 reactions are associated with increased cell-mediated immunoreactivity and a shift in the manifestations of the disease towards the tuberculoid side (upgrading). Type 2 reactions are episodes of increased inflammation in all organs that harbor ML, including peripheral nerves, and are much more generalized than Type 1 reactions. Type 2 reactions of the skin are expressed by papules or nodules and are designated erythema nodosum leprosum (ENL). Type 2 reactions were reported in 1969 to contain complexes of mycobacterial antigen, immunoglobulins and complement (Wemambu et al. 1969) and have since been considered as immune complex–mediated manifestations (Gelber 1995). It seems, however, that the mechanism underlying ENL is more complicated, as shifts in T cells in the lesions have also been reported (see section on Immunology).

Type 1 reactions occur most often in borderline forms of leprosy, occasionally in LL and perhaps in TT. They develop acutely or insideously and are notorious for the nerve damage they may induce. They may persist for months (BT leprosy) or even years (LL leprosy) (Rose and Waters 1991). Affected nerves may be tender on palpation and spontaneously painful, and loss of nerve function becomes manifest. The nerves most frequently affected are the ulnar, peroneal and facial nerves, but other nerves may also be affected. Existing skin lesions show swelling and increase of redness, and new lesions develop. There may be marked, sometimes unilateral edema of hands, feet or face. Type 1 reactions may complicate the clinical syndrome when leprosy is diagnosed, or may develop during anti-mycobacterial treatment or after treatment has been terminated. Risk factors have not been conclusively identified although case reports and uncontrolled observations indicate that BCG, extent of clinical disease, pregnancy and puerperium, and therapy, particularly of BT patients, should be considered as such. The problem is that there are no generally accepted diagnostic criteria for these reactions. Some authors feel that Type 1 reactions are 'upgrading' (see for instance Modlin and Rea 1994) or

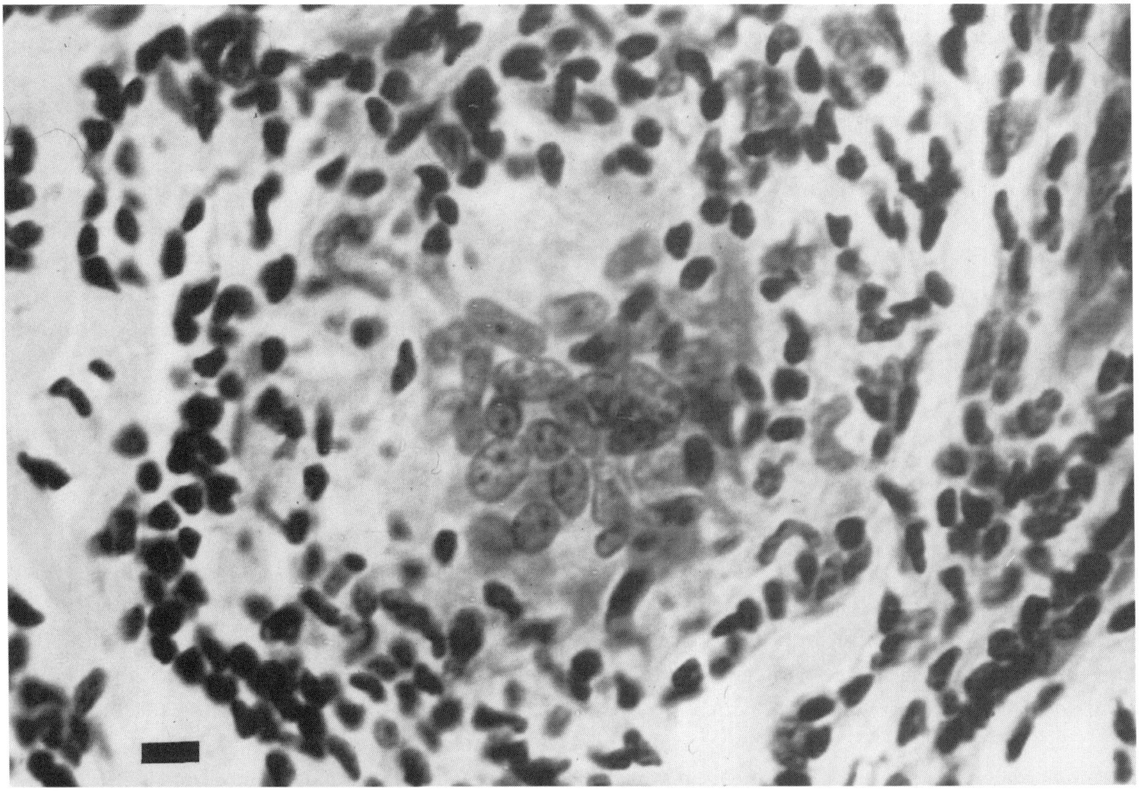

Figure 22.3 *Cryostat section, Hematoxylin stain. Borderline tuberculoid leprosy. Same biopsy as in Figure 22.5. Granuloma. Bar: 10 μm.*

prefer the designation 'reversal reactions' (Rose and Waters 1991). The latter term implies upgrading. Other authors (for instance Lienhardt and Fine, 1994; Gelber 1995) accept downgrading as a possible manifestation of Type 1 reactions.

Type 2 reactions are acute (Pfaltzgraff and Ramu 1994; Bloom and Ellner 1995) and occur in 11–54% of LL patients and in 2.7–23% in BL patients (Scollard et al. 1994; van Brakel Khawas 1994b). Various authors suggest they occur most often either within the first 2 years or in the second and third year after the onset of treatment. Type 2 reactions encompass an entire spectrum of manifestations including fever, erythema nodosum, neuritis, iritis, uveitis and episcleritis, orchitis, lymphnode swellings, distension of the face, hands and feet, digits, arthritis, etc. Nerve involvement is expressed by pain, spontaneous and on palpation, and some enlargement. Motor and sensory loss of nerve function are not usually very marked and less than in Type 1 reactions.

Pathology

General description

The pathological changes in the two opposite poles of leprosy differ in major aspects (Job 1994). The pathology of the tuberculoid forms is characterized by granulomatous infiltrates with mainly epitheloid cells and some Langhans cells in the center, and lymphocytes in the periphery (Figure 22.3). Granulomas are a typical feature of infections by intracellular organisms, in particular mycobacteria. The epitheloid cells are considered to be macrophage-derived and have well developed endoplasmic reticulum. They are believed to have a secretory function. Lymphocytes in the center are $CD4^+$ T helper (T_h) cells. $CD8^+$ T cells are found in the rim surrounding the center, which may become necrotic or caseous. Leprosy bacilli are rarely discovered. Leprosy granulomas in the skin, infiltrate cutaneous nerves. One or a few larger nerves in the vicinity may also be affected: some or all fascicles of a

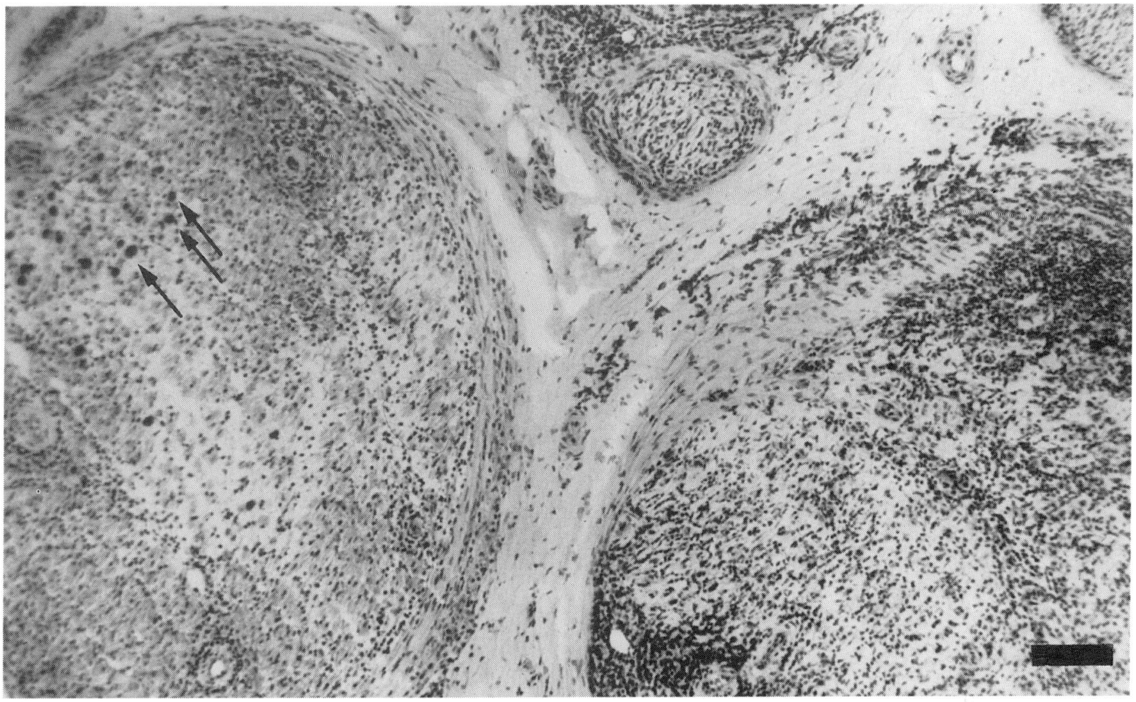

Figure 22.4 *Transverse cryostat section of sural nerve biopsy, Hematoxylin and eosin stain. Borderline tuberculoid leprosy. Inflammatory infiltrates in several fascicles. At some places myelinated fibres are still discernible (arrows). Bar: 100 μm.*

nerve are infiltrated and the nerve fibers in the fascicles disappear (Figure 22.4). In the borderline forms, the perineurial sheaths may show a variable degree of inflammation. Not infrequently one observes a caseous area in a nerve, surrounded by a rim of inflammatory and other cells, indicating that it is the endoneurial content of the fascicle that has become necrotic (Figure 22.5).

In the lepromatous forms of leprosy, cellular inflammatory infiltrates consist predominantly of macrophages but also contain plasma cells, mast cells and some lymphocytes, mainly $CD8^+$ T cells. Such infiltrates may form bands or strings immediately below the epidermis. The perineurial sheaths of the cutaneous nerves are infiltrated by macrophages and may appear thickened (Jacobs et al. 1993). The degree of infiltration of the endoneurial spaces is not great; it is mainly the number of macrophages which is increased (Shetty et al. 1988). Adequate staining reveals large numbers of bacilli, often arranged in so-called 'globi', in macrophages, Schwann cells of unmyelinated or less often myelinated fibers and to a lesser degree endothelial and perineurial cells, and other cells (Figures 22.6 and 22.7) (Shetty et al. 1988; Jacobs et al. 1993). Leprosy bacilli are occasionally seen in axons (Hirata and Harada 1994; Job 1994). A characteristic feature of the lepromatous forms of leprosy is the presence of heavily vacuolated, 'foamy' cells, mainly macrophages (Figure 22.8). This foamy appearance is thought to be related to products secreted by bacilli or to degeneration of the lipid-rich bacilli. LL is a generalized disorder and affects not only skin but also subcutaneous nerves and mixed motor-sensory nerves, as well as many other organs. In contrast to the tuberculoid form of leprosy neuritis where nerves may be entirely destroyed, nerves in the lepromatous forms of leprosy maintain their architecture and their myelinated nerve fibers for prolonged periods, even when the unmyelinated Schwann cells and macrophages are loaded with bacilli (Figure 22.6).

Large nerves in the limbs in long-standing, advanced, treated leprosy, be it of the borderline tuberculoid or lepromatous pole, are severely fibrosed, as shown in a study by Miko et al. (1993) of amputated

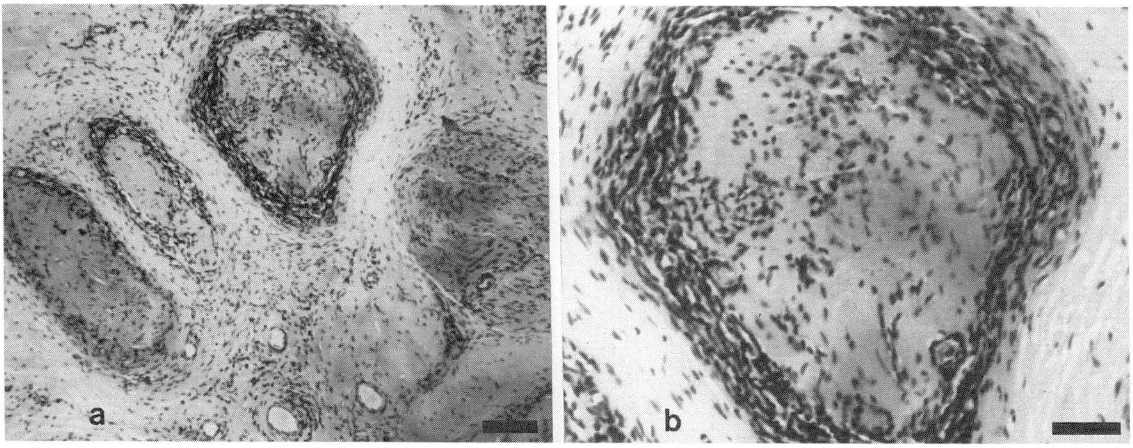

Figure 22.5 *Transverse cryostat sections of sural nerve biopsy, Hematoxylin stain. Borderline tuberculoid leprosy. Same biopsy as in Figure 22.3. (a) Three fascicles with inflammatory infiltrations of the perineurial sheaths. Bar: 100 μm. (b) Enlargement of the fascicle in the center of (a), showing that nerve fibers are not discernible. Bar: 50 μm.*

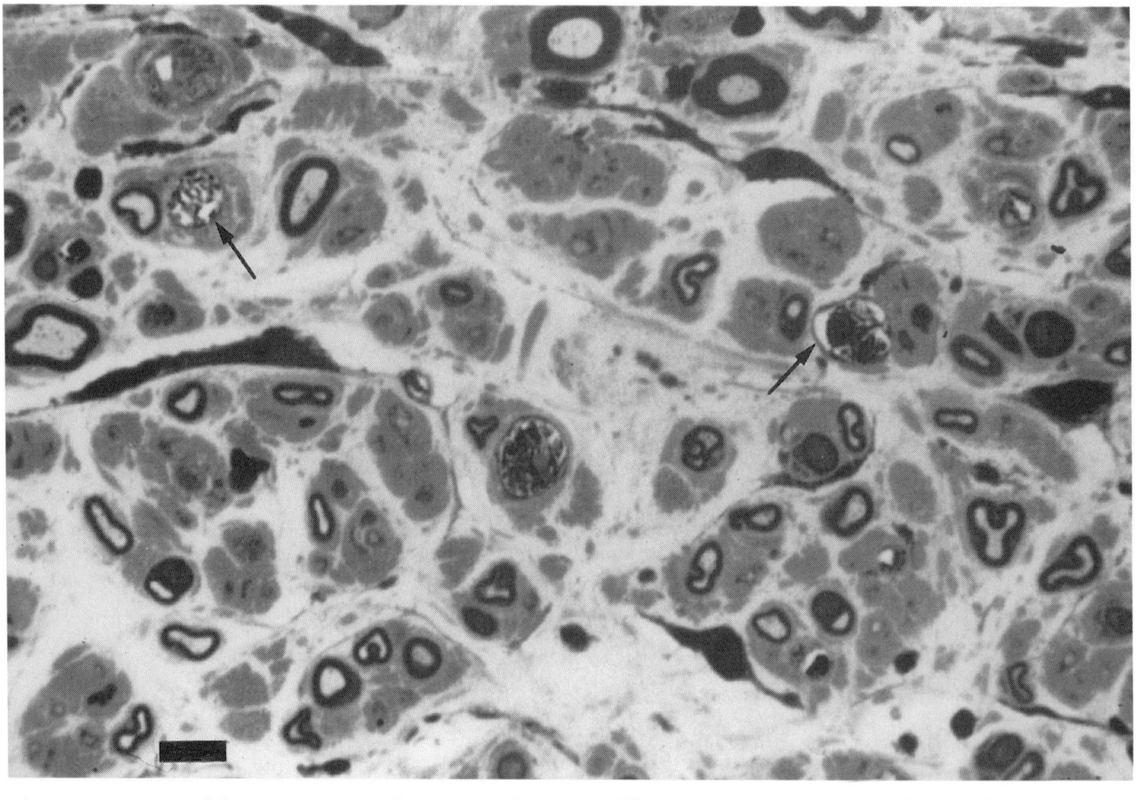

Figure 22.6 *Biopsy of the ramus superficialis of the radial nerve. Toluidine blue stained epon section. Lepromatous leprosy. Bacilli are discernible as fine black dots in several slightly vacuolated cells (arrows). Notice normal aspect of many myelinated fibers. Bar: 10 μm.*

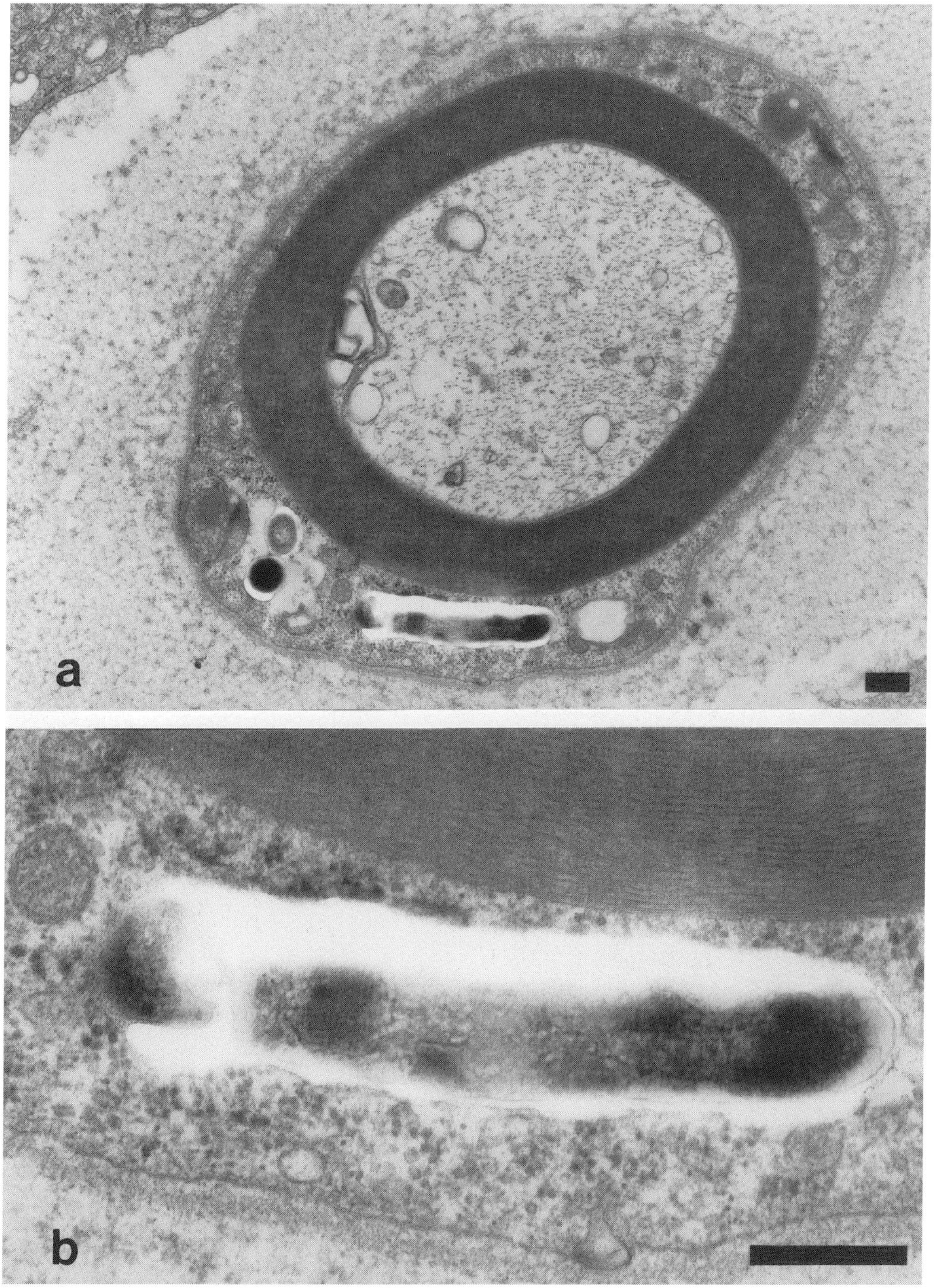

Figure 22.7 *Electron micrograph of myelinated nerve fiber. Same nerve biopsy as in Figure 22.6. (a) Two* Mycobacterium leprae *are present in Schwann cell cytoplasm: one is transversely sectioned and the other longitudinally. Bar: 1 μm. (b) Density of this longitudinally sectioned mycobacterium is irregular, indicating non-viability. Bar: 1 μm.*

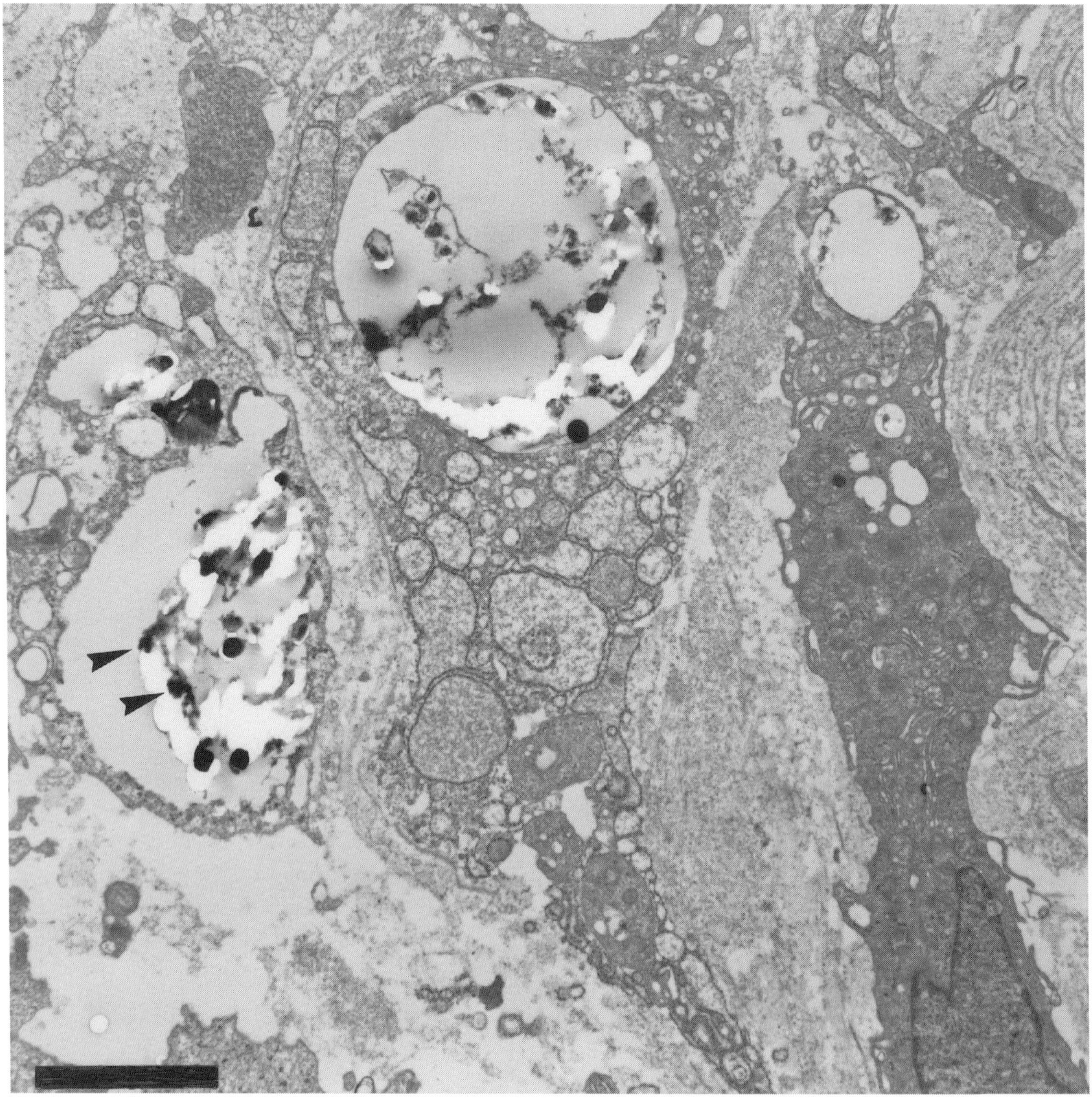

Figure 22.8 *Electron micrograph. Same nerve biopsy as in* Figure 22.7 *Several cell processi are vacuolated. Two vacuoles contain transversely sectioned* Mycobacterium leprae *(arrowheads). Bar: 3 μm.*

lower limbs. The changes become progressively more severe in a distal direction. The most distal nerves in the skin of the toes are often destroyed 'beyond recognition'. The plantar nerves contain some thin axons. There is some evidence of nerve fiber regeneration.

Pathology of Type 1 and 2 reactions

The main histological features of Type 1 reactions are an influx of mononuclear cells and an increase of edema, followed at a later stage by the appearance of epitheloid cells and giant cells (Job 1994). The histology of erythema nodosum leprosum is characterized by increase of inflammation of the dermis, superimposed on an already existing lepromatous infiltrate with deposition of immune complexes, vasculitis, infiltration by polymorphonuclear cells, some infiltration by $CD4^+$ T cells, necrosis and ulceration (Job 1994; Bloom and Ellner 1995).

Degeneration of nerve fibers: how and why?

The question is how, and for what reason do nerve fibers degenerate? Unmyelinated fibers in mildly affected nerves in cases of LL are reduced in density (Jacobs et al. 1993). This may in part be due to endoneurial edema but it is feasible that a proportion of these fibers degenerate and disappear by a process not yet elucidated, but caused by the accumulation of bacilli in the cytoplasm. Leprosy bacilli in axons and Schwann cells of myelinated fibers are rare but antigens from these bacilli could possibly play a role in the pathogenesis of myelinated fiber degeneration (Shetty et al. 1994). Axonal atrophy and paranodal demyelination of consecutive nodes of Ranvier, probably secondary to axonal atrophy or another axonal type of pathology, have been described (Jacobs et al. 1987, 1993; Shetty et al. 1988). Evidence pointing to axonal atrophy has been discovered both in early tuberculoid and lepromatous types of leprosy. This type of pathology is somewhat unexpected: atrophy of axons might conceivably be secondary to mechanical nerve damage (compression) proximal to the biopsy, or to degeneration of nerve fibers more distally (Jacobs et al. 1993). An iatrogenic cause (dapsone or thalidomide) might also be considered. At the site of cellular infiltrates whole internodes may be demyelinated, possibly due to myelinolytic factors released from the infiltrating cells (Jacobs et al. 1987). The marked loss of nerve fibers in tuberculoid forms of leprosy is related to the granulomatous inflammation in the immediate vicinity of the fibers. Loss of myelinated fibers in the lepromatous type of leprosy could be due to the presence of mycobacterial leprae specific antigens, and crossreacting antigens, in nerve fibers (Shetty et al. 1994). The reader will realize from these considerations that the exact causes of nerve fiber degeneration in the different forms of leprosy are at present not clearly understood.

Immunology

There is an exponential increase in the number of publications on the immunology of leprosy. We shall restrict ourselves in this section to a short discussion of four queries and the immunology of Type 1 and 2 reactions. The questions are: (1) how is protective immunity induced and which antigens are involved, (2) what is the effector mechanism of protective immunity, (3) is susceptibility for leprosy under genetic control, and (4) is the type of immune response under genetic control?

Which antigens induce protective immunity?

Intracellular mycobacteria secrete proteins into their environment. In animal models, protection against mycobacteria can only be induced by vaccination with live, not with dead attenuated mycobacteria. Dead mycobacteria do not secrete anymore. It has been suggested that protective immunity against mycobacteria is elicited by these secreted proteins. Most key proteins of *M. leprae* are now known and available for further investigations in the recombinant form (Young et al. 1992; Brennan 1994). *M. leprae* and other mycobacteria secrete a fibronectin *M. leprae*-binding 30–31 kDa protein complex, also referred to as antigen 85 or Ag 85. The *M. leprae* genes for this complex are approximately 85% homologous with the genes in *Mycobacterium tuberculosus* and *Mycobacterium bovis* BCG (Launois et al. 1993). In cultures of *Mycobacterium bovis* BCG (Bacille Calmette-Guérin), this protein complex is one of the major secreted proteins. The 30–31 kDa *M. leprae* protein is strongly immunogenic. T cells from household contacts of leprosy patients who develop a positive lepromin reaction, proliferate and produce IFN-gamma against the 30–31 kDa complex (Launois et al. 1993, 1995). This is not observed in household contacts that remain lepromin negative. The major *M. leprae* cytosolic protein, a 10 kDa heatshock protein is also strongly immunogenic. These two proteins could very well play a significant role in eliciting T cell-mediated protective immunity. Other antigens from other proteins or carbohydrates are at present being investigated with regard to their role in the immunological reactions; before long, a more complete picture is likely to emerge.

What is the effector mechanism of protective immunity?

Bacterial proteins, including the secreted proteins are broken down in the endosomal/lysosomal pathway, transported to the cell membrane and presented to the exterior by HLA class II molecules. These latter molecules are expressed by some macrophages and B cells but not by other somatic cells, unless induced by cytokines to do so. $CD4^+$ T cells recognize peptides presented by HLA class II molecules and can act in at least two ways. Some of the $CD4^+$ cells are cytotoxic and kill *Mycobacterium*-pulsed macrophages. They are apparently assisted in the killing process by $CD8^+$ cytotoxic cells, an unexpected recent finding (Ottenhoff 1994). How the $CD8^+$ cytotoxic cells become involved is not yet clear. Other $CD4^+$ T cells belong to the 'helper' category. At present two types of T helper cells can be distinguished: T_h1 and T_h2 (Paul and Seder 1994). T_h1 cells are defined by the production of interleukin 2 (IL-2) and interferon-gamma (IFN-gamma). IL-2 stimulates growth and differentiation of T cells and IFN-gamma is the major activator of macrophages. T_h1 cells promote cell-mediated immune reactions and play a key role in combating intracellular pathogens like mycobacteria. The T_h2 cells are defined by the production of IL-4, IL-5, IL-10 and IL-13. IL-4 and IL-5 stimulate B cells, eosinophils and mast cells and play a role in antibody production and humoral immunity. Antibodies are of little use in combating intracellular ML.

T cells from patients with tuberculoid leprosy which react with *M. leprae* are predominantly of the T_h1 phenotype (Yamamura et al. 1991). Cytokines of T_h1 cells, when injected in lesions from patients with LL, increase cell-mediated immunity and degradation of *M. leprae* (Kaplan et al 1989). Why this immune response should lead to TT leprosy in some exceptional individuals and to containment of infection in most others is unclear. In lesions from patients with LL, the mRNAs of T_h2 cells predominate over T_h1 cells. Some T cells in these patients suppress the response of T helper cells towards *M. leprae* (Ottenhoff 1994).

Is susceptibility to leprosy under genetic control?

The so-called *bcg* gene in mice appears to control innate resistance to mycobacteria. A similar gene might operate in humans and influence susceptibility for leprosy. Susceptibility in humans is not controlled by HLA linked genes (Vidal et al. 1993; Ottenhoff 1994).

Is the type of immune response under genetic control?

De Vries et al. and other groups (for a review see de Vries and Ottenhoff 1994) discovered an association of the type of immunopathology with HLA class II alleles. In some populations, TT is associated with HLA-DR and LL with HLA-DQ1. There is now some insight into the nature of these associations. It appears that dependent on the mode of presentation of an antigen by HLA class II molecules either T_h1 or T_h2 cells are activated (de Vries and Ottenhoff 1994; Mehra 1995). One of the most extensively investigated recombinant *M. leprae* proteins is hsp 65. This protein has 24 T cell epitopes which are presented on macrophage cell membranes by different HLA class II molecules. When restricted to HLA-DR2, DR5 and DR8, hsp65 induces a T_h1-like cytokine profile fitting a cell-mediated immune response and when restricted to HLA-DR1 or DR7 it induces a T_h2-like response.

Immunological aspects of Type 1 and 2 reactions

Type 1 or reversal reactions are due to an increase of cell-mediated immunity towards *M. leprae* and involve augmentation of $CD4^+$ T_h1 cell in infiltrates and elimination of leprosy bacilli. This, in itself favorable, reaction does, however, cause tissue damage, in particular neuritis. The cytokine pattern in lesions showing reversal reactions has characteristics similar to those in tuberculoid lesions and lepromin skin tests, only the level of the cytokine mRNAs is higher (Yamamura et al 1992). Messenger RNA of TNF-alpha is increased in reversal reactions in both nerve and skin biopsies (Khanolakar et al. 1995). TNF-alpha has a role in granuloma formation and contributes to the development of cell-mediated immunity. It also causes tissue damage and stimulates the production of reactive oxygen intermediate metabolites (Tracey et al. 1989). It is suggested that this cytokine might produce damage to peripheral nerves (Khanolakar-Young et al. 1995).

The cytokine pattern in ENL shows T_h2 characteristics (Yamamura et al. 1992) favoring humoral immune reactions. Tissue damage is suggested to be mediated at least in part by immune complex deposition and complement fixation (Modlin and Rea 1994).

Treatment

See Table 22.5.

Table 22.5 *Medical therapy in leprosy*

	Medication	Duration
Paucibacillary leprosy	Dapsone: 0.9–1.4 mg kg^{-1}, orally and daily. Rifampin: 10 mg kg^{-1}, orally, on empty stomach, under supervision, once a month.	6 months
Multibacillary leprosy	Dapsone: as in PB leprosy Rifampin: as in PB leprosy Clofazimine: 50 mg/day self-administered and 300 mg once a month under supervision.	Two years, or longer until smear negative
Type 1 reaction.		
A. with erythema, skin oedema	A. analgesics	
B. with other signs and symptoms	B. prednisone	40–60 mg per day, tapering when clinical signs react favorably, preferably no longer than 3 or 4 months
Type 2 reaction	A. prednisone B. thalidomide	A. as in Type 1 reactions B. advocated by many leprologists and some dermatologists, opposed by others. Daily dose at onset: 200 mg, twice daily, tapering after a few days. Maximum cumulative dose of 14 g.

Treatment of infections

Multidrug therapy (MDT) for leprosy was advised by the WHO in 1982. Monodrug therapy with dapsone, the current form of treatment at that time, had several drawbacks. Patient compliance during long-term treatment was poor and relapse rates were high. Most important of all, *M. leprae* became increasingly resistant to dapsone (Cartel et al. 1991). For PB leprosy, WHO advised to combine dapsone (daily dose 0.9–1.4 mg kg^{-1} orally, standard adult daily dose 100 mg) with rifampicin (10 mg kg^{-1} once a month, standard adult dose 600 mg or 450 mg when bodyweight is less than 45 kg, on an empty stomach and under supervision) for 6 months. Three drugs were recommended for MB leprosy: dapsone (same dose as in PB leprosy), rifampicin (again as in PB leprosy) and clofazimine (50 mg/day, self-administered and 300 mg once a month under supervision). Treatment of MB leprosy had to be continued for 2 years, or longer if after 2 years viable bacilli were still present in the skin smears.

The effect of this new form of treatment was initially not easy to establish. The clinical manifestations are not a sufficient measure in view of the chronicity of the disease. Relapse rates are a more clear-cut criterion but have to be differentiated from reactions which is not always easy. In MB leprosy the effect can be assessed by quantifying the viable bacilli in skin smears. Recent WHO data, collected in a 9-year follow-up period, indicate that relapse rates are overall less than 1% (Noordeen 1995). How long the follow-up period should be, before one can be sure that 'the disease will not come back' (Waters 1995) is not known. One should not be too optimistic too soon. Not all leprosy bacilli are necessarily killed, even after standard treatment. Replication of *M. leprae* is an extremely slow process. It may well take more than a decade before a sufficient number of bacilli has been generated to cause manifestations of LL.

Other points which have to be considered in assessing the success of therapy are the side-effects, the resistance of bacilli to the drugs and patient compliance (Jacobson 1994). Side-effects are uncommon and mild in dapsone and rifampin medication, but occasionally they are severe and life-threatening (exfoliative dermatitis, agranulocytosis, hepatotoxicity). Clofazimine has gastrointestinal pseudo-obstruction as the most severe, but rare complication. It is, however, infamous for the marked discoloration it induces, in particular of skin lesions. This is not a permanent effect, but it may take years for the discoloration to disappear completely. For light skin people, this may create a problem. In the USA, clofazimine is not prescribed and only dapsone and rifampin are given.

When the multidrug regimen was introduced, patient compliance generally improved, probably due to the much shorter treatment programs. Finally, the drug resistance problem was overcome by the multidrug approach. Up till now no major difficulties with resistant bacilli have been encountered.

Satisfactory treatment of infection does not mean that all bacterial remnants have been cleared. Leprosy reactions remain possible for years after treatment. During an 8-year period of observing 980 MB patients, all of whom had been treated until they were smear negative (with a high percentage of previously dapsone-treated patients), 11 patients (1.1%) had reactions. Most of these episodes (63%) occurred during the first 3 years of observation; one was noted after 7 years (Vijayakumaran et al. 1995). It is our impression that late reactions are more common in MB patients after 2 years of multidrug treatment.

Treatment of Type 1 and 2 reactions

Recommendations for treatment are with few exceptions predominantly based on retrospective studies or on personal experience of experts. Non-steroidal anti-inflammatory drugs (NSAIDs) and corticosteroids are both advocated and rest, splints and physiotherapeutic measures are considered important.

Corticosteroids are prescribed for their immunosuppressive effects and allow effective treatment of Type 1 and 2 reactions (Gelber 1995). Some authors recommend that corticosteroids are given only in cases with severe neuritis, ocular complications or extensive and inflamed skin lesions (Bhutani 1995). The best method to prevent disability is, however, to treat neuritis effectively, at an early stage (Miko et al. 1993; Pereira et al. 1993). Rose and Waters (1991) distinguish between mild reversal reactions with no more than mild erythema, skin edema and slight nerve tenderness which can be treated, according to these authors, with analgesics and which should resolve in a few weeks, and more severe reactions which should all be treated with corticosteroids. The effect of treatment on the nerves can be followed by several methods of sensory testing and manual muscle strength testing or nerve conduction studies. Gelber (1995) advises initiating treatment with prednisone, 40–60 mg daily, and tapering the dose according to the clinical signs. Treatment should be continued for 2–3 months to prevent relapse of reaction. The side-effects of corticosteroids are few when treatment is given for limited periods.

Thalidomide lowers tumor necrosis factor levels (Sampaio et al. 1991), slows polymorphonuclear leukocyte migration (Barnhill et al. 1984) and decreases IgM synthesis (Shannon et al. 1981). The favorable effect of thalidomide on ENL reactions is not disputed. In an editorial in *The Lancet*, Jakeman and Smith (1994) state that 'many trials of thalidomide have confirmed its usefulness in controlling erythema nodosum leprosum'. Its 'speed of action, bringing about subjective improvement within 24 hours in many cases, together with the steroid-sparing action, makes thalidomide the treatment of choice in serious ENL, despite numerous transient side-effects, such as mucosal dryness, rashes and constipation'. Thalidomide is known to cause a mainly sensory, distressing and disabling neuropathy with little tendency to recover (Le Quesne 1993). The effect of thalidomide on the autonomic nervous system has not been examined sufficiently. The incidence of this neuropathy was low, at the time that thalidomide was still being used as a hypnotic (the 1950s and early 1960s). Neuropathy was found to be frequent in patients receiving thalidomide in a daily dose of 400 mg for dermatological ailments (for a review see Critchley 1987). Clavelou et al. (1995) performed a prospective study in a group of 50 patients, who were all treated with thalidomide for dermatological reasons. Clinical evidence of neuropathy developed in 18 patients (36%). The chance of neuropathy increased when the age was over 56 years and the cumulative dose more than 14 g. Thalidomide is widely known and feared for its severe teratogenic effects and should not be given to women prior to the menopause. Recently it was reported that in a country which according to the government exerted strict controls on thalidomide, 47 thalidomide-damaged children had been born since the early 1960s when the use of the drug as a hypnotic was halted (Cutler 1994). There is a difference of opinion on the continued use of thalidomide in leprosy (Cutler 1994; Jones 1994; Gelber 1995; Jakeman and Smith 1994).

Recovery of lesioned nerves

The general experience in patients with severe axonal neuropathies is that recovery is partial and a degree of disability remains. Recovery of severe neuropathies progresses usually from proximal to distal: the borderline between hypoesthesia and anesthesia shifts in the distal direction. The most distal parts of the limbs (digits, footsoles) are the last to improve.

The extent of the problem created by leprosy can scarcely be overestimated: there are at present approximately three million or more patients with residual deformities due to leprosy and a considerable number of them have anesthetic footsoles. It is not clear what degree of spontaneous recovery can be expected in relation to the severity of neuropathy. In most patients, however, protective sensibility in anesthetic footsoles is not likely to return. Nerve decompression and neurolysis are ineffective (Bourrel 1991). Pereira et al.(1990) reasoned that nerve damage at the so-called predilection sites would be segmental and that fibrosis at these sites would block regeneration. Grafts of muscle tissue at these sites might therefore enhance regeneration. The question is how long are these damaged segments? Turkof et al. (1994) observed that swellings of the ulnar nerve extended from the distal part of the upper arm to halfway down the lower arm. Most authors feel that the length of grafts should not exceed, or be less than, 10 cm. Another problem is that muscle grafts for regeneration of mixed peripheral nerves appear not to be very successfull (Carder and Norris 1993).

There is hope that neurotrophic factors will prove to enhance the regenerating capacity of nerve fibers to a clinically relevant degree. Up till now, experimental investigations of these factors have concentrated mostly on traumatic nerve lesions, iatrogenic neuropathies and models of motor neuron disease. Similar investigations are now also feasible in animal models of leprosy.

For the first few years, rehabilitation will be the only therapy available to the patient handicapped by leprous neuropathy. A discussion of this subject is not within the scope of this chapter.

Acknowledgments

We thank Dr Aagje Jennekens-Schinkel for reading the manuscript. The first author acknowledges his introduction to clinical leprosy by Dr Wim Theuvenet.

References

Barnhill, R.L., Doll, N.J., Millikan, L.E., and Hastings, R.C. (1984). Studies on the anti-inflammatory properties of thalidomide: effects on polymorphonuclear leukocytes and monocytes. *J. Am. Acad. Dermatol.* **10**: 814–819.

Bell-Krotoski, J.A. (1991). Advances in sensibility evaluation. *Hand. Clin.* **7**: 527–546.

Bhutani, L.K. (1995). Medical management of leprosy. In Grand Round, report of a meeting of physicians and scientists at the All India Institute of Medical Sciences, New Delhi. *Lancet* **345**: 701.

Blake, L.A., West, B.C., Lary, C.H., and Todd, J.R. (1987). Environmental non-human sources of leprosy. *Rev. Inf. Dis.* **9**: 562–577.

Bloom, W.H. and Ellner, J.J. (1995). Immunology of mycobacterial infection. In *Principles and Practice of Infectious Diseases*, 4th edn, ed. G.L. Mandell, J.E. Bennet, and R. Dolin, pp. 1437–1449. New York: Churchill Livingstone.

Booth, R.J. and Watson, J.D. (1994). *M. leprae* antigens and the molecular biology of leprosy. In *Leprosy*, 2nd edn., ed. R.C. Hastings, pp. 123–135. Edinburgh: Churchill Livingstone.

Bourrel, P. (1991). Surgical rehabilitation. *Lepr. Rev.* **62**: 242–254.

Brennan, P.J. (1994). The microbiology of *Mycobacterium leprae*, Part II. *Int. J. Lepr.* **62**: 594–598.

Browne, S.G. (1975). Leprosy: clinical aspects of nerve involvement. In *Topics on Tropical Neurology*, ed. R.W. Hornabrook, p. 1. Philadelphia: F.A. Davis.

Carder, J.S. and Norris, R.W. (1993). Repair of mixed peripheral nerves using autografts: a preliminary communication. *Br. J. Plast. Surg.* **46**: 557–564.

Cartel, J.L., Boutin, J-P., Spiegel, A., Pilchart, R., and Roux, J.-F. (1991). Longitudinal study on relapses of leprosy in Polynesian multibacillary patients on dapsone monotherapy between 1940 and 1970. *Lepr. Rev.* **62**: 186–192.

Critchley, E.M.R. (1987). Neuropathies due to drugs. In *Handbook of Clinical Neurology*, vol. 51, ed. P.J. Vinken, G.W. Bruyn, H.L. Klawans, and W.B. Matthews, pp. 293–314. Amsterdam: Elsevier Science Publishers.

Clavelou, P., Colamarino, R., D'Incan, M., Deffond, D., Tournilhac, M., and Souteyrand, P. (1995). Thalidomide-related neuropathy: a prospective, clinical, electromyographic trial. *Neurology* **45**(suppl. 4)A: 168.

Cutler, J. (1994). Thalidomide revisited. *Lancet* **343**: 795.

Davey, T.F. and Rees, R.J.W. (1974). The nasal discharge in leprosy: clinical and bacteriological aspects. *Lepr. Rev.* **45**: 121–134.

Desikan, K.V. and Sreevatsa. (1979). Studies on viability of *M. Léprae* outside the human body. *Lepr. India* **51**: 588–589.

De Vries, R.R.P. and Ottenhoff, T.H.M. (1994). Immunogenetics of leprosy. In *Leprosy*, 2nd edn., ed. R.C. Hastings, pp. 113–121. Edinburgh: Churchill Livingstone.

Gelber, R.H. (1995). Leprosy (Hansen's disease). In *Principles and Practice of Infectious Diseases* 4th edn, ed. G.L. Mandell, J.E. Bennet, and R. Dolin, pp. 2243–2250. New York: Churchill Livingstone.

Gormus, B.J., Xu, K., Baskin, G.B., Martin, L.N., Bohm, R.P., Blanchard, J.L., Mack, P.A., Ratterree, M.S., McClure, H.M., Meyers, W.M., and Walsh, G.P. (1995). Experimental leprosy in monkeys. I. Sooty mangabey monkeys: transmission, susceptibility, clinical and pathological findings. *Lepr. Rev.* **66**: 96–104.

Hastings, R.C. (ed). (1994). *Leprosy.* Edinburgh: Churchill Livingstone.

Hirata, T. and Harada, N. (1994). Electron microscopic observations of small unmyelinated nerve tissue proper in a dermal lesion of a relapsed lepromatous patient. *Int. J. Lepr.* **62**: 619–622.

Jacobs, J.M., Shetty, V.P, and Antia, N.H. (1987). Teased fibre studies in leprous neuropathy. *J. Neurol. Sci.* **79**: 301–313.

Jacobs, J.M., Shetty, V.P., and Antia, N.H. (1993). A morphological study of nerve biopsies from cases of multibacillary leprosy given multidrug therapy. *Acta Neuropathol.* **85**: 533–541.

Jacobson, R.J. (1994). Treatment of leprosy. In *Leprosy*, 2nd edn, ed. R.C. Hastings, pp. 317–349. Edinburgh: Churchill Livingstone.

Jakeman, P. and Smith, W.C.S. (1994). Thalidomide in leprosy reaction. *Lancet* **343**: 432–433.

Jakeman, P., Jakeman, N.R.P., and Singay, J. (1995). Trends in leprosy in the Kingdom of Bhutan, 1982–1992. *Lepr. Rev.* **66**: 69–75.

Job, C.K. (1994). Pathology of leprosy. In *Leprosy*, 2nd edn, ed. R.C. Hastings, pp. 193–224. Edinburgh: Churchill Livingstone.

Job, C.K., Chehl, S.K., and Hastings, R.C. (1994). Transmission of leprosy in nude mice through thorn pricks. *Int. J. Lepr.* **62**: 395–398.

Jones, G.R.N. (1994). Thalidomide: 35 years on and still deforming. *Lancet* **343**: 1041.

Kaplan, G., Kiessling, R., Teklemariam, S., Hancock, G., Sabawork., Sheftel, G., Job, C.K., Converse, P., Ottenhoff, T.H.M., Becx-Bleumink, M., Dietz, M., and Cohn, Z.A. (1988). The reconstitution of cell-mediated immunity in the cutaneous lesions of lepromatous leprosy by recombinant interleukine 2. *J. Exp. Med.* **169**: 893–907.

Khanolakar-Young, S., Rayment, N., Brickell, P.M., Katz, D.R., Vinayakumari, S., Colston, M.J., and Lockwood, D.N.J. (1995). Tumour necrosis factor (TNF-alpha) synthesis is associated with the skin and peripheral nerve pathology of leprosy reversal reactions. *Clin. Exp. Immunol.* **99**: 196–202.

Launois, P., Niang N'Diaye, M., De Bruyn, J., Sarthou, J-L., Rivier, F., Drowart, A., Van Vooren, J.P., Milan, J., and Huygen K. (1993). The major secreted antigen complex (Ag 85) from *Mycobacterium bovis* Bacille Calmette-Guérin is associated with protective T cells in leprosy: a follow-up study of 45 household contacts. *J. Infect. Dis.* **167**: 1160–1167.

Launois, P., Niang N'Diang, M., Cartel, J.L., Mane, I., Drowart, A., Van Vooren, J.P., Sarthou, J.L., and Huygen K. (1995). Fibronectin binding antigen 85 and the 10–kilodalton GroES-related heatshock protein are the predominant Th-1 response inducers in leprosy contacts. *Infect. Immun.* **63**: 88–93.

Le Quesne, P.M. (1993). Neuropathy due to drugs. In *Peripheral Neuropathy*, 3rd edn, vol. 2, ed. P.J. Dyck, P.K. Thomas, J.W. Griffin, P.A. Low, J.F. Poduslo, pp. 1571–1581. Philadelphia: W.B. Saunders.

Lienhardt, C. and Fine, P.E.M. (1994). Type 1 reaction, neuritis and disability in leprosy. What is the current epidemiological situation? *Lepr. Rev.* **65**: 9–33.

Lumpkin III, L.R., Cox, G.F., and Wolf Jr, J.E. (1983). Leprosy in five armadillo handlers. *J. Am. Acad. Dermatol.* **9**: 899–903.

Mehra, N.K. (1995). Immunogenetics of leprosy. In: Grand Round, report of a meeting of physicians and scientists at the All India Institute of Medical Sciences, New Delhi. *Lancet* **345**: 699–701.

Meyers, W.M., Gomus, B.J., and Walsh, G.P. (1994). Experimental leprosy. In *Leprosy*, 2nd edn, ed. R.C. Hastings, pp. 385–408. Edinburgh: Churchill Livingstone.

Miko, T.L., Le Maitre, C., and Kinfu, Y. (1993). Damage and regeneration of peripheral nerves in advanced treated leprosy. *Lancet* **342**: 521–525.

Mistry, N.N. and Antia, N.H. (1993). Polymerase chain reaction and assessment of leprosy chemotherapy. *Lancet* **342**: 1060.

Modlin, R.L. and Rea, T.H. (1994). Immunopathology of leprosy. In *Leprosy*, 2nd edn, ed. R.C. Hastings, Edinburgh: Churchill Livingstone.

Noordeen, S.K. (1995). Elimination of leprosy as a public health problem: progress and prospects. *Bull. World Org.* **73**: 1–6.

Ottenhoff, T.H.M. (1994). Immunology of leprosy: lessons from and for leprosy. *Int. J. Lepr.* **62**: 108–121.

Paul, W.E. and Seder, R.A. (1994). Lymphocyte responses and cytokines. *Cell* **76**: 241–251.

Pereira, J.H., Cowley, S.A., Gschmeisser, S.E., Bowden, R.E.M., and Turk, J.I. (1990). Denatured muscle grafts for nerve repair: an experimental model of nerve damage in leprosy. *J. Bone Joint Surg. Br.* **72B**: 874–880.

Pereira, J.H, Bowden, R.E.M, Gschmeisser, S.E, and Narayankumar, T.S. (1993). Nerve damage in leprosy. *Lancet* **342**: 1060–1061.

Pfaltzgraff, R.E. and Ramu, G. (1994). Clinical leprosy. In *Leprosy*, 2nd edn, ed. R. C. Hastings, pp. 237–287. Edinburgh: Churchill Livingstone.

Pönnighaus, J.M., Fine, P.E.M., Sterne, J.A.C., Bliss, L., Wilson, R.J., Malema, S.S., and Kileta, S. (1994). Incidence rates of leprosy in Karonga district, Northern Malawi: patterns by age, sex, BCG status and classification. *Int. J. Lepr.* **62**: 10–23.

Rees, R.J.W. and Young, D.B. (1994). The microbiology of leprosy. In *Leprosy*, 2nd edn, ed. R.C. Hastings, pp. 49–53. Edinburgh: Churchill Livingstone.

Ridley, D.S. and Jopling, W.H. (1966). Classification of leprosy according to immunity: a five group system. *Int. J. Lepr.* **34**: 255–273.

Rose, P. and Waters, M.F.R. (1991). Reversal reactions in leprosy and their management. *Lepr.Rev.* **62**: 113–119.

Sabin, T.D., Swift, T.R., and Jacobson, R.R. (1993). Leprosy. In *Peripheral Neuropathy*, 3rd edn, vol. 2, ed. P.J. Dyck, P.K. Thomas, J.W. Griffin, P.A. Low, and J.F. Poduslo, pp. 1354–1379. Philadelphia: W.B. Saunders.

Sampaio, E.P., Sarno, E.N, Galilly, R. et al. (1991). Thalidomide selectively inhibits tumor necrosis factor alpha production by stimulated human monocytes. *J. Exp. Med.* **173**: 699–703.

Scollard, D.M., Smith, T., Bhoopat, L. Theetranont, C., Rangdaeng, S., and Morens, D.M. (1994). Epidemiological characteristics of leprosy reactions. *Int. J. Lepr.* **62**: 559–567.

Shannon, E.J., Miranda, R.O, Morales, M.J. et al. (1981). Inhibition of de novo IgM antibody synthesis by thalidomide as relevant mechanism of action in leprosy. *Scand. J. Immunol.* **13**: 553–562.

Shetty, V.P., Antia, N.H., and Jacobs J.M. (1988). The pathology of early leprous neuropathy. *J. Neurol. Sci.* **88**: 115–131.

Shetty, V.P., Uplekar. M.W., and Antia N.H. (1994). Immunohistological localization of mycobacterial antigens within the peripheral nerves of treated leprosy patients and their significance to nerve damage in leprosy. *Acta Neuropathol.* **88**: 300–306.

Thomas, D.A., Mines, J.S., Thomas, D.C., Mack, T.M., and Rea, T.H. (1987). Armadillo exposure among Mexican born patients with lepromatous leprosy. *J. Infect. Dis.* **156**: 990–992.

Tracey, K.J., Vlassara, V., and Cerami, A. (1989). Cachectin/tumour necrosis factor. *Lancet* **2**: 1122–1126.

Turkof, E., Tambwekar, S., Mansukhani, K., Millesi, H., and Mayr, N. (1994). Intraoperative spinal root stimulation to detect most proximal site of leprous ulnar neuritis. *Lancet* **343**: 1604–1605.

Van Brakel, W.H. and Khawas, I.B. (1994a). Silent neuropathy in leprosy: an epidemiological description. *Lepr. Rev.* **65**: 350–360.

Van Brakel, W.H. and Khawas, I.B. (1994b). Nerve damage in leprosy: an epidemiological and clinical study of 396 patients in West Nepal. Part 1: definitions, methods and frequencies. *Lepr. Rev.* **65**: 204–221.

Vidal, S.M., Malo, D., Vogan, K., Skamene, E., and Gros P. (1993). Natural resistance to infection with intracellular parasites: isolation of a candidate for bcg. *Cell* **73**: 469–485.

Vijayakumaran, P., Manimozzhi, N., and Jesudasan, K. (1995). Incidence of late leprae reaction among multibacillary leprosy patients after MDT. *Int.J. Lepr.* **63**: 18–22.

Waters, M.F.R. (1995). Relapse following various types of multidrug therapy in multibacillary leprosy. *Lepr. Rev.* **66**: 1–9.

Wemambu, S.N.C., Turk, J.L., Waters, M.F.R., and Rees, R.J.W. (1969). Erythema nodosum leprosum: a clinical manifestation of the Arthus phenomenon. *Lancet* **2**: 933–935.

Yamamura, M., Uyemura, K., Deans, R.J., Weinberg, K., Rea, T.H., Bloom, B.R., and Modlin, R.L. (1991). Defining protective responses to pathogens: cytokine profiles in leprosy lesions. *Science* **254**: 277–279.

Yamamura, M., Wang, X-H., Ohmen, J.D., Uyemura, K., Rea, T., Bloom, B., and Modlin, R.L. (1992). Cytokine patterns of immunologically mediated tissue damage. *J. Immunol.* **149**: 1470–1475.

Young, D.B., Kaufmann, S.H.E, Hermans, P.W.M., and Thole, J.E.R. (1992). Mycobacterial antigens: a compilation. *Mol. Microbiol* **6**: 133–145.

23 Neuropathies associated with herpes virus infections

I. Steiner and D. Wolf

Introduction

The herpes viruses are double-stranded DNA viruses with the unique ability to establish latent infection in their hosts and cause recurrent disease by reactivation. Of the human herpesviruses, herpes simplex virus type 1 and 2 (HSV-1 and 2) and varicella-zoster virus (VZV) are neurotropic, namely they establish latent infection in the peripheral nervous system (PNS) and the viral genome is maintained in peripheral sensory ganglia (PSG) for the entire life of the host. The PSG are the reservoir from which the neurotropic herpesviruses can reactivate and cause neurological and mucocutaneous disorders. Human cytomegalovirus (HCMV) can cause several PNS disorders, mainly in immunocompromised individuals. The aim of this review is to cover the phenomenology of PNS disorders associated with herpes viruses and to examine the molecular and cellular basis of latent herpes virus infection within PSG.

The three neurotropic herpes viruses vary in the clinical disorders they cause, and differ in the molecular basis that underlies them; however, they share several features that govern the biology of their infection in the human nervous system. (1) The primary infection involves the mucocutaneous surfaces which serve as the portal of entry of the viral particles into the PNS. (2) The primary and the infectious recurrent diseases caused by the same virus usually occur within the same cutaneous distribution. (3) Under normal (i.e. immunocompetent) conditions, the reactivation infection usually does not spread beyond the anatomic distribution and the vicinity of a single PSG. (4) While primary infection usually takes place during the first two to three decades of life, reactivation may occur throughout life, sometimes at a very advanced age. These features can be grouped under a unifying hypothesis that is now the dogma in herpes virology (Goodpasture 1929; Hope-Simpson 1965): Following primary infection, the virus gains access to axon endings within the mucocutaneous surfaces and is transported to the PSG. The viral genome is maintained within the PSG which serves as a reservoir for viral nucleic acids. Latent herpetic infection is a lifelong state. Under certain circumstances the virus can reactivate and travel to regions innervated by the respective PSG causing recurrent disease there.

Neurotropic herpes viruses: clinical syndromes

Varicella-zoster virus (VZV)

Primary infection

VARICELLA. VZV is the agent responsible for chickenpox (varicella) and herpes zoster ('shingles') (for reviews see Kennedy 1987; Gilden et al. 1992). Primary infection is an exanthematous, highly contagious disease, affecting young children (Preblud 1986). The incubation period lasts usually between 9 to 21 days (Grose 1981), and patients can transmit the virus from 2 days before the appearance of the rash until vesicles have crusted, usually a time span of 8 days. The rash consists of vesicular skin lesions with a characteristic distribution, affecting mainly the thorax and the face within the sensory supply of the ophthalmic branch of the trigeminal nerve. Several central nervous system (CNS) complications may follow chickenpox and include congenital varicella syndrome, acute cerebellar ataxia, meningoencephalitis, myelitis and Reye's syndrome. A detailed description of these entities is beyond the scope of this review.

ACUTE INFLAMMATORY DEMYELINATING POLYNEUROPATHY (AIDP, GUILLAIN-BARRÉ SYNDROME (GBS)). This accounts for about 7% of all the complications of varicella (Miller et al. 1956; Rab and Choudhury 1963). On the other hand, among all patients with varicella it is a rare complication (e.g. eight out of 2534 patients in the study by Bullowa and Wishik 1935), and none of the patients with fatal GBS extensively studied by Haymaker and Kernohan (1949), developed the disease following chickenpox. The interval between appearance of the rash and the neurological symptoms ranges from 7 to 20 days and there are no characteristic features to distinguish this postvaricella polyradiculopathy from any other AIDP which follows infection. AIDP variants such as cranial nerve palsies (extraocular nerve paralysis with diplopia, facial diplegia, bulbar involvement) or ataxia have also been reported (Miller et al. 1956; McKendell and Klawans 1978).

Reactivation: herpes zoster (shingles)

EPIDEMIOLOGY AND CLINICAL PICTURE. Herpes zoster is a disease of the elderly. People over 60 years of age have an eight to tenfold increased incidence of zoster compared to those under 60 years (Harnisch 1984). An exception are immunocompromised individuals (Schimpff et al. 1972; Mazur and Dolin 1978) including AIDS patients (van de Perre et al. 1988) who have an increased disease prevalence at a younger age. Although any level of the neuroaxis may be affected by zoster, it tends to involve the cutaneous sites where the highest burden of lesions containing viral particles was present during chickenpox: the thorax and the face within the distribution of the trigeminal nerve.

Typical zoster takes the form of vesicular eruptions distributed unilaterally within a dermatome. In immunocompetent individuals, zoster is usually a single episode and more than three recurrences are extremely rare. The vesicles are clear, become turbid and crust within 5–10 days. Resolution may leave scars. The main neurological complications include peripheral sensory disturbances, and in most cases no motor, CNS or systemic abnormalities occur. The condition might be preceded by paresthesias, itching and pain. The sensory symptoms may be severe enough to suggest an alternative cause, such as coronary ischemia or an abdominal condition (Gais and Abrahamson 1939). Pain and itching are usual concomitants of the eruption, and may also follow the rash and become a chronic, though self-limited disorder termed postherpetic neuralgia (PHN; see below). Dissemination of the eruption and the symptomatology to neighboring dermatomes may occur. Occasionally, a typical herpes zoster pain is not associated with skin lesions and is accompanied only by a rise in VZV antibody titers, a condition termed 'zoster sine herpetica'.

Herpes zoster may be associated with subtle signs of aseptic meningitis in up to 50% of patients (Appelbaum et al. 1962). These patients show mild cerebrospinal fluid (CSF) mononuclear pleocytosis with mild increase in protein levels; however, only seldom is this associated with isolation of the causative virus from the CSF.

PREDISPOSING FACTORS. Predisposing factors and triggers for the appearance of zoster infection include diabetes mellitus, surgery and other trauma, spinal anesthesia, exposure to ultraviolet light, malignancies and conditions associated with immune suppression such as lymphoma, steroid therapy, immunosuppressive agents

(Hope-Simpson 1965; Juel-Jensen 1970; Schimpff et al. 1972) and AIDS. Despite the increased incidence of zoster in cancer patients, apparently healthy individuals who develop zoster do not have an increased risk for an occult cancer, and therefore the cost-effectiveness of a thorough search for an underlying malignancy in patients with zoster without a diagnosed neoplasm is questionable (Ragozzino et al. 1982).

While varicella can follow exposure to zoster, the opposite, namely the occurrence of shingles following exposure to a patient with chickenpox, is extremely rare (Thomas and Robertson 1971; Morens et al. 1980), and the underlying mechanism unclear.

HERPES ZOSTER IN THE IMMUNOCOMPROMISED HOST. This is more prevalent than in the healthy population and takes a more severe course. Widespread dissemination which occurs in 2–10% of zoster patients is usually associated with malignancy or immunosuppression.

Patients who are HIV-positive, and suffer either from what was formerly termed AIDS-related complex (ARC) or from AIDS, have an increased incidence of herpes zoster, which is more protracted, tends to recur and might be complicated by dissemination, encephalitis and death. In the population at risk, the occurrence of herpes zoster raises the possibility of HIV infection and is regarded as a poor prognostic sign (Melbye et al. 1987; van de Perre et al. 1988).

Peripheral neurological complications of herpes zoster

The central neurological complications which follow herpes zoster, i.e. encephalomyelitis, isolated myelitis, granulomatous arteritis, optic neuritis, and multifocal leukoencephalitic syndromes are beyond the scope of this review. The PNS complications of zoster include the following.

POSTHERPETIC NEURALGIA (PHN). This is the most common neurological complication of zoster (Burgoon et al. 1957, Price 1981; Gilden et al. 1992). It is defined as pain in the distribution of the rash which persists beyond 4–6 weeks following shingles. The risk for PHN increases with age, and almost half of the patients over 60 years who suffer from zoster will develop it (Gilden et al. 1992), immunocompromised patients being more susceptible. The pain involves the affected dermatome and is usually severe, burning, lancinating and constant. In fact, it can be so disturbing as to lead to severe depression and even suicide. The pathogenesis of PHN is not well understood. Whether this syndrome is the outcome of persistence of the viral infection following zoster, as might be suggested by the presence of VZV-specific proteins in peripheral mononuclear cells of patients with PHN (Vafai et al. 1988), or is due to structural changes within the PSG following reactivation (Kennedy and Steiner 1994), is not clear. Treatment of PHN is usually very difficult and the pain in many cases may be intractable. The therapeutic regimen may consist of the combination of local application of cold, analgesics and carbamazepine and/or tricyclic antidepressants preferably amitriptyline (Max 1994). Topical application of capsaicin (Watson et al. 1993) or lidocaine (Rowbotham et al. 1995) may also have a temporary effect. When considering more drastic measures, such as surgery (i.e dorsal root entry zone operation or ganglionotomy), it should always be kept in mind that PHN is a self limited condition.

MOTOR INVOLVEMENT. Motor impairment in zoster is the exception, though its reported incidence varies (0.5–31%). It may follow shingles within 1 day to 4 months, and in 90% of cases it involves the same segment which is affected by the rash: peripheral facial weakness with zoster oticus and eruption within the ear canal and the adjacent skin (Ramsay–Hunt syndrome), ophthalmoplegia, mainly of the III cranial nerve (Thomas and Howard 1972), arm weakness in association with zoster within cervical dermatomes (also responsible sometimes for diaphragmatic paresis (Anderson and Keal 1969) and lumbosacral zoster leading to leg weakness. Neurogenic bladder and loss of anal sphincter control may follow sacral zoster (Jellinek and Tulloch 1976). The prognosis of the motor weakness is generally good and more than half of the patients regain full motor power (Grant and Rowe 1961; Gupta et al. 1969; Greenberg 1970; Thomas and Howard 1972). In another third the improvement is significant.

AIDP. Zoster has also been associated with a polyneuropathic syndrome which conforms with the diagnostic criteria of AIDP (Asbury et al. 1978). The interval between the rash and the neurological symptoms ranges from several days to months. The true incidence of this disorder is unknown as both herpes zoster and AIDP are quite common. It seems that AIDP following chicken-pox is more prevalent than AIDP following zoster. Several features distinguish AIDP postzoster from the condition that follows other infections. The shorter the interval between the herpes zoster infection and AIDP, the more severe the disease (Knox et al. 1961). Cranial nerve involvement is present in 50% of patients (Kennedy 1987). The mortality rate is exceptionally high, up to half of the cases (Dayan et al. 1972). This figure, however, is probably a reflection of an era prior to the advent of intensive and respiratory care, but nevertheless suggests that AIDP following zoster is a more severe disease. It seems likely that the polyneuropathic syndrome following zoster shares the same pathogenesis as AIDP and has an immune-mediated basis (Steiner and Abramsky 1985).

Diagnosis of VZV infections

The diagnosis of VZV infection is usually clinical; however, occasionally laboratory confirmation might be required. This may include an attempt (usually unsuccessful) to culture the virus from body fluids or the CSF by incubating fluid samples with susceptible human cell lines until cytopathic effect appears (Gold 1966). Additional techniques consist of immunofluorescent demonstration of viral antigens in biopsied lesions (Peters et al. 1979), electron microscopy (Steele et al. 1983), retrospective fourfold increase in antibody titer following infection (Bieger et al. 1977) and the indirect membrane immunofluorescence assay (Gershon et al. 1980). With the advent of molecular biology technology, polymerase chain reaction (PCR), a highly sensitive method to amplify nucleic acids, may become a fast and effective means to diagnose VZV infections (Nahass et al. 1995).

Treatment

Under normal immune surveillance, zoster infection is a self-limited condition. In immunocompromised patients and individuals over 60 years of age, acyclovir (alpha-cycloguanosine, see below) has been shown to reduce dissemination and shorten the course of herpes zoster (Peterslund et al. 1981; Bean et al. 1982; Balfour et al. 1983). Systemic administration of acyclovir may also shorten the course of the disease in immunologically intact individuals (Peterslund et al. 1981; Bean et al. 1982), while topical usage reduces the duration of the sensory symptomatology during the acute course of the disease. Both do not influence the incidence of PHN (Kennedy 1987). Steroid usage is controversial. They carry the risk of side-effects and complications, especially in the elderly population and under immune-compromised conditions, and therefore are not recommended by us.

Herpes simplex viruses type 1 and 2

Compared with VZV, PNS infections due to HSV-1 and 2 are of little clinical significance. Nevertheless, these viruses have been the focus of great biological interest (Steiner and Kennedy 1993) and the accumulated knowledge has now paid off with the recent advances in the arena of viral vectors for gene transfer and therapy. The clinical disorders caused by these two viruses are very different from those caused by VZV, and the molecular basis of their latent infection in the PNS is also different.

HSV-1 and 2 are closely related viruses which partially differ in their biochemical composition, cytopathic effect and genetic information as well as their neurotropic features. Nevertheless, their genetic material is homologous to a considerable extent and they share crossreactivity between their glycoproteins. Likewise, there is a great deal of similarity between the clinical manifestations of the disorders they cause, although they are usually transmitted via different routes and induce primary and recurrent disease in different parts of the body.

Primary infection

Mucocutaneous surfaces are the site of primary infection. Both viruses can cause genital and orofacial infections, which are clinically indistinguishable; however, the mouth and lips are the common site for HSV-1 primary infection which usually occurs prior to age 5 years and in most of the cases is asymptomatic (Cesario et al. 1969). When clinically apparent, gingivostomatitis and pharyngitis are frequent manifestations, and fever and cervical lymphadenopathy are then common. Following primary infection, an immune response with seroconversion is triggered.

As HSV-2 infections are usually acquired through sexual contact (Nahmias et al. 1969), primary infection is a feature of the second and third decades of life. Small grouped vesicles which ulcerate and coalesce to involve a larger genital surface are the usual manifestation.

PNS COMPLICATIONS. Primary HSV-1 infections are extremely rare and sometimes merit a special report. Thus, radiculomyelopathy following primary HSV-2 infection (Handler and Perkin 1982), and acute autonomic neuropathy with favorable prognosis following oral HSV infection (Neville and Sladen 1984) were recorded. Sacral radiculitis associated with pain and paresthesias has been reported in genital or rectal primary HSV-1 and 2 infection (Craig and Nahmias 1973; Handler and Perkin 1982). AIDP following both primary or reactivated HSV infection seems to be more prevalent (Olivarius and Buhl 1975; Black et al. 1983), but there are no exact clinical and epidemiological data to delineate this syndrome. Idiopathic peripheral facial nerve paralysis (Bell's palsy) following HSV infection is much less prevalent compared with its prevalence following VZV, ranging from 0 to 9% post-HSV compared with 14–25% in VZV (Kukimoto et al. 1988).

Reactivation

With both viruses, reactivations can be asymptomatic. e.g. viral shedding may not be associated with clinical disease. Reactivation at the orofacial or genital site is caused by the same virus type that caused the primary infection at the same site. This bears on the frequency of reactivations. In the genital region, HSV-2 has a much higher frequency of reactivations than HSV-1 (Reeves et al. 1981).

In the orofacial region, recurrent disease is almost always due to HSV-1 and it is triggered by exposure to sunlight, severe stress, trauma (such as neurosurgical manipulation) fever or menses. Herpes labialis or cold sores is an extremely frequent condition affecting between 30 to 61% of the population (Whitley 1990). Clinically, lesions are closely clustered vesicles which usually reoccur at the same site, tend to remain very localized and do not involve the entire dermatome. They take up to 10–14 days to heal. Some patients can anticipate the appearance of cold sores by mild sensory symptoms such as tingling or burning but only very rarely by neuralgia which is always transitory and is not associated with any permanent sensory deficit (Constantine et al. 1988; Gominak 1990).

The genital recurrent infection, mainly due to HSV-2, occurs in up to 60% of patients who have a latent genital herpetic infection (Chang et al. 1974), and is usually of shorter duration. HSV-2 has also been isolated from the urethra and urine of women and men without concomitant genital lesions with and without urethritis. Occasionally recurrent herpes genitalis is associated with radiculitis and meningitis (Craig and Nahmias 1972; Handler and Perkin 1982). When sphincter disturbances, such as urinary retention or difficulty in initiation of micturition occur, it may be difficult or even impossible to distinguish between polyradiculitis and low segmental myelitis. Most patients have pleocytosis in the CSF and elevated protein.

HSV may also reactivate under immunocompromised conditions, though to a lesser extent than VZV. Notably, HSV accounts for most viral infections in bone marrow recipient patients (Bustamante and Wade 1991; Momin and Chandrasekar 1995) causing hemorrhagic, oral or genital mucocutaneous lesions, esophagitis and sometimes pneumonia. In this setting, prophylactic therapy might be indicated (see below) .

Diagnosis

The standard laboratory procedure to diagnose HSV infection is to grow the virus from the lesions or fluids in tissue culture (Corey 1986). Cultures are positive in 60–90% of clinically suspected cases. Additional means may include cytology, histopathology of biopsied lesions and monoclonal antibodies directed against HSV-1 and HSV-2 (Goldstein et al. 1983). Serological diagnosis is not of great clinical value. PCR, in use for the diagnosis of herpes simplex encepalitis (Lakeman and Whitley 1995), may become also a useful diagnostic tool in the differential diagnosis of cutaneous lesions (Nahass et al. 1995).

Treatment

Acyclovir is an antiviral compound developed for use against herpes simplex infections. It is phosphorylated to its active form by the virus-specific thymidine kinase enzyme and prevents viral replication by inhibiting the viral (as well as the cellular) DNA polymerase. Topical, oral and parenteral preparations are available. It has been reported to be effective in controlling the recurrent HSV infection in immunocompetent (Douglas et al. 1984; Straus et al. 1984a) as well as immunocompromised patients (Straus et al. 1984b). This however, carries the risk of developing acyclovir-resistant viral strains, a concern especially in immunocompromised patients. In immunocompetent individuals, cessation of acyclovir leads to reactivation rates similar to those present prior to therapy, reflecting the fact that the viral reservoir itself is probably not affected by this mode of therapy.

Immunology of neurotropic herpes virus infections

Abundant information is gathered on the immunological concomitants of HSV infections. Animal models and humans have served to obtain data on the immunogenetic background, macrophages, specific T cell subpopulation, antibody formation and lymphokine response. The results and interpretation of the data vary with the route of infection, the animal model, the amount of viral load, the viral strain, etc., and the relevance of the information to both the incidence and the severity of the primary and recurrent HSV-1-induced disease in the immunocompetent host is sometimes questionable.

All three neurotropic herpesviruses possess the ability to produce recurrent infections in the presence of circulating antibodies. A defective immune system may render the individual more susceptible to VZV recurrent disease compared with HSV. Nevertheless, both HSV and VZV can cause severe recurrent disease under immunocompromised conditions.

Under experimental conditions, the immune system can influence HSV gene expression during the acute phase of infection. Antibodies have been shown to bind to HSV-1 infected neurons, thus suppressing viral replication (Birmanns et al. 1993; Oaks et al. 1984). CD8 cytotoxic T cells may terminate viral gene expression in neurons prior to cell destruction (Simmons and Tscharke 1992). Infected neurons fail to express major histocompatibility complex (MHC) antigens (Oldstone 1991). Indeed, it has recently been shown that an HSV-specific protein can bind to a cellular transporter associated with antigen processing, leading to the retention of MHC class I molecules within the cell, enabling the virus to evade the host immune response (Froh et al. 1995; Hill et al. 1995). While an intact immune system is not an absolute prerequisite for the establishment of HSV latent infection in experimental animals (Moriyama et al. 1992; Valyi-Nagy et al. 1992) it may still have an impact upon the efficacy of this process. Likewise, a competent immune response is not required for the maintenance of latent HSV-1 infection and prevention of reactivation in the same experimental animal models (Moriyama et al. 1992; Valyi-Nagy et al. 1992).

About 80% of adults are seropositive to VZV glycoproteins (Giller et al. 1989), but it is the cellular immune response that plays a key role in preventing recurrent VZV infection. Patients with impaired cell-mediated immunity, unlike those with a defective humoral response, are prone to develop disseminated and fatal VZV infection (Merigan and Stevens 1971). The decline in the VZV-specific T cell response that accompanies normal aging (Miller 1980) is probably responsible for the prevalence of herpes zoster in this age population (see below).

Molecular and cellular basis of latent herpetic infections in human peripheral sensory ganglia

Most of the information on the molecular concomitants of herpes virus latency stem from studies on HSV-1 because it is relatively easy to propagate this virus in cell cultures and it readily infects experimental animals. VZV on the other hand, is a species-specific virus and the molecular data are therefore limited mainly to human tissues obtained at post-mortem. Thus, the initial information was gathered on HSV-1 latency in experimental animals, confirmed by studies of human autopsy material, and then extrapolated, when feasible, to the other human neurotropic herpes viruses.

Herpes simplex virus

HSV-1 is a lytic virus. During replication in cells in culture the infected cell is destroyed. Replication at the peripheral site of primary infection or in the PSG is not mandatory for the establishment of latency (Steiner et al. 1990). Lack of replication carries obvious advantages for the virus as destruction of the host cell will prevent its ability to reside within the cell and to establish latent infection (Steiner and Kennedy 1991; Birmanns et al. 1993). The viral particles are transported from the peripheral site of primary infection to the PSG by retrograde axonal transport where they establish latent infection. During latent infection the viral DNA changes its form and becomes either circular or is present as a concatamer (Rock and Fraser 1983). During the same period the viral genome is maintained in a non-integrated (episomal) form in the neuronal host cell, thus avoiding unforeseen effects upon the host genetic material (Mellerick and Fraser 1987). Indeed, the function and metabolism of the infected host cell remain unaltered. Although theoretically the virus can reside latent in non-neuronal cells, all the information suggests that in PSG HSV-1 resides only in neuronal cells.

During latency, restricted viral gene expression takes place (Spivack and Fraser 1987; Stevens et al. 1987; Steiner et al. 1988). The genes expressed during latency differ from those which are expressed during HSV-1 replication in cells in culture (Spivack and Fraser 1988). Two types of RNA species are expressed during latent infection: more abundant RNAs termed latency-associated transcripts (LATs) and less abundant minor LATs (mLATs). The latency-associated gene expression of HSV-1 plays a role in viral reactivation from latent infection (Javier et al. 1988; Steiner et al. 1989; Trousdale et al. 1991). The exact DNA sequences which mediate this function and the potential gene products of the latency-associated genes are unknown and their mechanisms of action remain to be elucidated. HSV-1 reactivations, even when they are multiple and recurrent, are not associated with permanent sensory deficit. We have therefore suggested (Steiner and Kennedy 1991) that these events are not associated with neuronal cell destruction. It follows that HSV-1 does not replicate in PSG during reactivation in a similar fashion to that present during its replication in cultured cells.

As latency is established primarily, if not exclusively, in neurons, it appears that some host and cellular properties of the neuron might favour latency by arresting viral replication. Indeed, neurons, at least in culture, express factors which have an inhibitory effect upon HSV-1 replication at an early stage which is not yet associated with irreversible cell damage (Ash 1986; Kemp et al. 1990; Wheatley et al. 1991).

Varicella zoster virus

VZV DNA was identified in human PSG (Gilden et al. 1983; Mahalingam et al. 1990); however, there are no data on the organization and exact location of the latent VZV genome within the host cell. The levels of VZV DNA are much lower than the levels of HSV-1 during latent infection in human PSG (Mahalingam et al. 1993). Viral gene expression is restricted during VZV latency (Croen et al. 1988; Meier et al. 1993). Consistent with the observed differences in DNA amounts, there is evidence that the amounts of HSV-1 RNA present in latently infected PSG are considerably higher than the amounts of VZV RNA detected during latency (Croen et al. 1988; I. Steiner et al., unpublished observations). In situ hybridization has been used to study the cellular site of latent VZV in human PSG. Thus, during latent VZV infection, viral RNA was reported in some of the studies (Croen et al. 1988; Meier et al. 1993), but not all, to be present in non-neuronal cells immediately surrounding neurons. These findings conflict with those of another group (Gilden et al. 1987).

Since by contrast with HSV-1, sensory impairment accompanies and follows herpes zoster, neuronal loss is more likely to occur during VZV reactivation. Indeed, pathological studies of PSG during herpes zoster show extensive necrosis and neuronal destruction (Kennedy 1987). Reactivation following explantation of PSG from humans and experimental animals is readily achieved with HSV-1 but latent VZV can not be reactivated in this way.

Molecular model of HSV and VZV latent infections

Based on these differences we have proposed a model that might explain the differences between the reactivation phenotypes of the two viruses (Kennedy & Steiner 1994). If indeed VZV, at least in part, resides latently in non-neuronal cells, it has to reach the neurons within the PSG in order to be able to get via the axon to the periphery. Thus, viral replication during reactivation is mandatory for VZV reactivation in contrast to the lack of a full reactivation cycle during HSV-1 reactivation. Active VZV replication will release infectious particles that will spread to the entire ganglion and infect many neurons culminating in a peripheral disease within the distribution of the entire PSG. This will result in neuronal destruction with transient or permanent sensory loss on the one hand and depletion of cells capable of serving as reservoirs for future reactivations on the other. Moreover, unlike HSV-1, where reactivation takes place within one neuron, and is therefore more likely to evade the host immunological response, VZV reactivation involves spread of virus throughout the tissue and can be altered by cellular as well as humoral immune responses. This could also explain why the incidence of zoster increases with age as it has been shown that VZV-specific T cell responses diminish with advancing age (Miller 1980; Berger et al. 1981), and why zoster is so prevalent in immunocompromised individuals. This also explains the meningeal reaction with CSF pleocytosis due to the active infectious process. By contrast, as latent HSV-1 resides in neurons initially and viral replication within the PSG does not occur to any significant extent, the resulting cutaneous eruption is more restricted in area.

The amounts of herpes virus DNA and RNA present in the PSG during latent infection determine the ability of the virus to reactivate. It has been suggested (Roizman and Sears 1987) that a smaller copy number of viral genomes within latently infected nervous tissue cells is associated with the inability of the virus to initiate replication, while a larger copy number per cell will facilitate the viral ability to reactivate. This is further supported by the distribution of zoster within cutaneous surfaces where chickenpox lesions are abundant and therefore able to supply the PSG with a heavy load of viral particles, enough to enable potential reactivation. In any case, it follows that HSV-1 reactivation will be favoured compared with VZV as there is significantly more HSV-1 DNA and latency-associated gene expression present in the tissue prior to the reactivation stimulus. When VZV reactivates, it reduces the remaining amounts of virus within PSG, and it may, in a sense, undergo a form of 'burnout' regarding subsequent reactivations.

Peripheral nervous system disorders due to human cytomegalovirus

HCMV is the major cause of congenital viral infections in developed countries leading to severe birth defects. It is also the most common cause for an infectious mononucleosis syndrome not due to Epstein–Barr virus. In the last 20 years, HCMV has been identified as a major pathogen of immunocompromised patients (Alford and Britt 1990). In the context of immunosuppression it has also been implicated in a variety of PNS disorders.

AIDP in immunocompetent individuals

In immunocompetent individuals, HCMV and Epstein–Barr virus are considered among the most common pathogens associated with AIDP occurrence. This is based mainly on results of urine or throat cultures, and on serological evidence for recent infection in up to 15% and 8% of the cases, respectively (Dowling and Cook 1981). In the absence of evidence for direct PNS involvement by the virus, it seems likely that these viruses, like other systemic infections, might trigger an immune response culminating in damage to the myelin of peripheral nerves (Steiner and Abramsky 1985). It is noteworthy that a naturally occurring disease in chickens which simulates AIDP is caused by Marek's disease virus (MDV), a lymphotropic herpes virus (Pepose et al. 1981). The pathological lesions within the PNS in Marek's disease are similar to those of experimental allergic neuritis (EAN) (Lampert et al. 1977), an experimental animal model of AIDP, and both are considered to be mediated, in part, by cellular immune mechanisms.

HCMV-induced disease under immunosuppression

HCMV is being increasingly recognized as a cause of PNS damage in patients with advanced AIDS; however, the clinical and pathological spectrum of HCMV-induced peripheral neuropathies and the true incidence of HCMV-associated PNS disease has not yet been fully delineated. This is due to difficulty in antemortem diagnosis and the paucity of pre and postmortem pathological assessment of the peripheral diseased tissue (Simpson and Tagliati 1994; McCutchan

1995). Two distinct HCMV-induced peripheral nerve syndromes in AIDS patients have emerged: lumbosacral polyradiculopathy and mononeuritis multiplex.

Lumbosacral polyradiculopathy

The syndrome of lumbosacral polyradiculopathy (also termed polyradiculomyelopathy or myelomeningoradiculitis), in HIV-infected patients is characterized by a subacute onset (0.5–6 weeks; mean 2 weeks) of bilateral weakness of the lower extremities, associated with areflexia and variable sensory loss. This is frequently accompanied by sacral paresthesias and bladder and anal sphincter dysfunction. The disorder progresses as an ascending flaccid paraparesis that mimics AIDP clinically (Eidelberg et al. 1986; Behar et al. 1987; Miller et al. 1990; So and Olney 1994). Pathological studies reveal characteristic cytomegalic inclusions in Schwann cells and endoneurial fibroblasts in the ventral and dorsal roots of the cauda equina accompanied by marked inflammation and axonal breakdown (Eidelberg et al. 1986; Behar et al. 1987).

The diagnosis of HCMV-associated lumbosacral polyradiculopathy relies mainly on clinical and CSF findings. CSF examination usually reveals elevated protein, normal or slightly decreased glucose and hundreds to thousands of cells, predominantly polymorphonuclear leukocytes. Electrodiagnostic studies and magnetic resonance imaging (MRI) may serve as adjunctive diagnostic tools. Findings are those of acute motor axonal loss with reduced amplitude of the compound muscle action potentials and early appearance of fibrillation potentials in denervated muscles (So and Olney 1994). MRI may reveal enlargement of the conus medullaris, clumping of the lumbosacral roots or enhancement of the lower spinal cord leptomeninges with gadolinium (So and Olney 1994; McCutchan 1995). Viral cultures, though specific, are positive for HCMV in only half of the patients (Kim and Hollander 1993; So and Olney 1994), and may require prolonged propagation due to low viral titer. Similarly, rapid immunostaining procedures are often negative. Detection of HCMV DNA in CSF by PCR may become a sensitive and specific diagnostic method (Wolf et al. 1992). Detection of the HCMV lower matrix protein (pp65) in CSF polymorphonuclear leukocytes was shown to be of comparable diagnostic value in a small number of patients with polyradiculopathy (Revello et al. 1994).

The predilection of HCMV for the lumbosacral area and the marked pleocytosis, as well as the frequent association of the lumbosacral polyradiculopathy with ventriculoencephalitis has led credence to the suggestion that HCMV may disseminate in the nervous system via the CSF and be transported by polymorphonuclear cells. HCMV-related lumbosacral polyradiculopathy should be differentiated from other, less common causes of AIDS-associated progressive polyradiculopathy. A milder form that results in spontaneous clinical stabilization has been described and is associated with mononuclear pleocytosis. Additional rare causes include lymphomatous involvement of the lower spinal cord, toxoplasma myelitis, neurosyphilis and tuberculosis.

Mononeuritis multiplex

HCMV-induced mononeuritis multiplex, less common than lumbosacral polyradiculopathy, can present as multifocal asymmetrical sensorimotor deficits in the distribution of major peripheral or cranial nerves, including facial or laryngeal palsy (Said et al. 1991; Roullet et al. 1994). This syndrome typically occurs in the setting of severe immunosuppression with CD4 lymphocyte count below 0.05×10^9/L, and may coexist with HCMV encephalitis, polyradiculopathy or retinitis.

Electrophysiological abnormalities are those of axonal neuropathy including low motor and sensory amplitudes in an asymmetrical distribution. Biopsy, if obtained from an affected nerve, may establish the diagnosis by demonstrating multifocal necrotizing vasculitis of epineural arteries associated with intranuclear and intracytoplasmatic inclusion bodies, characteristic of HCMV, and presence of HCMV antigens in the tissue. Both conventional virological methods and nerve biopsy, although highly specific, are not sensitive tools for the diagnosis of HCMV-associated mononeuritis multiplex. CSF cultures are positive in only 15% of the cases and nerve biopsy frequently yields non-specific findings. By contrast, HCMV DNA has been detected in the CSF of 90% of the patients, further supporting the disseminated nature of this peripheral neuropathy syndrome (Roullet et al. 1994). Unless treated, the disease rapidly progresses to quadriparesis and death. At autopsy the lesions may also involve dorsal root ganglia.

A milder form in which sensory symptoms, with pain as a prominent feature, precede motor signs by weeks to months has been described (Roullet et al. 1994). Recently, a patient with necrotizing but also a demyelinating mononeuritis multiplex syndrome due to HCMV was reported (Morgello and Simpson 1994).

Distal painful neuropathy

The causative role of HCMV in the distal painful polyneuropathy of AIDS patients is still questionable (Fuller et al. 1993). This relatively common syndrome is characterized by a subacute onset of numbness and pain, accompanied by contact dysesthesia and mild symmetrical sensory loss. While the sensory symptomatology typically remains stable or improves spontaneously, progressive loss of ankle reflexes develops. CSF examination usually reveals increased protein concentration and electrophysiological studies are consistent with axonopathy. Concurrent systemic HCMV infection has been documented in several series in 80% of patients with distal painful neuropathy (Fuller et al. 1993, Mastroianni et al. 1994) and anecdotal reports correlate HCMV infection of dorsal root ganglion cells with the clinical syndrome. Sural nerve biopsies of these patients reveal only axonal atrophy without any signs of HCMV infection. Although it has been suggested that empirical antiviral therapy should be initiated in patients with distal painful neuropathy, the pathogenetic role of HCMV as well as the beneficial effect of such therapy have not been established.

Treatment

Two drugs are currently available for the treatment of HCMV peripheral neuropathy. Ganciclovir, a nucleoside analogue, is selectively activated in infected cells in a combined process. The initial phosphorylation to ganciclovir monophosphate is mediated by a viral kinase, encoded by the HCMV UL97 gene, and further phosphorylation is mediated by cellular kinases (Littler et al. 1992; Sullivan et al. 1992). The active form, ganciclovir triphosphate, is an effective inhibitor of the HCMV polymerase and of viral replication. Foscarnet inhibits the viral DNA polymerase at the pyrophosphate binding site. It does not require phosphorylation to exert its antiviral effect and is often active against ganciclovir resistant strains. Relatively little is known about the pharmacokinetics of ganciclovir and foscarnet in the human nervous system. Both cross the blood–brain barrier, although at variable rates, and limited studies suggest that drug levels achieved in CSF and brain at initiation of therapy exceed the ED_{50} for most HCMV isolates (McCutchan 1995).

At present, there are no established guidelines for the treatment of HCMV peripheral neuropathy due to the lack of prospective studies and the diverse nature of these syndromes. The institution of ganciclovir and foscarnet, alone or in combination, early in the course of HCMV-associated lumbosacral polyradiculopathy and mononeuritis multiplex can stabilize, and at times partially reverse, the clinical manifestations (Behar et al. 1987; Miller et al. 1990; Cohen et al. 1993; Kim and Hollander 1993; Roullet et al. 1994). Occasionally, initial worsening during the first 2 weeks of therapy was noted (So and Olney 1994). It was further suggested that recovery may be biphasic with the heavily damaged axons requiring months for remyelinization and regrowth. Despite improvement in 30–50% of treated patients, most patients remain with residual deficit. Moreover, prolonged antiviral therapy in advanced HCMV disease may lead to drug resistance, resulting from mutations in the viral UL97 gene and DNA polymerase. Indeed, ganciclovir-resistant HCMV genotypes have been detected in CSF of patients with lumbosacral polyradiculopathy on ganciclovir therapy (Wolf et al. 1995).

References

Alford, C.A., and Britt, W.J. (1990). Cytomegalovirus. In *Virology.* ed B.N. Fields, D.M. Knipe, R.M. Chanock, M.S. Hirsch, J.L. Melnick, T.P. Monath and B. Roizman, 2nd edn, pp. 1981–2010. New York: Raven Press.

Anderson, J.P. and Keal, E.E. (1969). Cervical herpes zoster and diaphragmatic paralysis. *Br. J. Dis. Chest.* **63:** 222–226.

Appelbaum, E., Kreps, S.I., and Sunshine, A. (1962). Herpes zoster encephalitis. *Am. J. Med.* **32:** 25–31.

Asbury, A.K., Arnason, B.G., Karp, H.R., and McFarlin, D.E. (1978). Criteria for diagnosis of Guillain-Barré syndrome. *Ann. Neurol.* **3:** 565–566.

Ash, R.J. (1986). Butyrate-induced reversal of herpes simplex virus restriction in neuroblastoma cells. *Virology* **155**: 584–592.

Balfour, H.H., Bean, B., Laskin, O.L., Ambinder, R.F., Meyers, J.D., Wade, J.C., Zaia, J.A., Aeppli, D., Kirk, L.D., Segreti, A.C., and Keeney, R.E. (1983). Burroughs Wellcome Collaborative Study Group: acyclovir halts progression of herpes zoster in immunocompromised hosts. *N. Engl. J. Med.* **308**: 1448–1453.

Bean, B., Braun, C., and Balfour, H.H. (1982). Acyclovir therapy for acute herpes zoster. *Lancet* **ii**: 118–121.

Behar, R., Wiley, C., and McCutchan, J.A. (1987). Cytomegalovirus polyradiculoneuropathy in acquired immune deficiency syndrome. *Neurology* **37**: 557–561.

Berger, R., Florent, G., and Just, M. (1981). Decrease of the lymphoproliferative response to varicella-zoster virus antigen in the aged. *Infect. Imm.* **32**: 24–27.

Bieger, R.C., van Scoy, R.E., and Smith, T.F. (1977). Antibodies to varicella zoster in cerebrospinal fluid. *Arch. Neurol.* **34**: 489–491.

Birmanns, B., Reibstein, I., and Steiner, I. (1993). Characterization of an in vivo reactivation model of herpes simplex virus from mice trigeminal ganglia. *J. Gen. Virol.* **74**: 2487–2491.

Black, D., Stewart, J., and Melmed, C. (1983). Sacral nerve dysfunction plus generalized polyneuropathy in herpes simplex genitalis. *Ann. Neurol.* **14**: 692.

Bullowa, J.G.M. and Wishik, S.M. (1935). Complications of varicella. I. The occurrence among 2534 patients. *Am. J. Dis. Child.* **49**: 923–926.

Burgoon, C.F., Burgoon, J.S. and Baldridge, G.D. (1957). The natural history of herpes zoster. *J. Am. Med. Assoc.* **164**: 265–269.

Bustamante, C.I. and Wade, J.C. (1991). Herpes simplex virus infection in the immunocompromised cancer patient. *J. Clin. Oncol.* **9**: 1903–1915.

Cesario, T.C., Poland, J.D., Wulff, H., Chin, T.D., and Wenner, H.A. (1969). Six years experience with herpes simplex virus in a children's home. *Am. J. Epidemiol.* **90**: 416–422.

Chang, T.W., Fiumara, N.J., and Weinstein, L. (1974). Genital herpes: some clinical and laboratory observations. J. Am. Med. Assoc. **229**: 544–545.

Cohen, B.A., McArthur, J.C., Grohman, S., Patterson, B., and Glass, J.D. (1993). Neurologic prognosis of cytomegalovirus polyradiculopathy in AIDS. *Neurology* **43**: 493–499.

Constantine, V.S., Francis, R.D., and Montes, L.F. (1988). Association of recurrent herpes simplex with neuralgia. *J. Am. Med. Assoc.* **205**: 181–183.

Corey, L. (1986). Laboratory diagnosis of herpes simplex virus infections. Principles guiding the development of rapid diagnostic tests. *Diag. Microbiol. Infect. Dis.* **4**: 111S–119S.

Craig, C. and Nahmias, A.J. (1973). Different patterns of neurologic involvement with herpes simplex virus type 1 and 2: isolation of herpes simplex virus type 2 from the buffy coat of two adults with meningitis. *J. Infect. Dis.* **127**: 365–372.

Croen, K.D., Ostrove, J.M., Dragovic, L.J., Smialek, J.E., and Straus, S.E. (1987). Latent herpes simplex virus in human trigeminal ganglia. Detection of an immediate early gene 'anti-sense' transcription by in situ hybridization. *N. Engl. J. Med.* **317**: 1427–1432.

Croen, K.D., Ostrove, J.M., Dragovic, L.J., and Straus, S.E. (1988). Patterns of gene expression and sites of latency in human nerve ganglia are different for varicella-zoster and herpes simplex viruses. *Proc. Natl Acad. Sci. USA* **85**: 9773–9777.

Dayan, A.D., Ogul, E., and Graveson, G.S. (1972). Polyneuritis and herpes zoster. *J. Neurol. Neurosurg. Psychiatry* **35**: 170–175.

Douglas, J.M., Critchlow, C., Benedetti, J., Mertz, G.J., Connor, J.D., Hintz, M.A., Fahnlander, A., Remington, M., Winter, C., and Corey, L. (1984). A double-blind study of oral acyclovir for suppression of recurrences of genital herpes simplex virus infection. *N. Engl. J. Med.* **310**: 1551–1556.

Dowling, P.C. and Cook, S.D. (1981). Role of infection in Guillain-Barré syndrome: laboratory confirmation of herpesvirus in 41 cases. *Ann. Neurol.* **9**(suppl.): 44–45.

Eidelberg, D., Sotrel, A., Vogel, H., Walker, P., Kleefield, J., and Crumpacker, C. (1986). Progressive polyradiculopathy in acquired immune deficiency syndrome. *Neurology* **36**: 912–916.

Froh, K., Ahn, K., Djaballah, H., Swmpe, P., van Endert, P.M., Tampe, R., Peterson, P.A., and Yang, Y. (1995). A viral inhibitor of peptide transporters for antigen presentation. *Nature* **375**: 415–418.

Fuller, G.N., Jacobs, J.M., and Guiloff, R.J. (1993). Nature and incidence of peripheral nerve syndromes in HIV infections. *J. Neurol. Neurosurg. Psychiatry* **56**: 372–381.

Gais, E.S. and Abrahamson, R.H. (1939). Herpes zoster and its visceral manifestation. *Am. J. Med. Sci.* **197**: 817–825.

Gershon, A., Steinberg, S., Greenberg, S., and Taber, L. (1980). Varicella-zoster-associated encephalitis: detection of specific antibody in cerebrospinal fluid. *J. Clin. Microbiol.* **12**: 764–767.

Gilden, D.H., Mahalingam, R., Dueland, A.N., and Cohrs, R. (1992). Herpes zoster: pathogenesis and latency. In *Progress in Medical Virology*, vol. 39, ed. L.J. Melnick, pp. 19–75. Basel: S. Karger.

Gilden, D.H., Rosenman, Y., Murray, R., Devlin, M., and Vafai A. (1987). Detection of varicella-zoster virus nucleic acid in neurons of normal human thoracic ganglia. *Ann. Neurol.* **22**: 377–380.

Gilden, D.H., Vafai, A., Shtram, Y., Becker, Y., Devlin, M., and Wellish, M. (1983). Varicella-zoster virus DNA in human sensory ganglia. *Nature* **306**: 478–480.

Giller, R.H., Winistorfer, S., and Grose, C. (1989). Cellular and humoral immunity to varicella zoster glycoproteins in immune and susceptible human subjects. *J. Infect. Dis.* **160**: 919–928.

Gold, E. (1966). Serologic and virus-isolation studies of patients with varicella or herpes zoster infections. *N. Engl. J. Med.* **274**: 181–185.

Goldstein, L.C., Corey, L., McDougall, J.K., Tolentino, E., and Nowinski, R.C. (1983). Monoclonal antibodies to herpes simplex viruses: use in antigenetic typing and rapid diagnosis. *J. Infect. Dis.* **147**: 829–837.

Gominak, S., Cros, D., and Paydarfar, D. (1990). Herpes simplex labialis and trigeminal neuropathy. *Neurology* **40**: 151–152

Grant, B.D. and Rowe, C.R. (1961). Motor paralysis of the extremities in herpes zoster. *J. Bone Joint Surg.* **43A**: 885–896.

Goodpasture, E.W. (1929). Herpetic infections with special reference to involvement of the nervous system. *Medicine* **8**: 223–243.

Greenberg, J. (1970). Herpes zoster with motor involvement. *J. Am. Med. Assoc.* **212**: 322.

Grose, C. (1981). Variation on a theme by Fenner: the pathogenesis of chickenpox. *Pediatrics* **68**: 735–737.

Gupta, S.K., Helal, B.H., and Kiely, P. (1969). The prognosis in zoster paralysis. *J. Bone Joint Surg.* **51B**: 593–603.

Handler, C.E. and Perkin, G.D. (1982). Radiculomyelopathy due to genital herpes. *Lancet* **ii**: 987–988.

Harnisch, J.P. (1984). Zoster in the elderly: clinical, immunologic and therapeutic considerations. *J. Am. Geriat. Soc.* **32**: 789–793.

Haymaker, W. and Kernohan, J.W. (1949). The Landry-Guillain-Barré syndrome. *Medicine* **28**: 59–141.

Hill, A., Jugovic, P., York, I., Russ, G., Bennink, J., Yewdell, J., Ploegh, H., and Johnson, D. (1995). Herpes simplex virus turns off the TAP to evade host immunity. *Nature* **375**: 411–415.

Hope-Simpson, R.E. (1965). The nature of herpes zoster: a long-term study and a new hypothesis. *Proc. R. Soc. Med.* **58**: 9–20.

Javier, R.T., Stevens, J.G., Dissette, V.B., and Wagner, E.K. (1988). A herpes simplex virus transcript abundant in latently infected neurons is dispensable for establishment of the latent state. *Virology* **166**: 254–257.

Jellinek, E.H. and Tulloch, W.S. (1976). Herpes zoster with dysfunction of bladder and anus. *Lancet* **ii**: 1219–1222.

Juel-Jensen, B.E. (1970). The natural history of shingles. Events associated with reactivation of varicella-zoster virus. *J. R. Col. Gen. Pract.* **20**: 323–327.

Kemp, L.M., Dent, C.L., and Latchman, D.S. (1990). Octamer motif mediates transcriptional repression of HSV immediate early genes and octamer-containing cellular promoters in neuronal cells. *Neuron* **4**: 215–222.

Kennedy, P.G.E. (1987). Neurological complications of varicella-zoster virus. In *Infections of the Nervous System*, ed. P.G.E Kennedy and R.T. Johnson, pp. 177–208. London: Butterworth.

Kennedy, P.G.E. and Steiner, I. (1994). A molecular and cellular model to explain the differences in reactivation from latency by herpes simplex and varicella-zoster viruses. *Neuropathol. Appl. Neurobiol.* **20**: 368–374.

Kim, Y.S. and Hollander, H. (1993). Polyradiculopathy due to cytomegalovirus: report of two cases in which improvement occurred after prolonged therapy and review of the literature. *Clin. Infect. Dis.* **17**: 32–37.

Knox, J.D.E., Levy, R., and Simpson, J.A. (1961). Herpes zoster and the Landry-Guillain-Barré syndrome. *J. Neurol. Neurosurg. Psychiatry* **24**: 167–172.

Kukimoto, N., Ikeda, M., Yamada, K., Tanaka, M., Tsurumachi H., and Tomita, H. (1988). Viral infection in acute peripheral facial paralysis: nationwide analysis centering on CF. *Acta Otolaryngol.* **446**(suppl.): 17–22.

Lakeman, F.D. and Whitley, R.J. (1995). Diagnosis of herpes simplex encephalitis: application of polymerase chain reaction to cerebrospinal fluid from brain-biopsied patients and correlation with disease. Collaborative Antiviral Study Group. *Natl Inst. Allergy Infect. Dis.* **171**: 857–863.

Lampert, P., Garrett, R., and Powell, H. (1977). Demyelination in experimental and Marek's disease virus-induced neuritis. Comparative electron microscopy studies. *Acta Neuropathol. (Berl)* **40**: 103–110.

Littler, E., Stuart, A.D., and Chee, M.S. (1992). Human cytomegalovirus UL97 open reading frame encodes a protein that phosphorylates the antiviral nucleotide analogue ganciclovir. *Nature* **358**: 160–162.

Mahalingam, R., Wellish, M., Lederer, D., Forghani, B., Cohrs, R., and Gilden, D. (1993). Quantitation of latent varicella-zoster virus DNA in human trigeminal ganglia by polymerase chain reaction. *J. Virol.* **67**: 2381–2384.

Mahalingam, R., Wellish, M., Wolf, W., Dueland, A.N., Cohrs, R., Vafai, A., and Gilden, D.H. (1990). Latent varicella-zoster viral DNA in human trigeminal and thoracic ganglia. *N. Engl. J. Med.* **323**: 627–631.

Mastroianni, C.M., Sebastiani, G., Folgori, F., Ajassa, C., Vullo, V., and Volpi, A. (1994). Detection of cytomegalovirus-matrix protein (pp65) in leukocytes of HIV-infected patients with painful peripheral neuropathy. *J. Med. Virol.* **44**: 172–175.

Max, M.B. (1994). Treatment of post herpetic neuralgia: antidepressants. *Ann. Neurol.* **35**: S50–S53

Mazur, M.H. and Dolin, R. (1978). Herpes zoster at the NIH: a 20 year experience. *Am. J. Med.* **65**: 738–743.

McCutchan, A. (1995). Cytomegalovirus infections of the nervous system in patients with AIDS. *Clin. Infect. Dis.* **20**: 747–754.

McKendell, R.R. and Klawans, H.L. (1978). Nervous system complications of varicella zoster virus. In *Handbook of Clinical Neurology*, vol. 34, ed. P.J. Vinken and G.W. Bruyn, pp. 161–183, Amsterdam North-Holland: Elesvier.

Melbye, M., Grossman, R.J., Goedert, J.J., Eyster, M.E., and Bigger, R.J. (1987). Risk of AIDS after herpes zoster. *Lancet* **i**: 728–731.

Meier, J.L., Holman, R.P., Croen, K.D., Smialek, J.E., and Straus, S.E. (1993). Varicella-zoster transcription in human trigeminal ganglia. *Virology* **193**: 193–200.

Mellerick, D.M. and Fraser, N.W. (1987). Physical state of the latent herpes simplex virus genome in mouse model system. Evidence suggesting an episomal state. *Virology* **158**: 265–275.

Merigan, T.C. and Stevens, D.A. (1971). Viral infections in man associated with acquired immunological deficiency states. *Fed. Proc.* **30**: 1858–1864.

Miller, A.E. (1980). Selective decline in cellular immune response in varicella-zoster in the elderly. *Neurology* **30**: 582–587.

Miller, H.G., Stanton, J.B., and Gibbons, J.L. (1956). Para-infectious encephalomyelitis and related syndromes. *Q. J. Med.* **25**: 427–505.

Miller, R.G., Storey, J.R., and Greco, C.M. (1990). Ganciclovir in the treatment of progressive AIDS-related polyradiculopathy. *Neurology* **40**: 569–574.

Mitchell, W.J., Deshmane, S.L., Dolan, A., McGeoch, D.J., and Fraser, N.W. (1990). Characterization of herpes simplex virus type 2 transcription during latent infection of mouse trigeminal ganglia. *J. Virol.* **64**: 5342–5348.

Momin, F. and Chandrasekar, P.H. (1995). Antimicrobial prophylaxis in bone marrow transplantation. *Ann. Intern. Med.* **123**: 205–215.

Morens, D.M., Bregman, D.J., West, M., Greene, M.H., Mazur, M.H., Dolin, R., and Fisher, R.I. (1980). An outbreak of varicella-zoster virus infection among cancer patients. *Ann. Intern. Med.* **93**: 414–419.

Morgello, S. and Simpson, D.M. (1994). Multifocal cytomegalovirus demyelinative polyneuropathy associated with AIDS. *Muscle Nerve* **17**: 176–182.

Moriyama, K., Mohri, S., Watanabe, T., and Mori, R. (1992). Latent infection of SCID mice with herpes simplex virus 1 and lethal cutaneous lesions in pregnancy. *Microbiol. Immunol.* **36**: 841–853.

Nahass, G.T., Mandel, M.J., Cook, S., Fan, W., and Leonardi, C.L. (1995). Detection of herpes simplex and varicella-zoster infection from cutaneous lesions in different clinical stages with the polymerase chain reaction. *J. Am. Acad. Dermatol.* **32**: 730–733.

Nahmias, A.J., Dowdle, W.R., Naib, Z.M., et al. (1969). Genital infection with type 2 herpes virus huminis. A commonly occurring venereal disease. *Br. J. Vener. Dis.* **45**: 294–298.

Neville, B.G.R. and Sladen, G.E. (1984). Acute autonomic neuropathy following primary herpes simplex infection. *J. Neurol. Neurosurg. Psychiatry.* **47**: 648–650.

Oaks, J.E. and Lausch, R.N. (1984). Monoclonal antibodies suppress replication of herpes simplex virus type 1 in trigeminal ganglia. *J. Virol.* **51**: 656–661.

Oldstone, M.B. (1991). Molecular anatomy of viral persistence. *J. Virol.* **65**: 6381–6386.

Olivarius, B.F., and Buhl, M. (1975). Herpes simplex virus and Guillain-Barré polyradiculitis. *Br. Med. J.* **i**: 192–193.

Pepose, J.S., Stevens, J.G., Cook, M.L., and Lampert, P.W. (1981). Marek's disease as an animal model for the Landry-Guillain-Barré syndrome. Latent infection restricted to neuronal supporting cells and accompanied by specific immune response to peripheral nerve myelin. *Am. J. Pathol.* **103**: 309–320.

Peters, A.C.B., Versteeg, J., Bots, G.T.A.M., Lindeman, J., and Smeets, R.E.H. (1979). Nervous system complications of herpes zoster: immunofluorescent demonstration of varicella zoster antigen in CSF cells. *J. Neurol. Neurosurg. Psychiatry* **42**: 452–457.

Peterslund, N.A., Setyer-Hansen, K., Ipsen, J., Esmann, V., Shonheyder, H., and Jukl, H. (1981). Acyclovir in herpes zoster. *Lancet* **ii**: 827–830.

Preblud, S.R. (1986). Varicella: complications and costs. *Pediatrics* **78**(suppl.): 728–735.

Price, R.W. (1981). Herpes zoster. *Neurol. Neurosurg. Update Series*, vol. 2, **21**: 1–8.

Rab, S.M. and Choudhury, G.M. (1963). Landry-Guillain-Barré syndrome after chickenpox. *N. Engl. J. Med.* **268**: 200–201.

Raggozino, M.W., Melton, L.J. III, and Kurland, L.T. (1982). Risk of cancer after herpes zoster: a population-based study. *N. Engl. J. Med.* **307**: 393–397.

Reeves, W.C., Corey, L., Adams, H.G., Vontver, L.A., and Holmes, K.K. (1981). Risk of recurrence after first episodes of genital herpes relation to HSV type and antibody response. *N. Engl. J. Med.* **305**: 315–319.

Revello, M.G., Percivalle, E., Sarasini, A., Baldanti, F., Furione, M., and Gerna, G. (1994). Diagnosis of human cytomegalovirus infection of the nervous system by pp65 detection in polymorphonuclear leukocytes of cerebrospinal fluid from AIDS patients. *J. Infect. Dis.* **170**: 1275–1279.

Roullet, E., Assuerus, V., Gozlan, J., Ropert, A., Said, G., Baudrimont, M., El Amrani, M., Jacomet, C., Duvivier, C., Gonzales-Canali, G., Kirsteffer, M. et al. (1994). Cytomegalovirus multifocal neuropathy in AIDS. Analysis of 15 consecutive cases. *Neurology* **44**: 2174–2182.

Rowbotham, M.C., Davies, P.S., and Foelds, H.L. (1995). Topical lidocaine gel relieves postherpetic neuralgia. *Ann. Neurol.* **37**: 246–253.

Rock, D.L. and Fraser, N.W. (1983). Detection of HSV-1 genome in the central nervous system of latently infected mice. *Nature* **302**: 523–525.

Roizman, B. and Sears, A.E. (1987). An inquiry into the mechanisms of herpes simplex virus latency. *Annu. Rev. Microbiol.* **41**: 543–571.

Said, G., Lacroix, C., Chemouilli, P., Goulon-Goeau, C., Roullet, E., Penaud, D., de Brouchet, T., Meduri, G., Vincent, D., Torchet, M. et al. (1991). Cytomegalovirus neuropathy in acquired immunodeficiency syndrome: a clinical and pathological study. *Ann. Neurol.* **29**: 139–146.

Schimpff, J., Serpick, A., Stoler, B., Rumack, B., Mellin, H., Joseph, J.M., et al. (1972). Varicella-zoster infection in patients with cancer. *Ann. Intern. Med.* **765**: 241–254.

Simmons, A. and Tscharke, D.C. (1992). Anti-CD8 impairs clearance of herpes simplex virus from the nervous system: implication for the fate of the virally infected neurons. *J. Exp. Med.* **175**: 1337–1344.

Simpson, D.M. and Tagliati, M. (1994). Neurologic manifestations of HIV infection. *Ann. Intern. Med.* **121**: 769–785.

So, Y.T. and Olney, R.K. (1994). Acute lumbosacral polyradiculopathy in acquired immunodeficiency syndrome: experience in 23 patients. *Ann. Neurol.* **35**: 53–58.

Spivack, J.G. and Fraser, N.W. (1987). Detection of herpes simplex type 1 transcripts during latent infection in mice. *J. Virol.* **61**: 3841–3847.

Spivack, J.G., and Fraser, N.W. (1988). Expression of herpes simplex virus type 1 latency-associated transcripts in the trigeminal ganglia of mice during acute infection and reactivation of latent infection. *J. Virol.* **62**: 1479–1485.

Steele, R.W., Keeney, R.E., Bradsher, R.W., Moses, E.B., and Soloff, B.L. (1983). Treatment of varicella-zoster meningoencephalitis with acyclovir: demonstration of virus in cerebrospinal fluid by electron microscopy. *Am. J. Clin. Pathol.* **80**: 57–60.

Steiner, I. and Abramsky, O. (1985). Immunology of Guillain-Barré syndrome. *Springer Semin. Immunopathol.* **8**: 165–176.

Steiner, I. and Kennedy, P.G.E. (1991). Herpes simplex virus latency in the nervous system: a new model. *Neuropathol. Appl. Neurobiol.* **17**: 433–440.

Steiner, I. and Kennedy, P.G.E. (1993). The molecular biology of herpes simplex virus type 1 latency in the nervous system. *Mol. Neurobiol.* **7**: 137–159.

Steiner, I., Spivack, J.G., Deshmane, S.L., Ace, C.I., Preston, C.M., and Fraser, N.W. (1990). A herpes simplex virus type 1 mutant containing a non-transinducing Vmw65 protein establishes latent infection in vivo in the absence of viral replication and reactivates efficiently from explanted trigeminal ganglia. *J. Virol.* **64**: 1630–1638.

Steiner, I., Spivack, J.G., Lirette, R.P., Brown, S.M., MacLean, A.R., Subak-Sharpe, J., and Fraser, N.W. (1989). Herpes simplex virus type 1 latency-associated transcripts are evidently not essential for latent infection. *EMBO J.* **8**: 505–511.

Steiner, I., Spivack, J.G., O'Boyle, D.R., Lavi, E., and Fraser, N.W. (1988). Latent herpes simplex virus type 1 transcription in human trigeminal ganglia. *J. Virol.* **62**: 3493–3496.

Stevens, J.G., Wagner, E.K., Devi-Rao, G.B., Cook, M.L., and Feldman, L.T. (1987). RNA complementary to a herpesvirus alpha gene mRNA is prominent in latently infected neurons. *Science* **235**: 1056–1059.

Straus, S.E., Rakiff, H.E., Seidlin, M. et al. (1984a). Suppression of frequently recurring genital herpes: a placebo-controlled double blind trial of oral acyclovir. *N. Engl. J. Med.* **310**: 1545–1550.

Straus, S.E., Seidlin, M., Rakiff, H., Jacobs, D., Bowen, D., and Smith, H.A. (1984b). Oral acyclovir to suppress recurring herpes simplex virus infections in immunodeficient patients. *Ann. Intern. Med.* **100**: 522–524

Sullivan, V., Talarico, C.L., Stanat, S.C., Davis, M., Coen, D.M., and Biron, K. (1992). A protein kinase homologue controls phosphorylation of ganciclovir in human cytomegalovirus infected cells. *Nature* **358**: 162–164.

Thomas, E.J. and Howard, F.M. (1972). Segmental zoster paresis. A disease profile. *Neurology* **22**: 459–466.

Thomas, M. and Robertson, W.J. (1971). Dermal transmission of virus as a cause of shingles. *Lancet* **ii**: 1349–1350.

Trousdale, M.D., Steiner, I., Spivack, J.G., Deshmane, S.L., Brown, S.M., MacLean, A.R., Subak-Sharpe, J.H., and Fraser, N.W. (1991). In vivo and in vitro reactivation impairment of a herpes simplex virus type 1 latency-associated transcript variant in a rabbit eye model. *J. Virol.* **65**: 6989–6993.

Valyi-Nagy, T., Deshmane, S.L., Raengsakulrach, B., Nicosia, M., Gesser, R.M., Wysocka, M., Dillner, A., and Fraser, N.W. (1992). Herpes simplex virus type 1 mutant strain in1814 establishes a unique, slowly progressing infection in SCID mice. *J. Virol.* **66**: 7336–7345.

Watson, C.P., Tyler, K.L., Bickers, D.R., Millikan, L.E., Smith, S., and Coleman, E. (1993). A randomized vehicle-controlled trial of topical capsaicin in the treatment of postherpetic neuralgia. *Clin. Ther.* **15**: 510–526.

Wheatley, S.C., Dent, C.L., Wood J.N., and Latchman, D.S. (1991). A cellular factor binding to the TAATGARAT DNA sequence prevents the expression of the HSV immediate-early genes following infection of non-permissive cell lines derived from dorsal root ganglion neurons. *Exp. Cell Res.* **194**: 78–82.

Whitley, R.J. (1990). Herpes simplex viruses, In *Virology.* ed B.N. Fields, D.M. Knipe et al., 2nd edn, pp. 1843–1886. New York: Raven Press.

Wolf, D.G. and Spector, S.A. (1992). Diagnosis of human cytomegalovirus central nervous system disease in AIDS patients by DNA amplification from cerebrospinal fluid. *J. Infect. Dis.* **166**: 1412–1415.

Wolf, D.G., Lee, D.J., and Spector, S.A. (1995). Detection of human cytomegalovirus mutants associated with ganciclovir resistance in cerebrospinal fluid of AIDS patients with central nervous system disease. *Antimicrob. Agents Chemother.* **39**: 2552–2554.

Vafai, A., Wellish, M., and Gilden, D.H. (1988). Expression of varicella-zoster virus in blood mononuclear cells of patients with postherpetic neuralgia. *Proc. Natl Acad. Sci. USA* **85**: 2767–2770.

Van de Perre, P., Bakkeres, E., Battungwanyo, J., Kestelyn, P., Lepage, P. et al. (1988). Herpes zoster in African patients: an early manifestation of HIV infection. *Scand. J. Infect. Dis.* **20**: 277–282.

PART V Therapy and management

24 Immunosuppression and immunomodulation

A. Brand

General aspects of immunosuppressive drugs and immunomodulatory treatment

Autoimmune diseases are treated with immunosuppressive drugs, either to inhibit a primary, recently amplified immune response or to reduce the intensity of a chronic ongoing immune response. Immunosuppressive drugs do not cure an autoimmune disease and have side-effects related to the toxicity of the drug and the immune suppression itself. For these reasons, research is focused on the induction of specific immunotolerance against the antigen eliciting the immune attack. Unfortunately, in most autoimmune diseases, the triggering (auto)antigens are unknown.

Immune-mediated tissue damage can be the result of autoantigen-specific T cells and/or antibodies. Both may show an extensive concomitant inflammatory reaction. An immune attack can be monophasic or self-limited, can have acute exacerbations and remissions or become chronic and slowly progressive. The selection of combinations of immune suppressive drugs for treatment of a particular disease is based on the presumed immunopathogenesis and characteristics of the disease.

Immunosuppressive drugs

Corticosteroids

Cytokine production

Corticosteroids induce multiple changes in many (interacting) cells of the immune system. Corticosteroids, like non-steroidal anti-inflammatory drugs (NSAIDs), affect prostaglandin metabolism by inhibition of cyclooxygenase. It was recently discovered that there exist two isoforms of cyclooxygenase (Cox), Cox 1 and 2, showing 60% amino acid homology. Cox 1 is constitutively expressed in most cell types whereas Cox 2 expression is induced by lipopolysaccharide (LPS) stimulation of monocytes and interleukin 1 (IL-1) treatment of fibroblasts. While NSAIDs affect either both enzymes or predominantly Cox 1, corticosteroids selectively inhibit Cox 2. Corticosteroids very effectively inhibit the synthesis of the proinflammatory cytokines, tumor necrosis factor-α (TNF-α) and IL-1β, produced by stimulated cells of the monocytic-macrophage lineage. Corticosteroids do not affect the gene-expression of these cytokines upon induction but reduce the efficiency of specific messenger (m)RNA translation for TNF-α or the stability of IL-1β mRNA in monocytes (Amano et al. 1993)(Table 24.1).

Tables 24.1 *Characteristics and application of immunosuppresive drugs*

Immunosuppressive pathways	Major side-effects	Toxicity	Application in immune-mediated neuropathies
Corticosteroids			
Anti-inflammatory (Cox 2 inhibitor) TNFα, IL-1β↓ Prevention of leucocyte adhesion *Anti-effector cells* ADCC inhibition *Immunoregulation* Inhibition TH-1 response	Masking bacterial infections Fungal infections	*Immediate effects* Weight gain Mental changes *Susceptible patients* Hypertension Diabetes *Late effects* Osteoporosis Myopathy Cataract Atherosclerosis	*CIDP* First line drug, induction 1 mg kg^{-1} 4–6 weeks; taper off in responding patients to lowest effective maintenance dose. Combine with other drugs if maintenance dose >0.2 mg kg^{-1} is necessary *Vasculitis* Induction dose 0.5–1 mg kg^{-1} in combination with second line drug. Life-threatening (systemic) vasculitis: pulse methylprednisolone and cyclophosphamide
Antimetabolites (azathioprine, methotrexate)			
(Precursor) B, T, NK cells	Leukocytopenia Virus-induced malignancies	Stomatitis, diarrhea (MTX) Megaloblastic anemia (AZA) Liver toxicity (MTX)	*CIDP* Second line corticosteroid-sparing drug (AZA or MTX) AZA: 1.5–2.5 mg kg^{-1} per day: effective after 2–3 months MTX: 7.5–15 mg m^{-2} per week: effective after 2–6 weeks *Vasculitis* AZA in combination with corticosteroids

Note:
AZA: azathioprine; CIDP: chronic inflammatory demyelinating polyneuropathy; MTX: methotrexate.

Leukocyte adhesion

Corticosteroids cause depletion of the mature peripheral blood lymphocytes trafficking to peripheral lymph nodes, resulting in redistribution to other compartments such as the bone marrow.

The onset of lymphocytopenia starts within 1 hour after administration of corticosteroids and is associated with a decrease in the number as well as the intensity of leukocyte-endothelial cellular adhesion molecule, L-selectin (LECAM-1) expressing cells and decrease of homing receptor (CD44) intensity. The changes in leukocyte adhesion proteins LECAM-1 and CD44 cannot be induced in vitro, which suggests accessory mechanisms in vivo. The reduction in adhesion proteins impairs the capacity of lymphocytes to adhere to inflamed endothelium, which is an important initial step in the inflammatory reaction. The corticosteroid-induced lymphocytopenia is transient and is restored within 24–48 hours after withdrawal, depending on the dose administered.

Lymphocyte interactions

Corticosteroids interact with CD4 inducer (helper) T cells, especially inhibiting the T helper 1 type (TH1) of response. This response leads to the production of interferon-γ and IL-2, stimulating cell-mediated immune responses, including delayed-type hypersensitivity (DTH), cytotoxic T cells (CTLs) and natural killer cells (NK). Compared with (TH1) T cells, B lymphocytes are resistant to corticosteroids, although after high (pulse) dosages, immunoglobulin concentrations decrease.

Phagocytosis and cytolysis

Corticosteroids also block phagocytosis by downregulation of Fcγ-receptors on monocytes and macrophages (Atkinson and Frank 1974). Furthermore, in high concentration, corticosteroids inhibit the release of lysosomal enzymes by monocytes, further decreasing the cytotoxic lysis of antibody-coated target cells.

In summary, corticosteroids have an immediate effect within hours on leukocyte-endothelial adhesion, blocking phagocytosis by Fcγ-receptor modulation followed by reduction of synthesis of proinflammatory cytokines (TNFα and IL-1β) and T (helper 1-type) cell inhibition. B cells are rather resistent to corticosteroids and only affected by high (pulse) dosages.

Experience in immune-mediated neuropathies

Guillain-Barré syndrome (GBS) does not respond to high-dose corticosteroids, even not to pulse therapy with methylprednisolone (Hughes 1991). This resistance to corticosteroids is shared with some septic and immunological conditions, in which the acute phase inflammatory reactions are already strongly activated and corticosteroids may even lead to undesired suppression of the subsequent natural feedback loop. One such feedback response is the production of IL-1 receptor antagonist (IL-1ra) by mononuclear cells in response to IL-1 secretion and inflammation (Granowitz et al. 1991).

Neuropathies in which IgM antibodies, which are considerably T cell independent, play a role, such as multifocal motor neuropathy (MMN) often associated with high-titered IgM anti-GM_1 antibodies and anti-MAG, anti-sulphatide and other anti-glycoconjugate associated neuropathies with IgM-monoclonal gammopathy, generally respond poorly to corticosteroids. In other acute and fulminant IgM-mediated autoimmune syndromes (cold antibody-induced hemolytic anemia), pulse methylprednisolone, probably due to interference with a secondary inflammatory reaction caused by activated complement components, may result in dramatic improvement (Meytes et al. 1985).

This refractoriness to corticosteroids supports the view that IgM antibodies against neural antigens do play a pathogenic role in these neuropathies with minor inflammatory manifestations.

The majority of patients with chronic inflammatory demyelinating polyneuropathy (CIDP), a disorder similar to GBS but with less obvious antecedent infections and less increased acute phase cytokines (Hartung et al. 1991) initially respond to corticosteroids. Long-term maintenance treatment is then necessary. The evaluation of the long-term management of corticosteroids as the sole treatment in CIDP is complicated by the occurrence of spontaneous remissions and relapses and dependency on high dosages of corticosteroids, with resultant side-effects (Dyck 1982; Pollard 1987; Vermeulen et al. 1993).

Neuropathies occur in almost any type of systemic vasculitis. In vasculitis of larger vessels, such as classical periarteritis nodosa (PAN), multiple mononeuropathies are found, whereas smaller vessel vasculitis may also cause symmetric peripheral polyneuropathy. Treatment for acute overwhelming vasculitis with severe (multi)system involvement includes pulse intravenous methylprednisolone and cyclophosphamide. After treatment of acute life-threatening attacks it is important to prevent relapses and improve final patient outcome. Corticosteroids and cyclophosphamide treatment for a limited period of 2 years is recommended (Hall and Conn 1995).

Toxicity

Corticosteroids have metabolic effects on mineral, bone and carbohydrate metabolism. They almost always and immediately cause weight gain, mental changes and sleep disturbance and, in high risk patients, diabetes and hypertension. Osteoporosis, myopathy, cataract, skin atrophy and atherosclerosis are late cumulative dose-dependent effects. Most observed infectious complications are candidiasis and unrecognized life-threatening bacterial infections. When doses above 0.5 mg kg^{-1} are used for prolonged periods, approximately 30% of patients develop these side-effects. Actual practice is to pulse with high dosages of methylprednisolone and then to aim at a maintenance dose of corticosteroids below 0.2 mg kg^{-1}. If too high a maintenance dose is required, corticosteroids are usually combined with other immunosuppressive drugs inhibiting T and/or B cell activation, proliferation and differentiation in order to lower the dose of corticosteroids. Some of such drugs are discussed below.

Purine and pyrimidine antimetabolites

Purine and pyrimidine antimetabolites are cytotoxic in the S-phase of the cell cycle and affect mainly cells that are dividing during exposure to the drug. The immunosuppressive effects are largely restricted to precursor lymphocyte populations and hardly affect mature (memory) cells (Dimitriu and Franci 1979). Both T cell dependent (IgG) and T cell independent (IgM) antibody responses are reduced. The peripheral blood lymphocyte numbers and T cell subsets remain normally distributed even after months of therapy with a slight reduction in $CD8^+$ lymphocytes (Trotter et al. 1982).

After years of treatment, FcRγ expressing lymphocytes, NK and CTL are reduced by ±50%, restoring slowly 2–3 months after withdrawal of therapy (Shih et al. 1982). Lymphokine production is not affected. Before cyclosporin was developed, methotrexate, 6-mercaptopurine (6-MP) and azathioprine were used as immunosuppressive drugs to prevent graft-versus-host disease after bone marrow transplantation and graft rejection after kidney transplantation.

In chronic autoimmune diseases, antimetabolites are administered as second line treatment in steroid-refractory or steroid-dependent rheumatoid arthritis, myasthenia gravis, autoimmune thrombocytopenia and Crohn's disease, allowing reduction of steroids. Azathioprine for autoimmune disease is generally administered in maintenance dosages of 1.5–2.5 mg kg^{-1} daily for 6–12 months and then reduced to the lowest effective dose. In many autoimmune diseases, it takes at least 6 weeks to 3 months before a beneficial effect is observed. Methotrexate is often given in schedules of one to three times weekly, intravenous, intramuscular or orally. Weekly intramuscular injections with 7.5–15 mg m^2 are well tolerated for prolonged periods of 1–2 years without major side-effects, while a beneficial effect can already be observed after 2–6 weeks, especially when the induction dose is combined with moderately high doses of prednisone (0.4–0.8 mg kg^{-1}).

Toxicity

Drug toxicity depends on dosage and duration of exposure and includes stomatitis, megaloblastic erythropoiesis, bone marrow depression, elevated liver enzymes and liver fibrosis, pancreatitis and gastrointestinal irritation. A striking increased risk of (virus-induced) malignancy such as human papilloma virus (HPV)-induced squamous skin cancers and other malignancies after long-term use is observed in transplant recipients. This risk seems substantially less in autoimmune diseases. In one study, cancer risk was not found to be increased (Connell et al. 1994). In another study four patients with malignancy were observed during long-term follow-up of 157 patients treated for inflammatory bowel disease (Bouhnik et al. 1996) in contrast to doubling of the risk for patients with rheumatoid arthritis after immunosuppressive (mainly azathioprine) treatment (Kinlen 1992). The occurrence of secondary malignancy in neurological diseases treated with maintenance azathioprine treatment is unknown. The incidence of neurological diseases treated for prolonged periods with these antimetabolites (e.g. myastenia gravis, chronic inflammatory demyelinating polyneuropathy) is low and information on this subject is difficult to obtain. Regular liver function studies are indicated and when abnormal, especially after cumulative doses of 1.5–2 g of methotrexate, a liver biopsy is advised. Increased aminotransferase levels occur in 50% of the patients shortly after initiation of methotrexate but are often transient and do not predict liver damage (Kremer et al. 1994). Folic acid substitution (1 mg daily) mitigates side-effects, but can mask vitamin B12 deficiency associated neural toxicity; therefore, screening B12 levels prior to therapy is suggested.

Alkylating agents

Cyclophosphamide, chlorambucil and melphalan cause disruption of DNA synthesis and block cellular division at the G2 phase of the cell cycle (Table 24.2). In addition, alkylating agents have various other effects on cell metabolism, RNA and protein synthesis. Cyclophosphamide is activated in vivo by the liver. For non-malignant or premalignant (monoclonal gammopathy) antibody-mediated autoimmune diseases, there is ample experience with cyclophosphamide. Most sensitive are B cells, precursors of suppressor T cells and amplifiers of suppressor cells. Depending on dosage and timing of administration of cyclophosphamide in relation to antigen priming in animal experiments, cyclophosphamide results in enhancement (when cyclophosphamide is given after immunization) or depression (when cyclophosphamide is given before immunization) of the delayed type hypersensitivity response.

This immunomodulatory effect of cyclophosphamide occurs at low dosages and is attributed to depletion of precursors of suppressor cells (Hengst and Kempf 1984). Moderate dosages ($\pm$10 mg kg^{-1} in one dose or 2–3 mg kg^{-1} per day for 4–5 days) deplete B cell-dependent areas of spleen and lymph nodes without measurable effects on T cell-mediated immune responses. Inhibition of in vitro IgM-plaque forming cells lasts up to 14 days after withdrawal of cyclophosphamide.

Inhibition of helper T cells and their precursurs is obtained with higher dosages and reversed by IL-2 (Ozer et al. 1982). Very high cytostatic dosages (20–40 mg kg^{-1}) also reduce cytotoxic T (CTL) cells and NK cells: an effect that restores within a week after drug cessation (Ozer et al. 1982). Cyclophosphamide and chlorambucil are used in the treatment of B cell lymphoproliferative diseases of low grade malignancy and melphalan is the major drug effective in multiple myeloma.

Experience in immune-mediated neuropathies

Multifocal motor neuropathy (MMN) is often associated with high-titer IgM anti-GM_1 antibodies and is resistant to corticosteroids. Responsiveness to alkylating agents is very likely for IgM-antibody mediated autoimmune diseases (Nydegger 1991). The IgM anti-GM_1 antibody titer was observed to decrease after treatment with cyclophosphamide in association with clinical improvement (Feldman et al. 1991). The clinical response associated with antibody reduction was superior after high dose intravenous cyclophosphamide induction therapy followed by intermittent monthly courses compared with chronic maintenance treatment with daily low dosages of cyclophosphamide (Pestronk et al. 1988).

In monoclonal IgM-associated autoimmune syndromes with autonomous B cell proliferation, alkylating agents are often given, either as intermittant courses with cyclophosphamide or as daily maintenance treatment with chlorambucil (0.1 mg kg^{-1}), with monitoring for leukocytopenia. Treatment for chronic low grade malignant B cell proliferative diseases is however not aimed at cure and a reduction of paraprotein level below 20% is rarely obtained. Thus, it is often difficult to prevent further nerve damage in these patients. Patients with Waldenström's disease (immunocytoma) may further benefit from courses of cyclophosphamide supported with intermittent plasmapheresis at 3-week intervals. Severe polyneuropathy associated with paraproteinaemia may benefit from courses of plasma exchange followed by cyclophosphamide and methylprednisone intravenously, a scedule reportedly successful in aggressive, transfusion dependent, cold hemolytic anemia (Nydegger et al. 1991).

For younger patients or patients in otherwise

Table 24.2 *Characteristics and application of immunosuppressive drugs*

Immunosuppressive pathways	Major immunosuppressive side-effects	Toxicity	Application in immune-mediated neuropathies
Alkylating drugs (cyclophosphamide, chlorambucil, melphalan)			
Low dose Precursor of suppressor cells Amplifiers of suppressor cells *Moderate dose* B cells *Intermediate dose* Helper T cells *Cytostatic dose* CTL and NK cells	Leukopenia Hypogammaglobulinemia	Bone marrow dysplasia and secondary leukemia (total dose dependent) Hemorrhagic cystitis (high dose-associated) Pneumonitis	*Multifocal motor neuropathy* Cyclophosphamide is first line drug (preferentially by intermittent courses) *Paraprotein* associated polyneuropathy: cyclophosphamide in monthly intervals or chlorambucil 0.1 mg kg^{-1} daily *POEMS* as second line drug: monthly courses as in myeloma treatment In severe *vasculitis*, daily cyclophosphamide maintenance is used in combination (or after pulsing) with corticosteroids
Cyclosporin			
CD4 T cell inhibition	High dose: viral infections virally-induced cancer	Nephropathy Hypertension Neurotoxicity	Third line treatment in CIDP

Note:
CIDP: chronic inflammatory demyelinating polyneuropathy; POEMS: polyneuropathy, organomegaly, endocrinopathy, monoclonal gammopathy and skin changes

good condition with low grade lymphoproliferative disease, more aggressive treatment aimed at eradication of the IgM producing clone or even cure of the disease can be considered (see Recent drugs). In POEMS syndrome (Broussole et al. 1991), if no solitary bone lesion or plasmacytoma is found, high dose corticosteroids and melphalan are options causing variable degrees of improvement in 30–50% of the cases.

Toxicity

The main toxicity of alkylating agents is leukopenia, prolonged treatment of cyclophosphamide leads to myelodysplastic hematopoiesis with the risk of secondary leukemia. Bladder toxicity often occurs after high dose (more than 1 g m^{-2}) intravenous cyclophosphamide used to condition for allogeneic bone marrow transplantation and is rarely observed in oral or intravenous treatment for autoimmune diseases or cancer, provided optimal hydration and diuresis is maintained.

Cyclosporin and related drugs

Cyclosporine has profound effects on T lymphocyte proliferation by blocking IL-2 gene transcription, which occurs after T cell activation by T cell receptor (TCR) and antigen-presenting cell (APC) interaction (Table 24.2). Cyclosporine binds to calcineurin and inhibit Ca^{2+}- dependent phosphatase activity involved in lymphokine expression, degranulation and apoptosis. Calcineurin is important in the signal transduction pathway leading to IL-2 expression and subsequent expression of early cytokines (IL-3, IL-4, TNF-α, GM-CSF and IFN-γ) which are produced 2–4 hours after initiation of T cell activation. Once mRNA of these early cytokines is expressed cyclosporin is ineffective. The inhibitory effect of cyclosporin can be reversed by exogenous administered IL-2.

Cyclosporin at moderate dosages of 3–7.5 mg kg^{-1}, an effective dose in some autoimmune diseases, selectively modulates the immunoregulatory responses of the T helper cell population, leaving T independent responses and established CTL responses unimpaired. At such moderate dosages, the susceptibility to bacterial, fungal and parasitic infections is not greatly increased. Higher dosages of cyclosporin, as given to prevent transplant rejection, inhibit CTL and NK responses and enhance susceptibility for viral infections and may be cancer (Nalesnik et al. 1988).

Experience in autoimmune diseases

Cyclosporin has been administered in all types of autoimmune disease (Fathman and Meyers 1992). Randomized studies have been performed in Behçet's disease, Crohn's disease, Graves ophthalmopathy, early onset type I diabetes and others. Clinical responses in uncontrolled studies in refractory autoimmune thrombocytopenia, myasthenia gravis, pemphigoid diseases and CIDP suggest a broad efficacy. Almost all clinical experience in autoimmune diseases shows a more favourable response compared with other drugs but frequent relapse after withdrawal. This is the main reason why cyclosporin is reserved as third or fourth line treatment in refractory patients.

Toxicity

Drug-related side-effects of cyclosporin are dose-related. At dosages of more than 10 mg kg^{-1} frequent side-effects are nephropathy (50%), hypertension (40%), neurotoxicity (20%), hepatic dysfunction (15%) and hyperglycemia. These figures are reported in transplant patients and reversible after dose reduction. Nephrotoxicity, tremors, paresthesias, gingival hyperplasia and trichinosis also occur at lower dosages (3–7 mg kg^{-1}) used in autoimmune diseases. The risk of neoplasia in kidney transplant recipients is not significantly different compared with conventional immunosuppressive therapy; after long-term treatment for autoimmune diseases this incidence is not known.

Recent drugs

For more than two decades the antimetabolites and alkylating agents discussed above were the exclusive first line drugs for (low-grade) malignant lymphoproliferative diseases and second line treatment in corticosteroid-refractory autoimmune diseases or as corticosteroid-sparing drugs. One of the newer drugs successfully used to treat patients with chronic lymphocytic leukemia (CLL) and other low-grade lymphoma's, including Waldenström's disease, is fludarabine monophosphate, an adenine analog resistant to adenosine deaminase.

The in vivo converted active metabolite of fludarabine is incorporated into DNA and assumed to accumulate in B cells, where the drug continues to be effective after cessation of treatment.

Fludarabine causes a decrease in ($CD4^+$) peripheral blood cells, and there is considerable bacterial and viral infectious toxicity (Keating et al. 1989). Fludarabine induces an acquired T cell immunodeficiency and may cause development or (temporary) enhancement of autoimmune hemolytic anemia in more than 20% of CLL patients (Myint et al. 1995). In other conditions, not like CLL associated with antibody mediated hemolytic anemia, induction of autoantibodies have not (yet) been observed, but precaution is warranted in antibody-mediated autoimmunity.

Two other purine nucleoside analogs currently investigated in clinical trials are 2-CdA (2-chlorodeoxyadenosine) and 2-deoxycoformycin or pentostatin. These three new anti-metabolites: fludarabine, 2-CdA and 2-Deoxycoformycin are increasingly administered to patients with low grade lymphoproliferative disorders, either in randomized studies with standard alkylating and/or antimetabolite treatment or in patients refractory to these treatments. Although the side-effects (neutropenia, fever and infections) are more severe than with the classical antimetabolites, causing infectious complications in up to 10% of treated patients, tumor reduction is more effective. Thus, these drugs should be considered in the future in severe neuropathies associated with plasma cell dyscrasia's.

Another very promising antimetabolite interfering with pyrimidine synthesis is Brequinar sodium. This drug was mainly tested in animal models for inhibition of (xeno)allograft reactivity. In these models, it appeared to be a potent suppressor of the secondary immune response at the cellular and humoral levels and able to reverse graft rejections and to reduce the presence of preformed (allo)antibodies despite ongoing antigenic stimulation (Woo et al. 1993). This seems extremely promising for chronic autoimmune diseases in which persistent antigenic stimulation occurs with considerable memory cell establishment.

Immunomodulation

Modification of the immune response in cancer, transplantation and autoimmune diseases can be obtained by a variety of immunomodulatory approaches. These include irradiation, plasmapheresis, administration of monoclonal antibodies or recombinant interleukins and even (HLA-shared) blood transfusions. Some of these approaches of possible relevance for immune-mediated neurological diseases are discussed.

Total nodal/lymphoid irradiation/total body irradiation

Experience with total lymph node irradiation (TLI) comes from treatment of Hodgkin's disease. Total lymphoid irradiation causes profound immunosuppressive effects on the proliferative capacity of lymphocytes and the delayed-type hypersensitivity response. In animal experiments, TLI induces severe T (helper) lymphocytopenia with doubling of B cells. The IgM antibody response restores quickly after TLI, but IgG (T cell dependent) antibody production is severely reduced, probably life-long. Shortly after TLI, lymphocyte repopulation occurs with immature cells which appear identical with 'natural' suppressor cells found in neonatal spleen and adult bone marrow (Slavin 1987).

This transient immaturity enhances the development of antigen-specific tolerance and chimerism of allogeneic cells (Strober et al. 1989).

After experience in animals with spontaneous autoimmune diseases (NZB mouse/MRL/1 mice) and induced autoimmune diseases (adjuvant arthritis), patients with intractable rheumatoid arthritis, drug-resistent systemic lupus erythematosus (SLE) and multiple sclerosis (MS) were, with encouraging results in some patients, treated with TLI (Tanay et al. 1984).

The side effects of TLI can be, depending on extension and dose fractionation, considerable (transient leuko- and thrombocytopenia, nausea, xerostomia, weight loss and frequent viral infections). Although the effects of TLI are, in contrast to immunosuppressive drugs, prolonged and not associated with major bacterial infections, this treatment will remain reserved for individual patients with severe therapy-resistant autoimmune diseases such as described for autoimmune thrombocytopenia or dermatomyositis (Kelly et al. 1988) of predominantly T helper cell-mediated or IgG autoantibody origin.

Plasmapheresis

In therapeutic plasmapheresis, multiple components such as antibodies, complement and cytokines are removed. Plasmapheresis, in contrast to corticosteroids, has been reported to be successful in meningococcal sepsis, microangiopathic hemolytic syndromes and overwhelming malaria infection, conditions attributed to increased TNF-α and IL-1 production. Although randomized studies were not performed in these critically ill patients, animal experiments have shown that plasma exchange reduces plasma IL-1 levels and improves survival after intravenous infusion with *Escherichia coli* (Røkke et al. 1993). In autoimmunity, plasmapheresis is most effective in immune-mediated diseases with a monophasic nature, generally of postinfectious origin, such as GBS and Goodpasture's syndrome. Also, acute exacerbations of chronic diseases, such as myasthenic crisis, can be succesfully reversed with plasmapheresis in combination with drugs to suppress the production of antibodies (Table 24.3).

For chronic autoimmune diseases, with either ongoing antigenic stimulation or autonomous B cell production, maintenance therapy with plasmapheresisis generally is not indicated. Exceptions exist, for example for patients with aggressive cryoglobulinemic vasculitis, therapy-resistent CIDP or acute GBS-like relapses and lymphoproliferative diseases with IgM autoantibody syndromes. Such patients may benefit from maintenance plasmapheresis at 1–3 weekly intervals in addition to treatment with cyclophosphamide or chlorambucil.

Side-effects of plasmapheresis in experienced centers are infrequent (less than 5%) and mortality is rare, less than 0.01% (Korach et al. 1993). Patients on angiotensin converting enzyme inhibiting drugs have an increased risk for anaphylactic or hypotensive reactions because of delayed clearance of bradykinins present in exchange fluids or released as a result from contact activation with extracorporeal circuits. It is advised to withhold these drugs 24 hours before apheresis (Owen and Brecher 1994). Chronic plasmapheresis results in iron deficiency and hypogammaglobulinemia. In combination with immunosuppressive drugs, the susceptibility to bacterial infections is increased.

Selective immunoadsorption

An apheresis technique recently more widely applied is selective immunoadsorption by the use of columns coated with hydrophobic substances (e.g. tryptophan) or with staphylococcal protein-A (Staph. A) or other ligands for selective ex vivo immunoglobulin removal. With protein-A columns dramatic responses have been observed in patients with various autoimmune diseases. Patients not responding to plasmapheresis can improve with column-apheresis. The incidence of adverse reactions however is higher than with plasmapheresis and occasionally life-threatening reactions have been reported (Smith et al. 1992).

In addition to adsorption of antibodies, other immunomodulatory effects are mediated by column-apheresis. It is postulated that immune complexes, idiotypic and anti-idiotypic antibodies and staphylococcal protein-A material may elute from the column and recirculate in the patient. Such eluates can stimulate in vivo B and T cell populations and interact with mononuclear cells (for a review see Rock 1993).

Experience in immune-mediated neuropathies

Plasmapheresis or high-dose intravenous immunoglobulin (IVIG), applied as soon as possible after manifestation of GBS, has been shown to be effective in controlled studies (Guillain-Barré Syndrome Study Group 1985; Ropper 1992; van de Meché et al. 1992). Plasmapheresis may be effective by removal of acute phase proteins and presumed pathogenic antibodies.

Early relapses of GBS after plasma exchange or IVIG treatment do occur however (Irani et al. 1993). In the randomized study of van de Meché et al. relapse incidence was similar after IVIG and plasma exchange. In case of relapse, treatment with plasmapheresis or IVIG must be reinstituted.

In GBS, assays to predict the severity of disease and to monitor disease activity and treatment response are lacking. It remains to be established whether measurements of cytokine profiles as in Kawasaki disease can be helpful in this respect.

Table 24.3 *Characteristics and application of immunosuppressive drugs*

Immunosuppressive pathways	Major immunosuppressive side-effects	Toxicity	Application in immune-mediated neuropathies
Plasmapheresis Removal of antibodies, complement and cytokines	Hypogammaglobulinaemia	Hypotension (cave ACE-inhibitors) Allergic reactions	*GBS* First line treatment (equally effective as IVIG) *CIDP*, *vasculitis* neuropathy, *Polyneuropathy with paraprotein* Third line, supporting other treatment modalities
Intravenous immunoglobulin *Anti-inflammatory* IL-1 ↓ IL-1ra ↑ *Anti-effector cells* ADCC ↓ NK ↓ Complement activation ↓ *Anti-id antibodies* Neutralization Regulation *Immunoregulation* Inhibition of TH1, Enhancement TH2 response *Antiproliferative effects?*	Not known	Headache, HCV-transmission Hemolytic anemia (anti-A and B) Aseptic meningitis Allergic reactions (in IgA-deficiency)	*GBS* First line treatment (equally effective as plasmapheresis) *CIDP* First line choice in selected cases of severe paralysis and/or children. *MMN* and *CIDP* Supporting other treatment modalities or in refractory patients

Note:
ACE: angiotensin converting enzyme; CIDP: chronic inflammatory demyelinating polyneuropathy; GBS: Guillain-Barré syndrome; MMN: multifocal motor neuropathy.

CIDP also responds to plasmapheresis and IVIG treatment (Dyck et al. 1986; van Doorn et al. 1990), but both are usually not a practical therapeutic option to treat this often chronic disease. Plasmapheresis or IVIG can be restricted to: (1) severely affected patients as induction-treatment followed by corticosteroids or other immunosuppressive drugs, (2) prepuberal children in which high maintenance-dose of steroids are contraindicated, (3) patients refractory to corticosteroids and other immune suppressive drugs, and (4) patients requiring high corticosteroid maintenance dosage, allowing dose reduction.

In a sham-apheresis controlled study on 39 patients Dyck et al. (1991) showed that patients with monoclonal gammopathy of undetermined significance (MGUS) associated neuropathy improved their neuropathy disability score. Patients with IgG and IgA gammopathy improved but patients with IgM-MGUS associated polyneuropathy showed no statistically significant improvement. IgM-associated neuropathies (of which 50% of the patients have antibodies against myelin-associated glycoprotein) represent a distinct entity. The duration of plasma exchange (six exchanges in 3 weeks) and the short follow-up may be not long enough to cause a favorable clinical response in these chronic, slowly progressing neuropathies.

In POEMS syndrome, a multisystem disease with plasma cell dyscrasia (PCD), no autoantibody activity of the monoclonal protein has been identified. Plasma exchange, applied in patients refractory to other therapies, has not been very successfull (Silberstein et al. 1985, Miralles et al. 1992).

Clinical experience with column immunoadsorption in neurological autoimmune diseases is limited. A preliminary study in six patients with paraneoplastic neurological syndromes recorded complete and durable responses in five of the six patients (Cher et al. 1995).

Photopheresis

In extracorporeal photochemotherapy, mononuclear cells are extracorporeally irradiated with ultraviolet light (UV-A) in the presence of a photosensitizing substance (often 8-methoxy-psoralen or 8-MOP). The patients are treated with 8-MOP orally and subsequently their peripheral blood lymphocytes are collected by lymphocytapheresis, irradiated with UV-A light and returned to the patients. It is also possible to add 8-MOP to the collected lymphocytes prior to UV-A exposure. Clinical experience with photoinactivation is originally based on treatment of cutaneous T cell lymphoma (mycosis fungoides).

Photochemotherapy with 8-MOP specifically acts on activated T cells. Murine and primate experimental models suggest that the 8-MOP photoinactivation approach is particularly effective against expanded clones of inducer T cells. It is postulated that lethally damaged but still antigenic photoinactivated cells evoke an immune response leading to subsequent destruction of the non-photoinactivated counterpart populations in vivo (Edelson et al. 1991).

In several centers worldwide, the effects of photopheresis on organ graft rejection, chronic graft versus host disease and selected autoimmune diseases (systemic sclerosis, pemphigus vulgaris, rheumatoid arthritis, multiple sclerosis, insulin-dependent diabetes mellitus) are being evaluated; however, conclusions have not yet been reached and the design of many of these studies has been criticised. Extracorporeal photopheresis has minimal side-effects, similar to large volume plasmapheresis and is well-tolerated by the patients. Upon reinfusion of treated cells, nausea and short-term febrile reactions are observed. Long-term systemic side-effects of extracorporeal irradiated lymphocytes have to be awaited.

Intravenous immunoglobulin (IVIG)

Intravenous immunoglobulin (IVIG) is prepared from plasma pools derived from 10 000 to 60 000 donors. It contains antibodies against environmental pathogens, postpregnancy and transfusion-induced alloantibodies, natural autoantibodies and regulatory anti-idiotypic antibodies and molecules of the immunoglobulin superfamily (HLA-molecules, CD4, CD8) and IFN-γ (Lam et al. 1993). Intravenous immunoglobulin affects all axes of the immune system, but it is unknown whether all these effects are mediated by a single or multiple components of IVIG. Considering the number of donors involved in a batch, IVIG is the safest of all blood products and HIV transmissions have not been observed.

Transmission of hepatitis C (HCV) has occurred

in approximately 450 recipients and was restricted to a limited number of batches. This is in contrast to HCV transmission to almost 100% of hemophilia patients treated by factor VIII products. However, since the elimination of HCV positive donors (after 1991), apparently eliminating protective antibodies, the observed HCV-RNA in IVIG and the reported incidence of hepatitis C by IVIG is increasing, necessitating additional virus inactivation steps such as solvent and detergent treatment. Serious allergic reactions can be seen in a proportion of patients with IgA deficiency. In a survey of complications of IVIG in neurological disease, minor adverse effects were frequently found (59%) and discontinuation because of side-effects occurred in 16% of cases. Mortality or persistent morbidity was not observed (Brannagan et al. 1996).

Modulation of Fc receptors and complement

Blocking of Fc-IgG receptors by IVIG is presumably the major mechanism resulting in an increase of platelets in autoimmune thrombocytopenia (ITP). After administration of IVIG the clearance of particulate immune complexes, such as IgG-coated red cells, is decreased (Fehr et al. 1982). Increase of platelets can also be obtained by other approaches that block or modulate macrophage and monocyte Fcγ-receptors (receptors for IgG). Such approaches are induction of hemolysis by the administration of anti-Rh-D immunoglobulin to Rh-D positive individuals or the infusion of a monoclonal antibody against the FcRγIII receptor (Clarkson et al. 1986). All Fcγ-receptors are expressed on macrophages (activated monocytes) and play a role in antibody dependent cytotoxicity (ADCC). FcγRs are also found on Schwann cells, perineurial cells and endoneurial macrophages. It is assumed that FcγRs in the nervous system, which are upregulated in inflammation (by IFN-γ), play a role in antigen-presentation and transport of IgG, a function Fcγ-receptors have in the placenta in transporting maternal IgG to the fetus.

IVIG contains monomeric and dimeric IgG (Roux and Tankersly 1990). Monomeric IgG preferentially binds to the FcγR-I (CD64) on monocytes/macrophages and has a moderate affinity for the FcR-IIIa (the phospholipid anchored transmembrane form of FcγR-III) present on macrophages and NK cells. IVIG also contains dimers which bind to the FcγR-II receptor and the FcR-IIIb (CD16, the phosphatidyl inositolglycan anchored form of FcγR-III). The FcγR-II (CD32) is also expressed on B cells and is induced by hematopoietic colony-stimulating growth factors, G-CSF and GM-CSF, on myeloid cells and has a high affinity for complexed IgG3. FcγR-IIIb, also a strong binder of IgG3 dimers, is expressed on granulocytes.

Besides a direct binding of IgG monomers, dimers and in vivo formed immune complexes to Fcγ-receptors, the Fc part of anti-HLA class I and II antibodies (present in IVIG) are also capable of blocking ADCC after binding to class I and II antigens on monocytes (Neppert et al. 1985).

Moreover, IVIG also inhibits the uptake of C3b and C4b onto red cells which carry the complement receptor CR1 (CD35) and increase survival of complement activating IgM-coated red cells (Basta et al. 1991). By the binding of monomeric and dimeric IgG in IVIG and the formation of immune complexes in vivo after binding of infused IVIG with recipient antigens, multiple Fcγ receptors on various cell types can be modulated. This results in a decrease of ADCC of IgG antibody targeted antigens and reduced cytotoxicity by NK cells, while by interaction between IVIG and activated complement components also IgM-antibody mediated effects are mitigated.

Cytokine interactions and anti-inflammatory effects of IVIG

In patients with the mucocutaneous lymph node syndrome or Kawasaki disease the effect of IVIG was demonstrated in a randomized study (Newburger et al. 1986). Children treated with IVIG and aspirin compared with aspirin only experienced a significant lower incidence (8% versus 23%) of coronary artery aneurysms. In this acute (presumably postinfectious) small and medium vessel multiorgan perivasculitis, high levels of IL-1, TNF-α and IFN-γ are secreted. Aneurysms still developed in IVIG treated patients who continued producing IL-1 but not in patients in whom IL-1 levels normalized (Leung et al. 1989). These findings in Kawasaki disease indicate that IVIG normalizes increased IL-1 levels in vivo. Induction of IL-1 is also a crucial factor in bacterial endotoxin-mediated complications and in case reports IVIG was considered life-saving in the treatment of septic shock syndrome (Barry et al. 1992).

There are several studies on in vitro, ex vivo and in vivo effects of IVIG on the (pro)inflammatory cytokine profile. In general, in vitro experiments with various antibodies show that complexed IgG, IgG-Fc-receptor binding and IgG-crosslinking induces production of TNF-α, IL-6 and IL-1 receptor-antagonist (IL-1ra) by monocytes and IFN-γ production by NK cells. In vitro and in vivo IVIG inhibits lipopolysaccharide-induced TNF-α and IL-1 production and results in induction of IL-1ra. After IVIG infusion to non-infected patients, a rapid increase, indicating release and not production, of IFN-γ, IL-6, IL-8, TNF-α and IL-1ra was observed (Aukrust et al. 1994).

The complete understanding of how IVIG inhibits inflammatory cytokines is unknown. IVIG contains antibodies against bacterial toxins, natural antibodies against cytokines including TNF-α, IL-1 and IL6 (Abe et al. 1994) and is contaminated with α2-macroglobulin, which binds a variety of cytokines (La Marre et al 1991). It is quite conceivable that IVIG can induce as well as suppress cytokine production in vivo, depending on the underlying disorder and the activation state of various (accessory) cells expressing costimulatory signals.

Anti-idiotypic antibodies

A clinical effect of IVIG by immediate reduction of pathogenic antibodies in vivo was first demonstrated in anti-FVIII-c autoantibodies causing an acquired bleeding disorder (Sultan et al. 1987). In a series of experiments, we found antibodies against a glycolipid determinant on neuroblastoma (NBL) cells, serving as a marker for immune-mediated demyelinating polyneuropathies (GBS and CIDP), which were neutralized in vivo and in vitro by IVIG. IVIG contains anti-idiotypic antibodies against these NBL-antibodies (Lundkvist et al. 1989). Spontaneous recovery from GBS without IVIG treatment was also associated with increase in such anti-idiotypic antibodies, whose activity resided in the $F(ab)_2$ fragment. Both IgG from recovered GBS patients and IVIG crossreact with other autoantibodies, including platelet antibodies, acetylcholine-receptor antibodies, antineutrophil cytoplasmatic antibodies (ANCA) and thyroglobulin antibodies. These findings suggest that active autoimmune disease is associated with reduction of anti-idiotypic antibodies and that recovery from autoimmune diseases might be the result of increase in anti-idiotypic antibodies. IVIG can restore this effect transiently. In IVIG, these crossreactive anti-idiotypic antibodies constitute approximately 1% of the total IgG (Lundkvist et al. 1993); however, decrease of auto-antibody titer does not always accompany improvement after IVIG in all autoimmune diseases. Patients with myasthenia gravis improving after IVIG treatment have not all shown reduction in anti-acetylcholine-receptor antibodies, nor do patients with CIDP who carry anti-GM_1 antibodies. The variable affinity of anti-idiotypic antibodies binding to antibodies of individual patients was also found in vitro (Lundkvist et al. 1993). Nevertheless, in these patients, the beneficial effect are likely attributed to other (e.g. anti-inflammatory) effects of IVIG.

Interaction with lymphocyte activation

Clinical observations have shown improvement for a longer interval than the transient effect related to the half-life of the infused IgG (van Doorn et al. 1990). This may be the result of downregulation of the production of pathogenic antibodies. In vitro, and ex vivo after IVIG treatment, reduced production of immunoglobulins by pokeweed (PWD)-stimulated lymphocytes has been demonstrated (Stohl 1986; Kondo et al. 1991). After administration of IVIG to patients and experimental animals a transient rise in IgM-production was observed. It is assumed that this IgM reflects anti-idiotypic antibodies. It has therefore been speculated that pooled human IgM is also effective in the treatment of antibody-mediated autoimmune diseases (for a review see Hurez et al. 1993).

An effect on antibody production can be the result of direct interactions between IVIG and B cells, for instance with the immunoglobulin idiotype on the B cell surface or the FcRγ-II (CD32) on B cells. IVIG also contains antibodies against the CD5 antigen expressed on a small population of B cells preferentially involved in autoimmune reactivity (Vassilev et al. 1993).

An effect on IgG production by T cell dependent B cells can also be explained by IVIG inhibition of T cell activation. IVIG contains antibodies against the constant and the variable regions of the β-chain of the T cell receptors (TCR) (Marchalonis et al. 1992) and antibodies against the CD4 epitope expressed on helper T cells. The TCR interaction with major histocompatibility complex (MHC) antigen-associated peptides may furthermore be influenced by antibodies against HLA antigens and antibodies against peptides presented by the HLA molecules (for a review see Kaveri et al. 1994).

Intravenous IgG preparations also influence the balance between the T helper type 1 and 2 activation. Depending on the nature of the antigenic challenge and subsequent cytokines induced, at least two CD4 helper populations can be activated. Typical TH1-cytokines are IFN-γ, IL-2 and IL-12. These enhance a cell-mediated immune response, such as delayed-type hypersensitivity (DTH), CTL and NK induction. TH2-cells produce IL-4, IL-6, IL-10 and IL-13 and provide help for B cell activation and antibody production and atopic responses. In transplantation immunology in the mouse, IL-2 and IFN-γ are increased in case of rejection while type 2 cytokines are associated with tolerance (Dalman 1993).

In vitro, IVIG enhances PWD-induced TH2-type lymphocyte proliferation and inhibits the allogeneic (TH1-type) lymphocyte response (Brand et al. 1996). These results in vitro strongly suggest that IVIG restores an imbalance between TH1 and TH2 by inhibition of the TH1 response and enhancement of the TH2 response. This dual effect explains the beneficial effect of IVIG in predominantly TH1-mediated autoimmune diseases which are often organ-specific, in transplantation immunology (rejection and graft-versus-host disease), and in bacterial superantigen-induced lymphocyte activation while, on the other hand, (IgM) antibodies are induced, as observed in animal models, with possible anti-idiotypic activity against autoantibodies.

Antiproliferative effects and nerve repair

In vitro, IVIG shows a dose dependent antiproliferative effect resulting in growth arrest of activated cells in the Go/G1 phase of the cell cycle preventing progression to the S phase. This effect is observed with almost any proliferating cell type when IVIG is present in concentrations between 10 and 20 g L^{-1}, a level reached in vivo after the usual high dose IVIG for autoimmune diseases (van Schaik et al. 1992). This antiproliferative effect is not cytokine-dependent, not Fcγ-receptor-mediated and not based on cytotoxic or apparant apoptotic effects of IVIG. We recently identified an immunoglobulin fraction in IVIG binding to a glycolipid shared by malignant cells and activated lymphocytes) (Vuist et al. in press).

It is unknown whether this growth arrest occurs in vivo. If so, this may have particular consequences for demyelinating neuropathies because after demyelination environmental factors may prevent or promote myelin synthesis. Immunoglobulin was shown to promote CNS remyelination in the Theiler's virus mouse (Rodriquez and Lennon 1990). IVIG inhibits proliferation of not only autonomous growing cells but many growing cells. An induction of growth arrest of fibroblasts in culture was associated with upregulation of a growth arrest specific gene (GAS-3) (I.N. van Schaik et al., personal communication). This gene also encodes for the peripheral myelin protein, the PMP-22 protein.

Further confirmation is needed with Schwann cell cultures, whether proliferation arrest by IVIG contributes to remyelination by induction of differentiation of Schwann cells and synthesis of myelin.

Sequence of events

IVIG in the empirically established dosages for autoimmune diseases of 2 g kg^{-1} body weight administered in 2–5 days has an immediate effect on the proinflammatory cytokine profile and increase of IL-1 receptor-antagonist within 6 hours. Other immediate effects are the neutralization of pathogenic autoantibodies, inhibition of FcγR-mediated ADCC and NK cell cytotoxicity and binding of activated complement components present on target cells.

Longer acting effects of IVIG may result from downregulation of the TH1-helper cell and enhancement of the TH2 response resulting in tolerance and stimulation of anti-idiotypic antibodies.

Experience in immune-mediated neuropathies

In a randomized trial in GBS patients IVIG was as effective as plasma exchange (discussed in the section Plasmapheresis). The combination of plasma exchange followed by IVIG offers no substantial benefits and is associated with more side-effects (Hughes for the Guillain-Barré Syndrome Support Group 1995). Recently a patient with a pure dysautonomic variant of GBS was presented showing rapid improvement after IVIG (Heafield et al. 1996).

The improvement obtained by IVIG in CIDP can be dramatic. After a prolonged period of paralysis patients can rapidly improve from the third treatment day onwards. The incidence of responders is not exactly known and according to a small series comprising 144 patients was 50% (range 20–100%) (reviewed by van Doorn 1994). Criteria for CIDP are not uniform although clinical factors are helpful to improve prediction of responsiveness to IVIG (van Doorn et al. 1991).

Unfortunately there is no laboratory assay for CIDP, either to confirm diagnosis or to select (IVIG)-responding patients and to monitor therapy. Antibodies to GM_1 are present in a minority of patients with predominantly motor manifestations and persist despite clinical improvement to IVIG (van Schaik 1994).

Patients with motor neuropathy, especially those without conduction block or in whom a conduction block has not been found, may not improve with cyclophosphamide despite a decrease in the anti-GM-1 titer. These patients usually show transient improvement after IVIG infusions without any change in the GM_1 antibody titers (Chaudry et al. 1993, Nobile Orazio et al. 1993). It is not determined whether IVIG responding multifocal motor neuropathy (MMN) patients did in fact have variants of CIDP.

Immune response modifiers

ALG/ATG

Antilymphocyte (thymocyte) globulin (ALG/ATG) contains a mixture of antibodies induced by immunizing horse, rabbit or goat with human lymphocytes or purified T cells. AGT/ALG contains antibodies against CD2, CD3, CD4 and CD8 antigens on T cells and CD19 and CD20 on B cells, in addition to non-lineage specific antibodies such as anti-HLA class I/II antibodies, antibodies against adhesion molecules CD11a/CD18 and against activation markers (IL-2 receptor or CD25). ATG, developed in the 1960s, is still used as immunosuppressive agent to prevent or reverse graft rejection in transplantation and for some autoimmune diseases, classically for aplastic anemia, and recently for ANCA-positive systemic vasculitis.

The biological effects depend on the doses. Administered in high dosages, blockade of T cell proliferation occurs, affecting the G2/S phase of the cell cycle. In contrast, low doses of ATG results in stimulation of T cells (Bonnefoy-Berard et al. 1994).

Monoclonal antibodies

Monoclonal antibodies are now available directed against families of lineage dependent and cell cycle-dependent differentiation antigens on activated immune cells or against interleukins. There is an expanding clinical experience; monoclonal anti-CD3 and IL-2-receptor antibodies are widely used in transplantation immunology (Koenes 1992). Preliminary results of monoclonal antibodies against TNF-α in rheumatoid arthritis are promising. The broad-reactive humanized Campath-1H (anti-CDW52) monoclonal antibody reacting against normal and malignant mononuclear cells has been incidently used for treatment of autoimmune thrombocytopenia (ITP) and ANCA-positive systemic vasculitis (Table 24.4).

In POEMS syndrome without lytic or sclerotic lesions or isolated plasmocytoma that can be irradiated or resected, the results of corticosteroids with or without melphalan are disappointing in most patients. High levels of IL-6 and IL-1β have been demonstrated in serum (Gherardi et al. 1996) and in the abnormal plasma cells or associated angiofollicular hyperplasia lesions (Gherardi et al. 1994). Chemotherapy, as in myeloma and lymphoma, does not totally eradicate tumor cells which continue to produce abnormal cytokines. A transient response was obtained in a patient treated with a monoclonal antibody against IL-6 (Beck et al. 1994).

α-Interferon

Peripheral neuropathy occurs in up to 20% of the patients with mixed (type II and III) cryoglobulinemias. Of particular interest is small vessel vasculitis in association with immune complexes and cryoglobulins and the presence of viral markers for hepatitis B and C. Anti-HBV and HCV antibodies and/or antigens are increasingly recognized in cryoglobulinemias and low grade lymphoproliferative diseases especially in areas with a

Table 24.4 *Characteristics and application of immunosuppressive drugs*

	Side-effects	Toxicity	Experimental application of immune-mediated neuropathies
Miscellaneous			
Polyclonal or monoclonal antibodies	Fever, serum sickness	Allergic reactions Nephrotoxicity	Vasculitis (Campath-1H, anti-TNF) POEMS Sy (anti-IL-6)
α-Interferon	Flu-like symptoms Leuko-/granulocytopenia	Diarrhea Mental disturbances	First line treatment in hepatitis B/C associated vasculitis
TBI/TLI	Viral infections Hypogammaglobulinemia	Thrombocytopenia Stomatitis	Fourth line treatment in various refractory autoimmune diseases

Note:
POEMS: polyneuropathy, organomegaly, endocrinopathy, monoclonal gammopathy and skin changes.

high prevalence of hepatitis B and C (HBV and/or HCV). Immunosuppressive vasculitis treatment with methylprednisolone and cyclophosphamide may enhance viral replication. HCV/HBV-positive vasculitis with or without cryoglobulins may be better treated with plasmapheresis and/or α-interferon. Also IVIG was shown to induce prolonged remission in cryoglobulinemic vasculitis. It is unknown whether this effect was the result of antibodies against environmental antigens present in IVIG. It is expected in the near future applying RNA/DNA amplification that persisting infections in low grade lymphomas and immune complex diseases (exemplified by *Helicobactor pylori* and HBV/HCV) are increasingly discovered. Treatment may then be individualized from antibiotic treatment, α-interferons to IVIG (IVIG produced after 1991 does not contain anti-HCV antibodies).

Conclusions

In immune-mediated neuropathies, clinical experience and knowledge of the pathogenesis results in the following suggestions. For acute inflammatory polyneuropathy (GBS), first line treatment should consist of plasma exchange or IVIG, with reinstitution of therapy for relapse. It has yet to be determined whether additional treatment with monoclonal antibodies directed against early released cytokines can improve the speed of recovery and final outcome of the disease. For chronic demyelinating neuropathies (CIDP) initial treatment with corticosteroids and/or IVIG must generally be followed by a corticosteroid maintenance treatment. Further dosage reduction can be obtained by combination with azathioprine, cyclophosphamide or cyclosporin. Plasmapheresis and IVIG as maintenance therapy are generally reserved for restricted conditions.

Patients with MNN associated with conduction block and with or without IgM-GM1 antibodies and patients with polyneuropathies associated with IgM-monoclonal gammopathies generally do not respond to corticosteroids but may respond to cyclophosphamide or chlorambucil. In non-responding patients with severe manifestation of MMN, intravenous IgG can be considered whereas in patients with therapy-resistant monoclonal IgM gammopathy, aggressive treatment with dexamethason or newer antimetabolites such as fludaribine or 2-CdA aimed at substantial reduction or even eradication of the aberrant clone can be considered. In POEMS syndrome without lytic or sclerotic lesions or isolated plasmocytoma's that can be irradiated or resected, the poor results of corticosteroids with or without melphalan also justify administration of more aggressive treatment. In the heterogeneous group of vasculitis neuropathies, those with cryoglobulins associated with viral markers, may improve with α-interferons.

There is a trend towards more aggressive therapy in chronic autoimmune diseases with or without underlying plasma dyscrasia's, instead of maintenance treatment. This will undoubtly be associated with increased toxicity in the short term (infections) and long-term (neoplasia). Experience with chemotherapy and immune response modifying therapy in malignant diseases showed that in-vitro studies can not predict the best therapeutical approach. However, while waiting for antigen identification in autoimmune diseases which will lead to specific immunomodulation in the future, the current day patient needs correct classification of the neuropathy and protocol-based evaluation of treatment.

References

Abe, Y., Horiuchi, A., Miyake, M., and Kimura, S. (1994). Anti-cytokine nature of natural human immunglobulin: one possible mechanism of the clinical effect of intravenous immunoglobulin therapy. *Immunol. Rev.* **139**: 5–19.

Amano, Y., Lee. S.W., and Allison, A.C. (1993). Inhibition by glucocorticoids of the formation of interleukin-1α, interleukin-1β and interleukin 6: mediation by decreased RNA stability. *Mol. Pharm.* **43**: 176–180.

Atkinson, J.P. and Frank, H.M. (1974). Complement-independent clearance of IgG-sensitized erythrocytes: inhibition by cortisone. *Blood* **44**: 629–637.

Aukrust, P., Froland, S.S., Liabakk, N.-B., Müller, F., Nordøy, I., and Haug, C., Espevik, T. (1994). Release of cytokines, soluble cytokine receptors and interleukin receptor antagonist after intravenous administration in vivo. *Blood* **84**: 2136–2143.

Barry, W., Hudgins, L., Donta, S.T., and Pesanti, E.L. (1992). Intravenous Immunoglobulin therapy for toxic shock syndrome. *J. Am. Med. Assoc.* **267**: 3315–3316.

Basta, M., Fries, L.F., and Frank, M.M. (1991). High doses of intravenous Ig inhibit in vitro uptake of C4 fragments onto sensitized erythrocytes. *Blood* **77**: 376–380.

Beck, J.T., Hsu, S-M., and Wijdenes, J., Bataille, R., Klein, B., Vesole, D., Hayden, K., and Barloqie, B. (1994). Alleviation of systemic manifestations of Castleman's disease by monoclonal anti-Interleukin 6 antibody. *N. Engl. J. Med.* 602–605.

Bonnefoy-Bérard, N., Genestier, L., and Flacher, M. (1994) Apoptosis induced by polyclonal antilymphocyte globulins in human B-cell lines. *Blood* **83**: 1051–1059.

Bouhnik, Y., Lémann, M., Mary, J.Y., Scemama, G., Tai, R., Matuchansky, C., Modigliani, R., and Ramboud, J. C. (1996). Long-term follow up of patients with Crohn's disease treated with azathioprine or 6-mercaptopurine. *Lancet* **347**: 215–219.

Brand, A., Vuist, W.M., van Schaik, I.N., and Vermeulen, M. (1996). In vitro investigation of immunoglobulin treatment mechanisms in autoimmune disease. *Clin. Exp. Rheumatol.* **14** (Suppl. 15): S27–S30.

Brannagan, T.H., Nagle, K.J., Lange, D.J., and Rowland, L.P. (1996). Complications of intravenous immune globulin treatment in neurologic disease. *Neurology* **47**: 674–677.

Broussolle, E., Vighetto, A., Bancel, B., Cónfavreux, C., Pialat, J., and Aimard, G. (1991). Poems syndrome with complete recovery after treatment of solitary plasmacytoma. *Clin. Neurol. Neurosurg.* **93**: 165–170.

Chaudhry, V., Corse, A.M., Cornblath, D.R., Kuna, R.W., Drachman, D.B., Freimer, M.L., Miller, R.G., and Griffin, J.W. (1993). Multifocal motor neuropathy: response to human immune globulin. *Ann. Neurol.* **33**: 237–242.

Cher, L.M., Hochberg, F.H., Teruya, J., Nitschke, M., Valenzuela, R.F., Schmahmann, J.D., and Stowell, C. (1995). Therapy for paraneoplastic neurologic syndromes in six patients with protein-A column immunoadsorption. *Cancer* **75**: 1678–1683.

Clarkson, S.B., Bussel, J.B., Kimberley, R.P., Valinsky, J.E., Nachman, R.L., and Unkeless, J.C. (1986). Treatment of refractory immune thrombocytopenic purpura with an Fc-receptor antibody. *N. Engl. J. Med.* **314**: 1236–1239.

Connell, W.R., Kamm, M.A., Dickson, M., Balkwill, A.M., Ritchie, J.K., and Lennerd-Jones, J.E. (1994). Long-term neoplasia risk after azathioprine treatment in inflammatory Dowell disease. *Lancet* **343**: 1249–1252.

Dallman, M.J. (1993). Cytokines as mediators of organ graft rejection and tolerance. *Curr. Opin. Immunol.* **5**: 788–793.

Dimitriu, A. and Franci, A.S. (1979). Differential sensitivity of human lymphocyte populations to azathioprine. *Transplant. Proc.* **11**: 878–881.

Dwyer, J.M. (1992) Manipulating the immune system with immune globulin. *N. Engl. J. Med.* **326**: 107–116.

Dyck, P.J., O'Brien, P., Oviatt, K.I. et al. (1982). Prednisone improves chronic inflammatory demyelinating polyradiculoneuropathy more than no treatment. *Ann. Neurol.* **11**: 136–141.

Dyck, P.J., Daube, J., O'Brien, P. et al. (1986). Plasma exchange in chronic inflammatory demyelinating polyneuropathy. *N. Engl. J. Med.* **314**: 461–465.

Dyck, P.J., Low, P.A., Windebank, A.J., Yaradeh, S.S., Gosselin, S., Bourque, P., Smith, E.E., and Kyle, R.A. (1991). Plasma exchange in polyneuropathy associated with monoclonal gammopathy of undetermined significance. *N. Engl. J. Med.* **325**: 1482–1486.

Edelson, R., Heald, P., Perez, M., Rook, A. (1991). Photopheresis update. *Prog. Dermatol.* **25**: 1–6.

Faed, J.M., Day, B., Pollock, M., Taylor, P.K. Nukada, H., and Hammond-Tooke, G.D. (1989). High-dose intravenous human immoglobulin in chronic inflammatory demyelinating polyneuropathy. *Neurology* **39**: 422–425.

Fathman, C.G. and Myers, B.D. (1992). Cyclosporine therapy for autoimmune diseases. *N. Engl. J. Med.* **326**: 1693–1695.

Fehr, J., Hofmann, V., and Kappeler, U. (1982). Transient reversal of thrombocytopenia in idiopathic thrombocytopenic purpura by high-dose intravenous gammaglobulin. *N. Engl. J. Med.* **306**: 1254–1258.

Feldman, E.L., Bromberg, M.B., Albers, J.W., and Pestronk, A. (1991). Immunosuppressive treatment in multifocal motor neuropathy. *Ann. Neurol.* **30**: 397–401.

Gherardi, R.K., Belec, L., and Fromont, G. (1994). Elevated levels of interleukin-1β (IL-1β) and IL-6 in serum and increased production of IL-1β mRNA in lymphnodes of patients with polyneuropathy, organomegaly, endocrinopathy, M protein and skin changes (POEMS) syndrome. *Blood* **83**: 2587–2593.

Gherardi, R.K., Bélec, L., Soubrier, M., Intrator, L., Degos, J.D., and Anthier, F.J. (1996). Overproduction of proinflammatory cytokines imbalanced by their antagonists in POEMS syndrome. *Blood* **87**: 1458–1465.

Guillain-Barré Syndrome Study Group. Plasmapheresis and acute Guillain-Barré syndrome. *Neurology* **1985**: 1096–1104.

Granowitz, E.V., Santos, A.A., Poutsiaka, D.D. et al. (1991). Production of interleukin 1 receptor antagonist during experimental endotoxaemia. *Lancet* **338**: 1423–1424.

Hall, S. and Conn, D.L. (1995). Immunosuppressive therapy for vasculitis. *Cur. Opin. Rheumatol.* **7**: 25–29.

Hartung, H.P., Reiners, K., Schmidt, B., Stoll, G., and Toyka, K.V. (1991). Seruminterleukin-2 concentrations in Guillain-Barré syndrome and chronic idiopathic demyelinating polyradiculo neuropathy: comparison with other neurological diseases of presumed immunopathogenesis. *Ann. Neurol.* **30**: 48–53.

Heafield, M.T.E., Gammage, M.D., Nightingale, S., and Williams, A.C. (1996). Idiopathic dysautonomia treated with intravenous gammaglobulin. *Lancet* **347**: 28–29.

Hengst, J.C.D. and Kempf, R.A. (1984). Immunomodulation by cyclophosphamide. *Clin. Immunol. Allergy* **4**: 199–216.

Hughes, R.A.C. (1991). Ineffectiveness of high dose intravenous methylprednisolone in Guillain-Barré syndrome. *Lancet*: 1138–1142.

Hurez, V., Kaveri, S.V., and Kazatchkine, M.D. (1993). Expression and control of the natural autoreactive IgG repertoire in normal human serum. *Eur. J. Immunol.* **23**: 783–788.

Irani, D.N., Cornblath, D.R., Chaudry, V., Borel, C., and Hanley, D.F. (1993). Relapse in Guillain-Barré syndrome after treatment with human immune globulin. *Neurology* **43**: 873–875.

Kaveri, S.V., Mouthon, L. and Kazatchkine, M.D. (1994). Immunomodulating effects of intravenous immunoglobulin in autoimmune and inflammatory diseases. *J. Neurol. Neurosurg. Psychiatry* **57** (suppl): 6–8.

Keating, M.J., Kantarjian, M., Redman, J., Freidrich, E.J., and McCredie, K.B. (1989). Fludarabine: a new agent with major activity against chronic lymphocytic leukaemia. *Blood* **74**: 19–25.

Kelly, J.J., Madoc-Jones, H., Addman, L.S., Andres, P.L., and Munset, T.L. (1988). Response to total body irradiation in dermatomyositis. *Muscle Nerve* **11**, 120.

Kinlen, L.J. (1992). Malignancy in autoimmune diseases. *Autoimmunity* **5**: 363–371.

Koenes, R.A.P. (1992). Immuno-suppression by T cell antibodies in renal transplantation. *Nephron* **61**: 383–392.

Kondo, N., Ozawa, T., Mushiake, K. (1991). Suppression of immunoglobulin production of lymphocytes by intravenous immunoglobulin. *J. Clin. Immunol.* **11**: 152–158.

Korach, J.M., Bussel, A., Annane, D., Gajdos, Ph., and the Registry Study Group. (1993). 1991 Registry of the French Society of Haemapheresis (SFH). Preliminary results for the first year of the on-line computer access file. *Transfus. Sci.* **14**: 281–285.

Kremer, J.M., Alarcón, G.S., Lightfoot, R.W., Dent, P.B. and Wynblatt, M.E. (1994). Methotrexate for rheumatoid arthritis: suggested guidelines for monitoring liver toxicity. *Arthritis Rheum.* **37**: 316–28.

Lam, L., Whitsett, C.F., McNicholl, J.M., Hodge, T.W., and Hooper, J. (1993). Immunological active proteins in intravenous immunoglobulin. *Lancet* **342**: 678.

La Marre, J., Wollenberg, G.K., Gonias, S.L., and Hayes, M.A. (1991). Cytokine binding and clearance properties of proteinase activated α2-macroglobulins. *Lab. Invest.* **65**: 3–14.

Leung, D.Y., Kurt-Jones, E., Newburger, J.W., Cotran, R.S., Burns, J.C., and Pober, J.S. (1989). Endothelial cell activation and high interleukin 1 secretion in the pathogenesis of acute Kawasaki disease. *Lancet* **ii**: 1298–1302.

Lundkvist, I., van Doorn, P.A., Vermeulen, M., van Lint, M., van Rood, J.J., and Brand, A. (1989). Regulation of autoantibodies in inflammatory demyelinating polyneuropathy: spontaneous and therapeutic. *Immunol. Rev.* **110**: 105–117.

Lundkvist, I., Van Doorn, P.A., Vermeulen, M., and Brand, A. (1993). Spontaneous recovery from the Guillain-Barré syndrome is associated with anti-idiotype antibodies recognizing a cross reactive cell line antibody. *Clin. Immunol. Immunopathol.* **67**: 192–198.

Marchalonis, J.J., Kaymaz, H., Dedeoglu, I., Slutter, S.F., Yocum, D.E., and Edmundson, A.B. (1992). Human autoantibodies reactive with synthetic autoantigens from T cell receptor B chain. *Proc. Natl. Acad. Sci. USA* **89**: 3325–3329.

Meytes, D., Adler, M., Virag, I., Feigh, D., and Levene, C. (1985). High-dose methyl prednisolone in acute immune cold hemolysis. *N. Engl. J. Med.* **312**: 318 (letter).

Miralles, G.D., O'Fallon, J.R., and Talley, N.J. (1992). Plasma cell dyscrasia with polyneuropathy. *N. Engl. J. Med.* **327**: 1919–1923.

Myint, H., Copplestone, J.A., Orchard, J. et al. (1995). Fludarabine-related autoimmune haemolytic anaemia in patients with chronic lymphocytic leukaemia. *Br. J. Haematol.* **91**: 341–344.

Nalesnik, M.A., Jaffe, R., and Starzl, T.E. (1988). The pathology of post-transplant lymphoproliferative disorders occurring in the settings of cyclosporin A-prednisone immunosuppression. *Am. J. Pathol.* **133**: 173–177.

Neppert, J., Marguard, F., and Muller-Eckhardt, C. (1985). Murine monoclonal antibodies and human alloantisera specific for HLA-inhibit monocyte phagocytosis of anti-D sensitized red blood cells. *Eur. J. Immunol.* **15**: 559–563.

Newburger, J., Takshashi, M., Burns, J., Rosen, F.S. and Melish, M.E. (1986). The treatment of Kawasaki syndrome with intravenous gammaglobulin. *N. Engl. J. Med.* **315**: 41.

Nobile-Orazio, E., Meucci, N., Barbieri, S., Carpo, M., and Scarlato, G. (1993). High-dose intravenous immunoglobulin therapy in multi focal motor neuropathy. *Neurology* **43**: 537–544.

Nydegger, U.E., Kazatchkine, M.D., and Miescher, P.A. (1991). Immunopathologic and clinical features of hemolytic anaemia due to cold agglutinins. *Semin.Hematol.* **28**: 66–77.

Owen, H.G. and Brecher, M.E. (1994). Atypical reactions associated with use of angiotensin-converting enzyme inhibitors and apheresis. *Transfusion* **34**: 891–894.

Ozer, H., Cowens, J.W., and Colvin, M. (1982). In vitro effects of 4-hydroperoxycyclophosphamide on human immunoregulatory T-subset function. *J. Exp. Med.* **155**: 276–290.

Pestronk, A., Cornblath, D.R., Iliyas, A.A., Aldersen, K., and Adams, R.N. (1988). A treatable multifocal motor neuropathy with antibodies to GM1 ganglioside. *Ann. Neurol.* **24**: 73–78.

Plasma Exchange/Sandoglobulin Guillain-Barré Syndrome Trial Group. (1995). Comparison of plasma exchange, intravenous immunoglobulin, and plasma exchange followed by intravenous immunoglobulin in the treatment of Guillain-Barré syndrome. *Ann. Neurol.* **38**: 972.

Pollard, J.D. (1987). A critical review of therapies in acute and chronic inflammatory demyelinating polyneuropathies. *Muscle Nerve* **10**: 214–221.

Rock, G. (1993). The application of protein A immunoadsorption to remove platelet alloantibodies. *Transfusion* **33**: 192–193.

Rodriguez, M. and Lennon, V.A. (1990). Immunoglobulin promote remyelination in the central nerve system. *Ann. Neurol.* **27**: 12–17.

Røkke, O., Rolf, S., Revhang, A., and Rekvig, O.P. (1993). Plasma exchange, but not extracorporeal recirculation nor removal of white blood cells, depressing plasma levels of IL-1 during severe gram-negative septicemia. *Transfus. Sci.* **14**: 173–182.

Ropper, A.H. (1992). The Guillain-Barré Syndrome. *N. Engl. J. Med.* **326**: 1130–1136.

Roux, K.H. and Tankersley, D.L. (1990). A view on the human idiotypic repertoire. Electron microscopic and immunologic analysis of spontaneous idiotype-anti-idiotype dimers in pooled human IgG. *J. Immunol.* **144**: 1387–1395.

Shih, W.W.H., Ellison, G.W., Meyers, L.W., Durkos-Smith, D., and Fahey, J.L. (1982). Locus of selective depression of human NK cells by azathioprine. *Clin. Immunol. Immunopathol.* **23**: 672–681.

Silberstein, L.E., Duggan, D. and Berkman, E.M. (1985). Therapeutic trial of plasma exchange in osteosclerotic myeloma associated with the POEMS syndrome. *J. Clin. Apheresis* **2**: 253–257.

Slavin, S. (1987). Total lymphoid irradiation. *Immunol. Today* **8**: 88–92.

Smith, R.E., Gottschall, J.L., and Pisciotta, (1992). Life-threatening reaction to staphylococcal protein A immunomodulation. *J. Clin. Apheresis* **7**: 4–5.

Strober, S., Dhillon, M., and Schubert, M. (1989). Acquired immune tolerance to cadaveric renal allografts. *N. Engl. J. Med.* **321**: 28–33.

Stohl, W. (1986). Cellular mechanisms in the in vitro inhibition of pokeweed mitogen-induced B cell differentiation by immunoglobulin for intravenous use. *J. Immunol.* **136**: 4407–4413.

Sultan, Y., Rossi, F., and Kazatchkine, M.D. (1987). Recovery from anti-VIIIc (anti-hemophilic factor) autoimmune disease is dependent on generation of anti-idiotypes against anti-VIII-c antibodies. *Proc. Natl Acad. Sci. USA* **84**: 828.

Tanay, A., Strober, S., Logue, G., and Schiffman, G. (1984). Use of total lymphoid irrediation (TLI) in studies of the T cell dependence of auto antibody production in rheumatoid arthritis. *J. Immunol.* **132**: 1036–1040.

Trotter, J.L., Rodey, G.E., and Gebil, H.M. (1982). Azathioprine decreases suppressor T cells in patients with multiple sclerosis. *N. Engl. J. Med.* **306**: 365–366.

Van Doorn, P.A. (1994). Patients with chronic inflammatory demyelinating polyneuropathy. *J. Neurol. Neurosurg. Psychiatry* **57**: (Suppl.): 38–42.

Van Doorn, P.A., Brand, A., Strengers, P.F.W., Meulstee, J., and Vermeulen, M. (1990). High dose intravenous immunoglobulin treatment in chronic inflammatory demyelinating polyneuropathy: a double blind placebo controlled crossover study. *Neurology* **40**: 209–212.

Van Doorn, P.A., Vermeulen, M., Brand, A., Mulder, P.H.G., and Busch, H.F.M. (1991). Intravenous immunoglobulin treatment in patients with chronic inflammatory demyelinating polyneuropathy. *Arch. Neurol.* **48**: 217–220.

Van der Meché, F.G.A., Schmitz, P.I.M., and Dutch Guillain-Barré Study Group (1992). A randomized trial comparing intravenous immuneglobulin and plasma exchange in Guillain-Barré syndrome. *N. Engl. J. Med.* **326**: 1123–1129.

Van Schaik I.N., Lundkvist I., Vermeulen M. and Brand A. (1992). Polyvalent immunoglobulin for intravenous use interferes with proliferation in vitro. *J. Clin. Immunol.* **12**: 1–10.

Van Schaik I.N., Vermeulen M., Van Doorn P.A., and Brand A. (1994). Anti-GM-1 antibodies in patients with chronic inflammatory demyelinating polyneuropathy treated with intravenous immunoglobulins. *J. Neuroimmunol.* **54**: 109–115.

Vassilev, T., Gelin, C., Kaveri, S.V., Zilber, M.T., Boumsell, L., and Kazatchkine, M.D. (1993). Antibodies to the CD5 molecule in normal human immunoglobulin for therapeutic use. *Clin. Exp. Immunol.* **92**: 369.

Woo, J.B., Lemster, K, Tamura, T., Starzl, E., and Thomson, A.W. (1993). The antilymphocyte activity of brequinar sodium and its potentiation by cytidine: effects on lymphocyte proliferation and cytokine production. *Transplantation* **56**: 374.

25 Management of paralytic neuropathy in the intensive care unit

C.F. Bolton

Introduction

This subject should be considered in two main clinical settings. First, patients presenting outside the intensive care unit (ICU) with severe, rapidly developing paralysis requiring immediate management in the ICU unit, the commonest polyneuropathy being Guillain-Barré syndrome (GBS), the immune-mediated, acute inflammatory demyelinating polyneuropathy (AIDP). Second, neuromuscular disorders developing after admission to the ICU when there was some other cause for the initial critical illness or injury. These are usually the neuromuscular complications of sepsis and multiple organ failure, the commonest being critical illness polyneuropathy (CIP). The differential diagnosis in both categories is broad and it may not be possible from the initial clinical assessment to determine whether the rapidly developing paralysis is due to a polyneuropathy or to disease of spinal cord, neuromuscular junction or muscle. Electrophysiological testing is of great value in this situation, but magnetic resonance imaging (MRI), muscle biopsy, and other tests may be necessary (Figure 25.1). After the diagnosis has been clearly established, appropriate treatment can be given, and a prognosis established.

Polyneuropathy developing before admission to the critical care unit

This category involves patients who present with rapidly developing paralysis, which includes the respiratory muscles, with endotracheal intubation and mechanical ventilation being necessary. The course may be so rapid that time is insufficient for an accurate diagnosis. Thus, investigations must proceed after admission to the ICU.

In this acutely developing situation, clinical signs may be confusing. The differential diagnosis should be systematically approached (Table 25.1) and the relevant conditions eliminated.

In acute disorders of the high cervical spinal cord, compression due to neoplasm or infection, or acute transverse myelitis, the traditional signs of localized spinal cord disease may be absent. Hyperreflexia is usually abolished by spinal shock and the sensory level may be difficult to determine, particularly in high cervical lesions. Thus, MRI imaging of the spinal cord on an emergency basis is often necessary.

Motor neuron disease may present, for the first time and initially undiagnosed, as severe respiratory insufficiency. The clinical signs of combined upper and

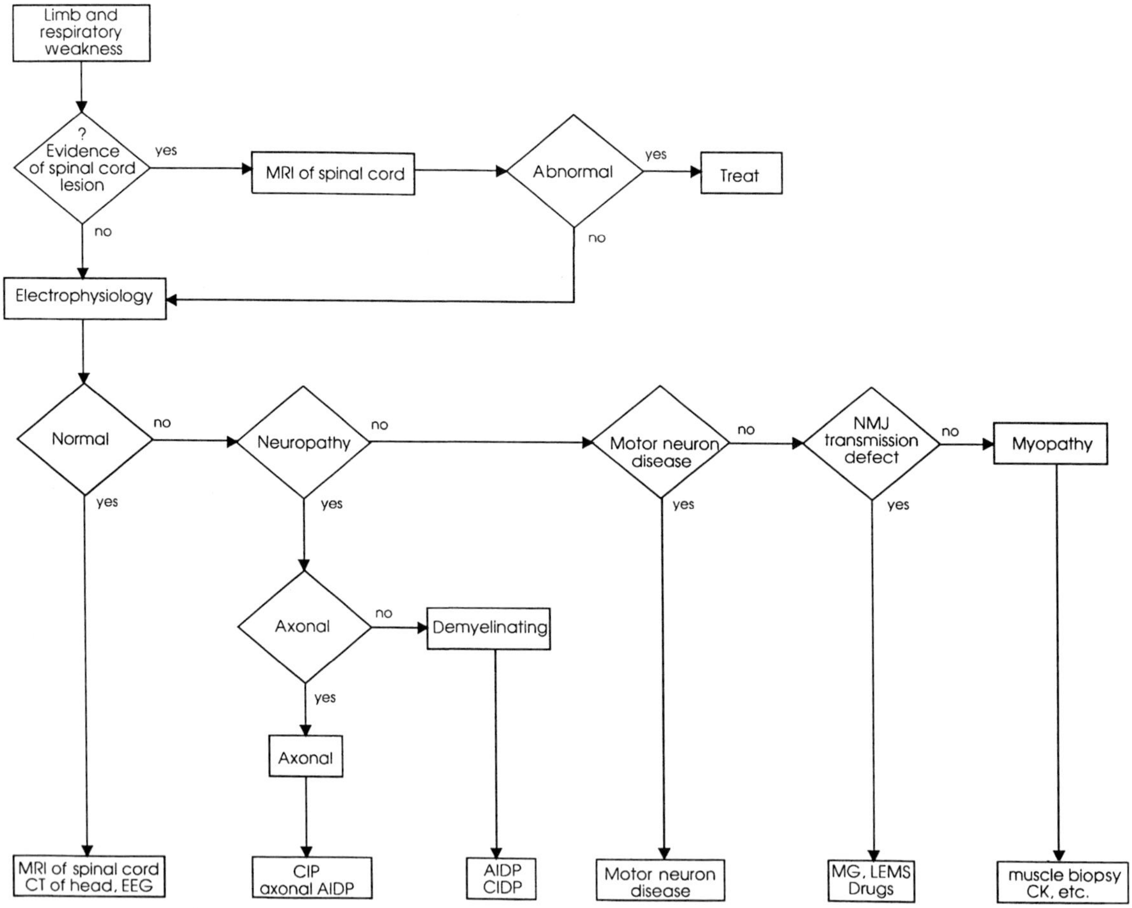

Figure 25.1 *Algorithm to show the decision making process in investigating patients presenting with limb and respiratory weakness, whether weakness presented before or after admission to the intensive care unit. If before, considerations of a spinal cord lesion and emergency MRI would be given higher priority than with weakness presenting after admission. Electrophysiological studies are most helpful, and are usually abnormal, with comprehensive testing, very early in the course of neuromuscular disease, often within 1–2 days in patients with AIDP. AIDP: acute inflammatory demyelinating polyneuropathy; CIDP: chronic inflammatory demyelinating polyneuropathy; CIP: critical illness polyneuropathy; CT: computed tomography; CK: creatine kinase; EEG: electroencephalography; LEMS: Lambert–Eaton myasthenic syndrome; MG: myasthenia gravis; MRI: magnetic resonance imaging; NMJ: neuromuscular junction.*

lower motor neuron signs, hypo- or hyperreflexia, muscle wasting and fasciculations, atrophy and fasciculations of the tongue, may not be clearly present. Electrophysiological studies, which would include phrenic nerve conduction and needle electromyography (EMG) of the chest wall and diaphragm, as well as comprehensive needle electromyography of limb muscles, will often strongly suggest the diagnosis. Even then, it may be necessary to proceed with MRI imaging. Atypical motor neuron disease, such as motor neuropathy with multifocal conduction block should be excluded (Preston and Kelly 1993).

Polyneuropathy is suspected in the presence of muscle weakness, hyporeflexia, distal sensory loss and the absence of upper motor neuron signs or bladder dysfunction, but, again, these signs may not always be clearly present. For example, bladder dysfunction is occasionally seen in GBS.

In acute inflammatory demyelinating polyneuropathy, the features are that of demyelination of

Table 25.1 *Different diagnosis of rapidly-developing paralysis involving respiratory muscles and requiring admission to the intensive care unit*

Disorders of the spinal cord
Acute epidural compression due to neoplasm, infection
Acute transverse myelitis
Motor neuron disease
Acute polyneuropathy
Acute inflammatory demyelinating polyneuropathy (AIDP)
Acute axonal form of AIDP
The acute motor neuropathy of youth
Other acute polyneuropathies: porphyria, organophosphate poisoning, etc.
Chronic polyneuropathies
Chronic inflammatory demyelinating polyneuropathy
Diabetic polyneuropathy
Neuromuscular transmission defects
Myasthenia gravis
Lambert–Eaton myasthenic syndrome
Hypocalcemia
Hypermagnesemia
Organophosphate poisoning
Wound botulism
Tick bite paralysis
Myopathy
Muscular dystrophy, myotonic dystrophy, etc.
Acute nectrotizing myopathy: myoglobinuria

peripheral nerve. In the initial stages conduction velocities may be only mildly depressed, but prolonged or absent F waves (Kimura 1978), evidence of conduction block, absence of abnormal spontaneous activity in muscle with remaining motor unit potentials firing rapidly, all suggest this diagnosis. Thus, even within hours of onset, the findings are often strongly suggestive of GBS.

Phrenic nerve conduction studies and needle EMG of the diaphragm are particularly valuable in establishing the type and severity of the involvement of phrenic nerve and diaphragm (Markand et al. 1984). Serial studies to follow the course of treatments, such as plasmapheresis, hyperimmune globulin or steroids, are valuable. In our experience symptomatic improvement may precede electrophysiological improvement.

The acute axonal form of GBS (Feasby et al. 1986, 1993) usually presents with a rapidly developing paralysis, which reaches completion within a matter of hours, and requires early admission to the critical care unit and full ventilatory assistance. All muscles of the body, including the cranial musculature, and even the eye muscles and pupils, may be totally paralyzed. Thus, clinically, the syndrome of brain death may be simulated but the electroencephalogram (EEG) is relatively normal. All peripheral nerves, including cranial nerves, may be unresponsive to electrical stimulation, even when the stimuli are of high voltage and long duration. Often sensory nerve, as well as muscle compound action potentials are reduced or absent. This may be an unusually severe form of GBS in which there is initially massive demyelination accounting for the unresponsiveness of the peripheral nerves on stimulation. Then, the axon is secondarily involved. Thus, denervation potentials may not appear in muscles for as long as 3–4 weeks following the onset of the polyneuropathy. Alternatively, it may represent a distinctive form of GBS in which the axon is primarily involved (Feasby et al. 1986, 1993). Recently, an association has been noted between this form of GBS (and occasionally the demyelinating form) and both *Campylobacter jejuni* enteritis and anti-GM or anti-GD^{1a} antibodies. This association may further explain the mechanism of the neuropathy (Editorial 1993).

Recovery from the polyneuropathy is extremely slow; however, the occasional patient will make a remarkably complete recovery. One of our patients has few disabilities and is even able to jog. Thus, despite the seemingly poor prognosis and great difficulties in management of these patients, a relatively full recovery is possible, and these patients should be given intensive and long-term management.

McKhann et al. (1991) have described the acute paralytic syndromes of children and young adults. It is characterized by a prodromal illness, symmetrical, ascending weakness over days, normal sensation, often preserved deep tendon reflexes and an increased cerebrospinal fluid (CSF) protein. The electrophysiological features are consistent with a pure motor dysfunction, a primary dysfunction of anterior horn cells or proximal axon. Muscle compound action potential amplitudes are reduced, but latencies are normal. Sensory conduction is normal. There are varying degrees of denervation of muscle. There may be significant respiratory paralysis. Good recovery eventually occurs. Whereas McKhann et al. (1991) made their observations in China, similar cases have been reported in the last 30 years in Mexico, Spain, India and, most recently, in three young men in the USA (Jackson et al. 1993). Cultures and serological studies for enteroviruses, including polio, have been negative. This may also be a variant of GBS and be related to *Campylobacter jejuni* enteritis and anti-GM1 antibodies.

Other polyneuropathies, such as acute porphyria, should also be considered and excluded when necessary. If there is any suspicion of Lyme disease, or human immunodeficiency virus (HIV) infection, appropriate antibody tests should be performed.

Occasionally, chronic polyneuropathies will evolve as rapidly developing respiratory insufficiency. While rare, it may occur in chronic inflammatory demyelinating polyneuropathy (CIDP) and diabetic polyneuropathy. In addition to the more typical clinical and electrophysiological signs of these polyneuropathies, it is worthwhile to carry out phrenic nerve conduction and needle EMG of the diaphragm to clearly show that the respiratory insufficiency is due to the neuropathy.

Defects in neuromuscular transmission are rare but present particular challenges in diagnosis. Both myasthenia gravis and the Lambert–Eaton myasthenic syndrome may present for the first time with respiratory insufficiency. Patients with myasthenia gravis may rarely present for the first time in respiratory failure. We have documented the findings in four patients. Muscle weakness tended to involve particularly the muscles of swallowing and breathing. Levels of aAChR antibodies were negative, a rare variant of myasthenia gravis (Burges et al. 1994) and repetitive nerve stimulation studies were often normal. Thus, the diagnosis rested on the presence of variability in the weakness of eye and facial muscles, a positive tensilon test and single fiber EMG. Phrenic nerve conduction and needle EMG studies of the diaphram indicated partial denervation of the diaphragm. These patients improved with immunosuppressive therapy, including weakness of the respiratory muscles. Typical presynaptic neuromuscular transmission defects, as in the Lambert–Eaton myasthenic syndrome, hypocalcemia, hypermagnesemia and wound botulism, are usually present, as determined electrophysiologically. In organophosphate poisoning, a repetitive discharge after a single electrical shock to a peripheral nerve is diagnostic. The effective maneuver in diagnosing tick bite paralysis is to carefully search for the tick and remove it.

Myopathies do not usually present a difficult diagnostic problem because, while respiratory muscles are occasionally involved, requiring intubation and admission to the ICU, the diagnosis is usually evident, having been established previously in chronic cases such as muscular dystrophy. In more acute myopathies, such as necrotizing myopathy with myoglobinuria, the diagnosis is clearly evident from the very high levels of creatine phosphokinase, at times myoglobinuria, and the evidence of muscle necrosis on muscle biopsy.

Once the correct diagnosis has been established and the patient does have a polyneuropathy, effective treatment can be instituted. As GBS, along with critical illness polyneuropathy, is commonest being polyneuropathy, managed in the ICU, all of the principles are embodied in relationship to GBS. Hence, its management will be discussed now.

Management of Guillain-Barré syndrome

This subject was recently reviewed by Ropper (1992). Seventeen percent of patients with GBS will require management in an intensive care unit (Andersson and Siden 1982). This incidence may be higher in large neuromuscular referral centres where more serious cases are referred.

Severe GBS is the most demanding problem presenting to the ICU staff. A multidisciplinary approach involving nursing, respiratory and physiotherapy staff, intensivists, neurologists and daily visits by the physician primarily responsible for the patient are essential. It is the general management of the patient which gives the best result and has resulted in a current mortality of only 1–2%. The particularly severe cases may be in the unit for months and there must be constant attention to the variety of complications that may arise.

Sepsis is perhaps the commonest of these. Culture surveillance should be part of the routine care. Chest radiographs should be performed at intervals to detect early infection. Temperature, heart and respiratory rate, blood pressure and estimates of urinary tract function should be regularly determined. Even in the absence of positive cultures, signs of sepsis should be treated with broad-spectrum antibiotics. It should be kept in mind that clouding of consciousness and worsening in the polyneuropathy may, in fact, be due to septic encephalopathy and critical illness polyneuropathy, rather than a complication of GBS.

Significant autonomic dysfunction occurs uncommonly but consists of cardiac arhythmias and wide swings in blood pressure and body temperature. Continuous monitoring of the heart rate and blood pressure are then important. Careful positioning will minimize acute postural changes in blood pressure. Only severe elevations of blood pressure will require specific treatment. Cardiac arhythmia may progress to complete heart block and require a pacemaker. Continuous cardiac monitoring should occur from the time of admission until the patient is stabilized and the neuropathy starting to improve. Dysautonomia of the bowel may progress to severe ileus and cecal rupture.

The syndrome of inappropriate anti-diuretic hormone secretion is a frequent complication, which may also be secondary to pulmonary sepsis or active mechanical ventilation. Judicious restriction of fluids, with gradual return of the serum sodium, usually gives the best results.

Deep venous thrombosis is common. Preventative measures, such as frequent moving of the patient, physiotherapy of the limbs, the use of support stockings and, if necessary, low-dose heparin treatment should be instituted.

The use of condom drainage or intermittent catheterization will help to minimize urinary tract infections. Daily mouth care and the use of methylcellulose eyedrops will enhance patient comfort.

There is risk of hypercalcemia due to prolonged recumbency, particularly after a number of weeks or months in patients who have persisting severe paralysis. If it is unnoticed, the patient may progress to a comatose state, particularly if serum calcium levels rise above 140 mg L^{-1}. Nausea, anorexia and increasing limb weakness may be early symptoms. Treatment consists of administration of calcitonin.

It is, unfortunately, not recognized that patients with GBS often experience severe pain. They must constantly be questioned regarding this disturbing complication. When present, narcotics should be used consistently and are quite effective. An intravenous morphine drip may be necessary. Patients should always be placed on a soft mattress and appropriate padding utilized to prevent pressure sores or compression of peripheral nerves.

These patients often become significantly depressed. Regular visits by relatives or support from patients who have successfully recovered from severe GBS are most helpful. Use of electronic equipment which can be manipulated by the patient's lips or chin, may greatly aid communication. A television set or listening to the radio by earphones will help ease the severe isolation imposed by the paralysis and sensory loss.

Physiotherapy is important in maintaining joint mobility, preventing pressure sores and phlebitis; however, it should not be too vigorous, as it may cause undue pain. Additional narcotic medication is often necessary at these times.

In an attempt to determine long-term prognosis, repeat electrophysiological studies are often helpful. If severe axonal degeneration persists, one can anticipate a very prolonged period of recovery. Clearcut signs of electrophysiological improvement suggest early recovery. These tests may be particularly painful in patients who have GBS and we have found that patients should be given adequate dosages of narcotics prior to this testing. Patients will then be more accepting of this important test.

Specific treatment of GBS is discussed in Chapter 6.

Polyneuropathy developing after admission to the intensive care unit

In large medical and surgical ICUs, at least 50% of patients have significant involvement of the nervous system. Neuromuscular problems are much more frequent than is generally recognized. Sepsis and multiorgan failure now occur in 20–50% of patients in a medical ICU (Tran et al. 1990) and 70% of such patients have CIP (Witt et al. 1991). Recent reports indicate neuromuscular blocking agents and steroids may cause further distinctive neuromuscular syndromes. Because of difficulties in clinically evaluating such patients, identification of neuromuscular problems can only be established through electrophysiological tests (Bolton 1987), at times supplemented by muscle, and rarely, nerve biopsy. These investigations aid in managing conditions such as difficulty in weaning from the ventilator and limb weakness during recovery. The subject has been recently reviewed (Bolton 1993a; Bolton et al. 1994).

Clinical evaluation

This is particularly difficult as a history may not be obtained from the patient and ICU charts are time-consuming to review (Bolton 1993a). It is best to get the history and other data from both the intensive care resident and nurse. Particular attention is paid to previous or current evidence of sepsis and multiorgan failure, medications that the patient may be on, particularly injections of neuromuscular blocking agents, the essential primary and secondary diagnoses and results of computed tomographic (CT) or magnetic resonance scans, myelography, electroencephalopathy (EEG) and examination of the CSF. Evidence of acquired immune deficiency syndrome, reaction to hepatitis B antigen, any bleeding tendency, and essential data about current methods of ventilation should all be obtained. Note procedures that have been carried out: insertion of Swan Ganz catheters, use of vasopressor agents, surgical procedures on the chest and abdomen, and insertion of balloon catheters through iliac vessels or the aorta.

The physical examination may be limited to general observations such as the strength of muscular movements induced by reflex activity or in response to painful stimulation and abnormalities of deep tendon reflexes and plantar responses. The patient may appear generally weak in a non-specific way, with flaccidity, reduced deep tendon reflexes, and absent plantar responses, as a result of conditions varying as widely as acute encephalopathy, acute myelopathy with spinal shock, polyneuropathy, defects in neuromuscular transmission and myopathy.

In regard to the respiratory system, rapid, shallow respirations have been traditional signs of neuromuscular respiratory insufficiency, at times accompanied by paradoxical trunk movements if there is a predominance of diaphragm or chest wall weakness. These signs are often altered by full ventilation. The pattern of respiration must then be observed when the triggering mechanism is removed and the patient is allowed to initiate his own respirations, but still being ventilated with pressure support. This may be performed later, during needle EMG of the diaphragm and chest wall muscles (Bolton 1993b).

Electrophysiological evaluation

Technical challenges that may arise in the ICU are interference from adjacent machines, poorly grounded plug-ins, inadequate shielding of cables and interference from other electrical devices. There should be adequate skin preparation to reduce skin resistance. The 60 cycle notch filter on the EMG machine may have to be used.

Case report

Management of a patient who developed limb weakness and difficulty in weaning from the ventilator after admission to the ICU.

A 65-year-old woman was admitted to the emergency department with multilobular pneumonia, confusion and hypotension. There was a previous history of hypertension and chronic obstructive pulmonary disease. Shortly after arrival, she suffered a respiratory arrest, requiring intubation and transfer to the critical care unit. Sputum and blood cultures grew *Streptococcus pneumoniae*. Over the next several days, although she was treated with penicillin G, tobramycin and cloxacillin, she developed the adult respiratory distress syndrome. Initial neurological examination shortly after admission disclosed encephalopathy and extensor plantar responses but normal motor power and tendon reflexes. A CT head scan and CSF were normal. An EEG revealed mild generalized suppression. Over the next several weeks, she developed elevated levels of serum amylase and hepatic enzymes, a pneumothorax, a bronchopleural fistula and phlebitis. She required several courses of aminoglycosides for recurrent infections and had mildly elevated trough levels of serum tobramycin.

Two months following admission, she was still unable to breathe independently but was able to complain of stabbing foot pain. She had developed heavy pigmentation, deafness (due to aminoglycosides), weakness in all limbs and areflexia. Median and common peroneal nerve conduction studies revealed normal conduction velocities and distal latencies but reduced amplitudes of compound muscle and sensory nerve action potentials. The sural nerve action potential was absent. The diaphragm potential was absent on bilateral phrenic nerve stimulation. Needle EMG showed numerous trains of fibrillation potentials and positive sharp waves in quadriceps femoris, medial gastrocnemius, first dorsal interosseus, right deltoid and right chest wall muscles. Studies of adrenal function were normal and the pigmentation was postulated to be secondary to elevated levels of catecholamines.

One month later, muscle strength had improved and pigmentation lessened, but she remained deaf, areflexic and ventilator dependent. Compound muscle action potential amplitudes had improved. Sural nerve potentials had returned and needle EMG revealed less abnormal spontaneous activity in various muscles.

Four months after admission, she was weaned from the ventilator. Tendon reflexes had returned in the arms. Compound muscle and sensory nerve action potentials had improved further and spontaneous activity had subsided with the appearance of polyphasic voluntary motor units. Six months following admission, she was discharged ambulatory, with a mild right foot drop and absent ankle jerks.

At a 2-year follow-up examination, she had normal skin pigmentation, was moderately deaf, had mildly weak dorsiflexion of the right foot and absent ankle jerks. Nerve conduction studies were normal. (Reprinted with permission, Zochodne et al. 1987).

Comment: This patient developed multilobar pneumonia as a primary illness but quickly suffered respiratory arrest and had to be admitted to the intensive care unit. The infecting organism was *Streptococcus pneumoniae* which was cultured from blood and sputum. She then developed the adult respiratory distress syndrome, septic encephalopathy and evidence of hepatic dysfunction. Thus, there was evidence of sepsis and multiorgan failure.

It was not until 2 months after admission, when she had recovered from the septic encephalopathy and the sepsis and multiorgan failure, that it was first noted that she was unable to breathe independently and had weakness and areflexia in all four limbs. Electrophysiological studies revealed a severe, axonal motor and sensory polyneuropathy, typical of critical illness polyneuropathy. Bilateral phrenic nerve conduction studies showed an absent response from both diaphragms and needle EMG of chest wall muscles revealed denervation, providing direct evidence that the polyneuropathy was the cause of difficulty in weaning from the ventilator. Subsequent to this report in the literature, we developed the technique of needle EMG of the diaphragm and now routinely perform that, in addition to phrenic nerve conduction studies, to further investigate the respiratory insufficiency in these patients. The electrophysiological studies in this patient indicated that there was likely to be a further prolonged period of inability to wean from the ventilator and weakness in the limbs.

Thus, it was not until 4 months from the time of the admission that she could be weaned from the ventilator and, at 6 months, was discharged from hospital, ambulatory, but with a mild, right foot drop. Clinical and electrophysiological studies at 2 years indicated, at that time, there had been almost complete recovery from the polyneuropathy.

These, and other cases of critical illness polyneuropathy, have shown only normal or mild elevations in creatinine phosphokinase. Hence, an associated, significant myopathy with muscle fiber necrosis is unlikely to be present in these patients. There would, thus, be no need for muscle biopsy.

In this patient, neuromuscular blocking agents and steroids were not given and, hence, there would be no need to do repetitive nerve stimulation studies to determine if there was a defect in neuromuscular transmission secondary to the use of neuromuscular blocking agents. Such studies should always be performed if the patient has been given neuromuscular blocking agents at any time during the course of their treatment. The effect of these agents may be prolonged over several days if there is concomitant renal failure.

The demonstration of critical illness polyneuropathy and its effect on strength of respiratory and limb muscles provided the intensivists with important information regarding prognosis, the likely need for prolonged ventilatory care, and subsequent physiotherapy for the chest and limbs. Rehabilitation is much more effective, knowing the underlying cause and prognosis for the limb muscle weakness. Recovery in this case occurred over a matter of months, whereas in milder cases of critical illness polyneuropathy recovery occurs in a matter of weeks.

It may not be possible to electrically stimulate certain nerves due to the presence of intravascular lines, surgical wounds and dressings, casts, splints, and so forth. There is also the remote possibility that cardiac arhythmias may be induced if an electrical stimulus is applied near an intravascular line whose target is near the heart. It may be wise to choose the opposite limb for nerve stimulation. The ground electrode should always be on the same side of the body that is being stimulated, to avoid transmission of the electrical impulse through the heart. The technique of needle EMG of the diaphragm can now be regarded as quite safe.

Disorders that can be tested by electromyographic techniques

Myelopathy

Myelopathies seen in the unit are traumatic; compressive due to neoplasm, hemorrhage, or infection in the epidural space, and vascular, such as spinal cord infarction secondary to surgical procedures on the aorta.

Motor conduction studies show decreased amplitudes of compound muscle action potentials due to anterior horn cell disease, if there has been at least 5 days since the injury. If sensory conduction is normal, and if clinical sensory loss is present, the lesion lies proximal to the dorsal root ganglion, usually indicating a myelopathy.

Needle EMG abnormalities will appear after a 10 to 20 day time interval, depending on the distance between the site of injury along the nerve and the muscle. The pattern of needle EMG signs of denervation should assist localization of the segmental level, whether it is unilateral or bilateral, and roughly the number of segments involved, although due to the considerable overlap, particularly in paraspinal muscle innervation, the results may not be precise.

In somatosensory evoked potential (SEP) studies, scalp recordings would reveal delayed or absent potentials. Normal peripheral nerve and T12 responses would localize the lesion to above the T12 level. Absent or delayed T12 responses would suggest the lesion is in the region of the cauda equina or lumbosacral plexus if limb peripheral nerve SEPs were normal. Unless the spinal cord lesion clearly involves the somasthetic pathways, SEP results may be normal in the presence of a spinal cord lesion of considerable size.

Lumbosacral or brachial plexopathies

These may be secondary to direct trauma, usually from motor vehicle accidents or surgery. Insertion of catheters into the iliac arteries or aorta may dislodge thrombi and the resulting embolization impair vascular supply to nerves and, in this manner, induce focal ischemic plexopathy (Wilbourn et al. 1983). Direct surgical trauma to vessels may also induce vascular insufficiency.

EMG studies should successfully demonstrate abnormalities on motor and sensory nerve conduction and, in particular, on needle EMG, that would localize the lesion to the brachial or lumbosacral plexus.

Mononeuropathies

If the patient's primary reason for admission to the unit was the postoperative state, the initial surgery may have induced a mononeuropathy when operating room equipment or perhaps the surgery itself, directly damaged peripheral nerves. Phrenic nerves, either bilaterally or unilaterally, may be damaged at the time of surgery by direct trauma or by the application of cold, as occurs in the hypothermia associated with cardiac surgery (Abd et al. 1989).

More distal nerves may be damaged as a result of impairment of nutrient blood supply through distal embolization. Thus, patients following cardiac or vascular surgery may manifest varying combinations of involvement of femoral or sciatic nerves. Electrophysiological studies show a relatively pure axonal degeneration of motor and sensory fibers.

Patients who are being anticoagulated run the risk of hemorrhage. A sudden rise in tissue pressure produces a 'compartment syndrome', the severe compression resulting in ischemia to nerve, as well as muscle. The compartments most commonly involved are the iliopsoas and gluteal, producing acute femoral or sciatic neuropathies (Matsen 1980). Fractures and soft tissue trauma may also induce compartment syndromes. An immediate CT scan should be ordered, which will show the location of the hemorrhage. Then, surgical decompression may successfully decompress the nerve. The situation is so acute and emergent that electrophysiological studies are of little value.

Critical illness polyneuropathies

This polyneuropathy is the commonest seen in the ICU and is a regular complication of the syndrome of sepsis and multiorgan failure (Bolton et al. 1984; Courturier et al. 1984; Zochodne et al. 1987; Bolton 1987). It is manifest as difficulty in weaning from the ventilator and varying degrees of limb weakness, just as the patient seems to be recovering from the sepsis syndrome. It may be the commonest cause of long-term ventilator dependence (Spitzer et al. 1989). Only severe polyneuropathies will cause obvious clinical signs but electrophysiological studies will show the presence of a pure, predominantly motor, and sensory polyneuropathy. Phrenic nerve conduction studies and needle EMG of the diaphragm (Bolton et al. 1991) and chest wall muscles will provide additional and more direct evidence of involvement of the neuromuscular respiratory system. Recovery occurs in a matter of weeks in milder cases and in a matter of months in more severe cases. Serial electrophysiological studies are often valuable in determining the ultimate prognosis and in gauging the rate of recovery. Unfortunately, patients with particularly severe polyneuropathies may not recover.

Neuromuscular transmission defects

Standard repetitive stimulation studies at slow and fast rates should be utilized to detect pre- or postsynaptic defects. Stimulation and assessment of the response by palpation, the 'train of four' technique of anesthetists is too inaccurate, and the method using force recordings, too cumbersome and time-consuming.

The commonest type of neuromuscular transmission defect to be seen in the ICUs is the use of neuromuscular blocking agents. The frequency of their use in ICUs varies considerably. They are used to lower metabolic demands, prevent shivering or 'fighting' with the ventilator, lower intracranial pressure and improve chest compliance (Partridge et al. 1990). In our unit, such drugs are used infrequently and systematic studies in critically ill patients by repetitive nerve stimulation studies have failed to reveal a defect in neuromuscular transmission, aside from the phenomenon of pseudofacilitation, a normal variation (Bolton et al. 1986). Instead, limb weakness and difficulties in weaning from the ventilator in critically ill patients were usually shown to be due to critical illness polyneuropathy (Zochodne et al. 1987).

Recent reports delineate three relatively distinct syndromes, in addition to critical illness polyneuropathy. In the first of these (Gooch et al. 1991; Hirano et al. 1992), a critically ill patient in the unit is placed on neuromuscular blocking agents, either vecuronium or pancuronium bromide, for longer than 48 hours to ease ventilation and when taken off the drug the patient is noted to be quadriplegic, and later cannot be weaned from the ventilator. Electrophysiological studies have shown a relatively pure axonal degeneration, varying elevations of creatinine phosphokinase and, on muscle biopsy, a mixed picture of denervation and muscle fiber necrosis. Recovery usually occurs over a matter of weeks or a few months, depending upon the severity. Many of these patients were septic and the pure axonal motor polyneuropathy may have been due to a combination of the effects of sepsis and the neuromuscular blocking agent. Repetitive stimulation studies in these patients may or may not have shown a defect in neuromuscular transmission.

In the second syndrome (Danon and Carpenter 1991; Lacomis et al. 1993), a previously healthy, usually younger person or child, develops severe asthma requiring large doses of steroids, neuromuscular blocking agents and full mechanical ventilation for several days. After discontinuation of this therapy, the patient is noted to be quadriplegic and cannot be weaned from the ventilator. Here, the electrophysiological studies often point to primary myopathy. Again, creatinine phosphokinase levels may be variably elevated; however, it is on muscle biopsy that the distinctive feature appears. Certain stains will reveal a loss of structure of muscle fibers centrally. Electron microscopy will show that this is due to a loss of the thick filaments. Thus, the syndrome has been called a thick filament myopathy. Again, spontaneous and relatively satisfactory recovery occurs.

In the third syndrome, pancuronium bromide or vecuronium are given in the presence of renal failure. This may prolong the neuromuscular blockade for several weeks after discontinuing the drug. Here, repetitive nerve stimulation studies will show a defect in neuromuscular transmission. Again, prompt recovery should occur (Segredo et al. 1992).

It should be emphasized that these three syndromes may occur in varying combinations, and in many the septic syndrome and critical illness polyneuropathy may be the key underlying factors. In practical terms, these neuromuscular blocking agents should not be continued beyond 48 hours and be used in the lowest possible dosages. Comprehensive electrophysiological studies, and often muscle biopsy, are necessary for accurate diagnosis.

Basic investigations have shown how the combinations of sepsis, neuromuscular blocking agents and steroids may theoretically produce these three syndromes, singly or in combination (Bolton et al. 1994).

Myopathies

Generalized wasting of muscle has traditionally been attributed to disuse atrophy or catabolic myopathy (Roussos and Macklem 1982; Penn 1986). While causing clear-cut muscle weakness and wasting, it is accompanied by normal electrophysiological results and normal levels of creatinine phosphokinase. Muscle biopsy may be normal or reveal type 2 muscle fiber atrophy. In our experience, the commonest cause of muscle wasting has been critical illness polyneuropathy. In addition to denervation atrophy, we have noted occasional scattered necrotic muscle fibers which may account for mild elevation in creatinine phosphokinase in a few of our patients who had sepsis and multiorgan failure.

A rare but distinct syndrome is panfascicular muscle fiber necrosis. It comes on acutely as a result of a variety of precipitating factors, including infection, drugs and fever, (Penn 1986). This condition would be expected to occur more commonly (because of the high incidence of infection and various medications in the ICU). Ramsay et al. (1993) have termed this a 'necrotizing myopathy of intensive care'. Patients will be noted to develop severe muscle weakness and tenderness. Creatinine phosphokinase elevations are quite high and there may be myoglobinuria. Electrophysiological studies may be normal or may show some abnormal spontaneous activity. The diagnosis is made by a muscle biopsy, which shows diffuse necrosis, possibly with some inflammatory reaction. Recovery usually occurs promptly but failed to do so in four of the five patients reported by Ramsay et al. (1993).

Electrophysiological studies of the respiratory system

We have recently developed the techniques of phrenic nerve condition, and needle EMG of the diaphragm (Bolton 1993). These have proven of great value in establishing that respiratory insufficiency is due to a neuromuscular disorder. The techniques will determine impairment of 'central drive' – a disturbance of the voluntary or automatic centers of respiration, or disorders of phrenic nerves, neuromuscular junction or muscle. For example, in patients with GBS, the degree of involvement of the phrenic nerves can be determined and will supplement measurements, including vital capacity in determining the need for respiratory assistance. Documenting the degree of axonal degeneration or demyelination of phrenic nerves aids in long-term prognosis.

In a recent study of 40 patients who had difficulty in weaning from the ventilator when a neuromuscular cause was suspected, 38 of 40 were shown to have such a disorder (Maher et al. in press). Most had critical illness polyneuropathy, but there were varying combinations of unilateral phrenic nerve damage, neuromuscular transmission defects and primary myopathies. Combined electrophysiological studies of limbs and the respiratory system were of great assistance in identifying these conditions and rendering a prognosis.

References

Abd, A.G., Braun, N.M.T., Baskin, M.I., O'Sullivan, M.M., and Alkaitis, D.A. (1989). Diaphragmatic dysfunction after open heart surgery: treatment with a rocking bed. *Ann. Intern. Med.* **111**: 881–886.

Andersson, T. and Siden, A. (1982). A clinical study of Guillain-Barré syndrome. *Acta Neurol. Scand.* **66**: 316–327.

Bolton, C.F. (1987). Electrophysiological studies of critically ill patients. *Muscle Nerve* **10**: 129–135.

Bolton, C.F. (1993a). EMG in the critical care unit. In *Clinical Electromyography*, 2nd edn, ed. W.F. Brown and C.F. Bolton, pp. 759–773. Boston: Butterworth-Heinemann.

Bolton, C.F. (1993b). Clinical neurophysiology of the respiratory system. AAEM Minimonograph no. 40. *Muscle Nerve* **16**: 809–818.

Bolton, C.F., Gilbert, J.J., Hahn, A.F., and Sibbald, W.J. (1984). Polyneuropathy in critically ill patients. *J. Neurol. Neurosurg. Psychiatry* **47**: 1223–1231.

Bolton, C.F., Laverty, D.A., Brown, J.D., Witt, N.J., Hahn, A.F., and Sibbald, W.J. (1986). Critically ill polyneuropathy: electrophysiological studies and differentiation from Guillain-Barré syndrome. *J. Neurol. Neurosurg. Psychiatry* **49**: 563–573.

Bolton, C.F., Grand'Maison, F., Parkes, A., and Shkrum, M. (1991). Needle electromyography of the diaphragm. *Neurology* **41**: 415.

Bolton, C.F., Young, G.B., and Zochodne, D.W. (1994). Neurological changes during severe sepsis. In *Current Topics in Intensive Care*, No. 1, pp. 759–773. Philadelphia: W.B. Saunders.

Burges, J., Vincent, A., Molenaar, P.C., Newsom-Davis, J., Peers, C., and Wray, D. (1994). Passive transfer of seronegative myasthenia gravis to mice. *Muscle Nerve* **17**: 1393–1400.

Courturier, J.C., Robert, D., Monier, P. (1984). Polynevrites compliquant des sejours prolonges en reanimation. A propos de 11 cas d'etiologie encore inconnue. *Lyon Med.* **252**: 247–249.

Danon, M.J. and Carpenter, S. (1991). Myopathy with thick filament (myosin) loss following prolonged paralysis with vecuronium during steroid treatment. *Muscle Nerve* **14**: 1131–1139.

Editorial. (1993). The Guillain-Barré syndrome at 75: the *Campylobacter* connection. *Ann. Neurol.* **34**: 125–127.

Feasby, T.E., Gilbert, J.J., Brown, W.F., Bolton, C.F., Hahn, A.F., Koopman, W.F., and Zochodne, D.W. (1986). Acute axonal form of Guillain-Barré polyneuropathy. *Brain* **109**: 1115–1126.

Feasby, T.E., Brown, W.F., Bolton, C.F., Gilbert, J.J., and Koopman, W.J. (1993). Severe axonal degeneration in acute Guillain-Barré syndrome; evidence of two different mechanisms? *J. Neurol. Sci.* **116**: 185–192.

Gooch, J.L., Suchyta, M.R., Balbierz, J.M., Petajan, J.H., and Clemmer, T.P. (1991). Prolonged paralysis after treatment with neuromuscular blocking drugs. *Crit. Care Med.* **19**: 1125–1131.

Hirano, M., Ott, B., Raps, E., Minetti, C., Lénnihan, L., Libbey, N.P., Bonilla, E., and Hays, A.P. (1992). Acute quadriplegic myopathy: a complication of treatment with steroids, nondepolarizing blocking agents, or both. *Neurology* **42**: 4082–4087.

Jackson, C.E., Barohn, R.J., and Mendell, J.R. (1993). Acute paralytic syndrome in three American men. *Arch. Neurol.* **50**: 732–735.

Kimura, J. (1978). Proximal versus distal slowing of motor nerve conduction velocity in the Guillain-Barré syndrome. *Ann. Neurol.* **3**: 344–350.

Lacomis, D., Smith, T.W., and Chad, D.A. (1993). Acute myopathy and neuropathy in status asthmaticus: case report and literature review. *Muscle Nerve* **16**: 84–90.

Maher, J., Rutledge, F., Remtulla, H., Parkes, A., Bernardi, L., and Bolton, C. Neuromuscular disorders associated with failure to wean from the ventilator. *Intens. Care Med.* (in press).

Markand, O.N., Kincaid, J.C., Pourmand, R.A., Moorthy, S.S., King, R.D., Mohamed, Y., and Brown, J.W. (1984). Electrophysiologic evaluation of diaphragm by transcutaneous phrenic nerve stimulation. *Neurology* **34**: 604–614.

Matsen, F.A. (1980). *Compartmental Syndromes*. New York: Grune & Stratton.

McKhann, G.M., Cornblath, D.R., Ho, T., Lo, C.Y., Bai, C.Y., Wu, H.S., Yei, D.F., Zhang, W.C., Zaori, Z., Jiang, Z., Griffin, J.W., and Asbury, A.K. (1991). Clinical and electrophysiological aspects of acute paralytic disease of children and young adults in northern China. *Lancet* **338**: 593–597.

Partridge, B.L., Abrams, J.H., Bazemore, C., and Rubin, R. (1990). Prolonged neuromuscular blockade after long-term infusion of vecuronium bromide in the intensive care unit. *Crit. Care Med.* **18**: 1177–1179.

Penn, A.S. (1986). Myoglobinuria. In *Myology*, 2nd edn, ed. A.G. Engel and B.Q. Banker, pp. 1792–1793. New York: McGraw-Hill.

Preston, D.C. and Kelly, J.J. (1993). A typical motor neuron disease. In *Clinical Electromyography*, 2nd edn, ed. W.F. Brown and C.F. Bolton, pp. 451–476. Boston: Butterworth-Heinemann.

Ramsay, D.A., Zochodne, D.W., Robertson, D.M., Nag, S., and Ludwin, S.K. (1993). A syndrome of acute severe muscle necrosis in intensive care unit patients. *J. Neuropath. Exp. Neurol.* **52**: 387–398.

Ropper, A.H. (1992). The Guillain-Barré syndrome. *N. Engl. J. Med.* 326: 1130–1136.

Roussos, C. and Macklem, P.T. (1982). The respiratory muscles. *N. Engl. J. Med.* **307**: 786–797.

Segredo, V., Caldwell, J.E., Matthay, M.A., Sharma, M.L., Gruenke, L.D., and Miller, R.D. (1992). Persistent paralysis in critically ill patients after long-term administration of vecuronium. *N. Engl. J. Med.* **327**: 524–528.

Spitzer, A.R., Maher, L., Awerbuch, G., and Bowles, A. (1989). Neuromuscular causes of prolonged ventilator dependence. *Muscle Nerve* **12**: 775.

Tran, D.D., Groeneveld, A.B.J., van der Meulen, J., Nauta, J.J.P., Strack van Schijndel, R.S.J.M., and Thijs, L.G. (1990). Age, chronic disease, sepsis, organ system failure, and mortality in a medical intensive care unit. *Crit. Care Med.* **18**: 474–479.

Wilbourn, A.J., Furlan, A.A.J., Hulley, W., and Ruschhaupt, W. (1983). Ischemic monomelic neuropathy. *Neurology* **33**: 447–451.

Witt, N.J., Zochodne, D.W., Bolton, C.F., Grand'Maison, F., Wells, G., Young, G.B., and Sibbald, W.J. (1991). Peripheral nerve function in sepsis and multiple organ failure. *Chest* **99**: 176–184.

Zochodne, D.W., Bolton, C.F., Wells, G.A., Gilbert, J.J., Hahn, A.F., Brown, J.D., and Sibbald, W.J. (1987). Critical illness polyneuropathy: a complication of sepsis and multiple organ failure. *Brain* **110**: 819–842.

26 Diagnosis and symptomatic therapy of nerve pain

Ch.J. Vecht and P.L.I. Dellemijn

Introduction

Neuralgia or nerve pain is due to nerve injury. This chapter will focus on the symptomatic therapy of neuralgia. To better understand the rationale of therapy, an introduction on types and causes of pain is given. The subject of pain and particularly of nerve pain is rife with synonyms. The nomenclature is not always unequivocal and may easily lead to misunderstandings. If relevant, we will shortly explain the terms that have more than one connotation and most terms are summarized in Table 26.1. The principles of nociceptive and non-nociceptive nerve pain are explained, including clinical characteristics and the mechanisms. Recommendations on symptomatic treatment with drugs are based on evidence provided by the outcome of controlled clinical trials.

Nociceptive pain

Nociceptive pain (inflammatory pain) refers to pain in response to activation of peripheral nociceptors by mechanical pressure, extreme high and low temperatures, or chemical mediators.

If these stimuli cause actual tissue damage, like trauma, surgery, infection or tumor, a local inflammatory reaction takes place. The inflammatory process includes the release and production of a number of chemical mediators and neuropeptides leading to sensitization, repeated and sustained depolarization of peripheral nociceptors. Any pain that is triggered by an acute damaging event or by ongoing tissue damage can be characterized as nociceptive pain. This pain originates from somatic structures like skin, periost, joints or muscles and is also referred to as somatic pain. The nociceptors have been recognized as nerve endings of thin myelinated and unmyelinated sensory nerve fibers. The thin myelinated or Aδ-fibers respond to noxious stimuli and are characterized by high threshold mechanoreceptors that respond to mechanical and thermal stimuli. The unmyelinated C-fibers respond to mechanical, thermal and chemical stimuli (polymodal nociceptors) (van Hees and Gybels 1981).

Nociceptive pain can also originate from structures in the thorax or abdomen and is then designated as visceral pain. One believes that visceral nociceptors are the free nerve endings of thin unmyelinated afferents travelling with sympathetic fibers. Referred pain, as a rule, originates from stimulation of primary

Table 26.1 *Terms used for nerve pain*

General terms	Nociceptive	Non-nociceptive
Nerve pain	Nociceptive nerve pain	Deafferentation pain
Neuralgia	Nerve trunk pain	Superficial dysesthetic pain
Neurogenic pain	Radicular pain	Peripheral neuropathic pain
Neuropathic pain	Malignant nerve pain Nerve compression pain Inflammatory nerve pain	Central pain Causalgia[a] Non-inflammatory nerve pain

Note:
[a] The term causalgia usually refers to nerve pain (often acutely following nerve damage) that is associated with sympathetic reflex dystrophy.

afferent nociceptors in other sites than the skin like the viscera, bony structures, ligaments and joints. These primary afferent nociceptors converge on or costimulate secondary sensory neurons in the dorsal horn (van Moll and Vecht 1994). Activation of these neurons will be perceived as pain in the area of the corresponding dermatome. A visceral lesion may thus produce visceral pain, referred pain or both.

Chemical mediators that accompany local inflammatory responses include the release of K^+ ions, histamine, 5-hydroxytryptamine, bradykinin and the formation of prostaglandins. All kinds of tissue injury like trauma (sprain, bruise or fracture, etc.), infectious disease, ischemia or hemorrhage or the presence of cancer activate peripheral nociceptors followed by an inflammatory response. Aδ and C nerve endings are stimulated by bradykinin, serotonin, K^+, H^+ or histamine. The nociceptors can be sensitized by PGE_1, PGE_2, PGI_2, $PGF_2\alpha$, 8R, 15S-diHETE, bradykinin, H^+ and adenosine. Stimulation of C-fibers will also lead to local release of substance P and calcitonin-gene related peptide that synergistically exert proinflammatory effects. The postganglionic sympathetic afferents release noradrenaline, ATP, adenosine, PGE_2, PGI_2, IL-1 and neuropeptide Y.

Depolarization of nociceptors evokes action potentials in primary afferent sensory neurons which have their cell body in the dorsal root ganglion. Transduction and transmission of the impulse will signal the message to secondary sensory neurons in the dorsal horn of the spinal cord. Stimulation of the secondary neuron results in signals that are carried through fibers of the spinothalamic and other ascending tracts that convey action potentials to the third sensory neuron in the thalamus. The thalamus gives its information to the sensory cortex resulting in perception and localization of pain. The system is modulated by the descending tracts and interneurons that influence incoming activity to secondary and third neurons. The ensuing balance determines the actual activity of the system and will determine the quality, severity and localization of the pain.

Non-nociceptive pain

Not all pain is nociceptive and other types are comprehensively contained by the term non-nociceptive pain. The essence of non-nociceptive (non-inflammatory) pain is the presence of pain without activation of the peripheral nociceptor by ongoing tissue damage or an inflammatory response. In general, non-nociceptive pain can be divided in neuropathic pain, reflex sympathetic dystrophy, psychogenic pain, and idiopathic pain (Table 26.2).

Although neuropathic pain is usually thought to represent a form of non-nociceptive pain, the concept that all neurogenic pain is neuropathic can be challenged. We will first discuss the general characteristics and diagnosis of nerve pain and subsequently the issue

Table 26.2 *Types of Pain*

Nociceptive (=inflammatory pain)	Non-nociceptive (=non-inflammatory pain)
Actual (somatic) pain	Neuropathic pain
Visceral pain	Reflex sympathetic dystrophy
Referred pain	Idiopathic pain
Nociceptive nerve pain	Psychogenic pain

of a nociceptive versus a non-nociceptive type of nerve pain, followed by the symptomatic treatment of nerve pain. Idiopathic pain and psychogenic pain shall not be discussed in this chapter.

Diagnosis of nerve pain

For a diagnosis of nerve pain, (1) pattern of localization, (2) pain characteristics, (3) signs of sensory disturbances, and (4) neurophysiological testing may all be required. There is no consensus whether all four conditions should be met for making a diagnosis of nerve pain, although the criteria (3) and (4) are probably the most convincing. Nerve pain may occur without other clinical manifestations of nerve injury, although there is not much clinical research on this issue.

Pattern of localization

The distribution of the pain in combination with signs of sensory dysfunction involving a peripheral nerve, plexus, nerve root or central pathway is usually the first indication for the presence of nerve pain. The pain may occur along the anatomical course of the affected nerve or over the skin served by the nerve. If the nerve contains motor fibers, the presence of concomitant weakness, muscle atrophy or reflex abnormalities will obviously help to determine the location of the nerve injury.

Pain characteristics

One often tries to characterize pain by three conditions: quality, time profile and pain intensity.

Quality of the pain

Nerve pain may have specific attributes like burning, stinging, hot or flashing. Studies using the McGill Pain Questionnaire, however, have shown that many nociceptive and neuropathic pains overlap substantially with labels initially felt to be characteristic for neuropathic pain (Boureau et al. 1990; Tearnan et al. 1990). Thus, analysing the quality of the pain by verbal sensory descriptors cannot reliably distinguish the type of pain.

Time profile

One often associates neuropathic pain with pain occurring in attacks or paroxysms based on the classical example of trigeminal neuralgia; however, many nociceptive and neuropathic pains are continuously present and the time profile is often not particularly helpful to distinguish a nociceptive from a neuropathic pain. Interestingly, in one series of patients with cancer of the head and neck nociceptive pain often occurred in attacks or paroxysms while neuropathic pain was continuously present (Vecht et al. 1992). Likewise, it is questionable whether a specific time profile can sufficiently be relied upon for diagnosing nerve pain.

Pain intensity

Like most medical conditions, pain can vary in intensity. This may inform us on the degree of suffering, but not so much on the type or the cause of the pain.

Clinical signs of nerve injury

Nerve injury may be recognized by sensory disturbances with an increased or decreased sensitivity to noxious (painful) or innoxious stimuli.

Allodynia

This is defined by pain produced by normally non-painful stimuli like stroking the skin. Pain evoked by lightly brushing or stroking the skin can be a prominent symptom of postherpetic neuralgia and painful neuropathy (Loh and Nathan 1978; Nurmikko 1994). Allodynia to a moving mechanical stimulus has also been labeled as dynamic mechanical hyperalgesia (Koltzenburg et al. 1994). Allodynia to moderate cool temperatures has been labeled as cold hyperalgesia.

Hyperalgesia

This is increased awareness of painfulness upon a noxious stimulus that is perceived more strongly than normally. For example, sharp, cold or heat stimuli can be perceived as extra painful following delivery of the stimulus. Mechanical hyperalgesia is defined as decreased threshold and increased magnitude of pain in response to mechanical stimuli (Ochoa and Yarnitsky 1993). Mechanical or static hyperalgesia for punctate noxious stimuli can be elicited when only C-fibers are stimulated (Kilo et al. 1994). Dynamic hyperalgesia is mediated by myelinated Aβ-fibers (Hansson and Lindblom 1992). Stimulation of A-Δ nociceptor units evoke a sensation of sharp pain that disappears during selective myelinated fiber block, while C-polymodal nociceptor units evoke a sensation of delayed, dull or burning pain, resistant to A-fiber block (Ochoa and Torebjörk 1989). Probably, C-fiber excitation results also in central sensitization at the level of the dorsal horn evoking Aβ-fiber mediated hyperalgesia. This implies that excitation of primary nociceptive afferents is an important cause of neuropathic pain and that the ensuing central mechanisms responsible for allodynia are a sequel of nociceptor activation (Ochoa and Yarnitsky 1993; Koltzenburg et al. 1994).

Hyperpathia

This is a complex of symptoms related to evoked pain to repetitive noxious skin stimulation: the stimuli are perceived delayed and more painful (summation) with spatial and temporal after sensations.

Apart from these types of abnormal sensory processing to evoked stimuli, an absolute or relative sensory deficit may be present to noxious stimuli, like hypalgesia to pin-prick, cold or heat, and non-noxious stimuli like cool hypesthesia, warm hypesthesia, diminished vibration sense. Furthermore, spontaneous painful sensory sensations like dysesthesias, or non-painful sensory sensations (paresthesias) may point to the diagnosis of nerve injury.

Neurophysiological evidence for nerve injury

As objective neurological signs may be absent with pain due to nerve injury, there is a great need for standardized testing of sensory disturbances for clinical, legal, and research purposes. Quantitative testing can be divided in electrophysiological studies and psychophysical tests. Electromyography (EMG) and nerve conduction studies (NCV), sensory evoked potentials of mixed motor-sensory nerves (SEP) or of specific dermatomes (dermatome SEP) may help to provide evidence of nerve injury. These electrophysiological methods preferentially test the thick large myelinated fibers, which are not necessarily involved in neuropathic pain. The function of cutaneous nociceptive C-fiber afferents can be assessed quantitatively by measurement of the axon reflex vasodilatation in response to histamine iontophoresis using laser Doppler flowmetry (Baron and Saguer 1995). Psychophysical quantitative tests are available to test both thick myelinated fibers with vibrametry or Von Frey hairs, and thin myelinated and unmyelinated fibers with thermotesting. Quantitative thermotesting assessing detection thresholds for warm sensation, cold pain and heat pain assesses unmyelinated C-fibers, whereas the cold detection threshold assesses thin unmyelinated Aδ-fibers. A number of distinct patterns in thermal thresholds have been identified in neuropathic pain syndromes (Verdugo and Ochoa 1992). Presently, quantitative sensory testing is developing into an indispensable tool for assessment and grading of nerve dysfunction (Peripheral Neuropathy Association 1993).

Nociceptive nerve pain

Mechanisms of nociceptive nerve pain

In 1984, Asbury and Fields proposed to distinguish two types of nerve pain. The first type was a nociceptive type of pain, that they labeled as nerve trunk pain. The other type is a non-nociceptive type of nerve pain that they labeled as neuropathic or superficial dysaesthetic pain. It was proposed that nociceptive nerve pain is associated with ongoing injury to the trunk of the nerve, i.e. to the nerve root or the plexus. One question that arises is how to explain the occurrence of nociceptive nerve pain. This may not be obvious as only sensory nerve endings contain the receptors for pain or other sensory modalities and the nerve itself seems to have no such receptors. Asbury and Fields pointed to the presence of the free unmyelinated nerve endings in the surrounding connective tissue of a nerve root and brachial or lumbar plexus: the nervi nervorum. The presence of nervi nervorum in root sheath and epi- and perineurium has been shown by a number of investigators (Hildebrand et al. 1988; Janig and Koltzenburg 1991; Olmarker 1991). At the level of the nerve roots, nervi nervorum run in the nerve sheath which are essentially an extension of the pia mater consisting of from three to four up to 12 layers of cells, and inclosing the endoneurium and the axonal fibers (Olmarker 1991). The axons of the peripheral nerves are enclosed by epi- and perineurium which contain the unmyelinated and myelinated fibers. If a nerve trunk is compressed or infiltrated, this will be accompanied by local inflammation and edema and the free nerve endings in the surrounding connective tissue of the nerve trunk become activated. Another not mutually exclusive explanation is that a local inflammatory process may change or sensitize the axonal membranes of sensory fibers that now may become susceptible for innoxious stimuli (Devor et al. 1992). The activation may then result in the awareness of irradiating pain. Lumbosacral disc herniation, for example, is often perceived by pain in the buttock or posterior upper leg. The straight leg rising sign represents the mechanical stimulus that leads to depolarization of sensitized nervi nervorum or inflamed axonal membranes at the site of the injured nerve root. Spinal nerve roots that show signs of inflammation are very sensitive to mechanical manipulation (Greenbarg et al. 1988). Another factor that is probably important in causing nociceptive nerve pain is compression of a nerve root at the level of the dorsal ganglion, which is located in the intervertebral foramen. Mechanical compression at that site leads to a heavy barrage of action potentials with severe accompanying pain (Gelfan and Tarlov 1956; Howe et al. 1977; Garfin et al. 1991).

Nociceptive nerve pain syndromes

Acute herpes zoster

The pain in acute herpes zoster is believed to result from activation of latent viral nucleic acid in the dorsal root ganglion. The viral particles are transported along the sensory nerves to the skin to produce the characteristic dermatomal rash (Figure 26.1). The pain may precede the vesicular rash and continue after healing of the skin lesions. The pain in herpes zoster results from inflammation of the dorsal root ganglion, nerve root, nervi nervorum in the surrounding connective tissue of the nerve, or portions of the skin served by the involved dermatome, and sometimes extending rostrally into the spinal cord. Afferents with small diameter fibers are predominantly affected during acute zoster (Baron and Saguer 1995). Risk factors for acute herpes zoster are older age, patients with hematological malignancies, and other immunocompromised patients, including those receiving immunosuppressive therapy (Portenoy et al. 1986).

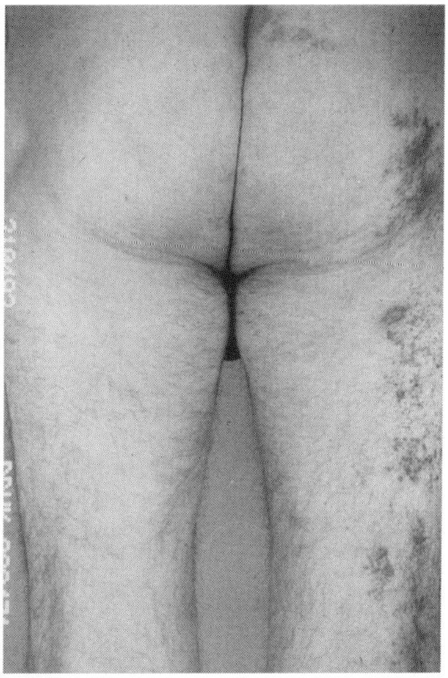

Figure 26.1 *Acute herpes zoster in distribution of S1 root. Example of nociceptive nerve pain.*

Other nociceptive nerve pains

Conditions like a herniated disc or vertebral metastasis may cause nociceptive pain by compression or inflammation of the nerve trunk. Other conditions that may give rise to an inflammed nerve are idiopathic plexus neuritis, diabetic amyotrophy and may all be considered to represent examples of nociceptive nerve pain (Table 26.3).

Diagnosis of nociceptive nerve pain

The concept of nociceptive nerve pain implies that the pain may be felt along the anatomical course of a particular nerve with or without spontaneous positive sensory phenomena like paresthesias or dysesthesias

Table 26.3 *Causes of nociceptive nerve pain*

Cranial nerve	
Symptomatic trigeminal neuropathy	
	Sjögren's disease, SLE, mixed connective tissue disease
	Other systemic disorders
	Metastatic cancer (bone metastasis, leptomeningeal cancer)
Infraorbital or mental neuropathy	
	Bone metastasis at foramen ovale or in mandibular bone
	Perineural tumor extension (head and neck cancer)
	Leptomeningeal cancer
Symptomatic glossopharyngeal neuropathy	
	Tumor
Nerve root	
	Herniated disc
	Vertebral metastasis
	Acute herpes zoster
	Guillain-Barré syndrome
	Perineural tumor extension
	Leptomeningeal cancer
	Lyme disease
Plexus, brachial or lumbar	
	Lymph node metastasis
	Diabetic amyotrophy
	Idiopathic plexus neuritis
	Psoas hematoma
	Retroperitoneal abscess
	Pancoast tumor (superior pulmonal sulcus tumor)
Peripheral nerve	
	Vasculitis
	Leprosy neuritis
	Nerve compression syndromes[a] (carpal tunnel, tarsal tunnel, ulnar neuropathy, etc.)

Notes:

a The pain in peripheral nerve compression syndromes may be different from compression pain of nerve roots of plexus, due to differences in surrounding connective tissue or nervi nervorum distribution.

SLE: systemic lupus erythematosus.

(pins and needles), and signs of diminished sensation in response to external stimuli like hypalgesia. Without a causative treatment of the pathological process responsible for the inflammatory response (herpes zoster, metastasis), degeneration or infiltration of sensory fibers in the nerve may lead to permanent nerve injury that persists long after the inflammatory response has waned as in postherpetic neuralgia. Thus, a nociceptive nerve pain may progress with development of signs and symptoms of permanent damage to the nerve. One reason to treat nerve compression by a hernia, tumor, etc. is to prevent potentially irreversible nerve damage. A nociceptive nerve pain that remains undiagnosed or untreated may result in a mixed nociceptive and non-nociceptive nerve pain.

Neuropathic pain

Neuropathic pain or non-nociceptive nerve pain is based on damage or dysfunction of peripheral sensory nerve fibers without inflammatory response.

The primary nociceptive afferents of damaged peripheral nerves have lowered thresholds (Cline et al. 1989; Laird and Bennett 1992) and increased expression of voltage-sensitive sodium channels (Devor et al. 1992, 1993). This may lead to chronic ectopic spontaneous electric impulse discharge and pacemaker activity from regenerating fibers or from a neuroma (Wall and Gutnick 1974). In painful diabetic neuropathy, sprouts from unmyelinated fibers may play a critical role in eliciting spontaneous action potentials and pain. The mechanisms of neuropathic pain include totally or partially deafferented dorsal horn cells which become disinhibited and hyperexcitable producing an increased spontaneous firing rate. Following deafferentation, noradrenergic perivascular axons may sprout around dorsal root ganglion sensory neurons and lead to hyperexcitability of primary sensory neurons (McLachlan et al. 1993). The hyperexcitability includes prolonged or enhanced susceptibility for incoming nociceptive afferent impulses. Local changes at the level of the damaged nerve may result in enhanced excitability of peripheral nerves by changes in morphology, local chemistry, and inducing nerve growth factor activity (Mohamed and Carr 1994) (Table 26.4). Spontaneous ectopic discharge and hypersensitization from a nerve stump, pacemaker activity originating from a neuroma together with desinhibition at the level of second order sensory neurons in the dorsal horn, all contribute to the pain after deafferentation (Devor 1994). Following

Table 26.4 *Mechanisms of neuropathic pain*

Peripheral mechanisms
Spontaneous depolarization
Ectopic impulse activity
Ephaptic discharge
Lowered threshold for depolarization
Noradrenergic hypersensitivity
Neuroma formation
Polymodal receptor development
Afferent C-fiber degeneration
Central mechanisms
Neuronal hyperexcitability
Spreading of firing field
Aβ-neuronal disinhibition
Central sprouting of myelinated afferents
C-polymodal overactivation

peripheral nerve injury, multiple messages are generated including release of the excitatory amino acids glutamate and aspartate from peripheral afferent nerve endings and acting at NMDA receptors. This produces both immediate and long-term changes in the dorsal horn of the spinal cord (Bennett and Laird 1992). This may include transsynaptic degeneration of inhibitory interneurons, leading to disinhibition of secondary order sensory neurons and central hyperexcitability with increased expression of C-fos proteins and dynorphin peptide (Ruda and Dubner 1992).

In some neuropathic pain syndromes like causalgia and reflex sympathetic dystrophy, the pain is accompanied with symptoms of dysregulation of the sympathetic nervous system. This has led to the concept that these pains are sympathetically maintained (Roberts 1986). Recently, the concept of relief following sympathetic blockade has been challenged (Schott 1986; Dellemijn et al. 1994a). Other mechanisms seem to be involved as one may deduce from observations that sympathectomy is not or only temporarily effective and that sympathetic overactivity would normally not enhance the susceptibility for pain. Other explanations for this type of pain include activation of low threshold mechanoreceptors which are enhanced by increased sympathetic efferent activity and are based upon overactivity or desinhibition in central pathways.

Another mechanism may be an artificial junction between efferent sympathetic and sensory fibers and the observation of increased noradrenergic sensitivity of unmyelinated nociceptive receptors (McLachlan et al. 1993). Sympathetic excitation or outflow may further enhance fiber sensitization by tissue injury and local inflammation. Subsequently, nociceptors become more excitable by the release of noradrenaline and other sympathetic mediators.

Neuropathic pain syndromes

Trigeminal neuralgia

The classical prototype of neuropathic pain is trigeminal neuralgia, which is so characteristic that it is hard to misdiagnose. The pain occurs in short and heavy bouts which can be elicited by tapping the face or by activities like chewing, laughing or shaving. Outside these unbearable pain attacks, the patient is free of pain, although he may live in fear of his next attack. The origin of trigeminal and other periodic neuropathic pains is probably based on sudden depolarization of thin myelinated and unmyelinated nerve fibers. Apart from spontaneous depolarization at the site of injury, ephaptic discharge may be another cause for a heavy barrage of action potentials once an axon has become depolarized. Ephaptic depolarization occurs when one action potential leads to transfer of depolarization to neighboring axons that normally make no contact with each other and act independently. One explanation for this phenomenon is the occurrence of a local and subtle damage that may arise at the site of contact between the trigeminal nerve and the superior cerebellar artery. This artery may become elongated and touch the fifth cranial nerve in the posterior fossa.

Postherpetic neuralgia

Postherpetic neuralgia (PHN) is a complication of acute herpes zoster related to irreversible damage to primary afferent C-nociceptors accompanied with morphological changes in the dorsal horn of the spinal cord (Baron and Saguer 1995; Watson et al. 1991). Thus, PHN is not a continuation of herpes zoster with persistent viral replication. Duration of pain in the affected dermatome of acute herpetic neuralgia longer than 3 months after the onset of herpes zoster is probably a conservative definition of PHN. PHN occurs in 10–15%

of patients (Ragozzino 1993). With increasing age, the incidence of postherpetic neuralgia increases up to 50% in those over 70 years (Demorgas and Kierland 1957; Rogers and Tindall 1971). Herpes zoster in the trigeminal distribution seems to predispose for postherpetic neuralgia.

Painful diabetic neuropathy

The common occurrence of diabetes mellitus in the population makes a painful diabetic polyneuropathy a frequent commodity. Pain, dysesthesias, and paresthesias in feet or legs were reported in 12% of insulin-dependent diabetics and in 32% of non-insulin-dependent diabetics (Zeigler et al. 1992; O'Hare et al. 1994). The symptoms of painful diabetic neuropathy consist of aching or stabbing sensations and burning paraesthesias, often worse at night and perceived in the feet or legs, often with allodynia. The pain can be continuous or occur in episodes and its onset is often associated with a period of weight loss. In diabetics with pain, the accompanying neuropathy is often clinically and pathologically mild (Llewelyn et al. 1991; Thomas, 1994).

Other neuropathic pain syndromes

Other polyneuropathies, particularly those associated with alcohol, human immunodeficiency virus (HIV), uremia, vitamin deficiencies, chemotherapy with cisplatin or vincristine, may be accompanied by pain, although in a minority as the prevailing complaint. Other frequently occurring examples of neuropathic pain syndromes are those occurring as remnants of earlier trauma or surgery to the peripheral nervous system. Well-known types include post-traumatic avulsion pain, phantom pain, and post-lymph node dissection pain after sacrificing a sensory nerve (Figure 26.2) (Table 26.5).

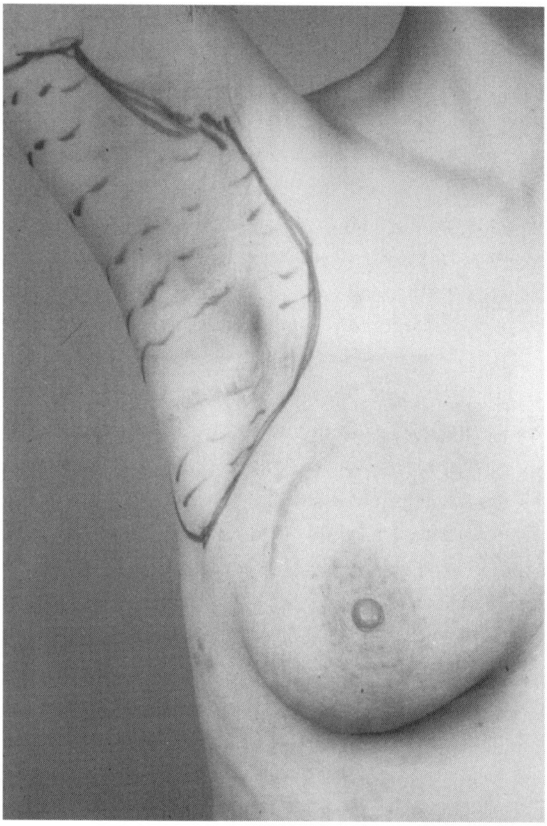

Figure 26.2 *Axillary post-dissection pain in the innervation area of intercostobrachial nerve following sacrificing this nerve during lymph node dissection. Example of non-nociceptive nerve pain (neuropathic pain).*

Diagnosis of neuropathic pain

In making a diagnosis of neuropathic pain the above-mentioned diagnostic characteristics of nerve pain can be used. Absence of local ongoing tissue damage recognized by no clinical signs of inflammatory reaction and normal neuroimaging studies combined with a knowledge of specific neuropathic pain syndromes will usually lead to the accurate diagnosis.

The specific nature of trigeminal and glossopharyngeal neuralgia have made them the arch examples for neuropathic pain; however, this association is somewhat unfortunate as this profile may have become an obstacle to recognizing more frequent types. The most common characteristic of neuropathic pain is a continuous, steady pain that may fluctuate over the day, though will not go away. Sometimes, possibly because of a circadian rhythm, the pain may get worse in the afternoon or evening hours. In fact, nerve pain may have any quality like aching, boring, burning, hot, cold, knife-like, toothache, tight or heavy feeling etc. Superimposed on the continuous pain, pain attacks may occur and may last seconds, minutes or hours. Like with any medical condition, the severity of the pain can be mild, moderate, severe or excruciating, although this will not inform us on the type or cause of the pain.

Causalgia and reflex sympathetic dystrophy

Causalgia is usually characterized as an acute nerve injury associated with signs of reflex sympathetic dystrophy. In reflex sympathetic dystrophy evidence of acute nerve injury may be absent. The pain usually begins with spontaneous local burning pain together with evoked pain like hyperpathia and allodynia to mechanical touch and cold days to weeks after the injury. The localization of the pain may spread beyond the originally injured part of the limb in a non-dermatomal distribution. Pain may vary in intensity and is associated with autonomic abnormalities like vasoconstriction, vasodilatation, piloerection and disturbances of sweating. In long-standing cases, trophic abnormalities of deeper tissues including bone is present. Often the skin shows trophic changes by a glossy, often reddish shine and the skin may feel cold or warm and dry.

Differences between nociceptive and non-nociceptive nerve pain

Clinically, these two types of nerve pain are not always easy to distinguish. Attention to the time profile and to the presumed underlying cause of the pain may help to distinguish the type of nerve pain. Nociceptive nerve pain is pain of de novo origin. The importance of any new pain is that apart from the patient's suffering, it should direct our attention to the underlying damage to the body. Usually a new pain that a patient will bring to the attention of the doctor elicits history taking, physical and neurological examination and further testing to reveal the cause of that pain. Any pain that follows trauma, infection or ischemia is by definition a nociceptive pain as the injury activates peripheral nociceptors by mechanical pressure, by noxious heat or cold or by chemical mediators of an inflammatory process. Also, any new pain without antecedent or clear previous injury is usually a nociceptive pain. A new irradiating pain in a limb points to radicular pain of nociceptive nature if there is no known previous injury or operation to which the pain can be linked. If a patient tells us that the irradiating pain in his leg gets worse on sitting, we may associate this with a herniated disc. If the pain gets worse on lying down, particulary at night, one's thoughts will rather drift to the presence of cancer. Neuroimaging may support the diagnosis by establishing proof of a compressed cranial nerve, root, plexus or peripheral nerve.

Not all pains are new. Some pains follow sooner or later the occurrence of nerve injury or at a time when a local inflammatory process has ceased. Postherpetic neuralgia may occasionally occur in a L5 or S1 distribution and if this continues after the blisters have healed we are confronted with sciatica of non-nociceptive or neuropathic nature. In this way both the time course and nature of the underlying cause guide us to the type of pain.

Interestingly, the clinical phenomena distinguishing nociceptive from non-nociceptive nerve pain may also be represented in experimental models. Loose ligation of a rat's sciatic nerve will result in edema and swelling of the nerve together with hyperalgesia to thermal stimuli and guarding behaviour of the afflicted paw in the rat (Bennett and Xie 1988). Dexamethasone administration results in reduction of the inflammatory response together with disappearance of guarding behaviour or hyperalgesia (Clatworthy et al. 1995). Another model is represented by the so-called autotomy behavior of the rat following axotomy by complete cutting of the ischiatic nerve and several lines of evidence point that this behaviour represents neuropathic pain. In this model, the rat shows behaviour of licking, nibbling and sometimes damaging the nails and fingers of the anesthetic though painful leg (anesthesia dolorosa) (Wall et al. 1979). The autotomy behaviour starts up to 3 weeks after axotomy and remains continuously present, while the hyperalgesia following loose ligation of the sciatic nerve starts instantaneously and disappears within a few weeks. These observations are compatible with the notion that autotomy model represents a non-nociceptive type of nerve pain and that loose ligation together with thermal hyperalgesia and guarding behavior may represent nociceptive nerve pain (Clatworthy et al. 1995).

Although both types of pain have joint characteristics, they may have different neuropeptide expression profiles at the level of the dorsal horn (Hokfelt et al. 1994). A number of neuropeptides are involved in transmission of the peripheral sensory response to secondary sensory neurons. Substance P is an undecapeptide colocalizing with the neurotransmitter calcitonin-gene related peptide (CGRP) in dorsal root ganglion (DRG) cells and can be observed in numerous terminals of the spinal dorsal horn. Following noxious stimuli and inflammation, there is C-fiber mediated increase of the release of substance P and CGRP from nerve endings with subsequent depolarization of secondary sensory neurons in lamina I and II of the dorsal horn.

Experimental peripheral axotomy represent mechanisms involved in deafferentation or neuropathic pain and under these conditions these neuropeptides react differently. Both substance P and CGRP in the nerve endings from substance P- and CGRP-containing primary sensory neurons become gradually depleted. Galanine (GAL) and vasoactive intestinal polypeptides (VIP) are other neuropeptides that can be found in a minority of DRG neurons, and are hardly present under normal conditions (Hokfelt et al. 1994). GAL antagonizes the effects of substance P and CGRP and is upregulated after axotomy. C-fiber activity is inhibited and spinal analgesic effects of morphine are enhanced, resulting in hyperpolarization of dorsal horn cells. GAL is able to counteract the excitatory effects of VIP, which is also increased following axotomy. Upregulated VIP seems to replace substance P and CGRP, while GAL potentiates the analgesic effect of morphine and antagonizes VIP. In contrast, in conditions of peripheral trauma and inflammation, both substance P and CGRP show increased concentrations in the nerve endings in the dorsal horn (Maggi 1995).

Table 26.5 *Causes of neuropathic pain*

Following trauma
Brachial plexus avulsion
Phantom pain
Following surgery
Occipital neuralgia (following suboccipital craniotomy)
Postneck dissection pain
(in distribution of auriculotemporal, transversi colli or suprascapular nerve)
Postaxillary dissection pain
intercostobrachial nerve
Post-inguinal dissection pain
obturator nerve
lateral femoral cutaneus nerve
Post-thoracotomy pain
intercostal nerve
Phantom pain
Stump pain
Following neuro-ablative procedures
Anaesthesia dolorosa of the trigeminal nerve following Sweet, Kirschner or Dandy procedure
Postrhizotomy (nerve roots)
Postchordotomy pain
Following infection
Postherpetic neuralgia
Post-Lyme pain
Following chemotherapy
Cisplatin neuropathy
Vincristine neuropathy
Taxol/taxotere neuropathy
Painful polyneuropathies
Alcohol
Diabetes
Uremia
Hypothyroidism
Vitamin deficiencies
Fabry disease
Human immunodeficiency virus

Symptomatic therapy of nociceptive nerve pain

The mechanism of inflammatory nerve pain makes it plausible that non-steroidal inflammatory agents and glucocorticoids can be expected to provide pain relief. These approaches have indeed been studied to some extent for acute herpes zoster, sciatic pain secondary to disc herniation and to a lesser degree for malignant nerve pain. Both conditions will be discussed here.

Acute herpes zoster

The antiviral agent acyclovir halves the duration of time for pain relief, may prevent scarring of skin lesions, and can reduce the intensity of the pain (Bean et al. 1982). In two double-blind trials, 800 mg acyclovir was compared with 400 mg per day five times a day for 7–10 days. The higher dose resulted in a significantly shortened period of viral shedding. The duration and pain intensity was less in acyclovir recipients compared with placebo (McKendrick et al. 1986, 1989; Huff et al. 1988). In acute herpes zoster ophthalmicus, oral acyclovir 600 mg fives times a day for 10 days resulted in reduced incidence and severity of keratitis and uveitis. Zoster-related pain was reduced during the acute phase of the disease, while it had no effect on incidence, severity or duration of postherpetic neuralgia (Cobo et al. 1986).

Acyclovir probably should be given to every patient with acute herpes zoster, but is mandatory in immunocompromised patients to prevent the dissemination of zoster infection.

Thus, acyclovir represents an effective analgesic therapy for acute herpes zoster and results in more rapid pain relief and less ocular complications, but does not prevent postherpetic neuralgia (McKendrick et al. 1989; Wood et al. 1994). The recommended dose is 800 mg five times a day for 7–10 days or 10 mg kg^{-1} given as 1 hour long intravenous infusion every 8 hours for 7 days.

Symptomatic analgesic therapy in acute herpetic zoster may also be attempted with NSAIDs, opioids, glucocorticoids, or local anaesthetic blocks, although the efficacy is not clearly established (Table 26.6).

Sciatica

Radicular pain as the consequence of compression and inflammation by a herniated disc of L5 and S1 roots is the most common example of nerve pain. A number of controlled clinical trials have been conducted on this subject; however, most studies lack sufficient statistical power. Another problem is that either acute or chronic back pain with or without acute or longstanding sciatica are often not clearly distinguished and that the time points for pain relief differ between 1 week to months or sometimes years. For acute low back pain that is usually associated with sciatica, one controlled study showed that a bedrest as short as 2 days is equally effective as 1 week (Deyo et al. 1986). Rest alone is often insufficient for sciatic pain and administration of non-steroidal anti-inflammatory drugs (NSAIDs) such as indomethacin or piroxicam seem to produce only moderate or insufficient relief (Bell and Rothman 1984).

There are no trials documenting the efficacy of opioids in sciatica. The analgesic effect of epidural steroids has been studied more extensively. Several studies (Dilke et al. 1973; Breivik et al. 1976; Ridley et al. 1988; Bush and Hillier 1991) reported pain relief from injections of 80 mg epidural methylprednisolone after 2 weeks compared with placebo. Other controlled studies (Snoek et al. 1977; Cuckler et al. 1985) and open label studies (Klenerman et al. 1984; Matthews et al. 1987) show contrasting results. A randomized trial with oral dexamethasone for 1 week starting at 64 mg per day for radicular pain due to disc herniation showed a significant effect ($p<0.05$) although the authors reported otherwise (Hedeboe et al. 1982). Another trial using the same regimen showed improvement of straight-leg raising with dexamethasone, but not of resting pain (Haimovic and Beresford 1986). Diffuse enhancement of nerve roots by herniated disc compression has clearly been shown since the introduction of MR- and CT-scanning. Interestingly, the degree of swelling correlates with the severity of root pain as indicated by Lasègue's positive sign on straight-leg raising (Gillstrom and Ehrnberg 1985). The presence of a positive Lasègue test may be a clinical sign for the presence of inflammatory nerve pain.

Presently, we believe that the issue of administering NSAIDs and oral or epidural glucocorticoid administration needs better designed trials of sufficient power and proper definition of acute or chronic low back pain and of sciatica with or without positive straight-leg raising test (Toyone et al. 1993) (Table 26.7).

Malignant nerve pain

Clinical experience suggests that glucocorticoids exhibit analgesic efficacy in nerve pain secondary to cancer (Foley 1979; Weissman 1988; Vecht et al. 1989). In metastatic spinal cord compression, a radiculopathy often contributes to the severity of the pain and in this situation dexamethasone is remarkably effective within 3 hours after administration in a dose of 10 mg intravenously, followed by 16 mg per day (Vecht et al. 1989).

Opioids have been found to be effective in radiating nerve pain secondary to tumor compression in an open label study (Vainio and Tigerstedt 1988). In a placebo-controlled explanatory trial in 20 patients with malignant nerve pain, the NSAID naproxen in a dose of 1500 mg/day appeared at least as effective as slow-release

Table 26.6 *Acute herpes zoster*

Reference	Drug studied	Dose/day (mean or median)	No. of patients	Type of study	Placebo-controlled	Percentage positive responders	Magnitude of pain relief (%)	Overall effect (significance)	Duration of therapy	Other remarks
Keczkes and Basheer (1980)	Prednisolone Carbamazepine	40 mg 400 mg	40	Parallel group		85 (17/20) 35 (7/20)		Significant	4 weeks	Significantly smaller incidence of PHN with prednisolone
McKendrick et al. (1986)	Acyclovir	4000 mg for 7 days	205	Double-blind	+	40 (10/25) 0 (0/30) in acute phase		0.03	1 week	Acylovir also arrested new lesion formation
McKendrick et al. (1989)	Acyclovir	Same study	376			No difference in PHN incidence at 3 and 6 months		NS		No effect of acyclovir on development of PHN
Huff et al. (1988)	Acyclovir	2000 mg vs 4000 mg vs placebo for 10 days	252	Double-blind	+		7.8 days vs 10.0 days	0.03	10 days	Shorter duration of acute pain on 'high-dose' acyclovir No effect on development of PHN at 6 months
Huff et al. (1993)	Acyclovir Placebo	4000 mg for 7 days	187	Double-blind parallel	+		20 days vs 62 days	0.02	1 week	Significant earlier cessation of pain
Hoang-Xuan et al. (1992)	Acyclovir 7 days vs 14 days	4000 mg	86	Double-blind parallel	+		43 50	NS	1 week vs 2 weeks	Study in acute herpes ophth. 13% developed PHN

Notes:
PHN: postherpetic neuralgia; NS: not stated.

Table 26.7 *Sciatica*

Reference	Drug studied	Dose/day (mean or median)	No. of patients	Type of study	Placebo-controlled	Percentage positive responders	Magnitude of pain relief (%)	Overall effect (significance)	Duration of therapy	Other remarks
Dilke et al. (1973)	Methylprednisolone Saline	80 mg	100	Double-blind parallel	+	46 (16/35) methylprednisolone 11 (4/36) saline		<0.01		Assessment during admission period
Breivik et al. (1976)	Methylprednisolone Bupivacaine	80 mg 0.25%	35	Double-blind crossover	–	59 (17/29) methylprednisolone 25 (6/24) bupivacaine		<0.05		
Snoek et al. (1977)	Methylprednisolone Saline	80 mg	51	Double-blind parallel	+	58 methylprednisolone 52 saline		NS		
Klenerman et al. (1984)	Depomedrone Bupivacaine	80 mg 0.25%	63	Open	+	79 depomedrol 68 bupivacaine 83 acupuncture 68 saline		NS		Time of evaluation is not given
Cuckler et al. (1985)	Methylprednisolone Procaine	80 mg	73	Double-blind parallel	+	32 (7/22) methylprednisolone 36 (5/14) placebo	40 methylprednisolone 44 placebo	NS		Evaluation at 24 hours
Haimovic and Beresford (1986)	Dexamethasone	64 mg down to 0 mg in 7 days	33	Double-blind parallel	+	42 (8/19) 17 (1/6)		0.05		Improvement within 7 days
Hedeboe et al. (1982)	Dexamethasone	64 mg down to 0 mg in 7 days	39	Double-blind parallel	+	68 (13/19) 35 (7/20)		<0.02		Evaluation at day 9; duration of pain reduced from 62 to 20 days
Ridley et al. (1988)	Methylprednisolone	80 mg	39	Double-blind parallel	+	90 (17/19) methylprednisolone 17 (3/16) placebo		<0.005		Evaluation at 2 weeks

Table 26.7 *(cont.)*

Reference	Drug studied	Dose/day (mean or median)	No. of patients	Type of study	Placebo-controlled	Percentage positive responders	Magnitude of pain relief (%)	Overall effect (significance)	Duration of therapy	Other remarks
Bush and Hillier (1991)	Methylpred-nisolone	80 mg	23	Double-blind parallel	+	58 (7/12)		<0.02		
	Procaine	0.5%				27 (3/12)				
Weber et al. (1993)	Piroxicam	20–40 mg	208	Double-blind parallel	+		45 42	NS		Evaluation at 2 weeks

Note:
NS: not stated.

morphine 60 mg/day (Dellemijn et al. 1994b). Intravenous lidocaine seems ineffective in malignant nerve pain (Ellemann et al. 1989; Bruera et al. 1992).

In nociceptive nerve pain due to cancer epidural clonidine showed a significant effect as an adjunct to morphine in a double-blind randomized trial in 85 patients, while it was ineffective in somatic and visceral pain (Eisenach et al. 1995).

Thus, there is evidence from controlled trials on malignant nerve pain for efficacy of NSAIDs, opioids, and epidural clonidine as adjunct, while clinical experience supports the use of glucocorticoids as well.

In malignant radiculopathy due to vertebral metastasis, radiotherapy or other types of anti-tumor therapy can lead to complete and longstanding pain relief.

Symptomatic therapy of neuropathic pain

Trigeminal neuralgia

The prototype of lancinating neuropathic pain is essential trigeminal neuralgia. For this type of pain the use of anticonvulsants is well known and clearly established. A number of placebo-controlled clinical trials have been carried out with the use of carbamazepine. Five of six studies showed carbamazepine to be effective, resulting in approximately 50% relief in 50–75% of patients (Campbell et al. 1966; Killian and Fromm 1968; Nicol, 1969; Vilming et al. 1986; Lindstrom and Lindblom 1987; Lechin et al. 1989) (Table 26.8). Of interest is the analgesic effect of the neuroleptic drug pimozide compared with carbamazepine in one trial (Lechin et al. 1989). Baclofen can also be effective (Fromm et al. 1984).

Postherpetic neuralgia

PHN represents a neuropathic pain syndrome, secondary to permanent nerve injury without the presence of inflammatory response. Tricyclic antidepressants have been studied in some well-designed trials (Table 26.9). The analgesic effect is independent of antidepressive action, i.e. pain relief occurs to the same degree in patients who are depressed or not (Watson et al. 1982; Max et al. 1988b). Amitriptyline has analgesic efficacy in a median daily dose of 65–100 mg which is lower than that commonly used to treat depression and leads to a significant relief of 25–50% in about two-thirds of patients (Watson et al. 1982, 1992; Max et al. 1988b). Maprotiline seems somewhat less effective (Watson et al. 1992). The selective noradrenergic agent desipramine results in substantial relief in more than half the patients (Kishore-Kumar et al. 1990).

The alpha-adrenergic drug clonidine might produce some efficacy in a dose of 0.2 mg/day, although this may be a consequence of sedation (Max et al. 1988a). Intravenous infusion of lidocaine 180 mg is about as effective as morphine (0.3 mg kg^{-1}) and significantly superior to placebo, producing about 40% pain reduction after 1 hour (Rowbotham et al. 1991). Clinical studies on local applications for PHN are of recent interest. Trials with topical capsaicin in PHN can hardly be blinded because of its burning effect (Watson 1995). Lidocaine administered in a 5% transdermal gel may produce significant reduction when applied under occlusion. Skin thickness and vascularity affect the onset and duration of analgesia. On continued use of topical lidocaine gel, about two-thirds of patients report sustained relief at blood levels that are below the minimum anti-arrhythmic concentration (Rowbotham et al. 1995). Local side-effects are infrequent and consist of mild and transient skin reddening. Application of local anaesthetic agents as 5% lidocaine-prilocaine creme (EMLA) (Stow et al. 1989) or 5–10% lidocaine (Kissin et al. 1989) and of topical application of NSAIDs, particular aspirin in different vehicles, such as chloroform (King 1988), ether (DeBenedittis et al. 1992), or vaseline intensive care solution (Kassirer et al. 1988) have been advocated in PHN.

Transcutaneous electrical neurostimulation (TENS) is usually not helpful, but essentially harmless and may be applied. There seems no convincing role for somatic or sympathetic neurolytic blockade or ablative surgery in postherpetic neuralgia (Table 26.9).

Painful diabetic neuropathy

Painful diabetic neuropathy has been extensively tested for a variety of agents. Most trials investigated the effect of tricyclic antidepressants, often in double-blind, placebo-controlled fashion (Table 26.10). Amitriptyline is effective in about three-quarters of patients with painful diabetic neuropathy producing a

Table 26.8 *Trigeminal neuralgia*

Reference	Drug studied	Dose/day (mean or median)	No. of patients	Type of study	Placebo-controlled	Percentage positive responders	Magnitude of pain relief (%)	Overall effect (significance)	Duration of therapy	Other remarks
Campbell et al. (1966)	Carbamazepine	600–800 mg	77	Double-blind crossover	+	60 (15/24) 10 (7/70)	58 26	<0.01	2 weeks ×2	
Killian and Froman (1968)	Carbamazepine	400–1000 mg	30	Open crossover	+	65 (19/27) 0 (0/27)		Significant	5 days ×2	
Nicol (1969)	Carbamazepine	800 mg	44	Double-blind crossover	+	75 (15/20) 25 (6/24)		Significant	3 weeks ×2	
Vilming et al. (1986)	Carbamazepine tizanidine	900 mg 18 mg	12	Double-blind parallel group	–	66 (4/6) 20 (1/5)		NS	3 weeks	
Lindstrom and Lindblom (1987)	Carbamazepine tocainide	max tolerated dose 20 mg/kg	12	Double-blind crossover	+		53 carba 51 toca	Carbamazepine ≈ tocainide significantly better than placebo	2 weeks ×2	
Lechin et al. (1989)	Carbamazepine pimozode	900 mg 12 mg	40	Double-blind cross-over	+	56 carbamaz 100 pimozide	50 70	<0.001	8 weeks ×2	
Fromm et al. (1984)	Baclofen	900 mg	10	Double-blind crossover	+	70 (7/10) 20 (2/10)		<0.05	1 week ×2	Results confirmed in open follow-up study

Note:
NS: not stated.

Table 26.9 *Postherpetic neuralgia*

Reference	Drug studied	Dose/day (mean or median)	No. of patients	Type of study	Placebo-controlled	Percentage positive responders	Magnitude of pain relief (%)	Overall effect (significance)	Duration of therapy	Other remarks
Watson et al. (1982)	Amitriptyline	75 mg	24	Double-blind crossover	+	67 (16/24)		<0.001	3 weeks ×2	
Watson et al. (1992)	Amitriptyline Maprotiline	100 mg 100 mg	32	Double-blind crossover	–	72 (23/32) 66 (21/32)	47 (15/32) 38 (12/32)	<0.01	5 weeks ×2	
Max et al. (1988b)	Amitriptyline Lorazepam Placebo	65 mg 0.5–3 mg	41	Double-blind crossover	+	47 (19/41) amitryptyline 15 (6/41) lorazepam 16 (7/41) placebo	38% amitrip-tyline	<0.01	6 weeks ×2	Lorazepam not effective, can induce severe depression (4 patients)
Kishore-Kumar et al. (1990)	Desipramine	167 mg/day	19	Double-blind crossover	+	63 (12/19) 11 (2/19)		<0.001	6 weeks ×2	
Gerson et al. (1977)	Carbamazepine Clomipramine vs. TENS	800 mg 10–75 mg/day 15 min/wk	29	Parallel group	–	92 (11/12)	62	<0.05	8 weeks	
Rowbotham et al. (1991)	Lidocaine Morphine	180 mg iv 0.3 mg/kg iv	19	Double-blind parallel	+		39 lidocaine 39 morphine	<0.06 lidocaine <0.01 morphine	1 hour	
Rowbotham et al. (1995)	Lidocaine Transdermal	5% gel	39	Double-blind	+		26 27	Significant <0.05	8–24 hr	Effective for cranial and for limb and torso postherpetic neuralgin
DeBenedittis et al. (1992)	Topical aspirin diethylether mixture	1000 mg tid	11	Crossover	+	Not stated	70	Positive 0.05		Indomethacin diclopfenac not effective
Max et al. (1988a)	Clonidine Codeine Ibuprofen Placebo	0.2 mg 120 mg 800 mg	40	Double-blind crossover	+		80 50 38 41	Clonidine vs placebo <0.01	6 hours	Association of pain relief and side-effects with clonidine

Table 26.10 *Symptomatic treatment of painful diabetic neuropathy*

Reference	Drug studied	Dose/day (mean or median)	No. of patients	Type of study	Placebo-controlled	Percentage positive responders	Magnitude of pain relief (%)	Overall effect (significance)	Duration of therapy	Other remarks
Max et al. (1987)	Amitriptyline	90 mg	29	Double-blind crossover	+	79 (23/29) 3 (1/29)	>50 in most respon-ders	<0.001	6 weeks ×2	
Max et al. (1991)	Desipramine	200 mg	20	Double-blind crossover	+	55 (11/20) versus 10 (2/20)	32 relief	<0.01	6 weeks ×2	
Max et al. (1992)	Amitriptyline Desipramine	105 mg 111 mg	38	Double-blind crossover	+	74 (28/38) amitriptyline 61 (23/38) desipramine	38 31	<0.05 <0.05	6 weeks ×2	No change for depression or not
	Fluoxetine Placebo	40 mg	46	Double-blind crossover	+	48 (22/46) fluoxetine 41 (19/46) placebo	27 22	Not stated	6 weeks ×2	
Gomez-Perez et al. (1995)	Nortriptyline with fluphenazine	60 mg 3 mg	18	Double-blind crossover	+	83 (15/18) 50 (9/18)	38 25	<0.01	4 weeks ×2	
Kvinesdal et al. (1984)	Imipramine	100 mg	12	Double-blind crossover	+	58 (7/12) imipramine 0 (0/12) placebo	60–100 imipramine 0–25 placebo	<0.02	5 weeks ×2	
Sindrup et al. (1990)	Imipramine Paroxetine Placebo	200 mg 40 mg	19	Double-blind crossover	+		67 64	<0.0002 <0.004	2 weeks ×3	
Sindrup et al. (1992)	Imipramine Mianserin Placebo	60 mg 150 mg	18	Double-blind crossover	+		imipramine ±40 mianserine ±5	<0.03 for imipramine not for mianserin	2 weeks ×3	
Sindrup et al. (1992)	Citalopram Placebo	40 mg	15	Double-blind crossover	+			<0.02	3 weeks ×2	
Rull et al. (1969)	Carbamazepine	600	30	Double-blind crossover	+	93 (28/30) 63 (19/30)		Significant	3 weeks ×2	
Saudek et al. (1977)	Phenytoin	mean plasma conc. 12.±118 mg L^{-1}	12	Double-blind crossover	+			Not stated	23 weeks ×2	
Chadda and Mathur (1978)	Phenytoin	300 mg	38	Double-blind crossover	+	74 (28/38) versus 26 (10/38)		Significant	2 weeks ×2	

Byas-Smith et al. (1995)	Clonidine	0.3 mg	41	Double-blind	+	29 (12/41)	20	Positive	1 week ×2	
Zeigler et al. (1992)	Clonidine transdermal	0.3 mg	24	Double-blind crossover	+	54 (13/24) 33 (8/24)	13	Not stated	6 weeks ×2	Positive subgroup responds positively following rechallenge
Stracke et al. (1992)	Mexiletine	450 mg	95	Double-blind placebo	+		44 mexiletine 13 placebo	0.02	5 weeks	
Dejgard et al. (1988)	Mexiletine 10 mg kg^{-1}	10 mg kg^{-1}	16	Double-blind crossover	+		47 versus −11	<0.01	10 weeks ×2	
Capsaicin Study group (1991)	Capsaicin transdermal	0.075% cream	252	Double-blind parallel	+	69.5 (84/121) 53.4 (70/131)	38.1 versus 27.4	0.01	8 weeks	Gradually increasing effect over 8 weeks
Capsaicin Study Group (1992)	Capsaicin Placebo	0.075% cream four times daily	219	Double-blind parallel	+	71 (156/219) capsaicin 51 (112/219) placebo	70 capsaicin 53 placebo	0.012	8 weeks	% improved gradually increased, at 6 weeks maximally
Tandan et al. (1992)	Topical capsaicine	0.075% cream	22	Double-blind parallel	+			Cold threshold <0.04	8 weeks	No clear effect on pain
Cohen and Harris (1987)	Ibuprofen Sulindac Placebo	600 mg three times daily 200 mg twice daily	18	Double-blind	+	44 (8/18) 44 (8/18)	Not stated	<0.01 <0.01	8 weeks ×1	
Young et al. (1983)	Sorbinol	200 mg	15	Double-blind crossover	+	85 (5/6) 0 (0/7)	Not stated	<0.01	4 weeks ×2	
Diabetic Control and Complications Trial Research Group (1993)	Insulin external pump Insulin injections		1441	Randomized	−	3 neuropathy 10 neuropathy	69↓ at 5 years	<0.006	6.5 years	
Cohen and Matthews (1991)	Pentoxifylline	400 mg three times daily	40	Double-blind	+	Not stated	39 versus 41	Not stated	6 months	

relief of approximately 50% (Max et al. 1987, 1992). The noradrenergic agent desipramine has milder anticholinergic actions and may thus lead to lesser complaints of a dry mouth or dizziness that are often a troublesome side-effect of amitriptyline. Desipramine is effective in about 60% of patients producing approximately one-third pain relief, and is usually administered in doses of 100–200 mg per day (Kishore-Kumar et al. 1990; Max et al. 1992). Other tricyclic antidepressants with mixed serotonergic and noradrenergic actions like imipramine or nortriptyline produce relief in about half the patients with painful diabetic neuropathy (Kvinesdal et al. 1984; Sindrup et al. 1990; Max et al. 1992). The serotinergic reuptake blocker citalopram and paroxetine have also been found to be effective, in contrast to fluoxetine (Sindrup et al. 1990, 1992; Max et al. 1992). The analgesic effects of antidepressants seem most effective for combined serotonergic and noradrenergic reuptake blockers like amitriptyline and are, as in postherpetic neuralgia, independent of the antidepressant effect.

Anticonvulsants are well known analgesics for neuropathic pain, primarily based on their proven efficacy in trigeminal neuralgia (Kvinesdal et al. 1984). Carbamazepine can be effective in painful diabetic neuropathy as observed in one double-blind cross-over trial with placebo (Rull et al. 1969). In a controlled study of 38 patients phenytoin was effective, whereas a smaller trial failed to show significant effects (Saudek et al. 1977; Chadda and Mathur 1978).

The alpha-adrenergic agent clonidine has been tested in a number of painful neuropathic conditions. In diabetic neuropathy, it is effective in about 30% of patients, although of a limited magnitude (Byas-Smith et al. 1995). One study on transdermal clonidine did not produce convincing relief (Zeigler et al. 1992). The vasodilatating agent pentoxifylline seems ineffective in painful diabetic neuropathy (Cohen and Mathews 1991). Capsaicin depletes substance P and other peptides from primary afferent nociceptors resulting in burning pain; however, continuous application of capsaicin can produce analgesic effects. In painful diabetic neuropathy, it provides approximately 30% pain relief in about 70% of patients (Capsaicin Study Group 1991, 1992; Tandan et al. 1992). Interestingly, the number of patients exhibiting a good response increased over time. This would make it advisable to continue application of capsaicin at least over more than 8 weeks.

The anti-arrhythmic agent mexiletine can be helpful in doses of 5–10 mg kg^{-1} in about two-thirds of patients producing about 40–50% pain relief (Dejgard et al. 1988; Stracke et al. 1992)

Two studies on the effect of NSAIDs in painful diabetic neuropathy showed no response with ibuprofen and sulindac (Cohen and Harris 1987; Max et al. 1988a). It has long been asserted that the appropriate regulation of blood glucose levels in diabetes mellitus will lead to a better chance on prevention of diabetic neuropathy. A long-lasting controlled study over more than 5 years showed that insulin administration via an external pump clearly produced less neuropathy and less pain compared with patients randomized to three daily injections (The Diabetes Control and Complications Trial Research Group 1993).

The administration of the aldose reductase inhibitor sorbinol leads to less neuropathic pain after 4 months of treatment (Young et al. 1983).

Most of these controlled trials included a limited number of patients. Although this implies low statistical power, establishing a significant analgesic effect in these conditions makes the results the more convincing, particularly as most studies had a similar outcome and were well designed.

Symptomatic therapy of causalgia and reflex sympathetic dystrophy

It is believed that one way to prevent the development of sympathetic reflex dystrophy is early mobilization of the affected limb, together with psychiatric maneuvers and securing sufficient venous return of spalked or splinted limbs following injury or fracture. A noradrenergic depletor may be effective by administration of guanethidine or by a partial agonist/antagonist adrenergic drug like clonidine.

In a placebo-controlled study, Verdugo and Ochoa (1992) challenged the concept of sympathetically maintained pain based on repeatedly negative effects of phentolamine. Interestingly, in phentolamine responders they observed pain relief from administration of placebo. This study raises the question whether reflex sympathetic dystrophy (SMP) is associated with α-1-adrenergic receptor activity or not. There are other reasons why temporarily blocking of the sympathetic nervous system may relieve pain independent of a sympatholytic effect (Dellemijn et al. 1994b). In painful neuropathy without signs of sympathetic dystrophy, α1 and α2-blocker phentolamine produced relief in a placebo-controlled study (Vilming et al. 1986). Phentolamine may block ATP-regulated potassium ion channels in addition to alpha-adrenergic receptors. At present, there are no controlled trials which report convincing effects of sympathetic blockade in reflex sympathetic dystrophy or sympathetically maintained pain.

Table 26.11 *Antidepressants in neuropathic pain*

Mixed noradrenergic/ serotonergic	Selective noradrenergic	Selective serotonergic
Amitriptyline+	**Desipramine**+	**Clomipramine**+
Nortriptyline (in comb. with fluphenazine+)	**Maprotiline**+	Trazodone
Imipramine+		Nefazodone
		Zimelidine
		Fluoxetine −
		Fluvoxamine
		Sertraline

Note: bold: tested in controlled trial with neuropathic pain; + significantly effective; − not effective.

Discussion of individual drugs

Anticonvulsants

Carbamazepine is particularly effective for paroxysmal types of neuropathic pain or for the paroxysmal component of ongoing neuropathic pain. The efficacy and dosing schedule is similar when used as an anticonvulsant. In order to avoid side-effects like drowsiness or dizziness, it is advisable to gradually increase the dose starting with 100 or 200 mg to a total dose of 600–800 mg/day over 3–4 weeks unless pain control is achieved at a lower dose. If necessary, the use can be gradually pushed higher (not faster than 100 mg/day in 1 week) until the level of toxicity is reached, usually evident by vertigo, double vision or drowsiness. In that case, lowering the dose with 100 or 200 mg is often sufficient to get rid of these effects. Less than 10% of patients develop a generalized skin allergy that necessitates discontinuation of the drug.

Effective doses of phenytoin can be administered promptly. If one wishes to achieve rapidly an effective serum level for pain, 1000 mg orally can be administered the first day followed by the maintenance dose of approximately 5 mg kg^{-1}. The therapeutic window of phenytoin is limited showing an effective dose range of 10–20 μg L^{-1} phenytoin in serum. Signs of toxicity are drowsiness, ataxia, double vision, tremor, paroxysmal dyskinesias and liver abnormalities.

There are no controlled studies on the use of valproic acid for neuropathic pain, but it may be worth a trial particularly in those patients resistant to antidepressants or other anticonvulsants.

Antidepressants

Amitriptyline is a tricyclic antidepressant with extensive side-effects, but it seems the most effective drug for neuropathic pain. Doses should be started low, e.g. 10 mg amitriptyline, and initially increased every 4–7 days by similar amounts up to 50 mg/day unless cumbersome toxicity or sufficient pain relief occurs. Many patients do not need more than 50 mg per day (McQuay et al. 1992; Bowsher, 1995; Watson, 1995). The response of amitriptyline correlates with plasma levels of 50–300 mg ml^{-1}. If necessary, the dose of amitriptyline can be increased up to doses higher than 150 mg day or serum levels of over 100 mg L^{-1}, representing the cumulative concentration of amitriptyline and the active metabolite nortriptyline.

Desipramine has lesser anticholinergic side-effects and may thus be preferable if the patient cannot tolerate a dry mouth, has glaucoma, or suffers from prostatism. The effective dose is somewhat higher than for amitriptyline: approximately 100 mg/day. Other tricyclics that can be used are nortriptyline or imipramine. Serotinergic reuptake blockers are usually less effective for neuropathic pain. Tricyclic antidepressants that combine noradrenergic and serotonergic reuptake blocking effects seem the most effective for neuropathic pain as compared with selective noradrenergic or selective serotinergic drugs.

Opioids for nerve pain

In recent years, there has been controversy about the use of opioids for chronic non-malignant pain and particularly for neuropathic pain. The idea of administering opioids in neuropathic pain is based on observations that neuropathic pain cannot sufficiently be controlled in a substantial percentage of patients, despite the use of tricyclic antidepressants or anticonvulsants.

The more ready availability of opioids in cancer pain over the last 20 years without observations of significant dependence or addiction may be an underlying drive for this view. Besides, a subset of patients with neuropathic pain seem to do well on stable doses of opioids (Watson et al. 1988; Watson 1995). Several controlled trials showed the efficacy of acute intravenous dosing of opioids in neuropathic pain (Portenoy et al. 1990; Rowbotham et al. 1991; Jadad et al. 1992), while others could not corroborate such an effect (Arner and Arner 1985; Arner and Meyerson 1988). If the proven analgesic efficacy of opioids with instantaneous dosing holds true, the chronic use of opioids for neuropathic pain remains still to be seen. Interestingly, in two studies the majority of good responders had nerve pain secondary to cancer (Portenoy et al. 1990; Jadad et al. 1992; Cherny et al. 1994), which seems to imply a substantial nociceptive component. These observations concur with other studies examining the effects of opioids on malignant nerve pain. In an open label trial, Vainio and Tigerstedt (1988) observed a good response in patients with radicular pain associated with cancer. Dellemijn et al. observed favourable responses in malignant nerve pain, both with naproxen and opioids (Dellemijn et al. 1994b).

Conversely, a placebo-controlled trial on truly neuropathic pain (non-nociceptive and not associated with cancer) did not show convincing effects of opioids, although doses used were quite small (Arner and Meyerson 1988; Kupers et al. 1991). In opioid mediated-analgesia individual dose titration is mandatory to obtain the optimal effect. Another controlled trial failed to show an analgesic effect on the sensory dimension of neuropathic pain, although there was a positive affective dimension (Kupers et al. 1991).

Overall, we conclude that on the currently available evidence opioids are effective for nerve pain associated with active cancer, and of doubtful merit in non-nociceptive nerve pain (neuropathic pain). Further studies on the value of the distinction between nociceptive and non-nociceptive nerve pain seem warranted, in particular whether this distinction would determine the proper symptomatic regimen.

For the present time, we recommend treating nociceptive nerve pain according to the guidelines given for nociceptive pain (Vecht et al. 1992), i.e. applying a phase I drug (paracetamol or NSAID) followed, if insufficient, by a phase II drug (codeine or tramadol) for non-malignant nerve pains like sciatica or other disc-dependent radiculopathies, idiopathic brachial plexus neuritis and Lyme radiculoneuritis.

For malignant nerve pain we would advise starting with a phase I drug and, if insufficient, followed by phase III drugs, i.e. orally or transdermally administered strong opioids. When necessary, parenterally administered opioids (via subcutaneous, intravenous, epidural or intrathecal route) can be given representing phase IV of the WHO recommendations on cancer pain. If opioid titration leads to intolerable side-effects and inadequate pain relief, choosing another opioid or changing the route of administration may provide adequate relief. Concurrent administration of a glucocorticoid can be helpful, especially if side-effects can be kept minimal by limiting the treatment period to 3 weeks or shorter with cumulative doses of 400 mg dexamethasone or less.

Thus, the symptomatic treatment of malignant nerve pain essentially corresponds to the WHO guidelines on therapy of nociceptive pain in cancer.

Acknowledgments

We thank Janet van Vliet for her help in preparing the manuscript.

References

Arner, S. and Arner, B. (1985). Differential effects of epidural morphine in the treatment of cancer-related pain. *Acta Anaesthesiol.Scand.* **29**: 32–36.

Arner, S. and Meyerson, B.A. (1988). Lack of analgesic effect of opioids on neuropathic and idiopathic forms of pain. *Pain* **33**: 11–23.

Asbury, A.K. and Fields, H.L. (1984). Pain due to peripheral nerve damage: a hypothesis. *Neurology* **34**: 1587–1592.

Baron, R. and Saguer, M. (1995). Mechanical allodynia in postherpetic neuralgia: evidence for central mechanisms depending on nociceptive C-fiber degeneration. *Neurology* **45** (suppl. 8): S63–S65.

Bean, B., Braun, C., and Balfour, H.H. (1982). Acyclovir therapy for acute herpes zoster. *Lancet* **2**: 118–121.

Bell, G.R. and Rothman, R.H. (1984). The conservative treatment of sciatica. *Spine* **9**: 54–56.

Bennett, G.J. and Xie, Y.K. (1988). A peripheral mononeuropathy in rat that produces disorders of pain sensation like those seen in man. *Pain* **33**: 87–107.

Bennett, S.J. and Laird, J.M.A. (1992). Central changes contributing to neuropathic hyperalgesia. In *Hyperalgesia and Allodynia*, ed. W.D. Willis Jr, pp. 305–310. New York: Raven Press.

Boureau, F., Doubrere, J.F., and Luu, M. (1990). Study of verbal description in neuropathic pain. *Pain* **42**: 145–152.

Bowsher, D. (1995). Pathophysiology of postherpetic neuralgia: towards a rational treatment. *Neurology* **8** (suppl.): S56–S57.

Breivik, H., Hesla, P.E., Molnar, I., and Lind, B. (1976). Treatment of chronic low back pain and sciatica: comparison of caudal epidural injections of bupivacaine and methylprednisolone with bupivacaine followed by saline. In *Advances in Pain Research and Therapy*, ed. J.J. Bonica and D. Albe-Fessard, pp. 927–932. New York: Raven Press.

Bruera, E., Ripamonti, C., Brenneis, C., and et al., (1992). A randomized double-blind cross-over trial of intravenous lidocaine in the treatment of neuropathic cancer pain. *J. Pain Sympt.Man.* **7**: 138–140.

Bush, K. and Hillier, S. (1991). A controlled study of caudal epidural injections of triamcinolone plus procaine for the management of intractable sciatica. *Spine* **16**: 572–575.

Byas-Smith, H.G., Max, M.B., Muir, J., and Kingman, A. (1995). Transdermal clonidine compared to placebo in painful diabetic neuropathy using a two-stage enriched enrollment phase. *Pain* **60**: 267–274.

Campbell, F.G., Graham, J.G., and Zilkha, K.J. (1966). Clinical trial of carbamazepine (Tegretol) in trigeminal neuralgia. *J.Neurol.Neurosurg.Psychiatry* **29**: 265–267.

Capsaicin Study Group. (1991). Treatment of painful diabetic neuropathy with topical capsaicin. *Arch.Intern.Med.* **151**: 2225–2229.

Capsaicin Study Group. (1992). Effect of treatment with capsaicin on daily activities of patients with painful diabetic neuropathy. *Diabetes Care* **15**: 159–165.

Chadda, V.S. and Mathur, M.S. (1978). Double-blind study of the effects of diphenylhydantoin sodium on diabetic neuropathy. *J.Assoc.Physicians India* **26**: 403–406.

Cherny, N.I., Thaler, H.T., Friedlander-Klar, H., et al. (1994). Opioid responsiveness of cancer pain syndromes caused by neuropathic or nociceptive mechanisms: a combined analysis of controlled single-dose studies. *Neurology* **44**: 857–861.

Clatworthy, A.L., Illich, P.A., Castro, G.A., and Walters, E.T. (1995). Role of peri-axonal inflammation in the development of thermal hyperalgesia and guarding behavior in a rat model of neuropathic pain. *Neurosci.Lett.* **184**: 5–8.

Cline, M.A., Ochoa, J., and Torebjörk, H.E. (1989). Chronic hyperalgesia and skin waning caused by sensitized C nociceptors. *Brain* **112**: 621–647.

Cobo, L.M., Foulks, G.N., Liesegang, T., et al. (1986). Oral acyclovir in the treatment of acute herpes zoster ophthalmicus. *Ophthalmology* **93**: 763–770.

Cohen, K.L. and Harris, S. (1987). Efficacy and safety of nonsteroidal anti-inflammatory drugs in the therapy of diabetic neuropathy. *Arch.Intern. Med.* **147**: 1442–1444.

Cohen, S.M. and Mathews, T. (1991). Pentoxifylline in the treatment of distal diabetic neuropathy. *Angiology* **42**: 741–746.

Cuckler, J.M., Bernini, P.A., Wiesel, S.W., Booth, R.E., Rothman, R.H., and Pickens, G.T. (1985). The use of epidural steroid in the treatment of lumbar radicular pain. *J.Bone Joint Surg.* **67A**: 63–66.

DeBenedittis, G., Besana, F., and Lorenzetti, A. (1992). A new topical treatment for acute herpetic neuralgia and post-herpetic neuralgia: the aspirin/diethyl mixture. An open label-study plus a double-blind controlled clinical trial. *Pain* **48**: 383–390.

Dejgard, A., Petersen, P., and Kastrup, J. (1988). Mexiletine for treatment of chronic painful diabetic neuropathy. *Lancet* **i**: 9–11.

Dellemijn, P.L.I., Fields, H.L.K., Allen, R.R., McKay, W.R., and Rowbotham, M.C. (1994a). The interpretation of pain relief and sensory changes following sympathetic blockade. *Brain* **117**: 1475–1487.

Dellemijn, P.L.I., Verbiest, H.B.C., Van Vliet, J.J., Roos, P.J., and Vecht, Ch.J. (1994b). Medical therapy of malignant nerve pain. A randomized double-blind explanatory trial with naproxen versus slow-release morphine. *Eur.J.Cancer* **30**: 1244–1250.

Demorgas, J.M. and Kierland, R.R. (1957). The outcome of patients with herpes zoster. *Arch.Dermatol.* **75**: 193–196.

Devor, M. (1994). Textbook of Pain. In *Pathophysiology of Injured Nerve*, ed. P. Wall and L. Melzack. Edinburgh: Churchill Livingstone.

Devor, M., Govrin-Lippmann, R., and Angelides, K. (1993). Na^+ channel immunolocalization in peripheral mammalian axons and changes following nerve injury and neuroma formation. *J.Neurosci.* **13**: 1976–1992.

Devor, M., White, D.M., Goetzl, E.J., and Levine, J.D. (1992). Eicosanoids, but not tachykinins, excite C-fiber endings in rat sciatic nerve-end neuromas. *NeuroReport* **3**: 21–24.

Deyo, R.A., Diehl, A.K. and Rosenthal, M. (1986). How many days of bed rest for acute low back pain? A randomized clinical trial. *N.Engl.J.Med.* **315**: 1064–1070.

Diabetes Control and Complications Trial Research Group. (1993). The effect of intensive treatment of diabetes on the development and progression of long-term complications in insulin-dependent diabetes mellitus. *N.Engl.J.Med.* **329**: 977–986.

Dilke, T.F.W., Burry, H.C., and Grahame, R. (1973). Extradural corticosteroid injection in management of lumbar nerve root compression. *Br.Med.J.* **2**: 635–637.

Eisenach, J.C., DuPen, S., Dubois, M., and Miguel, R. (1995). Epidural clonidine analgesia for intractable cancer pain. *Pain* **61**: 391.

Ellemann, K., Sjögren, P., Banning, A.M., Jensen, T.S., Smith, T. and Geertsen, P. (1989). Trial of intravenous lidocaine on painful neuropathy in cancer patients. *Clin.J.Pain* **5**: 291–294.

Foley, K.M. (1979). Management of pain of malignant origin. In *Current Neurology*, ed. H.R. Tyler and P. Dawson, pp. 279–301. Boston: Houghton Mifflin.

Fromm, G.H., Terrence, C.F., and Chattha, A.S. (1984). Baclofen in the treatment of trigeminal neuralgia: double blind study and long term follow up. *Ann.Neurol.* **15**: 240–244.

Garfin, S.R., Rydevik, B.L., and Brown, R.A. (1991). Compressive neuropathy of spinal nerve roots. A mechanical or biological problem? *Spine* **16**: 162–166.

Gelfan, S. and Tarlov, J.M. (1956). Physiology of spinal cord, nerve root, and peripheral nerve compression. *Am.J.Physiol.* **185**: 217–229.

Gerson, G.R., Jones, R.B., and Luscombe, D.K. (1977). Studies on the concomitant use of carbamazepine and clomipramine for the relief of postherpetic neuralgia. *Postgrad. Med. J.* **53**: 104–109.

Gillstrom, P. and Ehrnberg, A. (1985). Long-term results of autotraction in the treatment of lumbago and sciatica: an attempt to correlate clinical results with objective parameters. *Arch.Orthop.Trauma Surg.* **104**: 294–298.

Gomez-Perez, F.J., Rull, J.A., Dies, H., Rodriquez-Rivera, J.G., Gonzalez-Barranco, J., and Lozano-Castaneda, O. (1985). Nortriptyline and fluphenazine in the symptomatic treatment of diabetic neuropathy: a double-blind cross-over study. *Pain* **23**: 395–400.

Greenbarg, P.E., Brown, M.D., Pallares, V.S., Tompkins, J.S., and Mann, N.H. (1988). Epidural anesthesia for lumbar spine surgery. *J.Spin.Disord.* **1**: 139–143.

Haimovic, I.C. and Beresford, H.R. (1986). Dexamethasone is not superior to placebo for treating lumbosacral radicular pain. *Neurology* **36**: 1593–1594.

Hansson, P. and Lindblom, U. (1992). Hyperalgesia assessed with quantitative sensory testing in patients with neurogenic pain. In *Hyperalgesia and Allodynia*, ed. W.D. Willis Jr, pp. 335–343. New York: Raven Press.

Hedeboe, J., Buhl, M., and Ramsing, P. (1982). Effects of using dexamethasone and placebo in the treatment of prolapsed lumbar disc. *Acta Neurol.Scand.* **65**: 6–10.

Hildebrand, C., Oscarsson, A., and Risling, M. (1988). Fibre composition of the feline trochlear and abducens nerves. *Brain Res.* **453**: 401–407.

Hoang-Zuan, T., Buchi, E.R., Herbort, C.P., Denis, J., Frot, P., Thenault, Said Buliqueu, Y. (1992). Oral acyclovir for herpes zoster ophthalmicus. *Ophthalmology* **99**: 1062–1071.

Hokfelt, T., Zhang, X., and Wiesenfeld-Hallin, Z. (1994). Messenger plasticity in primary sensory neurons following axotomy and its functional implications. *TINS* **17**: 22–30.

Howe, J.F., Loeser, J.D. and Calvin, W.H. (1977). Mechanosensitivity of dorsal root ganglia and chronically injured axons: a physiological basis for the radicular pain of nerve root compression. *Pain* **3**: 25–41.

Huff, J.C., Bean, B., Balfour, H.H., et al. (1988). Therapy of herpes zoster with oral acyclovir. *Am.J.Med.* **85** (suppl. 2A): 84–89.

Huff, J.C., Drucker, J.L., Clemmer, A., Laskin, O.I., Connor, J.D., Bryson, Y.J., and Balfour, H.H. (1993). Effect of oral acyclovir on pain resolution in herpes zoster: a reanalysis. *J. Med. Virol.* **1P**: 93–96.

Jadad, A.R., Carroll, D., Glynn, C.J., Moore, R.A., and McQuay, H.J. (1992). Morphine responsiveness of chronic pain: double-blind randomised crossover study with patient-controlled analgesia. *Lancet* **339**: 1367–1371.

Janig, W. and Koltzenburg, M. (1991). Receptive properties of pial afferents. *Pain* **45**: 77–85.

Kassirer, M.R., King, R.B., and Robert, A. (1988). Concerning the management of pain associated with herpes zoster and postherpetic neuralgia. *Pain* **35**: 368–369.

Keczkes, K. and Basheer, A.M. (1980). Do corticosteroids prevent post-herpetic neuralgia? *Br. J. Dermatol.* **102**: 551–555.

Killian, J.M. and Fromm, G.H. (1968). Carbamazepine in the treatment of neuralgia. Use and side-effects. *Arch.Neurol.* **19**: 129–136.

Kilo, S., Schmelz, M., Koltzenburg, M., and Handwerker, H.O. (1994). Different patterns of hyperalgesia induced by experimental inflammation in human skin. *Brain* **117**: 385–396.

King, R.B. (1988). Concerning the management of pain associated with herpes zoster and postherpetic neuralgia. *Pain* **33**: 73–78.

Kishore-Kumar, R., Max, M.B., Schafer, S.C., et al. (1990). Desipramine relieves postherpetic neuralgia. *Clin.Pharm.Ther.* **47**: 305–312.

Kissin, I., McDanal, J., and Xavier, A.V.(1989). Topical lidocain for relief of superficial pain in postherpetic neuralgia. *Neurology* **39**: 1132–1133.

Klenerman, L., Greenwood, R., Davenport, H.T., White, D.C., and Peskett, S. (1984). Lumbar epidural injections in the treatment of sciatica. *Br.J.Rheumatol.* **23**: 35–38.

Koltzenburg, M., Torebjörk, H.E., and Wahern, L.K. (1994). Nociceptor modulated central sensitization causes mechanical hyperalgesia in acute chemogenic and chronic neuropathic pain. *Brain* **117**: 579–591.

Kupers, R.C., Konings, H., Adriaensen, H., and Gybels, J.M. (1991). Morphine differentially affects the sensory and affective pain ratings in neurogenic and idiopathic forms of pain. *Pain* **47**: 5–12.

Kvinesdal, B., Molin, J., Froland, A., and Gram, L.F. (1984). Imipramine treatment of painful diabetic neuropathy. *JAMA* **251**: 1727–1730.

Laird, J.M.A. and Bennett, G.J. (1992). Dorsal root potentials and afferent input to the spinal cord in rats with an experimental peripheral neuropathy. *Pain Res.* **584**: 181–190.

Lechin, F., van der Dijs, B., Lechin, M.E., et al. (1989). Pimozide therapy for trigeminal neuralgia. *Arch.Neurol.* **46**: 960–963.

Lindstrom, P. and Lindblom, U. (1987). The analgesic effect of tocainide in trigeminal neuralgia. *Pain* **28**: 45–50.

Llewelyn, J.G., Gilbey, S.G., Thomas, P.K., King, R.H.M., Muddle, J.R., and Watkins, P.J. (1991). Sural nerve morphometry in diabetic autonomic and painful sensory neuropathy. *Brain* **114**: 867–892.

Loh, L. and Nathan, P.W. (1978). Painful peripheral states and sympathetic blocks. *J.Neurol.Neurosurg.Psychiatry* **41**: 664–671.

Maggi, C.A. 1995. Tachykinins and calcitonin gene-related peptide (CGRP) as co-transmitters released from peripheral endings of sensory nerves. *Progr. Neurobiol.* **45**: 1–98.

Matthews, J.A., Mills, S.B., Jenkins, V.M., et al. (1987). Back pain and sciatica: controlled trials of manipulation, traction, sclerosant and epidural injection. *Br.J.Rheumatol.* **26**: 416–423.

Max, M.B., Kishore-Kumar, R., Schafer, S.C., Meister, B., Gracely, R.H., Smoller, B., and Dubner, R. (1991). Efficacy of desipramine in painful diabetic neuropathy: a placebo-controlled trial. *Pain* **45**: 3–9.

Max, M.B., Culnane, M., Schafer, S.C., et al. (1987). Amitriptyline relieves diabetic neuropathy pain in patients with normal or depressed mood. *Neurology* **37**: 589–596.

Max, M.B., Lynch, S.A., Muir, J., Shoaf, S.E., Smoller, B., and Dubner, R. (1992). Effects of desipramine, amitriptyline, and fluoxetine on pain in diabetic neuropathy. *N.Engl.J.Med.* **326**: 1250–1256.

Max, M.B., Schafer, S.C., Culnane, M., Dubner, R., and Gracely, R.H. (1988a). Association of pain relief with drug side effects in postherpetic neuralgia: a single-dose study of clonidine, codeine, ibuprofen, and placebo. *Clin.Pharmacol.Ther.* **43**: 363–371.

Max, M.B., Schafer, S.C., Culnane, M., Smoller, B., Dubner, R., and Graceley, R.H. (1988b). Amitriptyline, but not lorazepam, relieves postherpetic neuralgia. *Neurology* **38**: 1427–1433.

McKendrick, M.W., McGill, J.I., White, J.E., and Wood, M.J. (1986). Oral acyclovir in acute herpes zoster. *Br.Med.J.* **293**: 1529–1532.

McKendrick, M.W., McGill, J.I., and Wood, M.J. (1989). Lack of effect of acyclovir on postherpetic neuralgia. *Br.Med.J.* **298**: 431.

McLachlan, E.M., Janig, W., Devor, M., and Michaelis, M. (1993). Peripheral nerve injury triggers noradrenergic sprouting within dorsal root ganglia. *Nature* **363**: 543–546.

McQuay, H.J., Carroll, D., and Glynn, C.J. (1992). Low dose amitriptyline in the treatment of chronic pain. *Anaesthesia* **47**: 646–652.

Mohamed, S.A. and Carr, D.B. (1994). Pain during herpes zoster (shingles) and long after. *Pain Clin. Updates* **II**: 1–4.

Nicol, C.F. (1969). A four year double blind study of tegretol in facial pain. *Headache* **9**: 54–57.

Nurmikko, T. (1994). Touch, temperature and pain in health and disease: mechanisms and assessments. In *Progress in Pain Research and Management*, ed. J. Boivie, P. Hansson and J. Lindblom, pp. 133–141. Seattle: IASP Press.

O'Hare, J.A., Abuaisha, F., and Geoghegen, M. (1994). Prevalence and forms of neuropathic morbidity in 800 diabetics. *Irish.J.Med.Sci.* **163**: 132–135.

Ochoa, J.L. and Torebjörk, H.E. (1989). Sensations evoked by selective intraneural microstimulation of identified C nociceptors fibres in human skin nerves. *J.Physiol.* **415**: 583–599.

Ochoa, J.L. and Yarnitsky, D. (1993). Mechanical hyperalgesias in neuropathic pain patients: Dynamic and static subtypes. *Ann.Neurol.* **33**: 465–472.

Olmarker, K. (1991). Spinal nerve root compression. Nutrition and function of the porcine cauda equina compressed in vivo. *Acta Orthop.Scand.* **62** (suppl. 242): 1–27.

Peripheral Neuropathy Association. (1993). Quantitative sensory testing: a consensus report. *Neurology* **43**: 1050–1052.

Portenoy, R.K., Duma, C., and Foley, K.M. (1986). Acute herpetic and postherpetic neuralgia: clinical review and current management. *Ann.Neurol.* **20**: 651–664.

Portenoy, R.K., Foley, K.M., and Inturrisi, C.E. (1990). The nature of opioid responsiveness and its implications for neuropathy pain: new hypotheses derived from studies of opioid infusions. *Pain* **43**: 273–286.

Ragozzino, M.W. (1993). The epidemiology and natural history of herpes zoster and postherpetic neuralgia. In *Herpes Zoster and Postherpetic Neuralgia*, ed. C.P.M. Watson, pp. 27–36. Amsterdam: Elsevier.

Ridley, M.G., Kingsley, G.H., Gibson, T., and Grahame, R. (1988). Outpatient lumbar epidural corticosteroid injection in the management of sciatica. *Br.J.Rheumatol.* **27**: 295–299.

Roberts, W. (1986). A hypothesis on the physiological basis for causalgia and related pains. *Pain* **24**: 297–311.

Rogers, R.S. and Tindall, J.P. (1971). Geriatric herpes zoster. *J.Am.Geriatr.Soc.* **19**: 495–503.

Rowbotham, M.C., Davies, P.S., and Fields, H.L. (1995). Topical lidocaine gel relieves postherpetic neuralgia. *Ann.Neurol.* **37**: 246–253.

Rowbotham, M.C., Reisner-Keller, L.A., and Fields, H.L. (1991). Both intravenous lidocaine and morphine reduce the pain of postherpetic neuralgia. *Neurology* **41**: 1024–1028.

Ruda, M.A. and Dubner, R. (1992). Molecular and biochemical events mediate neuronal plasticity following inflammation and hyperalgesia. In *Hyperalgesia and Allodynia*, ed. W.D. Willis Jr, pp. 311–325. New York: Raven Press.

Rull, J.A., Quibrera, R., Gonzalez-Millan, H., and Lozano Castaneda, O. (1969). Symptomatic treatment of peripheral diabetic neuropathy with carbamazepine (Tegretol): Double blind crossover trial. *Diabetologica* **5**: 215–218.

Saudek, C.D., Werns, S., and Reidenberg, M.M. (1977). Phenytoin in the treatment of diabetic symmetrical polyneuropathy. *Clin.Pharmacol.Ther.* **22**: 196–199.

Schott, G.D. (1986). Mechanisms of causalgia and related clinical conditions: the role of the central and of the sympathetic nervous systems. *Brain* **109**: 717–738.

Sindrup, S.H., Bjerre, U., Dejgaard, A., Brosen, K., Aaes-Jorgensen, T., and Gram, L.F. (1992). The selective serotonin reuptake inhibitor citalopram relieves the symptoms of diabetic neuropathy. *Clin.Pharmacol.Ther.* **52**: 547–552.

Sindrup, S.H., Gram, L.F., Brosen, K., Eshoj, O., and Mogensen, E.F. (1990). The selective serotonin reuptake inhibitor paroxetine is effective in the treatment of diabetic neuropathy symptoms. *Pain* **42**: 135–144.

Snoek, W., Weber, H., and Jorgensen, B. (1977). Double blind evaluation of extradural methyl prednisolone for herniated lumbar discs. *Acta Orthop.Scand.* **48**: 635–641.

Stow, P.J., Glynn, C.J., and Minor, B. (1989). EMLA cream in the treatment of post-herpetic neuralgia. Efficacy and pharmacokinetic profile. *Pain* **39**: 301–305.

Stracke, H., Meyer, U.E., Schumacher, H.E., and Federlin, K. (1992). Mexiletine in the treatment of diabetic neuropathy. *Diabetes Care* **15**: 1550–1555.

Tandan, R., Lewis, G.A., Badger, B.A., and Fries, T.J. (1992). Topical capsaicin in painful diabetic neuropathy. *Diabetes Care* **15**: 15–18.

Tearnan, J., Blake, H., and Cleeland, C.S. (1990). Unaided use of pain descriptors by patients with cancer pain. *J.Pain.Sympt.Man.* **5**: 228–232.

Thomas, P.K. (1994). Painful diabetic neuropathy: mechanisms and treatment. *Diab.Nutr.Metab.* **7**: 359–368.

Toyone, T., Takahashi, K., Kitahara, H., Yamagata, M., Murakami, M., and Moriya, H. (1993). Visualisation of symptomatic nerve roots. Prospective study of contrast-enhanced MRI in patients with lumbar disc herniation. *J.Bone Joint Surg.* **4**: 529–533.

Vainio, A. and Tigerstedt, I. (1988). Opioid treatment for radiating cancer pain: oral administration vs. epidural techniques. *Acta Anaesthesiol.Scand.* **32**: 179–185.

Van Hees, J. and Gybels, J. (1981). C nociceptor activity in human nerve during painful and non painful skin stimulation. *J.Neurol.Neurosurg.Psychiatry* **44**: 600–607.

Van Moll, B.J.M. and Vecht, Ch.J. (1994). Referred pain to the face by chest tumours. *Pain Clin.* **7**: 35–38.

Vecht, Ch.J., Haaxma-Reiche, H., Van Putten, W.L.J. et al. (1989). Initial bolus of conventional versus high-dose dexamethasone in metastatic spinal cord compression. *Neurology* **39**: 1255–1257.

Vecht, Ch.J., Hoff, A.M., Kansen, P.J., De Boer, M.F., and Bosch, D.A. (1992). Types and causes of pain in cancer of the head and neck. *Cancer* **70**: 178–184.

Verdugo, R. and Ochoa, J.L.K. (1992). Quantitative somatosensory thermotest. A key method for the evaluation of small calibre afferent channels. *Brain* **115**: 893–913.

Vilming, S.T., Lyberg, T., and Lataste, X. (1986). Tizanidine in the management of trigeminal neuralgia. *Cephalgia* **6**: 181–182.

Wall, P.D., Devor, M., Inbal, R., et al. (1979). Autotomy following peripheral nerve lesions: Experimental anesthesia dolorosa. *Pain* **7**: 103–113.

Wall, P.D. and Gutnick, M. (1974). Ongoing activity in peripheral nerves. The physiology and pharmacology of impulses originating from a neuroma. *Neurology* **24**: 580–593.

Watson, C.P., Chipman, M., Reed, K., Evans, R.J., and Birkett, N. (1992). Amitriptyline versus maprotiline in postherpetic neuralgia: a randomized, double-blind, crossover trial. *Pain* **48**: 29–36.

Watson, C.P., Evans, R.J., Reed, K., Merskey, H., Goldsmith, L., and Warsh, J. (1982). Amitriptyline versus placebo in postherpetic neuralgia. *Neurology* **32**: 671–673.

Watson, C.P., Watt, V.R., Chipman, M., Birkett, N., and Evans, R.J. (1991). The prognosis with postherpetic neuralgia. *Pain* **46**: 195–199.

Watson, C.P.M., Evans, R.J., Watt, V.R., and Birkett, N. (1988). Postherpetic neuralgia: 208 cases. *Pain* **35**: 289–297.

Watson, C.P.N. (1995). The treatment of postherpetic neuralgia. *Neurology* **45** (suppl. 8): S58–S60.

Weber, F., Holme, I., and Amlie, E. (1993). The natural course of acute sciatica with nerve root symptoms in a double-blind placebo-controlled trial evaluating the effect of piroxicam. *Spine* **18**: 1433–1438.

Weissman, D.E.(1988). Glucocorticoid treatment for brain metastases and epidural spinal cord compression. *J.Clin.Oncol.* **6**: 543–551.

Wood, M.J., Johnson, R.W., McKendrick, M.W. et al., (1994). A randomized trial of acyclovir for 7 days or 21 days with and without prednisolone for treatment of acute herpes zoster. *N.Engl.J.Med.* **330**: 896–900.

Young, R.J., Ewing, D.J., and Clarke, B.F. (1983). A controlled trial of sorbinol, an aldose reductase inhibitor in chronic painful diabetic neuropathy. *Diabetes* **32**: 938–942.

Zeigler, D., Lynch, S.A., Muir, J., Benjamin, J., and Max, M.B. (1992). Transdermal clonidine versus placebo in painful diabetic neuropathy. *Pain* **48**: 403–408.

27 Medical rehabilitation

G.W. van Dijk, N.C. Notermans and J. Gerritsen

Introduction

Although treatments are available nowadays for patients with immunological disease of peripheral nerves, physical impairments often persist in spite of these: patients with peripheral neuropathies can be left with muscle weakness, sensory and autonomic disturbances. The physical impairments in these patients may sometimes lead to permanent disability, as the disease has consequences for carrying out activities of daily living (ADL); however, a large number of patients with immune-mediated neuropathies remain independent in ADL and mobility. In addition to physical impairments and disability, peripheral neuropathies may cause handicaps. They may have a severe personal, emotional, social and vocational impact on the patients and their families. Rehabilitation is a process involving the combined expertise of an interdisciplinary team that considers the functional consequences of the disease and helps the patient to lead as normal a life as possible within the limits of functional abilities. The aim is to function at the most independent level possible. The rehabilitation process also considers the prevention or minimization of anticipated complications. Furthermore, patients and families are counselled regarding the prognosis, based upon the current residual function and the anticipated disease course.

The underlying pathology that leads to nerve degeneration is an important factor that plays a role in the outcome of the neuropathy. Roughly two types of pathological reactions of nerves can be distinguished: segmental demyelination and axonal degeneration. In severe inflammatory processes, Wallerian degeneration of axon and myelin sheath may also occur. In demyelinating neuropathies, recovery is possible when ongoing demyelination can be stopped and the cause eliminated. Remyelination by proliferating Schwann cells may lead to full recovery. Recovery from axonal degeneration, when possible, is often incomplete and takes much more time.

Some immune-mediated neuropathies have a relatively good prognosis, but others may prove to be incapacitating. In Guillain-Barré syndrome (GBS), where treatments are available and the course of disease is characterized by spontaneous improvement, many patients continue to have minor problems such as foot-drop or distal numbness, that do not interfere with ADL (Ropper 1992; Arnason and Soliven 1993). Permanent disability (due to weakness, ataxia, paresthesias or sensory loss) occurs in only 5–10%, occasionally leading to wheelchair dependency (Pleasure et al. 1968; Winer et al. 1985; Ropper 1986). Chronic inflammatory demyelinating polyradiculoneuropathy (CIDP) is not a self-limiting disease, but when treated appropriately, up to 30% make a complete recovery. In a large series of 92 of these patients (mean follow-up of 6.5 years), 34% had minimal or no disability, 31% had mild motor and sensory signs, 24% were moderately disabled and 3% required assistance in daily activities (McCombe et al. 1987). In vasculitic neuropathy (occurring in connective tissue diseases or on its own), and in neuropathies associated with monoclonal gammopathy, large controlled trials have not been performed and little is known about the long-term outcome (Kelly and Latov 1987; Chalk et al. 1993; Kyle and Dyck 1993). In multifocal motor neuropathy, treatment with cyclophosphamide or high-dose intravenous immunoglobulins may lead to improvement of muscle strength, although little is known of the prognosis and long-term effect of treatment (Chaudry et al. 1993; Pestronk et al. 1994). The outcome in infective neuropathies depends on the causative organism. In Lyme disease, antibiotics improve symptoms, prevent progression to later stages and eradicate the infection in nearly all patients (Steere 1989). Leprosy can be conquered by multidrug therapy, but it does result in severe disabilities caused by insensitive skin areas which lead to mutilations and deformities. Patients suffering from leprosy, in whom treatment was initiated some time after the onset of the disease do need extensive rehabilitation, but often this is not available in countries where leprosy is widespread (Jamil et al. 1993). In the course of human immunodeficiency virus (HIV) infection, all types of neuropathy can occur at any stage (Barohn et al. 1993). The course of the neuropathy is slowly progressive; spontaneous remissions are rare. In one case, treatment resulted in mild improvement (Dalakas et al. 1988).

Evaluation and rehabilitation plan

A rehabilitation plan is established based on accurate evaluation of function and considers the anticipated disease course of the neuropathy. The course in immune-mediated neuropathies can be acute or subacute, slowly progressive or relapsing. Anticipation of the disease course is very important in the rehabilitation program because the various natural histories of disease and treatment options require different therapeutic approaches. Evaluation is the first phase in rehabilitation management and focuses on the functional consequences of the neuropathy for the patient. Usually evaluation starts in the clinic where the (rehabilitation) physician may be consulted to determine a patient's need for rehabilitation services. During this consultation a proper patient history and physical examination is carried out to assess the impairments that have resulted from the neuropathy and to assess the remaining capabilities, taking preexisting and concurrent medical problems into account. The levels of assistance for functional independence in ADL are assessed (Table 27.1) (Grainger et al. 1986; Erickson and McPhee 1988). Furthermore, the patient's support system is investigated. It is essential to take this into account when deciding whether the rehabilitation program will take place in the family home or whether the patient requires institutional care.

After the evaluation, the data are summarized and a problem list and rehabilitation plan are constructed. The rehabilitation plan considers in particular the disabilities and handicaps that result from the disease. Physical impairments (weakness, contractures, pain) are treated to improve function and to prevent progression. Furthermore, remaining capabilities are trained to ameliorate their function. When necessary, functional dependency can be compensated for by aids and environmental adaptations (i.e. in the home, at the work place). Learning how to use these aids in an appropriate way is an essential part of the rehabilitation program. Depending on the goals and objectives of the rehabilitation plan, patients have to call on the help of the different members of the rehabilitation team (physician, nurse, physio- occupational- recreation- therapist, orthotist, psychologist and medical social worker). Not every patient with an immune-mediated neuropathy will need all of the above mentioned disciplines.

Let us now turn to the individual physical and functional impairments of patients with immune-mediated peripheral neuropathies and how to manage these from a rehabilitation point of view.

Table 27.1 *The functional independence measure*

1. Feeding
2. Grooming
3. Bathing
4. Dressing: upper body
5. Dressing: lower body
6. Using the toilet
7. Bladder management
8. Bowel management
9. Transfer: bed, chair, wheelchair
10. Transfer: toilet
11. Transfer: bath, shower
12. Walk/wheelchair
13. Stairs
14. Communication: comprehension
15. Comprehension: expression
16. Social interaction
17. Problem solving
18. Memory

Levels of assistance for the functional independence measure

7. Complete independence (timely, safely)
6. Modified independence (aid)
5. Modified dependence: supervision
4. Minimal assistance
3. Moderate assistance
2. Maximal assistance
1. Total assistance

Source: Granger et al. (1986).

Motor impairment

Appropriate motor function requires muscle strength, endurance and coordination. All of these functions can be impaired in patients with neuropathy. Here we will consider the management of weakness and endurance. The management of coordination, which is an integral part of motor re-education, is discussed in the paragraph on sensory disturbances and ataxia.

Weakness is often a predominant finding in patients with peripheral neuropathies. The extent and severity of weakness may range from total paralysis requiring mechanical ventilation to slight paresis of foot dorsiflexors or intrinsic hand muscles. In some neuropathies weakness is irreversible and progressive caused by ongoing denervation as a consequence of axonal degeneration. In other neuropathies demyelination may cause temporary weakness followed by improvement due to remyelination of motor nerve fibers. These different prognoses have to be taken into account and require different therapeutic approaches.

Exercise for strength and endurance

Therapeutic exercise by a physiotherapist is the most commonly used modality in treating weakness. When improvement of strength occurs after a period of paralysis, patients are retaught how to contract individual muscles or groups of muscles. This process of so-called motor re-education can employ different techniques that have evolved over the past years (Stillwell and Thorsteinsson 1993). Contraction of muscles can be encouraged by facilitatory techniques in which the therapist strokes or taps the skin overlying the muscle, hereby stimulating the sensory nerve endings in tendons, muscle and joints, and facilitating the firing of alpha motor neurons (Berger and Schaumberg 1988). Electrical stimulation of the innervating nerve can be applied if the nerve is sufficiently intact to produce muscle response after stimulation, so that the resulting movement produced by the stimulated muscles can be taught to the patient. Another technique that can be used in motor re-education is biofeedback. This technique encourages muscle contraction by visual or auditory feedback to the patient (Basmajian 1989).

When voluntary contraction has developed and patients are able to produce movement, an active exercise program should be implemented to build up strength and endurance. Increase in strength is achieved by exercise that increases tension in the muscle fiber (Goldberg et al. 1975). Tension production in the greatest number of muscle fibers is established by contractions in which a muscle must work maximally requiring maximum recruitment of motor units. If the muscle is not strong enough to move the limb, assistance can be provided manually by the therapist, by counterbalancing with weights, by eliminating the force of gravity, or by reducing friction, for example moving an arm on a table, with the arm lying on a skateboard. Once strength has increased, assistance is less necessary and exercise can be performed more actively by moving the limbs against the force of gravity, by the therapist applying manual resistance, by lifting weights, etc. Generally, increase in strength is achieved by repeating an exercise a few times against heavy resistance. Some recommend that high resistance weight training programs should begin as soon as muscle weakness develops (Milner-Brown and Miller 1988). Patients with muscle weakness due to denervation, however, do not always benefit from weight training programs. In some patients, strenuous exercise may lead to a decrease in strength. This so-called 'overwork weakness' has been reported many times in patients with neuromuscular disease, for example poliomyelitis, GBS, peripheral nerve lesions, amyotrophic lateral sclerosis and in progressive muscular dystrophies (Bennet and Knowlton 1958; Bensman 1970; Herbison et al. 1983; Feldman 1985; Fowler 1988). Therefore, muscle strength must be thoroughly evaluated during the exercise program at regular intervals and when a decrease in muscle strength is observed exercise activities should be limited to avoid further exercise-induced muscle damage (Herbison et al. 1983; Ropper et al. 1991).

Patients with slowly chronic progressive neuropathies and mild weakness do not need intensive strengthening exercises or a special motor re-education program. It is sufficient to keep these patients as active as possible by encouraging normal daily activities (Berger and Schaumberg 1988). If possible, exercise should consist of functional activities (walking, swimming, cycling), as these do not only achieve an increase in strength, but also endurance, control (coordination) and a range of motion.

Exercise for endurance will improve the cardiovascular condition and increase local muscle endurance. Generally, endurance exercise consists of many repetitive movements against light resistance. The load and number of repetitions or duration of the exercise are not critical, as long as the exercise is taken to the stage of fatigue (Delateur et al. 1976). Any of the methods used for strength development can be used to develop endurance, with suitable modification. Exercise for endurance can be done daily, but a 4–5 days training course during the week is usually sufficient (Dudley et al. 1982). Detailed exercise descriptions (Delateur 1982; Joynt 1988) considering the type of contractions (isotonic-isometric-isokinetic), the number of series of contractions and the number of repetitions are beyond the scope of this chapter.

Electrical stimulation

Electrical stimulation for improvement of strength is not often used in patients with polyneuropathy. The majority of investigators have not found a difference in strength during electrical stimulation or a voluntary exercise program when training healthy individuals (Kramer 1989). There are no controlled studies of electrical stimulation in patients with denervated muscle due to polyneuropathy. Atrophy can be retarded in denervated muscle in animals by strong electrical stimulation three or four times every day (Gutman and Gutman 1942; Pollock et al. 1951). In a physiotherapy department, for practical reasons stimulation can only be applied twice a day for 5 days; this is not likely to help retard atrophy (Stillwell and Thorsteinsson 1993). As it is not possible to stimulate many muscles for long periods of time, electrical stimulation is not appropriate in patients with polyneuropathy (Stillwell and Thorsteinsson 1993). Electrical stimulation can be used in single nerve lesions when reinnervation is likely to occur after a long period of time. If reinnervation occurs within 100 days, the recovery of function of the muscle is not modified by electrical stimulation (Stillwell and Thorsteinsson 1993). Besides the effect of electrostimulation on denervated muscle and prevention of atrophy, one would expect electrical stimulation to enhance reinnervation. It appears that electrical stimulation is of questionable value in improving reinnervation because of the difficulty with patient compliance; more importantly, it did not actually enhance reinnervation (Herbison et al. 1973, 1983).

Orthoses

Orthoses may be used when muscle weakness persists in a certain region. They may also be used temporarily when patients are recovering and mechanical support is required to start ambulation (Ragnarsson 1988). Ankle-foot orthoses provide support in patients with weakness of foot dorsiflexors, plantarflexors, invertors or evertors (Halan and Cardenas 1987). When it is only the foot dorsiflexion which is weak, a lightweight spring wire brace can prevent foot drop during the swing phase of gait. When weakness is more severe and the feet tend to pronate or supinate, the support of a double-upright steel brace may be needed. It is impor-

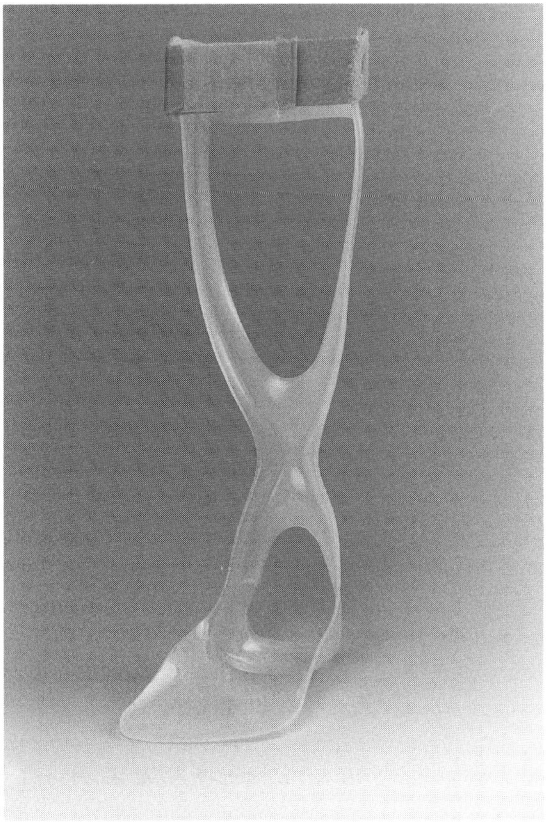

Figure 27.1 *Light-weight plastic ankle-foot orthosis fitting inside the shoe.*

tant to consider with this type of steel orthoses that they are heavy, which can be disadvantageous in patients with muscle weakness. Light-weight plastic ankle-foot orthoses (Figure 27.1) are often used at present and have the advantage of fitting inside the shoe (Lehneis 1972).

In case of weakness of the quadriceps muscles, knee-ankle-foot orthoses are available to support the knee during the stance phase of gait (Merrit 1987; Krebs et al. 1988). These braces are fastened to the shoes and extend up to the thigh, almost to the ischial tuberosity. They often have a knee joint that can be unlocked if the patient wants to sit down. Some patients with mild quadriceps weakness who are able to walk without orthotic support tend to hyperextend the knee during the stance phase of gait. Genu recurvatum may be progressive leading to pain when it reaches 15–20 degrees of hyperextension. In these cases, the knee can be braced by an orthosis that prevents hyperextension and allows normal flexion.

Some of the problems due to muscle weakness can also be overcome by orthopedic shoes, making other orthoses unnecessary. In the case of mild weakness of foot dorsiflexors, a shoe can be constructed with carbon fiber-strengthened uppers to correct a foot drop. Weakness of the intrinsic muscles of the foot may lead to serious deformities such as pes cavus in combination with claw or hammer toes and varus of the hind foot. It may cause pressure sores, especially in the plantar region of the metatarsophalangeal joints. These pressure problems can be solved by making a shoe wide enough for the metatarsophalangeal joints and by using an inlay that distributes pressure over the whole sole of the foot. The combination of muscle weakness and sensory disturbances makes push off and unrolling during walking difficult. Shoes with a surface or concealed bar may well correct the walking pattern.

Orthoses for the upper limbs are not prescribed as often in patients with muscle weakness due to peripheral neuropathies (Long 1966). In peripheral neuropathies, weakness in the upper limbs is often located in the intrinsic muscles of the hand and in the muscles around the wrist. A wide variety of wrist-hand orthoses can be prescribed depending on the residual hand functions and the support needed (Irani 1987). Wrist-drop orthoses made from malleable plastics are commonly used and can easily be applied and removed by the patient. They can be secured to the volar or dorsal aspect of the arm. Orthoses for support of the shoulder and elbow are complex and not very satisfactory. When proximal shoulder weakness is severe, a sling should support the arm that prevents the humeral head from subluxation in the shoulder joint.

Sensory disturbances and ataxia

Sensory disturbances may consist of loss of sensation (hypesthesia, hypalgesia), the occurrence of abnormal sensations (paresthesia, dysesthesia) or pain. In some immune-mediated neuropathies there are only sensory disturbances or the sensory symptoms and signs predominate over motor involvement. These are neuropathies associated with infectious disease (leprosy, HIV infections, Lyme disease), paraneoplastic syndromes, monoclonal gammopathies, autoimmune disease (e.g. Sjögren's syndrome) and sometimes patients with CIDP or GBS (Asbury and Brown 1990; Smith 1992). In these patients, the neurological examination may identify which populations of sensory neurons are affected (large, small or both).

Patients with distal hypesthesia are taught to inspect their feet regularly to look for breakdown of the skin and are advised not to walk on bare feet. Dysesthesia or pain may be the invalidating symptoms in patients with neuropathy. Some may have mild, uncomfortable dysesthesia, whereas others have severe, unbearable pain. When pain is associated with chronic neuropathy or when it persists after recovery, the rehabilitation team can offer multidisciplinary treatment by a physician, physiotherapist and when necessary a psychologist. The management of neuropathic pain is further discussed in Chapter 26.

In large diameter fiber loss, patients may have disturbances of proprioceptive sensations, sometimes leading to severe sensory ataxia and resulting in significant functional impairment. Sensory ataxia is most prominent in the sensory neuronopathies in Sjögren's syndrome, in malignancies or in idiopathic cases (Smith 1992).

Exercise for control and coordination

In patients with sensory ataxia the sensory feedback is disturbed, which makes the development of new sensory engrams more difficult. Furthermore, prolonged immobilization may result in sensory receptor degeneration (Weddell 1961). The peripheral sensory nervous system does, however, have a regenerative capacity, as sensory receptors can be effectively reinnervated after long periods of time and degenerated receptors may regrow (Wynn Parry 1981). Stimulation of (partially) denervated sensory receptors might enhance reinnervation and differentiation of these receptors (Stillwell and Thorsteinsson 1993). In patients with sensory ataxia, a sensory re-education program can be applied. Training consists of frequently repeating movements or certain tasks (Joynt 1988). For instance, the blind-folded patient receives different sensory stimuli. Afterwards, the patient is allowed to look at the stimulus in order to correlate this with visual cues. Sensory re-education in particular concerns the training of adequate hand function.

In practice, many patients with sensory ataxia have to learn to cope with this disabling symptom, and special attention is then paid to improvement of safety during walking to prevent patients from falling. When gait ataxia is present, balance exercises can be prescribed, gait aids may be necessary or patients may even become wheelchair-bound. Patients may benefit from shoes with a broadened heel and good stabilization around the ankle (Figure 27.2).

Ataxia of the upper limbs may cause severe problems in performing ADL. One of the main concerns is interference with normal feeding. Mechanical devices have been developed to aid people with severe ataxia of the upper limbs, but these devices are complex and often not acceptable for practical or social reasons (Broadhurst and Stammers 1990; Michaelis 1993). Patients with sensory ataxia have to rely on their visual feedback and this should be encouraged in the therapy. Refraction abnormalities should be corrected for. In situations where visual control is impossible, for example washing hair under a shower, impairment of control might become apparent. Instructions such as sitting on a chair when showering and washing hair are important to prevent patients from falling.

Contractures

Patients with pareses are at a high risk of developing contractures because they cannot voluntarily move their joints through the full range of motion. Contractures have a great impact on mobility and ADL and may limit the rehabilitation process, especially when present in the weight-bearing joints. Joints that are most likely to develop contractures are the shoulders, elbows, fingers, hips, knees and ankles. In patients with severe pareses or paralyses as in the acute stage of GBS, prevention is the best treatment for contractures and is one of the main treatment goals in physical therapy management in the acute stage of the disease (Eugen and Bell 1988). In these patients, contractures are prevented by: (1) proper positioning in bed (see also Chapter 25), (2) active or assisted exercise providing full range of motion in the joints, and (3) mobilization out of bed as soon as the medical conditions allow (Eugen and Bell 1988).

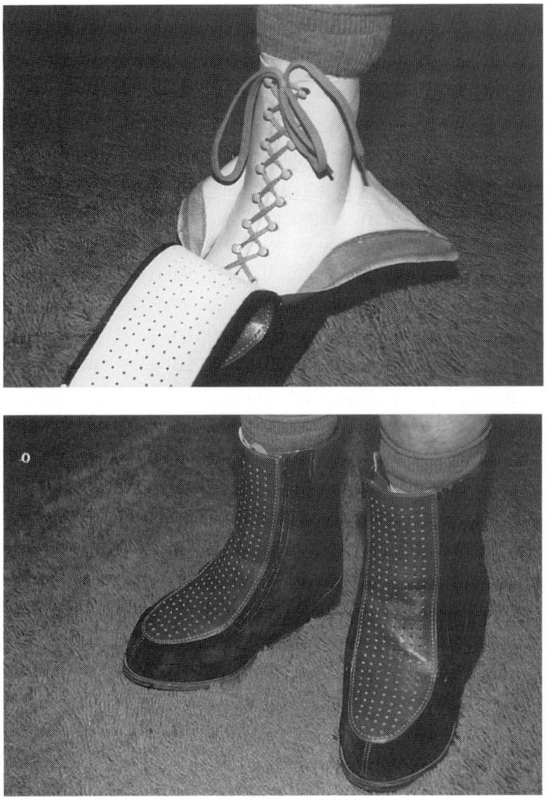

Figure 27.2 *Custom-made shoes with extra stabilization around the ankle.*

Positioning

Proper positioning of bedridden patients prevents not only the occurrence of contractures, but also of decubitus ulcers and of pressure on peripheral nerves (Ropper et al. 1991). The positioning of the patient starts with the selection of an adequate bed and mattress. The mattress should be firm to avoid hip flexion contractures. Pillows placed under the knees should be removed from time to time to prevent flexion contractures of the knee. According to these contractures, the prone position in bed would be advantageous in maintaining hip and knee extension, but most patients do not tolerate this position. Soft rolls may be placed under the trochanters to prevent exorotation contractures of the hips and to prevent pressure on the peroneal nerve at the fibular head. Plantar flexion contractures of the ankles can be prevented by removable ankle splints, which have to be worn at night and for a few hours per day. An important disadvantage of these splints is the risk of developing pressure ulcers. Placing the feet against a foot board has limited value, as this is only effective in the supine position and patients will seldom be able to maintain their feet close to the board for a long time during the day. To prevent shoulder contractures, arm positions are alternated from a neutral position (some 60 degrees shoulder abduction and slight internal rotation) to a position in exorotation with the help of pillows (Brown and Opitz 1970). The elbows alternate between a 90-degree flexed or an extended position. Wrists are extended and thumbs abducted over a handroll, or a palmar splint can be supplied (Berger and Schaumberg 1988).

Exercise for range of motion

To prevent contractures, joints are moved actively by the patient or assisted by the therapist over their full range of motion. These exercises should be performed daily (twice a day) (Berger and Schaumberg 1988). When contractures have developed, joints have to be stretched mildly for 20 minutes twice a day (Kottke et al. 1966). Stretching is carried out carefully with increasing intensity and avoiding severe pain. Angular movements of limbs during stretching can be attended with distraction of the joint to prevent impingement of periarticular tissue and to prevent compression of articular surfaces. Brisk movements will provoke a stretch reflex and should be avoided. Although stretching will almost always cause some pain, severe pain is to be avoided as this may increase the tension in the shortened muscles. The use of a passive range of motion machines may accompany manual stretching and range of motion exercises. These machines have the advantage that they stretch the joint over a longer period of time during the day (Mays 1990; Draznin and Rosenberg 1993). Heat applied to the tendon or joint capsule that has to be stretched will improve results from the stretching exercises. This improvement is based upon the effect of heat on viscosity of connective tissue (Krusen et al. 1971). Apart from this effect, heat may also add the benefit of reducing pain. The most used modality in heating is ultrasound, which allows local therapeutic heating of 40°C up until 43°C (Gersten 1955).

Orthoses can be used to correct contractures by the use of serial casting and dynamic splinting, which is particularly useful in contractures of the ankle and knee (Herbison et al. 1983).

Pressure ulcers

Pressure ulcers may occur in any patient with restricted mobility who lies or sits in the same position for too long. The most important factor in the formation of pressure ulcers is increased (unrelieved) pressure leading to ischemia of the skin and subcutaneous tissues. Furthermore, the rate of skin breakdown is increased by shearing forces, friction and moisture. Other factors that promote pressure ulcers are urinary and fecal incontinence and poor nutritional state (leading to hypoalbuminemia) (Frankel 1988; Tiernan and Lee 1990). Particularly at risk are the areas over bony prominences, e.g. ischial tuberosity, greater trochanter, sacrum, malleoli, heels and occiput.

Obviously, prevention is the best way of managing pressure ulcers. Prevention starts with the recognition of a patient at high risk. Those at high risk are patients with marked immobility, impaired sensation, lowered consciousness, or those receiving sedative or analgesic drugs (Berger and Schaumberg 1988). High risk areas should be examined several times a day for evidence of breakdown and special attention must be given to the nutritional state (adequate protein and vitamin intake). In bedridden patients, relief of pressure can be established by intermittently turning the patient (at least every 2 hours) and good positioning, as described before. Different pressure relief devices can be used, e.g. gel pads, sheepskin, special beds and mattresses and special wheelchair cushions.

Manifest ulcers are classified into five grades: grade I is an inflammatory response involving the intact epidermis, grade II a break or blistering in the epidermis, grade III an ulcer extending through the dermis, grade IV an ulcer extending through the full thickness of the skin into the deep fascia and muscle, and grade V a severe ulcus penetrating the underlying bone causing osteomyelitis (Shea 1975). Grade I and II ulcers are basically reversible, which stresses the importance of regular inspection of the skin areas at high risk. In higher grade ulcers, debridement is necessary to promote wound healing. Chemical debridement can be achieved by solvents in ointments. In severe cases surgical debridement and closure is necessary. Infected wounds are cultured and when systemic signs of infection or sepsis are present, adequate antibiotic treatment should be installed. In patients without signs of systemic infective illness, antibiotics are not necessary (Tiernan and Lee 1990).

Edema

In patients with neuropathy leading to immobilization, distal edema may develop because of decreased muscle activity resulting in venous pooling. Moreover, the venous circulation of the legs can be compromised by sitting for long periods at a time. Patients with a non-optimal venous system (e.g. varicosis) are especially at risk. When edema is present, other causes apart from venous pooling due to inactivity should be ruled out. Special attention is paid to the serum albumin value, which when below 25–30 g L^{-1} promotes the development of edema. Deep venous thrombosis should be regarded as a cause of edema, when edema is more prominent in one leg than in the other. Antithrombotics should be given in a period of immobilization for prevention of deep venous thrombosis. Edema causes increased local tissue pressure, which compromises tissue perfusion and increases the risk of developing pressure ulcers. Edema also increases the risk of developing contractures, especially in the upper limbs where contractures of the fingers can develop in patients with edema of the hands.

The non-pharmacological treatment of edema involves elevation of the affected limbs, compression with elastic stockings and when possible active exercises regularly during the day with the affected extremities. When a low sodium diet and/or diuretics are given in the treatment of edema, attention should be paid to potassium depletion. Furthermore, a decrease in plasma volume may cause or aggravate orthostatic hypotension, which should be taken care of.

Autonomic disturbances

Neuropathies affecting the autonomic nerve fibers give rise to various clinical syndromes (see also

Chapter 9). For some autonomic disturbances, patients can appeal for help to the rehabilitation team. These disturbances are bladder, bowel and sexual dysfunction. Independence in bladder and bowel management is one of the main goals of the rehabilitation program. Autonomic neuropathy may impair the nerve supply to the lower urinary tract, leading to lower motor neuron bladder dysfunction. In these patients bladder sensation is diminished so they do not recognize when it is distended. Furthermore, the bladder muscles are unable to contract to evacuate the organ owing to denervation. In severe cases the consequence can be overflow voiding, which may be complicated by abdominal pain, frequent infections of the lower urinary tract and skin complications with urinary incontinence (Opitz et al. 1988). Micturition can be supported by cholinergic medications, e.g. carbachol (4 mg every 6 hours). When bladder dysfunction is severe, patients may attend a bladder retraining program. We will emphasize that other urological complications (such as urinary tract infection, or urinary tract stones) should be ruled out first, before embarking on the bladder training program. The details of a bladder training are beyond the scope of this chapter and described elsewhere (Opitz et al. 1988). Impaired autonomic innervation of the bowel may cause decreased gastrointestinal motility, leading to obstipation (McLeod and Tuck 1987). The immobility in these patients will make them even more susceptible to obstipation. Food with a high dietary fiber content and adequate fluid intake is advised. If possible, anticholinergic drugs should be avoided and cholinergics (carbachol) can be used to stimulate bowel evacuation (Comarr 1958).

Sexual dysfunctions are often seen in patients with autonomic neuropathy. Although sexual desire remains intact, the genital responses (erection in men and lubrication in women) may be disturbed leading to problems with intercourse. The loss of sensation in the genital area may enhance these problems. Management of these problems can be an integral part of the rehabilitation program (Ducharme et al. 1988).

Orthostatic hypotension can also be a prominent and incapacitating feature of autonomic disturbances. In patients who have been bedridden for a period of time, postural dizziness may occur when mobilization out of bed begins. In these patients, orthostatic hypotension is present, not from autonomic neuropathy, but as a result of not having been upright for a long period of time. The complaints of dizziness when moving into an upright position will usually subside in a few days. When these complaints are severe, patients can be carefully customized to the vertical position with the help of a tilt table.

Functional training

Medical rehabilitation may help patients with immune-mediated peripheral neuropathies to gain functional recovery. Furthermore, in chronic progressive neuropathies the rehabilitation program may delay functional impairments and improve independence in ADL. Functional training is integrated in the rehabilitation program and is initiated as soon as possible. It includes training of ADL and ambulation (e.g. wheelchair mobility). The physiotherapist plays an important role in ambulation, especially in gait training. Patients who are recovering from a period of paralysis in whom improvement may occur, may temporarily require the support of appliances; training is aimed at gradual progression in ambulation from standing and walking in parallel bars to walking with crutches and canes, including climbing stairs, carrying shopping bags, and so on. Disabled patients with chronic neuropathy who are not likely to improve are trained in the use of their aids. The occupational therapist can contribute to the training of patients with ADL (i.e. training in self-care: feeding, grooming, toileting, transfers, ambulation). The occupational therapist may also help in assessing and using orthotic devices, adaptations in the home environment and the use of special devices to facilitate manipulation. Patients who are wheelchair-bound are taught how to drive their wheelchair safely, how to transfer from the chair into the car, how to drive the car when adjustments in the car have been carried out, etc.

When handicaps are present, patients are assisted in coping with their new role in the family, at work and in the community. If indicated, a medical social worker or psychologist can visit patients and his or her relatives in this new situation.

References

Arnason, B.G.W. and Soliven, B. (1993). Acute inflammatory demyelinating polyradiculoneuropathies. In *Peripheral Neuropathy* ed. P.J. Dyck, P.K. Thomas, E.H. Lambert and R. Bunge, pp. 1437–1497. Philadelphia: W.B. Saunders.

Asbury, A.K. and Brown, M.J. (1990). Sensory neuronopathy and pure sensory neuropathy. *Curr. Opin. Neurol. Neurosurg.* **3**: 708–711.

Barohn, R.J., Gronseth, A., LeForce, B.R. et al. (1993). Peripheral nervous system involvement in a large cohort of HIV-infected individuals. *Arch. Neurol.* 167–171.

Basmajian, J.V. (1989). Biofeedback for neuromuscular rehabilitation. *Crit. Rev. Phys. Rehabil. Med.* **1**: 37.

Bennet, R.L. and Knowlton, G.C. (1958). Overwork weakness in partially denervated skeletal muscle. *Clin. Orthop*, **12**: 22–29.

Bensman, A. (1970). Strenuous exercise may impair muscle function in Guillain-Barré patients. *JAMA* **214**: 468–469.

Berger, A.R. and Schaumberg, H.H. (1988). Rehabilitation of peripheral neuropathies. *J. Neurol. Rehabil.* **2**: 25–36.

Broadhurst, M.J. and Stammers, C.W. (1990). Mechanical feeding aids for people with ataxia: design considerations. *J. Biomed. Eng.* **12**: 209–214.

Brown, J.R. and Opitz, J.L. (1970). Treatment of neuropathies. In *Handbook of Clinical Neurology*, vol 8, ed. P.J. Vinken and G.W. Bruyn, pp. 373–411. New York: American Elsevier.

Chalk, C.H., Dyck, P.J., and Conn, D.L. (1993). Vasculitic neuropathy. In *Peripheral Neuropathy*, ed. P.J. Dyck, P.K. Thomas, E.H. Lambert and R. Bunge, pp. 1424–1436. Philadelphia: W.B. Saunders.

Chaudry, V., Corse, A.M., Cornblath, D.R. et al. (1993). Multifocal motor neuropathy: response to intravenous immunoglobulin. *Ann. Neurol.* **33**: 237–242.

Comarr, A.E. (1958). Bowel regulation for patients with spinal cord injury. *JAMA* **167**: 18–21.

Dalakas, M.C., Yarchoan, R., Spitzer, R. et al. (1988). Treatment of HIV-related polyneuropathy with 3′azido-2′,3′-dideoxythymidine. *Ann. Neurol.* **23**: S92–S97.

Delateur, B.J., Lehman, J.F., and Gianconi, R. (1976). Mechanical work and fatigue: their roles in the development of muscle work capacity. *Arch. Phys. Med. Rehabil.* **57**: 319–324.

Delateur, B.J. (1982). Therapeutic exercise to develop strength and endurance. In *Krusen's Handbook of Physical Medicine and Rehabilitation*, ed. F.J. Kottke, G.K. Stillwell and J.F. Lehman. Philadelphia: W.B. Saunders.

Draznin, E. and Rosenberg, N.L. (1993). Intensive rehabilitative approach to eosinophilia myalgia syndrome associated with severe polyneuropathy. *Arch. Phys. Med. Rehab.* **74**: 774–776.

Ducharme, S., Gill, K., Biener-Bergman, S., and Fertitta, L. (1988). Sexual functioning: medical and psychological aspects. In *Rehabilitation Medicine: Principles and Practice*, ed. J.A. DeLisa, pp. 519–536. Philadelphia: J.P. Lippincott.

Dudley, G.A., Abraham, W.M., and Terjung, R.L. (1982). Influence of exercise intensity and duration on biochemical adaptations in skeletal muscle. *J. Appl. Physiol.* **53**: 844–850.

Erickson, R.P. and McPhee, M.C. (1988). Clinical evaluation. In *Rehabilitation Medicine: Principles and Practice*, ed. J.A. DeLisa, pp. 25–65. Philadelphia: J.P. Lippincott.

Eugen, M.H. and Bell, K.R. (1988). Contracture and other deleterious effects of immobility. In *Rehabilitation Medicine: Principles and Practice*, ed. J.A. DeLisa, pp. 448–455.

Feldman, R.M. (1985). The use of strengthening exercises in post polio sequelae. *Orthopedics* **8**: 889–890.

Fowler, W.M. (1988). Management of musculoskeletal complications in neuromuscular diseases: weakness and the role of exercise. In *Advances in the Rehabilitation of Neuromuscular Diseases*, ed. W.M. Fowler, p. 497. Philadelphia: Hanley & Belfus.

Frankel, D.L. (1988). Nutrition. In *Rehabilitation Medicine: Principles and Practice*, ed. J.A. DeLisa, pp. 556–557. Philadeliphia: J.P. Lippincott.

Gersten, J.W. (1955). Effect of ultrasound on tendon extensibility. *Am. J. Phys. Med.* **34**: 360–362.

Goldberg, A.L., Etlinger, J.D., Goldspink, D.F., and Jablecki, C. (1975). Mechanism of work-induced hypertrophy of skeletal muscle. *Med. Sci. Sports* **7**: 185–198.

Granger, C.V. et al. (1986). Advances in functional assessment for medical rehabilitation. *Top. Geriat. Rehabil.* **1**: 59.

Gutmann, E. and Gutmann, L. (1942). Effect of electrotherapy on denervated muscles in rabbits. *Lancet.* **1**: 169–171.

Halan, E. and Cardenas, D. (1987). Ankle-foot orthosis: clinical implications. *Phys. Med. Rehabil.* **1**: 45.

Herbison, G.J., Teng, C., and Gordon, E.E. (1973). Electrical stimulation of reinnervating rat muscle. *Arch. Phys. Med. Rehabil.* **54**: 156–160.

Herbison, G.J., Jaweed, M.M., and Ditunno, J.F. (1983). Exercise therapies in peripheral neuropathies. *Arch. Phys. Med. Rehab.* **64**: 201–205.

Irani, K.D. (1987). Wrist and hand orthosis. *Phys. Med. Rehabil.* **1**: 137.

Jamil, S., Keer, J.T., Lucas, B. et al. (1993). Use of polymerase chain reaction to assess efficacy of leprosy. *Lancet* **342**: 264–268.

Joynt, R.L. (1988). Therapeutic exercise. In *Rehabilitation Medicine: Principles and Practice*, ed. J.A. DeLisa, pp. 346–371. Philadelphia: J.P. Lippincott.

Kelly, J.J. and Latov, N. (1987). *Polyneuropathies Associated with Plasma Cell Dyscrasias.* Boston: Martinus Nijhof.

Kottke, F.J., Pauley, D.L., and Ptak, R.A. (1966). The rationale for prolonged stretching for correction of shortening of connective tissue. *Arch. Phys. Med. Rehabil.* **47**: 345–352.

Kramer, J.F. (1989). Muscle strengthening via electrical stimulation. *Crit. Rev. Phys. Rehabil. Med.* **1**: 97–133.

Krebs, D.E., Edelstein, J.E., and Fishman, S. (1988). Comparison of plastic/metal and leather/metal knee-ankle-foot orthoses. *Am. J. Phys. Med. Rehabil.* **67**: 175.

Krusen, F.H., Kottke, F.J., and Ellwood, P.M. (eds) (1971). *Handbook of Physical Medicine and Rehabilitation.* Philadelphia: W.B. Saunders.

Kyle, R.H. and Dyck, P.J. (1993). Neuropathy associated with the monoclonal gammopathies. In *Peripheral Neuropathy*, ed. P.J. Dycke, P.K. Thomas,

E.H. Lambert and R. Bunge, pp. 1275–1287. Philadelphia: W.B. Saunders.

Lehneis, H.R. (1972). New developments in lower-limb orthotics through bioengineering. *Arch. Phys. Med. Rehabil.* **53**: 303–310.

Long, C. (1966). Upper limb bracing. In *Orthotics, Et cetera.* ed. S. Licht and H.L. Kamenetz, p. 152. New Haven.

Mays, M.L. (1990). Incorporating continuous passive motion in the rehabilitation of a patient with Guillain-Barré syndrome. *Am. J. Occup. Ther.* **44**: 750–754.

McCombe, P.A., Pollard, J.D., and McLeod, J.G. (1987). CIDP. A clinical and electrophysiological study of 92 cases. *Brain* **110**: 1617–1630.

McLeod, J.G. and Tuck, R.R. (1987). Disorders of the autonomic nervous system: Part 1. Pathophysiology and clinical features. *Ann. Neurol.* **21**: 419–430.

Merrit, J.L. (1987). Knee-ankle-foot orthotics: long leg braces and their practical applications. *Phys. Med. Rehabil.* **1**: 67.

Michaelis, J. (1993). Mechanical methods of controlling ataxia. *Baillières Clin. Neurol.* **2**: 121–139.

Milner-Brown, H.S. and Miller, R.G. (1988). Muscle strengthening through high-resistance weight training in patients with neuromuscular disorders. *Arch. Phys. Med. Rehab.* **69**: 14–19.

Opitz, J.L., Thornsteinsson, G., Schutt, A.H., Barret, D.M., and Olson, P.K. (1988). Neurogenic bladder and bowel. In *Rehabilitation Medicine: Principles and Practice*, ed. J.A. DeLisa, pp. 492–518. Philadelphia: J.P. Lippincott.

Pestronk, A., Lopate, G., Cornberg, A.J. et al. (1944). Distal tower motor neuron syndrome with high titers of IgM anti-GM1 antibodies: improvement following immunotherapy with monthly plasma exchange and intravenous cyclophosphamide. *Neurology* **44**: 2027–2031.

Pleasure, D.E., Lovelace, R.E., and Duvoisin, R.C. (1968). The prognosis of acute polyradiculoneuritis. *Neurology* **18**: 1143–1148.

Pollock, L.J., Arieff, A.J., Sherman, I.C. et al. (1951). Electrotherapy in experimentally produced lesions of peripheral nerves. *Arch. Phys. Med. Rehabil.* **32**: 377–387.

Ragnarsson, K.T. (1988). Orthotics and shoes. In *Rehabilitation Medicine: Principles and Practice*, ed. J.A. DeLisa, pp. 307–328. Philadelphia: J.P. Lippincott.

Ropper, A.H. (1986). Severe acute Guillain-Barré syndrome. *Neurology* **36**: 543–549.

Ropper, A.H., Wijdicks, E.F.M., and Truax, B.T. (1991). Guillain-Barré syndrome. Outcome and rehabilitation. *Contemp. Neurol. Series* **34**: 263–281.

Ropper, A.H. (1992). The Guillain-Barré syndrome. *N. Engl. J. Med.* **326**: 1130–1136.

Shea, J.D. (1975). Pressure sores: classification and management. *Clin. Orthop.* **112**: 89–100.

Smith, B.E. (1992). Inflammatory sensory polyganglionopathy. In *Peripheral Neuropathy: New Concepts and Treatments*, ed. P.J. Dyck, *Neurol. Clin.* **10**: 735–759.

Steere, A.C. (1989). Lyme disease. *N. Engl. J. Med.* **321**: 586–596.

Stillwell, G.K. and Thorsteinsson, G. (1993). Rehabilitation procedures. In *Peripheral Neuropathy*, ed. P.J. Dyck, P.K. Thomas, E.H. Lambert and R. Bunge, pp. 1692–1708. Philadelphia: W.B. Saunders.

Tiernan, P. and Lee, B.Y. (1990). Pathogenesis and management of pressure ulcers. *J. Neurol. Rehabil.* **4**: 129–136.

Weddell, G. (1961). Receptors for somatic sensation. In *Brain and Behavior*, ed. M.A.R. Brizier. Washington DC: American Institute of Biological Sciences.

Winer, J.B., Hughes, R.A.C., Greenwood, R.J. et al. (1985). Prognosis in Guillain-Barré syndrome. *Lancet* **1**: 1202–1203.

Wynn Parry, C.B. (1981). *Rehabilitation of the Hand.* London: Butterworths.

Index

Note: abbreviations and acronyms used in subheadings are: CEAN, chronic experimental allergic neuritis; CIDP, chronic inflammatory demyelinating polyneuropathy; CMV, cytomegalovirus; EAN, experimental allergic neuritis; GBS, Guillain–Barré syndrome; HMSN-1, hereditary motor and sensory neuropathy-1; ICU, intensive care unit; IVIG, intravenous immunoglobulin; LEMS, Lambert–Eaton myasthenic syndrome; MGUS, monoclonal gammopathies of undetermined significance; POTS, postural orthostatic tachycardia syndrome.

acquired immune deficiency syndrome *see* AIDS
acquired neuromyotonia *see* neuromyotonia
acrylamide, toxicity 150
acute autonomic neuropathies
  botulism 149, 248
  cholinergic 148
  classification 144–5
  drug-associated 149–50
  Guillain–Barré syndrome 148–9
  idiopathic (pandysautonomia) 144–7
  porphyria 149
  and sensory 133–4
  toxic 120, 149–50
acute autonomic and sensory neuropathy 133–4, 135
acute cholinergic neuropathy 148
acute inflammatory demyelinating polyneuropathy *see* Guillain–Barré syndrome
acute sensorimotor neuropathies 65, 219–20
acute sensory neuronopathy 126–7, 132–5
  and autonomic 133–4
  clinical features 132–4
  diagnostic algorithm 65
  differential diagnosis 135
  laboratory features 134
  pathogenesis 134–5
  pathological features 134
  prognosis 134
  therapy 134
acyclovir 398–9, 400
Adie's syndrome 128, 129, 151–2
adrenergic function, autonomic neuropathies 142–3
adrenoleucodystrophy 120
AIDS (acquired immune deficiency syndrome) 285
  autonomic neuropathy 297
  cytomegalovirus 289, 347–8, 349
  demyelinating neuropathy 290, 295
  distal painful neuropathy 349
  facial palsies 295
  and herpes zoster 341, 342
  HIV-infection staging 285–6
  polyradiculopathy 296, 348
  prevalence of neuropathy 286–9
  relative incidence of neuropathy 288
  sensory neuropathies 61–2, 286, 288, 289–91
  toxic neuropathies 296–7
AIDS related complex (ARC) 285, 288
  facial palsies 295
  herpes zoster 342
  toxic neuropathies 296–7
alkylating agents 175–6, 197, 198, 361–3
allodynia 391
amantadine, post-polio syndrome 281
amiodarone polyneuropathy 120, 150
amitriptyline 408, 409
amyloid neuropathies 152–4
  classification 152
  epidemiology 31–2
  familial 86–7, 135, 152, 153–4
  immunopathology 86–8
  myelomatous 86–7, 226
  nerve enlargement 324
  sporadic primary 152, 153
amyotrophic lateral sclerosis 191, 208
  see also motor neuron disease

angiocentric lymphoproliferative disorders 162
anticholinesterase, post-polio syndrome 280
anti-chondroitin sulfate C antibodies 170, 178, 205
anticonvulsants
  nerve pain 403, 404, 405, 406, 408, 409
  neuromyotonia 242
antidepressants, nerve pain 403, 405, 406, 408, 409–10
anti-ganglioside antibodies 88–9, 190–200
  anti-ganglioside titers 194
  and anti-sulfatide 203
  CIDP 196–7
  definitions 190–1
  differential diagnosis 196–7
  electrophysiology 193–4
  experimental data 195–6
  Guillain–Barré syndrome 104–6, 238–9
  histology 194–5
  IgG reactivity 238–9
  IgM reactivity 88, 170, 180–2, 204–5, 359
  immunological aspects 191–2
  lower motor neuron syndromes 192, 193, 195, 197–8
  motor neuropathy with conduction block 192–3, 194–5, 196–7
  therapy 197–8, 359, 361
anti-Hu antibodies 90–1, 130, 146, 216, 218
anti-idiotypic antibodies, IVIG 369
antilymphocyte globulin (ALG) 371
anti-MAG neuropathy 33, 34, 169–78
  and anti-sulfatide antibodies 203
  experimental 48, 177–8
  immunopathology 83–4
antimetabolites 242, 358, 360–1, 363–4
  see also azathioprine
anti-sulfatide antibodies 170, 178–80, 201–4
  axonal neuropathy 202–3
  demyelinating sensorimotor neuropathy 203
  immunopathology 89–90
  inflammatory demyelinating polyneuropathy 203
  neuropathy pathogenesis 201–2, 203–4
  polyneuropathy 201–2, 203
antithymocyte globulin (ATG) 371
areflexia 61
arsenic, toxicity 150
ataxia 61, 68, 420
atrophy, muscle 58
autonomic neuropathies 138–57
  acute
    botulism 149, 248
    cholinergic 148
    classification 144–5
    drug-associated 149–50
    Guillain–Barré syndrome 148–9
    idiopathic 144–7
    pandysautonomia 144–7
    porphyria 149
    and sensory 133–4, 135
    toxic 120, 149–50
  autonomic examination 139–40
  autonomic tests 140–3
  chronic
    amyloid 152–4
    classification 144
    diabetic 154
    distal small fiber 150–1
    POTS 138–9, 147–8
    pure cholinergic 151–2
  classification 143–5
  clinical evaluation 61, 138–9
  HIV-related 288, 289, 297
  orthostatic hypotension 138–9, 142–3, 147
  paraneoplastic 221
  rehabilitation 422–3
  sudomotor function 139, 140–2, 151
axonal neuropathies
  anti-sulfatide antibodies 202–3
  chronic idiopathic 118–19
  diagnostic algorithm 65, 66–7
  distal sensory 219
  electrophysiology 64, 75, 76, 78
  Guillain–Barré syndrome 89, 101–2, 113, 379
  immunopathology 85, 87, 88, 89, 90
azathioprine 360, 361
  CIDP 122
  LEMS 248
  neuromyotonia 242
  osteosclerotic myeloma 233
AZT (zidovudine) 295, 296, 300

Bannwarth's syndrome (meningoradiculoneuritis) 311, 315
bedridden patients 421, 422, 423
  see also paralytic neuropathy
biliary cirrhosis 135
biopsies *see* muscles, biopsy; nerve biopsy studies
bladder dysfunction 423
blood pressure, autonomic neuropathies 139, 142–3
blood–nerve barrier 6, 41–3
Borrelia burgdorferi 308, 309, 310, 312, 313–14, 316
botulism 149, 248
brachial neuritis, HIV infection 295
brachial plexopathies, ICU care 384
breast implants, silicone 259–62
Brequinar sodium 364

calcium channels, LEMS 238, 245–7
Campylobacter jejuni infection 13, 30–1, 89, 100, 103, 104–5, 379, 380
cancer patients
  antimetabolite toxicity 360–1
  cisplatin 135, 149
  nerve pain 399, 403, 410
  vincristine 150
  see also Lambert–Eaton myasthenic syndrome; multiple myeloma; neuromyotonia; paraneoplastic neuropathies
capsaicin, nerve pain 403, 407, 408
carbamazepine
  nerve pain 403, 404, 405, 406, 408, 409
  neuromyotonia 242
cardiovagal function tests 142
carpal tunnel syndrome 256, 313
causalgia 60, 395, 397, 408–9
2-CdA (2-chlorodeoxy-adenosine) 364
cellular immune system 8–11
  EAN 8–9, 37, 38, 46
central nervous system
  CIDP 118
  necrotizing arteritis 159–60
  paraneoplastic neuropathies 210
cerebrospinal fluid
  AIDS patients 290
  anti-MAG IgM reactivity 173
  CIDP 114
  Lyme neuropathy 314
  osteosclerotic myeloma 230
Chagas' disease 48–9, 152
Charcot–Marie–Tooth neuropathy 64, 76, 121, 324
chickenpox 341, 342, 343
Chinese paralytic syndrome 13, 101, 104, 105, 379–80
chlorambucil 198, 361, 362
2-CdA (2-chlorodeoxy-adenosine) 364
cholinergic neuropathies
  acute 148
  pure 144, 151–2
    see also Adie's syndrome; Lambert–Eaton myasthenic syndrome
chondroitin sulfate C 170, 178, 202–3, 205
chronic autonomic neuropathies
  amyloid 152–4
  classification 144
  diabetic 154
  distal small fiber 150–1
  POTS 138–9, 147–8
  pure cholinergic 151–2
chronic experimental allergic neuritis (CEAN) 46–7
chronic idiopathic anhidrosis 151–2
chronic idiopathic axonal neuropathy 118–19
chronic inflammatory demyelinating polyneuropathy (CIDP) 111–25
  animal model (CEAN) 46–7

chronic inflammatory demyelinating polyneuropathy (CIDP) (*cont.*)
anti-ganglioside antibodies 196–7
anti-sulfatide antibodies 203
clinical features 59–60, 61, 62, 113
and cytomegalovirus 295–6
differential diagnosis 118–21
epidemiology 31
Guillain–Barré syndrome compared 100, 112–13, 116–17
in HIV infection 295–6, 297, 300
immunopathology 9, 89
laboratory analysis 113–16
pathogenesis 116–17
rehabilitation 416
respiratory insufficiency 380
temporal profile 62, 100, 112, 116
therapy 113, 121–3, 373
corticosteroids 121–2, 358, 359
IVIG 123, 367, 371
plasmapheresis 122, 367
variants 117–18
chronic sensorimotor polyneuropathy 220–1
chronic sensory neuronopathy 126, 127–32
anti-sulfatide antibodies 179, 202–3
clinical features 127–9
differential diagnoses 135
electrophysiology 129
idiopathic 127, 129
laboratory study 130
MRI study 130
pathology 131–2
prognosis 132
with sicca syndrome 127–8, 129
with Sjögren's syndrome 127–9, 130, 131–2, 135
therapy 132
Churg–Strauss syndrome 158
cisplatin, toxicity 135, 149
clinical evaluation of neuropathies 55–72
autonomic nerve function 61
deficit measurement 64–8
differential diagnosis 63–4
disability scales 68
handicap measurement 64–8
motor function 56–62, 64–7
reflexes 61–2
sensory function 59–61, 67–8
skeletal deformities 65
systemic disease 62–3
temporal profile 62
clonidine, nerve pain 403, 408
complement 15–18
blood–nerve barrier 7
CIDP 114
EAN 18, 41, 44
humoral immune system 12
immunopathological studies 82, 83–5, 88, 89, 91–2
IVIG 368
compound muscle action potential (CMAP)
CIDP 115, 116
conduction block 74–5, 116
conduction velocity 76
demyelination criterion 77
experimental allergic neuritis 45
Guillain–Barré syndrome 103
LEMS 244
conduction *see* electrophysiological studies
contractures
clinical evaluation 63
rehabilitation 420–2
corticosteroids 357–60
anti-MAG IgM 174–5
chronic sensory neuronopathy 132
CIDP 121–2, 358, 359
cytokine production 357
cytolysis 359
experimental allergic neuritis 46
Guillain–Barré syndrome 107, 359
HIV-related neuropathies 300
idiopathic autonomic neuropathy 147
in immune-mediated neuropathies 359–60
LEMS 248
leprosy 335, 336
leukocyte adhesion 359
lymphocyte interactions 359
motor neuropathy with conduction block 197
neuromyotonia 242
osteosclerotic myeloma 233
phagocytosis 359
post-polio syndrome 280–1
sciatica 399, 401–2
toxicity 360
vasculitic neuropathies 165, 358, 360
cramp-fasciculation syndrome 242
cramps, clinical evaluation 56, 57
cranial neuropathy
causes of nerve pain 394
Lyme disease 311
Miller Fisher syndrome 58, 61, 102, 104, 105, 238–9
muscle weakness 58–9
sarcoidosis 63
critical illness polyneuropathies 385, 386
Crow–Fukase syndrome 234
cryoglobulinemia
classification 158–9
clinical evidence 63
with HIV infection 294
and IgM reactivity 169, 182
IVIG 373
α-interferon 371, 373
cyclophosphamide 361, 362
anti-MAG IgM 175
lower motor neuron syndromes 198
motor neuropathy with conduction block 197
cyclosporin 363
cytokines 19–20, 21
blood–nerve barrier 6, 7
cellular immune system 8–9, 10, 11
complement 18
corticosteroids 357, 359
cyclosporin 363
experimental allergic neuritis 18, 38, 46
Guillain–Barré syndrome 104, 108
HIV infection 298–9
IVIG 368–9
leprosy 334
plasmapheresis 365
post-polio syndrome 278, 280, 281
cytolysis, corticosteroids 359
cytomegalovirus (CMV) neuropathies 347–9
Guillain–Barré syndrome 30, 347
in HIV infection 289, 291, 294, 295–6, 298, 300, 347–9
mononeuritis multiplex 294, 348
polyradiculopathy 296, 348, 349
therapy 349
cytoskeletal proteins, IgM reactivity 170, 180

dapsone, toxicity 297
deficit measurement 64–8, 416
Dejerine–Sottas neuropathy 324
demyelinated fibers, conduction in 74
demyelinating neuropathies
acute inflammatory *see* Guillain–Barré syndrome
anti-MAG IgM 177–8
anti-sulfatide antibodies 179–80, 203
chronic inflammatory *see* chronic inflammatory demyelinating polyneuropathy
diagnostic algorithm 65, 66
electrophysiology 64, 75, 76, 77
HIV-related 288, 290, 295–6, 297, 300
immunopathology 81, 83–4, 85, 88, 89
osteosclerotic myeloma 232
paraneoplastic 210, 217
temporal dispersion 75, 116
demyelination
experimental allergic neuritis 37, 38–9, 41–6
experimental Chagas' disease 48–9
experimental paraprotein neuropathy 48
2-deoxycoformycin 364
deprenyl, post-polio syndrome 281
desipramine, nerve pain 406, 408, 409–10
diabetic neuropathy 154

cellular immune system 10–11
disability scale 68
painful 396, 403, 406–8
respiratory insufficiency 380
sudomotor function 142
vasculitic lesions 163
3,4-diaminopyridine (3,4-DAP), LEMS 248
didanosine (ddI), toxicity 287, 296–7
disability scales 68
distal painful polyneuropathy, AIDS 348
distal sensory neuropathy, cancer 219
distal small fiber neuropathy (DSFN) 150–1
distal symmetrical neuropathy (DSN) in HIV 286, 287, 288, 289–90, 291, 296
distal symmetrical polyneuropathy (DSP) in HIV 289, 296
DNA
herpes virus infections 346, 347
HIV infection 298
drug-associated neuropathies 120, 149–50
ganglioside-associated GBS 258–9
guanethidine 257–8
in HIV infection 286, 287, 296–7
neuromyotonia 239–40
dynamometry 64, 67
dysesthesia
clinical evaluation 60
rehabilitation 420
dysproteinemic polyneuropathies 31–4
see also amyloid neuropathies; monoclonal gammopathies; multiple myeloma; osteosclerotic myeloma

edema 422
electrical stimulation 418
electromyography 74–6, 77, 379
Guillain–Barré syndrome 103
in ICU 384–7
LEMS 244–5, 247–8
neuromyotonia 240–1
osteosclerotic myeloma 229–30, 232
post-polio syndrome 275
electroneurography 74–6, 77
electrophysiological studies 64, 73–80
acute sensory neuronopathy 133
anti-MAG IgM reactivity 174
chronic sensory neuronopathy 129
conduction block 74–5, 116
conduction velocity 76
demyelinated fibers 74
electrodiagnostic protocols 76–8
axonal degeneration 78
CIDP 78, 114–16
demyelination 77
MMN 78
electroneurography 74–6, 77
experimental allergic neuritis 45
fasciculations 57
Guillain–Barré syndrome 101–2, 103
HIV infection 287–8
motor neuron syndromes 57, 193–4
myelin-associated glycoprotein 174
nerve pain 392
normal fibers 73–4
paralytic neuropathy 380, 381, 382–7
temperature 76
temporal dispersion 74–5, 116
vasculitic neuropathies 160
see also electromyography
eosinophilia-myalgia syndrome (EMS) 252–4
Epstein–Barr virus 347
erythema migrans 63, 308, 310
see also Lyme neuropathy
erythema nodosum leprosum (ENL) 327, 332
exercise
for control 420
post-polio syndrome 281
for range of motion 421–2
for strength 417–18
experimental allergic encephalitis (EAE) 11
experimental allergic neuritis (EAN) xiv–xviii, 36–47, 117
blood–nerve barrier 41–3
cellular immunity 8–9, 38, 46
clinical features 37
complement 18, 41, 44
cytokines 18, 38, 46
electrophysiology 45
humoral immunity 39, 41, 46
immunopathology 37
synthesis 43–5
therapy 45–6
experimental Chagas' disease 48–9
experimental data
anti-ganglioside antibodies 195–6
anti-MAG IgM 48, 177–8
anti-sulfatide antibodies 203–4
eosinophilia-myalgia syndrome 253–4
guanethidine-induced neuropathy 257–8
nerve pain 397
silicone neurotoxicity 262
experimental paraprotein neuropathy 47–8

facial palsies
in HIV infection 295
Lyme disease 311
familial amyloid neuropathies (FAP) 152, 153–4
differential diagnosis 135
immunopathology 86–7
type I 153–4
type II (Rukavina, Indiana) 154
type III (van Allen, Iowa) 154
type IV 154
fasciculations, clinical evaluation 56–7
Fc receptors, IVIG 368
filum terminale, tumor of 121
fludarabine 176, 363–4
focal neuropathy
paraneoplastic 221
preceding CIDP 117–18
foscarnet
CMV-related neuropathy 349
HIV-related neuropathy 300

galactosylceramide *O*-sulfate *see* sulfatide
ganciclovir
CMV-related neuropathy 349
HIV-related neuropathy 300
gangliosides 190–1
associated neuropathies 88–9, 190–200
Guillain–Barré syndrome 104–6, 238–9, 258–9
IgM reactivity 88, 170–1, 180–2, 204–5
see also anti-ganglioside antibodies
CEAN 47
humoral immune system 12–13
post-polio syndrome 278, 280
glycolipids 5–6
CEAN 47
cellular immune system 9–10
see also gangliosides; sulfatide
glycoproteins
cellular immunity 8, 9
and cytokines 19–20
experimental allergic neuritis 41
molecular organization 4–5
gold therapy, rheumatoid arthritis 57
guanethidine-induced neuropathy 257–8
Guillain–Barré syndrome (GBS) 99–110, 148–9
or acute sensory neuronopathy 135
animal model *see* experimental allergic neuritis
anti-sulfatide antibodies 203
autonomic dysfunction 61, 102
axonal form 89, 101–2, 113, 379
and *C. jejuni* infection 30–1, 89, 100, 101, 103, 104–5, 379, 380
cancer patients 219
cellular immune system 9, 10
children 107
Chinese paralytic syndrome 13, 101, 104, 105, 379–80
CIDP compared 100, 112–13, 117
clinical description 57, 58, 59, 60, 61, 100–3
complement 17
cranial nerve variants 102
Miller Fisher syndrome 58, 61, 102, 104, 105, 238–9
diagnosis 102–3

Guillain–Barré syndrome (GBS) (*cont.*)
  electrophysiology 101–2, 103
  epidemiology 30–1
  functional grading 68
  future developments 108
  humoral immune system 13, 14
  ICU management 106, 148–9, 378–9, 380–1
  immunopathology 89
  Lyme disease 312–13
  parenteral ganglioside-associated 258–9
  pathogenesis 89, 103–6, 116–17
  prognosis 103, 415–16
  rehabilitation 415–16, 420
  temporal profile 62, 100, 116
  therapy 100, 106–7, 108, 359, 365, 370–1, 373
  and viral infections
    cytomegalovirus 30, 347
    HIV 295, 297, 300
    humoral immune system 14
    swine flue 31
    varicella zoster 341, 342–3

handicap measurement 64–8, 416
heart rate, autonomic neuropathies 139, 142
heavy metals, toxicity 150
hepatitis infection 162, 367–8
hereditary neuropathies
  familial amyloid 86–7, 135, 152, 153–4
  liability to pressure palsies (HNPP) 197
  motor 191
  motor and sensory 119
  sensory and autonomic 135
herpes virus infections 340–53
  cytomegalovirus 340, 347–9
    Guillain–Barré syndrome 30, 347
    in HIV infection 289, 291, 294, 295–6, 298, 300, 347–9
    lumbosacral polyradiculopathy 296, 348, 349
    mononeuritis multiplex 294, 348
    therapy 349
  herpes simplex 340, 343–5
    cellular basis 345–6
    diagnosis 344
    immunology 345
    molecular basis 345, 346–7
    neurological complications 344
    primary infection 343–4
    reactivation 344
    therapy 344–5
  and HIV 287, 296, 341
  varicella zoster 340, 341–3
    Guillain–Barré syndrome 341, 342–3
    herpes zoster pain 393, 398–9, 400
    herpes zoster radiculitis 296
    immunology 345
    molecular basis 345, 346–7
    motor involvement 342
    neurological complications 341, 342–3
    nociceptive nerve pain 393, 398–9, 400
    postherpetic neuralgia 342, 395–6, 403, 405
    primary infection 341
    reactivation 341–2
    therapy 343
HIV-related neuropathies 285–307
  autonomic 288, 289, 297
  brachial neuritis 295
  classification 285–6
  cranial nerve dysfunction 59
  and cytomegalovirus 289, 291, 294, 295–6, 298, 300, 347–9
  demyelinating 288, 290, 295–6, 297, 300
  distal symmetrical 286, 287, 288, 289–90, 296
  facial palsies 295
  and herpes zoster 287, 296, 342
  meralgia paresthetica 295
  mononeuritis multiplex 289, 291–5, 348–9
  pathogenesis 297–300
  polyradiculopathy 296, 300, 348
  prevalence 286–9
  rehabilitation 416
  relative incidence 288
  sensory axonal 287, 288, 289–91, 299, 300
  staging 285–6
  temporal profile 62
  therapy 300
  toxic 286, 287, 296–7
  and vasculitic 162, 291–4, 300
Hodgkin's disease 216, 219
Hu antibody 90–1, 130, 146, 216
human cytomegalovirus *see* cytomegalovirus
human immunodeficiency virus *see* HIV-related neuropathies
human immunoglobulin therapy *see* intravenous immunoglobulin
human lymphocyte antigen (HLA)
  humoral immune system 13
  leprosy 333–4
humoral immune system 11–15
  experimental allergic neuritis 39, 41, 46
hypalgia, clinical evaluation 60
hyperalgesia 392
hyperpathia 392
hypertrophy, clinical evaluation 57–8
hypesthesia
  clinical evaluation 60
  rehabilitation 420
hyporeflexia, clinical evaluation 61–2
hypothyroidism 120–1
hypotonia, clinical evaluation 57
idiopathic autonomic neuropathy (IAN) 144–7
  course 147
  differential diagnosis 146–7
  laboratory investigations 146
  management 147
  pathogenesis 146–7
  prognosis 147
idiopathic axonal neuropathy 118–19
idiopathic sensory neuronopathy 127, 129
IgA, humoral immune system 12
IgA MGUS
  epidemiology 33, 34
  immunopathology 85
  non-malignant 235
  plasmapheresis 367
IgE, humoral immune system 12
IgG
  complement cascade 15–16
  humoral immune system 12, 13
  immunoabsorption 46
  IVIG 368, 369–70
  LEMS 245
  paraneoplastic neuropathies 90–1
  post-polio syndrome 278, 279, 280
IgG MGUS 33, 34
  immunopathology 85
  non-malignant 235
  plasmapheresis 367
  temporal profile 62
IgM
  humoral immune system 11–13
  post-polio syndrome 278, 279
IgM monoclonal gammopathies 168–9
  associated neuropathies 169
    anti-chondroitin sulfate C 170, 178, 205
    anti-ganglioside 88, 170, 180–2, 204, 205, 359, 361
    anti-MAG 83–4, 169–78
    anti-sulfatide 89–90, 170, 178–80, 201, 202, 203
    cytoskeletal proteins 170, 180
    epidemiology 33
    experimental paraprotein 48
    humoral immune system 13–14
    IgM non-reacting forms 182–3
    therapy 174–6, 178, 180, 181, 182, 183, 359, 361–2
  and CIDP 113
  of undetermined significance (MGUS) 83–5, 168–9, 235, 367
  see also Waldenström's macroglobulinemia
immobilized patients 421, 422, 423
  see also paralytic neuropathy
immune interactions 3–28
  blood–nerve barrier 6
  cellular immune system 8–11

complement 15–18
cytokines 19–20
humoral immune system 11–15
immune response modifiers 371–3
antilymphocyte globulin 371
α-interferon 371, 373
monoclonal antibodies 371
immunofluorescence 82–3
immunoglobulin *see* IgA; IgG; IgM; intravenous immunoglobulin
immunomodulation 364–73
immune response modifiers 371–3
IVIG 367–71
photopheresis 367
plasmapheresis 365–7
total lymph node irradiation 364–5
immunopathological studies 81–95
anti-sulfatide antibodies 89–90
autoantibodies to GM1 88–9
experimental allergic neuritis 37
methodology 82–3
monoclonal gammopathy 83–5
paraneoplastic neuropathies 90–1
primary amyloidosis 86–8
vasculitic neuropathies 91
immunostaining 82
immunosuppressive drugs 357–64, 372, 373
alkylating agents 175–6, 197, 198, 361–3
antimetabolites 360–1, 363–4
cyclosporin 363
fludarabine 176, 363–4
see also corticosteroids
impairment measurement 64–8, 416
Indiana familial amyloid neuropathy 154
infection-related neuropathies 269–353
C. jejuni and GBS 13, 30–1, 89, 100, 103, 104–5, 379, 380
leprosy 319–39
Lyme disease 60, 61, 63, 308–18
with necrotizing arteritis 162
post-polio syndrome 269–84
see also herpes virus infections; HIV-related neuropathies
inflammatory demyelinating neuropathies
acute *see* Guillain–Barré syndrome
chronic *see* chronic inflammatory demyelinating polyneuropathy
inflammatory pain *see* nerve pain, nociceptive
intensive care unit (ICU) 377–88
brachial plexopathies 384
critical illness polyneuropathies 385, 386
electrophysiology 380, 381, 382–7
GBS 106, 148–9, 378–9, 380–1
lumbosacral plexopathies 384
mononeuropathies 384–5
myelopathies 384
myopathies 380, 386
neuromuscular transmission defects 385–6
paralysis after admission 381–4
paralysis before admission 377–80
respiratory system evaluation 386–7
interferon
immune response modification 371, 373
post-polio syndrome 280
intracellular adhesion molecule (ICAM) 6–7, 91
intravenous immunoglobulin (IVIG) 367–71
anti-idiotypic antibodies 369
anti-inflammatory effects 368–9
anti-MAG IgM 174–5
antiproliferative effects 370
CIDP 123, 367, 371
complement modulation 368
cryoglobulinemia 373
cytokine interactions 368–9
Fc receptor modulation 368
in GBS 100, 101, 107, 365, 370–1
HIV-related neuropathies 300
LEMS 248
lower motor neuron syndromes 198
lymphocyte activation 369–70
motor neuropathy with conduction block 197
nerve repair 370
neuromyotonia 242
sequence of events 370–1
vasculitic neuropathy 166, 373
Iowa familial amyloid neuropathy 154
ischemic neuropathy 160–1, 166
isoniazid, toxicity 297

Kaposi's sarcoma 295

Lambert–Eaton myasthenic syndrome (LEMS) 208, 238, 242–8
cancer associations 242, 243–4, 246–7
case study 243
clinical features 242–3
diagnosis 247–8
electromyography 244–5, 247–8
etiology 245
future developments 248
immunological associations 244
pathology 213, 216, 243–4
respiratory insufficiency 380
synaptotagmin antibodies 246
therapy 248
VGCC antibodies 238, 245–7
lamivudine, toxicity 296
leprosy 319–39
borderline borderline (BB) 323, 327
borderline lepromatous (BL) 323, 327, 328
borderline tuberculoid (BT) 323, 326, 327
classification 323–4
distribution 323
epidemiology 322–3
erythema nodosum leprosum 327, 332
genetic control 334
indeterminate 324, 325
lepromatous (LL) 323, 324, 326–7, 328, 329, 334
Lucio phenomenon 324
mid-borderline (BB) 323, 327
Mycobacterium leprae 319
antibiotics 335, 336
biochemistry 320
heat shock protein antigens 14
immunohistochemical test 322
immunology 333–4
lepromin tests 322
replication 320
Schwann cells 11
skin smears 320–2
structure 320
temperature range 320
transmission 322
viability 320
nerve fiber degeneration 332
neurological examination 325
neurological manifestations 324–5
outcomes 337
pathology 328–33
prevalence 323
pure neuritic 324, 327
rehabilitation 416
therapy 335–7
transmission 322–3
tuberculoid (TT) 323, 325, 327, 329, 334
Type 1 reactions 324, 327–8, 332, 334, 336
Type 2 reactions 324, 327, 328, 332, 334, 336
leukocytes
corticosteroid action 359
endothelial barriers 6
see also lymphocytes
lower bulbar variant of GBS 102, 104, 105–6
lower motor neuron syndromes 191, 192, 193, 195, 197–8
lumbosacral plexopathies 120, 384
lumbosacral polyradiculopathy, HIV infection 296, 348, 349
Lyme borreliosis 308
see also Lyme neuropathy
Lyme neuropathy 308–18
carpal tunnel syndrome 313
case studies 314–15
clinical features 309–10
CNS manifestations 310–11
cranial 310
definition 308
diagnosis 313

Lyme neuropathy (*cont.*)
disseminated infection 310
epidemiology 309
erythema chronicum migrans 63
future developments 316–17
Guillain–Barré syndrome 312–13
history 308–9
laboratory study 313–14
local infection 309–10
myositis 313
natural history 309
paresthesias 60
pathogenesis 315–16
polyradiculopathy 312, 315
prevention 317
radiculoneuritis 311–12, 315
reflexes 61
rehabilitation 416
therapy 316
lymphadenopathy syndrome (LAS) 285, 286, 287
lymphocytes
blood–nerve barrier 6
cellular immune system 8–11
and complement 18
corticosteroids 359
EAN 37, 38, 43–4, 45, 46
IVIG 369–70
post-polio syndrome 278
lymphoid irradiation 364–5
lymphoma, and mononeuritis multiplex 294–5
see also paraneoplastic neuropathies

macrophages
cellular immune system 10, 11
and complement 16, 18
EAN 37, 38, 44, 46
HIV infection 298–9
humoral immune system 12
mast cells, EAN 46
medical rehabilitation 415–25
autonomic disturbances 422–3
contractures 420–2
edema 422
electrical stimulation 418
evaluation 416, 417
exercise
for control 420
for range of motion 421–2
for strength 417–18
functional training 423
independence measures 416, 417
motor function 417–19
orthoses 418–19, 420–1
plan 416
pressure ulcers 421, 422
sensory function 419–20
melphalan 233, 361, 362
meningoradiculoneuritis (Bannwarth's syndrome) 311, 315
meralgia paresthetica, HIV infection 295
mercury, toxicity 150
Mestinon, post-polio syndrome 280
methotrexate 242, 360, 361
MHC molecules
blood–nerve barrier 6, 7
cellular immune system 8, 11
microscopic polyangiitis 158
migrant sensory neuritis of Wartenberg 291
Miller Fisher syndrome 58, 61, 102, 104, 105, 238–9
monoclonal antibodies 371
monoclonal gammopathies
autonomic dysfunction 61
epidemiology 32–3, 34
experimental 48
immunopathology 83–5
pain 59, 60
POEMS syndrome 234
proprioception 61
reflexes 61
temporal profile 62
see also IgA MGUS; IgG MGUS; IgM monoclonal gammopathies; multiple myeloma; osteosclerotic myeloma; Waldenström's macroglobulinemia
mononeuritis multiplex
CMV-induced 348–9
cellular immune system 11
clinical evaluation 55
in HIV infection 291–5, 300, 348–9
paresthesias 60
mononeuropathies
clinical evaluation 55
ICU management 384–5
motor function
evaluation 56–62, 64–7
rehabilitation 417–19
motor neuron disease (MND)
differential diagnoses
CIDP 78, 120
motor neuropathy 180–1, 191, 192, 193, 197
immunopathology 88–9
muscle atrophy 58
paraneoplastic damage 217–18
motor neuron injury, post-polio syndrome 273–9
motor neuropathies 191
anti-GM1 ganglioside antibodies 180–1, 182, 190–200
anti-gangliosides titers 194
and anti-sulfatide 203
conduction block 192–3, 194–5, 196–7
definitions 190–1
differential diagnosis 196–7
electrophysiology 193–4
experimental data 195–6
histology 194–5
immunological aspects 191–2, 239
lower motor neuron syndromes 192, 193, 195, 197–8
therapy 197–8
with conduction block 192–3, 194–5, 196–7
diagnostic algorithm 65–7
fasciculations 57
immunopathology 88–9
IVIG 371
multifocal *see* multifocal motor neuropathy
paraneoplastic 217–18
rehabilitation 417–19
upper motor neuron dysfunction 191
see also sensorimotor neuropathies
MRI study
acute sensory neuronopathy 134
chronic sensory neuronopathy 130
multifocal demyelinating neuropathy with persistent conduction block 118
multifocal motor neuropathy (MMN)
anti-GM1 antibodies 239
conduction velocity 76
rehabilitation 416
therapy 359, 361, 371, 373
multifocal paraneoplastic neuropathies 221
multiple mononeuritis *see* mononeuritis multiplex
multiple myeloma (MM) 225–34
amyloidosis of 86–7, 226
epidemiology 31
immunopathology 85
lytic 225–6, 233
management 233
osteosclerotic *see* osteosclerotic myeloma
peripheral neuropathies 48, 225
therapy 233
multiple sclerosis lesions 118
muscles
biopsy in necrotizing arteritis 160, 163
motor function 56–9, 64–7, 417–18
myasthenia gravis 238, 239–40, 241, 242, 248, 380
Mycobacterium leprae 319
antibiotics 335, 336
biochemistry 320
heat shock protein antigens 14
immunohistochemical test 322
immunology 333–4
lepromin tests 322
replication 320
and Schwann cells 11
skin smears 320–2
structure 320

temperature range 320
transmission 322
viability 320
myelin 4–5
cellular immune system 9, 10
complement 16–17, 18
humoral immune system 12–14
see also demyelinated fibers; demyelinating neuropathies; demyelination
myelin-associated glycoprotein (MAG) 4
anti-MAG IgM 169–78
animal models 177–8
and anti-sulfatide antibodies 203
clinical findings 171–3
electrophysiology 174
epidemiology 33, 34
immunopathology 83–4
laboratory findings 173–4
pathogenesis 176–8
pathology 174
therapy 174–6
cytokines 19–20
experimental paraprotein neuropathy 48
myeloma neuropathy *see* multiple myeloma; osteosclerotic myeloma
myelopathies, ICU management 384
myokymia, clinical evaluation 57
see also neuromyotonia
myopathies, ICU management 380, 386
myositis, Lyme neuropathy 313
myotonia, clinical evaluation 57

necrotizing vasculitis 158, 159
clinical aspects 159–61
diagnosis 164
in the elderly 163
electrophysiology 160
in HIV infection 291, 292–3
immunopathology 91
morphology 160–1
and multisystem disorder 62–3, 161–2, 163
non-systemic 163
pathophysiology 164–5
nerve biopsy studies 82–3
CIDP 116
HIV-associated neuropathies 290
motor neuropathy with conduction block 194–5
necrotizing arteritis 160, 163
osteosclerotic myeloma 230–1
nerve conduction *see* electrophysiological studies
nerve pain 59–60, 389–414
allodynia 391
causalgia 60, 395, 397, 408–9
diagnosis 391–2, 393–4, 396
distribution 391
electrophysiology 392
hyperalgesia 392
hyperpathia 392
intensity 391
neuropathic *see* nerve pain, non-nociceptive
nociceptive 389–90
acute herpes zoster 393, 398–9, 400
causes 394
diagnosis 393–4
due to cancer 399, 403
mechanisms 392–3, 397–8
non-nociceptive compared 397–8
sciatica 399, 401–2
therapy 398–403, 410
non-nociceptive 390–1, 394–7
anticonvulsants 409
antidepressants 409
diabetic neuropathy 396, 403, 406–8
diagnosis 396, 397–8
mechanisms 394–5
nociceptive compared 397–8
opioids 409
post-lymph node dissection 396
postherpetic neuralgia 342, 395–6, 403, 405
therapy 403–10
trigeminal neuralgia 395, 396, 403, 404
quality 391
reflex sympathetic dystrophy 395, 397, 408–9
time profile 391
neuralgia *see* nerve pain
neurofibromatosis 324
neuromyotonia (NMT) 238, 239–42
case study 240
clinical features 56, 57, 239–40
diagnosis 242
electromyography 240–1
etiology 241
future developments 242
therapy 240, 241, 242
VGKC antibodies 238, 241–2
neuropathic nerve pain *see* nerve pain, non-nociceptive
nociceptive pain *see* nerve pain, nociceptive
non-systemic vasculitic neuropathy 121, 129, 162
NSAIDS, nerve pain 399, 403, 408
nucleoside analogues 287, 296–7

occupational therapy 423
ocular symptoms
autonomic neuropathies 139, 151–2
herpes zoster 399
lepromatous leprosy 327
opioids, nerve pain 399, 403, 405, 409
organic solvents, toxicity 150
orthoses 418–19, 420–1
orthostatic hypotension 138–9, 142–3, 147, 423
osteosclerotic myeloma (OSM) 85, 226–34
case study 231
or CIDP 119–20
clinical features 226–8
epidemiology 31
future directions 233–4
immunopathology 85
laboratory features 228–31
bone marrow 228
cerebrospinal fluid 230
electromyography 229–30, 232
endocrinology 229, 232
nerve biopsy 230–1
radiography 229
management 233
pathogenesis 231–3
pathology 231–3
POEMs syndrome 119–20, 226, 234
therapy 233

pain *see* nerve pain
pandysautonomia (IAN) 144–7
paralytic Chinese syndrome *see* Chinese paralytic syndrome
paralytic neuropathy, ICU management 377–88
brachial plexopathies 384
critical illness 382–4, 385
electrophysiological evaluation 380, 381, 382–7
Guillain–Barré syndrome 106, 378–9, 380–1
lumbosacral plexopathies 384
management algorithm 378
mononeuropathies 384–5
myelopathies 384
myopathies 380, 386
neuromuscular transmission defects 385–6
paralysis after admission 381–4
paralysis before admission 377–80
respiratory system evaluation 386–7
paraneoplastic neuropathies 208–24
or acute sensory neuronopathy 135
autonomic 221
causes 208, 209
classification 209–10
diagnosis 216–17
focal 221
history 209
humoral immune system 14
or idiopathic autonomic neuropathy 146
immunopathology 90–1
motor 217–18
multifocal 221
pathology 210

paraneoplastic neuropathies (*cont.*)
  pathophysiology 213–16
  prevalence 210, 211–12
  sensorimotor 90, 219–21
  sensory 59–60, 61, 62, 126, 218–19, 225–6
  see also IgM monoclonal gammopathies; Lambert–Eaton myasthenic syndrome; multiple myeloma; neuromyotonia
parenteral ganglioside-associated GBS 258–9
paresthesias 60
peptide-T, HIV-related neuropathy 300
perhexiline maleate neuropathy 150
phagocytosis, corticosteroids 359
pharyngeal cervical brachial variant of GBS 102, 104, 105–6
phentolamine 408–9
phenytoin
  nerve pain 406, 409
  neuromyotonia 242
photopheresis 367
physiotherapy 417–18, 420, 421, 423
plasmapheresis 365–7
  anti-MAG IgM 174–5
  chronic sensory neuronopathy 132
  CIDP 122, 367
  experimental allergic neuritis 46
  Guillain–Barré syndrome 100, 101, 106–7, 365, 370–1
  HIV-related neuropathy 300
  immune-mediated neuropathies 365, 367
  LEMS 245, 248
  motor neuropathy with conduction block 197
  neuromyotonia 240, 241, 242
  selective immunoadsorption 365
cis-platinum, toxicity 135, 149
plexopathies 120, 384
POEMS syndrome 119–20, 226, 234–5
  therapy 363, 367, 371, 373
polio *see* post-polio syndrome
polyarteritis nodosa 62, 158–9, 161, 164–5, 360
polyradiculopathy
  HIV-associated 296, 300, 348, 349
  Lyme disease-associated 312, 315
porphyria 149
postherpetic neuralgia (PHN) 342, 395–6, 403, 405
post-polio syndrome (PPS) 269–84
  diagnosis 269–70
  incidence 273
  musculoskeletal symptoms 57, 270–1
  outcome 272–3
  pathogenesis 273–9
  post-poliomyelitis progressive muscular atrophy (PPMA) 270–2
    pathogenesis 276–8
    progression 272, 273
    respiration 271–2
    sleep apnea 272
  prevalence 273
  progression 272–3
  risk factors 272
  role of polio virus 274, 279–80
  treatment 280–1
postural orthostatic tachycardia syndrome (POTS) 138–9, 147–8
potassium channels, neuromyotonia 238, 241–2
prednisolone
  LEMS 248
  neuromyotonia 242
prednisone
  anti-MAG IgM 174–5
  CIDP 121–2
  idiopathic autonomic neuropathy 147
  leprosy 335, 336
  motor neuropathy with conduction block 197
  osteosclerotic myeloma 233
  post-polio syndrome 280
  vasculitic neuropathies 165
pressure ulcers 421, 422
proprioception 60–1
pure cholinergic neuropathies 144, 151–2
  see also Adie's syndrome; Lambert–Eaton myasthenic syndrome
purine antimetabolites 360–1
pyridoxine toxicity 135
pyrimidine antimetabolites 360–1, 364

quantitative sudomotor axon reflex test (QSART) 140–1, 151

radiation-induced lumbosacral plexopathies 120
radiculoneuritis, Lyme disease 311–12, 315
Rankin scale, modified 68
reflex sympathetic dystrophy 257, 395, 397, 408–9
reflexes, clinical evaluation 61–2
Refsum's disease 324
rehabilitation *see* medical rehabilitation
rheumatoid arthritis
  gold therapy 57
  and necrotizing arteritis 161–2
RNA
  herpes virus infections 346, 347
  HIV infection 298
  leprosy 334
  post-polio syndrome 278–9, 280
Ross syndrome 129, 151, 152
Rukavina familial amyloid neuropathy 154

sarcoidosis 63
Schwann cells 3–4
  complement 16, 17, 18
  cytokines 19–20
  experimental allergic neuritis 44–5
  pathogenic invasion 11
sciatica 399, 401–2
selective immunoadsorption 365
sensorimotor neuropathies
  anti-sulfatide antibodies 203
  diagnostic algorithm 65–7
  HMSN-1 119
  multiple myeloma patients 225, 226, 233
  paraneoplastic 90, 210, 219–21
sensory function
  clinical evaluation 59–61, 67–8
  rehabilitation 419–20
sensory neuropathies
  anti-GD1b antibodies 204–5
  anti-sulfatide antibodies 179, 202–3
  cancer patients 59–60, 61, 62, 126, 210, 218–19, 225–6
  diagnostic algorithm 65–7
  function quantification 67–8
  HIV patients 286, 288, 289–91
  multiple myeloma patients 225–6
  temporal profile 62
  see also acute sensory neuronopathy; chronic sensory neuronopathy; sensorimotor neuropathies
sexual dysfunction 139, 423
shingles (herpes zoster) 287, 296, 341–3
  nerve pain 393, 398–9, 400
sicca syndrome 127–8, 129
silicone neurotoxicity 259–62
  assessing causation 259–60
  clinical features 260–1
  epidemiology 260
  experimental data 262
  future developments 262
Sjögren's syndrome 62–3, 127–9, 130, 131–2, 135, 162
skeletal deformities 63
spinal muscular atrophy (SMA) 191, 197
sporadic primary amyloid neuropathy 152, 153
stavudine (d4T), toxicity 287, 296
subacute idiopathic demyelinating polyradiculoneuropathy 62, 112
subacute motor neuropathy 217–18
subacute sensorimotor neuropathy 219, 220–1
subacute sensory neuropathy 59–60, 61, 126, 218–19, 220
sudomotor function 139, 140–2, 151
sulfagalactosylceramide *see* sulfatide
sulfatide 201
  associated neuropathies 170, 178–80, 201–4

axonal 202–3
and chondroitin sulfate C 202–3, 205
demyelinating sensorimotor 203
immunopathology 89–90
inflammatory demyelinating 203
pathogenesis 201–2, 203–4
polyneuropathy 201–2, 203
sulfogluceronyl paragloboside (SGPG) 47
swine flu vaccination 30
synaptotagmin antibodies, LEMS 246
systemic disease, clinical evidence 62–3

temporal dispersion 74–5, 116
temporal profile, neuropathy 62
thalidomide, leprosy 335, 336–7
thallium, toxicity 150
therapeutic exercise 417–18, 420, 421–2
total lymph node irradiation (TLI) 364–5
toxic oil syndrome (TOS) 254–6
toxicity
alkylating agents 363
antimetabolites 360–1
corticosteroids 360
cyclosporin 363
toxin-induced neuropathies 126, 149–50, 251–62
or chronic sensory neuronopathy 135
eosinophilia-myalgia syndrome 252–4
ganglioside-associated GBS 258–9
guanethidine-induced 257–8
HIV-associated 286, 287, 296–7
neuromyotonia 239–40
silicone 259–62
toxic oil syndrome 254–6
trigeminal neuralgia 395, 396, 403, 404
trophic function 139–40
Trypanosoma cruzi 48–9, 152
tryptophan 252, 253
tumor of the filum terminale 121

vacor-associated autonomic neuropathy 150
Valsalva maneuver 142, 143
van Allen familial amyloid neuropathy 154
varicella zoster virus (VZV) 341–3
Guillain–Barré syndrome 341, 342–3
herpes zoster radiculitis 296
immunocompromised hosts 342
immunology 345
infection diagnosis 343
molecular basis 345, 346–7
motor involvement 342
neurological complications 341, 342–3
nociceptive nerve pain 393, 398–9, 400
postherpetic neuralgia 342, 395–6, 403, 405
primary infection 341
reactivation 341–2
therapy 343
vasculitic neuropathies 55, 158–67
autonomic dysfunction 61
classification 158–9
clinical aspects 58, 59, 60, 159–60
complement 17
in diabetes mellitus 163
diagnosis 164
in the elderly 163, 165
electrophysiology 160
in HIV infection 162, 291–4, 300
humoral immune system 14–15
immunopathology 91
ischemic neuropathy 160–1, 166
morphology 160
non-systemic 121, 129, 162
paresthesias 60
pathophysiology 164–5
rehabilitation 416
systemic 62–3, 161–2
temporal profile 62, 163
therapy 165–6, 358, 360, 373
vasomotor function 139–40
vincristine, toxicity 150, 297
viral infections
humoral immune system 14
with necrotizing arteritis 162
see also herpes virus infections; HIV-related neuropathies; post-polio syndrome
voltage-gated calcium channels, LEMS 238, 245–7
voltage-gated potassium channels, neuromyotonia 238, 241–2

Waldenström's macroglobulinemia (WM) 168, 169, 182
clinical diagnosis 33
immunopathology 83
weakness
clinical evaluation 58–9, 64, 67
rehabilitation 417–18
Wegener's granulomatosis 158, 159, 165
Western blot assays 314

X adrenoleucodystrophy 120
X-linked HMSN 119

zalcitabine (ddC) 287, 296, 297
zidovudine (AZT) 295, 296, 300